Clinical
Ophthalmology

Clinical
Ophthalmology

Professor **V. Kalevar** FAMS
Indore

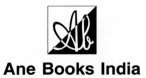

Ane Books India

New Delhi ◆ Chennai ◆ Mumbai
Bangalore ◆ Kolkata ◆ Thiruvananthapuram ◆ Lucknow

Clinical Ophthalmology

© Author, 2008

Published by

Ane Books India

Head Office	4821, Parwana Bhawan, 1st Floor, 24 Ansari Road, Darya Ganj, New Delhi - 110 002, INDIA Tel.: +91(011) 23276843-44, Fax: +91(011) 23276863 e-mail: kapoor@anebooks.com, Website: www.anebooks.com
Chennai	Avantika Niwas, 1st Floor, 19 Doraiswamy Road, T. Nagar, Chennai - 600 017 Tel.: +91(044) 28141554, 28141209 e-mail: anebooks_tn@airtelbroadband.in
Mumbai	G-012, Ground Floor, Jui Nagar Railway Station Building, Jui Nagar (East), Navi Mumbai - 400 706 Tel.: +91(022) 64522840, 64522841 e-mail: anebooksmum@gmail.com
Bangalore	38/1, 1st Floor, Model House, First Street, Opp. Shamanna Park, Basavannagudi, Bangalore - 560 004 Tel.: +91(080) 41681432 e-mail: anebang@airtelbroadband.in
Kolkata	Flat No. 16A, 220 Vivekananda Road, Maniktalla, Kolkata - 700 006 Tel.: +91(033) 23547119 e-mail: anekol@vsnl.net
Thiruvananthapuram	# 6, TC 25/2710, Kohinoor Flats, Lukes Lane, Ambujavilasam Road, Thiruvananthapuram - 01, Kerala Tel.: +91(0471) 4068777, 4068333 e-mail: anebookstvm@airtelbroadband.in
Lucknow	C-26, Sector-A, Mahanagar, Lucknow - 226 006 Mobile - +91 93352 29971

ISBN (10) : 81-8052-148-6

ISBN (13) : 978-81-8052-148-5

Printed at A.P. Offset Pvt. Ltd., India

Dedicated to

Professor RP Dhanda

Professor P Siva Reddy   *Professor G Venkataswami*

Foreword

I have considered it a privilege and an honour to have been asked to write a foreword for this lively new book on "Clinical Ophthalmology".

Dr. Kalevar has dealt with the entire vast subject of Ophthalmology with ease and fluency. Each section of the book begins with a delightful historical introduction and goes on in a systematic manner to deal with the basic matter of the topic. The treatment of some of the more prosaic aspects of Ophthalmology for example Strabismus and Refraction have been made simple to understand and easy to remember by very well formulated tables. She has provided the readers with concise tables for quick reference and flow charts for treatment modalities. The chapters on Uvea and Retina are quite refreshing.

The addition of a chapter on Prognostication lends a new concept to the outcome of diseases of the eye and the ultimate result of treatment. This certainly gives the young students of Ophthalmology something to think about when he deals with patients with poor vision and difficult diagnosis. The book will be very useful for both MBBS and Diploma students besides the general ophthalmology practitioners. It is a stimulating work and encourages further reading.

Dr. Sudha Sutaria
Past President
All India Ophthalmological Society

Preface

The objective of this book, *'Clinical Ophthalmology'* is to provide basic clinical knowledge of Ophthalmology to undergraduate students. It is expected that post-graduate students too will consider it useful as initial reading.

History of Ophthalmology has been compiled to make the reader aware of work put in over last centuries for Ophthalmology to have reached the stage that it enjoys today. It is important to acknowledge these efforts and obligatory to pay homage to the by gone stalwarts who understood Physio-pathology of the eye diseases and designed equipments and instruments.

It is natural that no one book can provide everything in today's world of specialties and super specialties. Sir Duke-Elder had written enormous volumes, each of over 1500 pages in that era when advances in understanding Physio-pathology and Technology were not at the level as it is today.

Throwing away old techniques and accepting newer ones is the trend. However, let us remember that old foundation is necessary scaffolding for building a new edifice. The book is an attempt in this direction and particularly takes the reader to bedside clinics by those teachers of olden times. There lies the significance of chapters on "Ocular Symptomatology" and "Clinical Examination of the Eye".

Detailed embryology of the eye and developmental anomalies provide an insight necessary to understand ocular pathology. The author has tried to include though briefly, the newer advances in technology and therapeutics.

Confidence and satisfaction gained by a correct diagnosis made on history, symptoms and meticulous clinical examination is incomparable to anything that can be attained after elaborate and expensive investigations. Investigations should be used as supportive and confirmative measures. They can not and should not replace clinical acumen of the Clinician. The book may have more to offer to the person who consults it as a guide to his own knowledge.

Lastly, the general attitude of the reader is more important than any of the specific and concrete functions of the book which is neither a commandment nor a holy writ but a reference work also for practising Ophthalmologists for clinical revisal and perhaps to solve a problem.

The author believes that "Science without Art is likely to be ineffective and Art without Science is likely to be inaccurate."

V. Kalevar

Acknowledgements

The author owes so much to the opportunities that came her way right from day one of her ophthalmic career. Having selected Ophthalmology as the first and only choice for post-graduation in 1960, there was no looking back.

Teachers in medical college and ophthalmology department provided all the incentive that was needed to develop clinical acumen, inclination towards research and teaching. In spite of the scepticism of a first girl joining ophthalmology for the first time in the institution (MGM Medical College and MY Hospital, Indore), Dean, Dr BC Bose, Superintendent, Dr R Bhattacharya and Prof. BK Dhir encouraged and helped. One person stands out above all, Prof. RP Dhanda whose advice and encouragement has gone a long way during the years of residency. This manuscript would not have seen the light of day if his guidance over the decades in preparation of presentations, teaching material and to a certain extent this manuscript also, had not been available. The implicit belief that he placed and often expressed, helped develop a confidence that never waned.

The author sincerely acknowledges her association with internationally recognised ophthalmologists, Prof. AE Maumenee, Dr JR Duke, Prof. Frank Walsh, Dr CH Dohlman, Dr MF Rafojo and Dr PK Basu during the periods of "Fight for Sight" and "NIH" fellowships in USA. Back home, Prof. DN Gupta, a well known pathologist who trained me in corneal histopathology, Prof. G Venkataswamy, Dr P Siva Reddy, Dr WP Thatte, Prof. SRK Malik, Dr BT Maskati, Prof. RK Mishra always had a word of encouragement and appreciation.

I am grateful to Dr Sudha Sutaria for readily agreeing to go through the manuscript and write foreword. She also suggested some inadvertent omissions and additions.

A lot has been drawn from communication with colleagues in India. Their experience has greatly helped preparation of this manuscript.

Dr Rajiv Chaudhary's help can not be mentioned in words. He was ready to support and advise whenever asked for. He willingly agreed to record and document every interesting case and also provide photographs of procedures on the equipments in his hospital. Quite a few photographs are from his hospital OPD patients.

Dr Tanuja Kate, consultant in Dr Chaudhary's Rajas hospital and a dear colleague, has been ever ready to help particularly for placing figures and photographs in the text.

Dr Tarakanth Shetty, PhD Biochemistry at NIMHANS, Bangalore, provided material for the introductory chapter on Immunology. It would not have been otherwise possible to touch the subject.

Ophthalmic colleagues over the last decades, Dr SR Khasgiwala helped presentation of intricate details for strabismus chapter. Dr SK Parwani, Dr Shreya Thatte and Dr Sudha Bhatia have been a moral support.

My mother, late Sanjivanibai Kalevar would have been happy today as she was the one who instilled the desire to take up medical career.

Last but certainly not the least, I thank the publishers M/s Ane Books India, who approached me last year with the proposal to write this book. I would not have taken up this huge a task at this stage of life but for Mr Sunil Saxena, Mr Jai Raj Kapoor and their Staff. I particularly thank Mr Majumdar for his help and persistence. I am immensely happy to have worked with Ane Books India.

To the Almighty, I offer my prayers and thank HIM for this journey through ophthalmology and a very satisfying innings indeed.

V. Kalevar

Contents

List of Colour Figures

PLATE 1

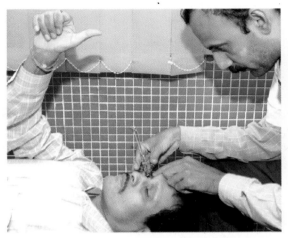

Fig. 6.3: Tonometry—showing intra-ocular tension record with Schiotz tonometer

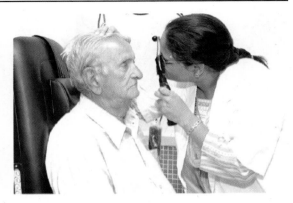

Fig. 6.6: Direct ophthalmoscopy

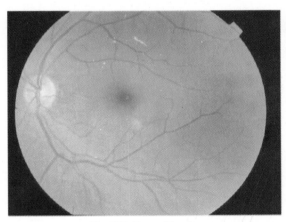

Fig. 6.7: Normal fundus

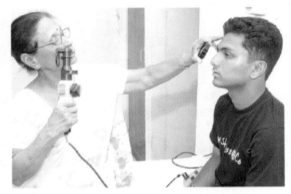

Fig. 6.9: Indirect ophthalmoscope—Monocular (Bonoscope)

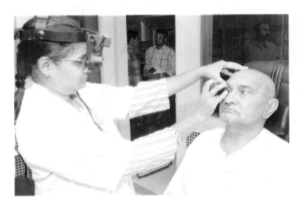

Fig. 6.10: Indirect ophthalmoscopy with Binocular

PLATE 2

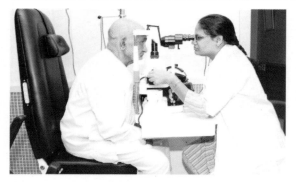

Fig. 6.11B: Slit lamp exam

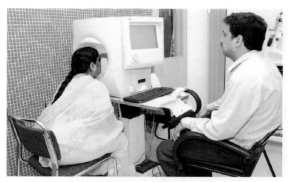

Fig. 6.16: Perimetry—automated equipment

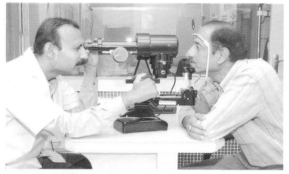

Fig. 6.17: Keratometry on automated equipment

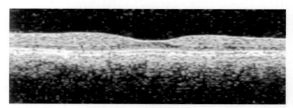

Fig. 6.23: OCT image—macular area

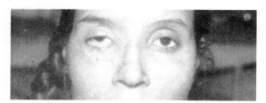

Fig. 7.3B: Atropine allergy—lid skin

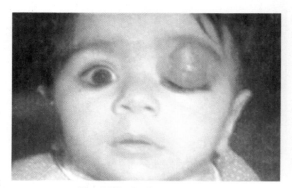

Fig. 7.5A: Angioma upperlid

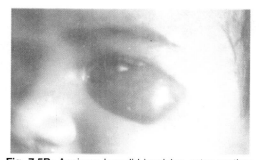

Fig. 7.5B: Angioma lowerlid involving outer canthus

PLATE 3

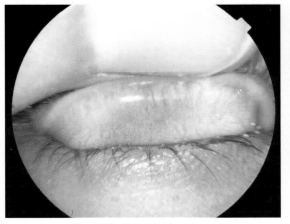

Fig. 8.2B: Everted lid—normal

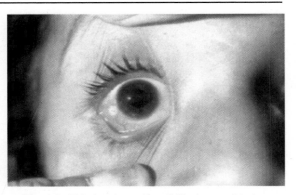

Fig. 8.6: Phlyclenular conjunctivitis. Large phlycten

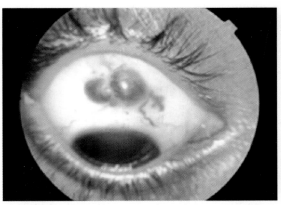

Fig. 8.10: Conjunctinal haemangioma

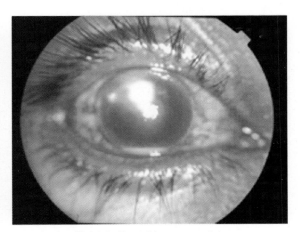

Fig. 9.6: Fungal hypopyon ulcer

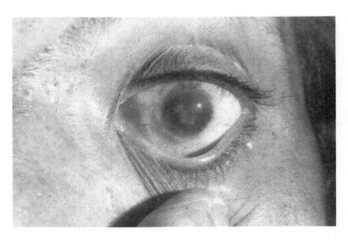

Fig. 9.8: Dendritic viral ulcer

PLATE 4

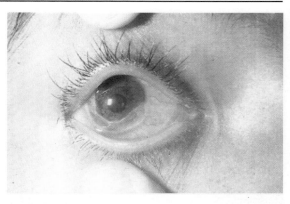

Fig. 9.9A: Early Marginal ulcer

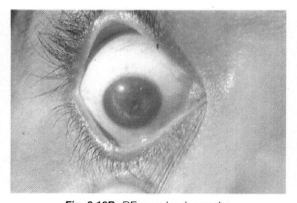

Fig. 9.9B: Marginal ulceration involving two-thirds of circumference

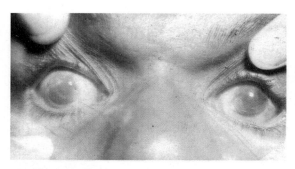

Fig. 9.10: Trachomatous cornea—Healed stage

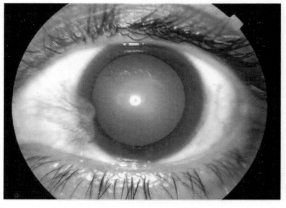

Fig. 9.11: Typical and true primary ptergium in the Horizontal inter-marginal area nasally

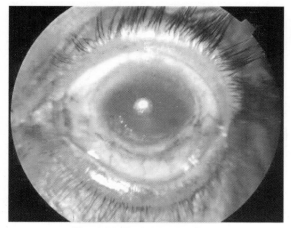

Fig. 9.17: Lattice dystrophy

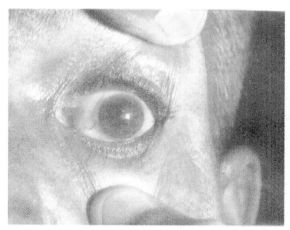

Fig. 9.18B: RE macular dysprophy

PLATE 5

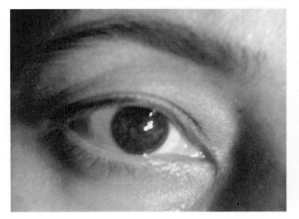

Fig. 9.18C: RE macular dystrophy

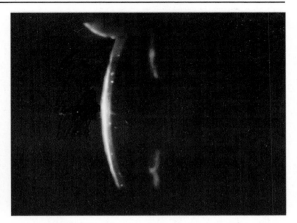

Fig. 9.18D: Macular dystrophy on slit lamp

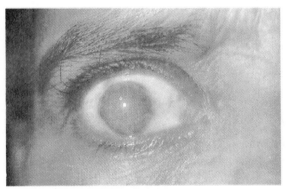

Fig. 9.19: Fuchs' dystrophy

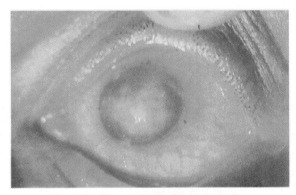

Fig. 9.20: Pseudophakic decompensation

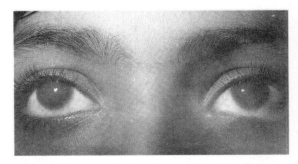

Fig. 9.21: Congenital hereditary endothelial dystrophy (CHED)

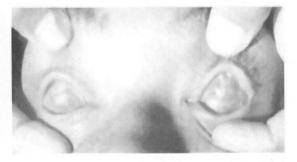

Fig. 9.27: Chemical burn—Totally opaque vascularised cornea BE

PLATE 6

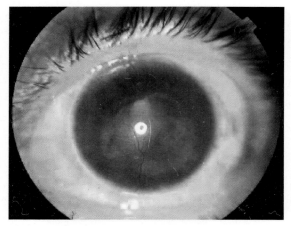

Fig. 9.29B: Vascularised corneal opacity

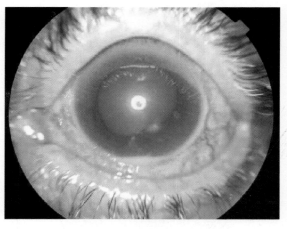

Fig. 10.2: Hypopyon—endophthalmitis due to perforating injury with splinter

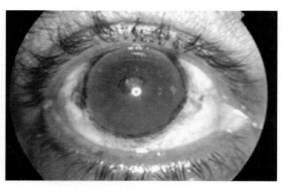

Fig. 11.4B: Posterior synechia

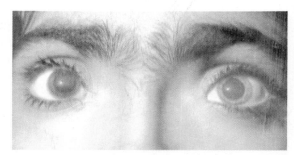

Fig. 11.8: Heterochromia iris. Note the dark brown iris in right eye and light blue iris in left eye

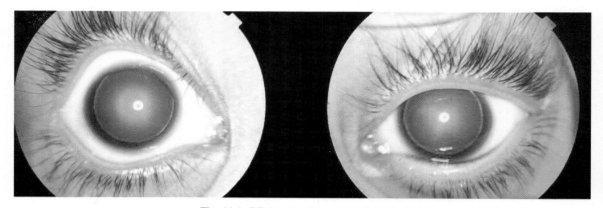

Fig. 11.9: BE Aniridia—lens equator visible

PLATE 7

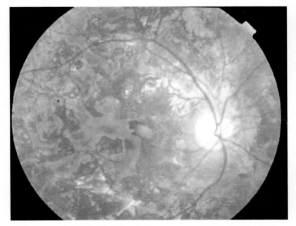

Fig. 11.11C: Disseminated healed choroiditis

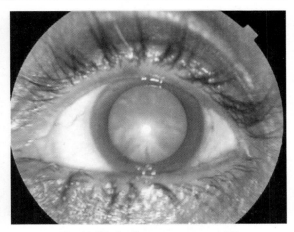

Fig. 12.5B: Senile mature cataract LE

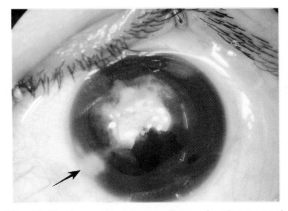

Fig. 12.12: Traumatic cataract after perforating corneal injury. Note membranous cataract with pigmentation down and in scar of injury arrow

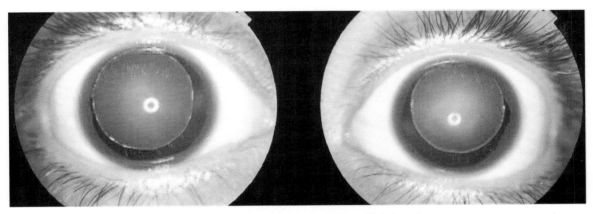

Fig. 12.15: Bilateral subluxation of lens-dilated pupil

PLATE 8

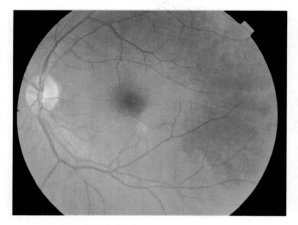

Fig. 13.2B: Normal optic nerve head

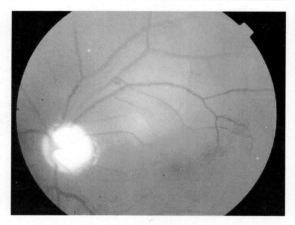

Fig. 13.3B: Optic nerve head with deep cupping. Note deviation of blood vessels as they come up on surface

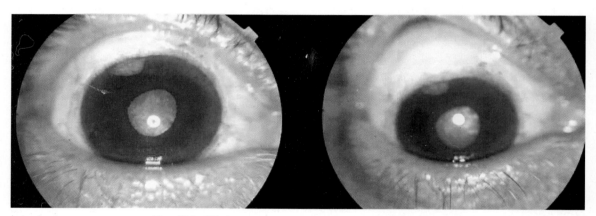

Fig. 13.8: RE glaucoma surgery done. Note mature cataract

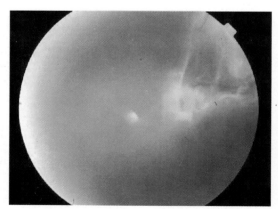

Fig. 14.2: Vitreous haemorrhage with proliferating membranes

PLATE 9

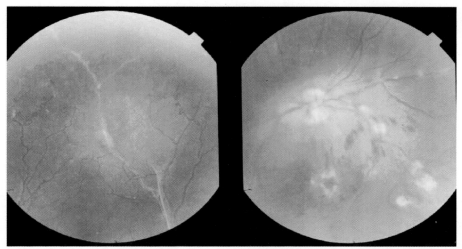

Fig. 15.2: Eales' disease. Rt—Central fundus involvement, Lt—Peripheral sheathing and cork-screw vessels

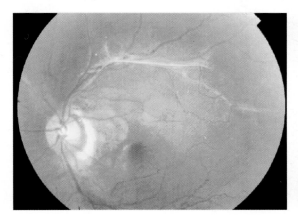

Fig. 15.3: Silver wire sheating of vessels

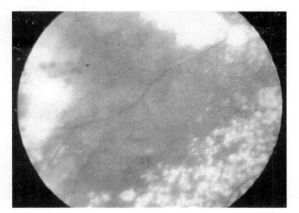

Fig. 15.4: Coat's exudative retinopathy

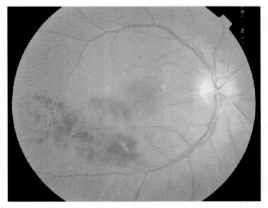

Fig. 15.5: Central art occlusion

PLATE 10

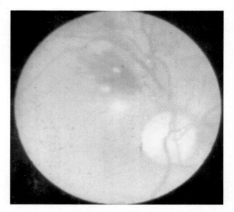

Fig. 15.6A: Thrombosis of retinal vein involving superior temporal branch showing haemorrhages in localised area

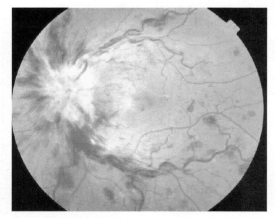

Fig. 15.6B: Central vein trunk thrombosis

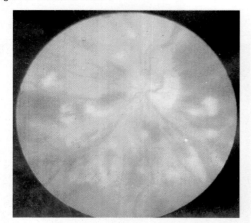

Fig. 15.6C: Central vein branch thrombosis

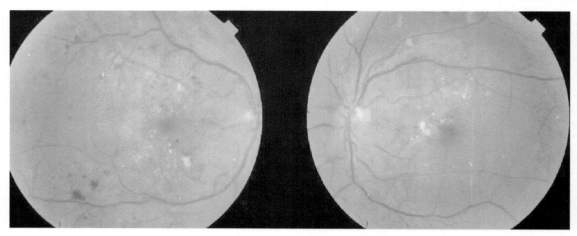

Fig. 15.7: Diabetic retinopathy haemorrhages and exudates

PLATE 11

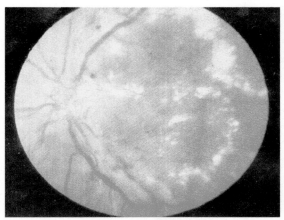

Fig. 15.9: Diabetic retinopathy–predominantly exudative showing early proliferative changes like neo-vasularisation on the disc

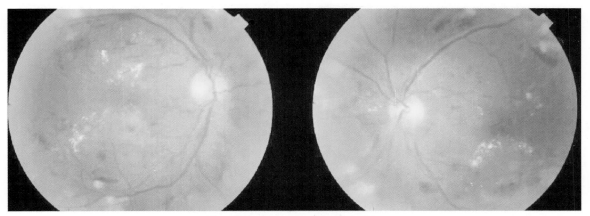

Fig. 15.11: Hypertensive retinopathy

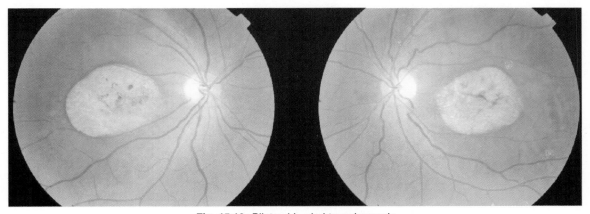

Fig. 15.12: Bilateral healed toxoplasmosis

PLATE 12

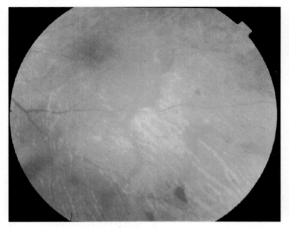

Fig.15.14: Retinitis pigmentosa—changes in mid periphery

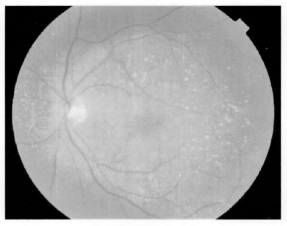

Fig. 15.15A: Dry AMD

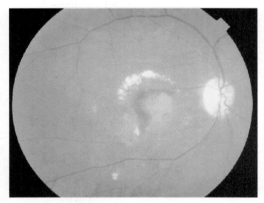

Fig. 15.15B: Exudative wet AMD

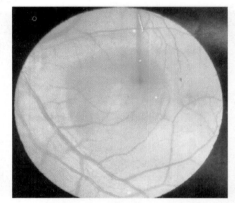

Fig. 15.16: CSR, circumscribed lesion

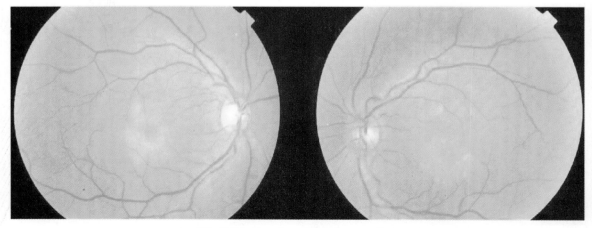

Fig. 15.18: Heredo-macular degenerations

PLATE 13

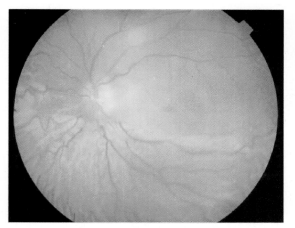

Fig. 15.19: Lower detachment of retina

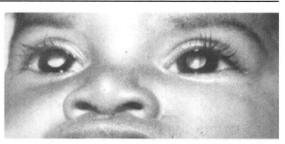

Fig. 15.21: Bilateral retrobulbar mass. Retino blastoma stage II appearance of cat's amaurotic eye

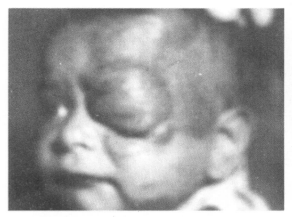

Fig. 17.5B: Extensive angioma involving scalp and part of face, may later lead to secondary glaucoma (Sturge-Weber Syndrome)

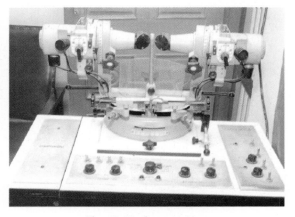

Fig. 18.28: Synoptophore

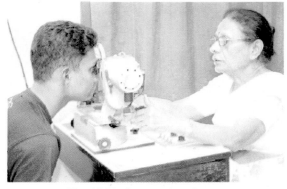

Fig. 18.29: Synoptophore in use

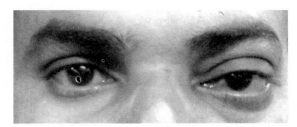

Fig. 20.4A: LE proptosis with dilated episcleral vessels (Courtsy Dr. Soraj Gupta)

PLATE 14

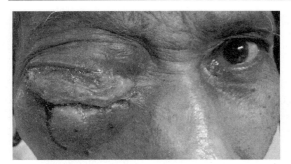

Fig. 20.7: Right orbital tumour involving lower lid and lateral nasal side *(Courtsy Dr. Shreya Thatte)*

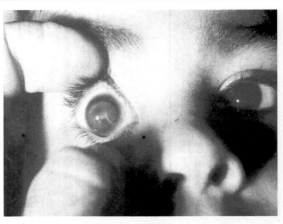

Fig. 21.2: Blood staining of cornea RE after Hyphaemna due to injury

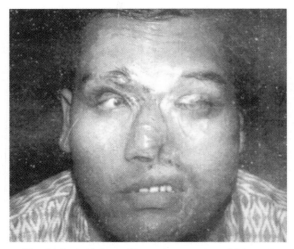

Fig. 21.4: Acid Burn. (Extensive scarring of lids and face. RE rehabilitated after penetrating keratoplasty

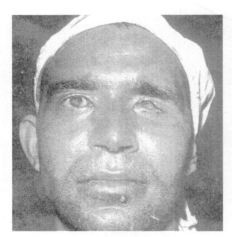

Fig. 21.5: Blast injury

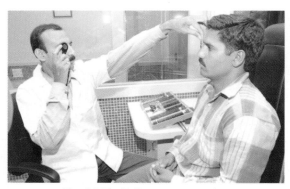

Fig. 24.3A: Retinoscopy procedure

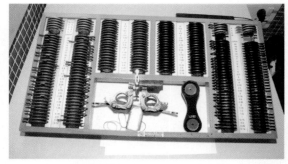

Fig. 24.3B: Standard trial case with full range of spheres, cylinders, prisms, maddox rod, red and green filters and a trial frame

PLATE 15

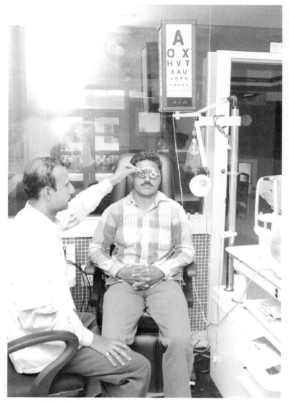

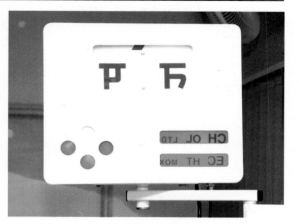

Fig. 24.4B: Sliding reverse vision chart with Duochrome Test

Fig. 24.4A: Sliding reverse vision chart with provision for duochrome and Worth's Four-dot Tests

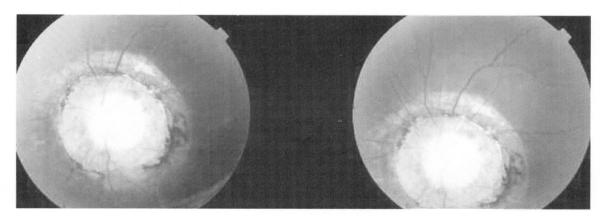

Fig. 25.1: Optic nerve coloboma

History of Ophthalmology

History is a fascinating subject. We all want to know all about our ancestors even if they belonged to an age we would not like to live in. Who does not want to know what seeds were sown from which grew the present industrial and scientific revolution? We ophthalmologists would like to know which of our ancestors' efforts have given us major successes in cataract surgery, corneal surgery, retinal surgery and vitreous surgery.

The happiest part of the history of ophthalmology is the origin of Indian ophthalmology from vedic times, the writings of Emperor Shen Nung of China 3700 years BC and the code of Hammurabi, founder of the Babylonian empire in Egypt, about 2000 BC.

Sushruta is recognised as the father of Indian medicine; even the father of medicine as such. It is Indian medicine which passed the knowledge of medicine on to the Greeks, the Romans, the Muslims and later on to the Western world. Sushruta had dealt with eye diseases and it was on the basis of his writings about 1000 BC that ophthalmology continued to be practised for centuries. He described 76 varieties of eye diseases, 51 of which were considered operable.

The technique of cataract operation of Sushruta continued to be practised till as late as 1745. Sushruta's description of the pterygium operation is no less exciting.

A few more references may be interesting.

The Atharva veda referred to the sun as the supreme lord of the eyes (Surya chakshunam Adhipati). The RIG VEDA dating back to 4500 BC mentions healing of the blind by removal of the eyes replaced by artificial ones. Charak, a contemporary of Sushruta, has been mentioned in Latin books and Sushruta's works have been translated into Latin.

The Takshila University Medical Centre was visited by a Chinese prince for eye treatment.

Egyptian ophthalmology has been mentioned in the writings of the old kingdom around 2600 BC but their therapeutics developed better around 1900 BC.

Greek ophthalmology is considered an ancient science starting about 1000 BC. The Hippocratic oath and the code of medical ethics were enunciated in 400 BC. Aristotle and Plato developed the understanding of vision but medicine, thereafter, fell into oblivion in the Alexandrian period.

Roman ophthalmic contributions were from the writings of Celsus AD 50 and Galen AD 250. Their writings are considered to be the only original documents to survive the ravages of time.

In spite of these developments from time to time in the primitive and prehistoric era, the eye continued to be associated with superstition, mysticism and legends. The eye was considered a representative of deities and gods. A glance could cause death and that is how the eye became a symbol of force. This negative approach continued without much development through the early Christian era and the Islamic period. Some change from medieval to modern medicine however came about from the 14th to 16th centuries AD.

The first ever book of ophthalmology was written by George Bartische in German in 1583. He laid down the following qualities for an oculist:

1. Religious parents
2. Religious nature
3. Knowledge of Latin
4. Work experience with an oculist
5. Healthy young age
6. Fine subtle hands
7. Nimble with both hands
8. Able to sketch instruments
9. Not be greedy for money
10. Not be a drunkard.

The eighteenth and nineteenth centuries were periods during which the foundations of recent ophthalmology were laid. Daviel, a French eye surgeon, performed the first cataract extraction on a hermit in 1747 and published the result in a French journal in 1753. The nineteenth century was a period of quicker developments, both in cataract and glaucoma. Helmholtz devised the ophthalmoscope in 1850. Graefe designed the knife for cataract section. The basics of ophthalmic physiology and pathology were better understood. Fuchs wrote a comprehensive book on ophthalmology, a masterpiece, again in German which was translated into English many years later.

Modern developments in ophthalmology were mostly concentrated in the last five decades, after the Second World War. With the advances in technology, machines have acquired more attention than man. The last thirty years have provided investigative and curative facilities beyond expectations. The fact however remains that the edifice of modern ophthalmology is based on yesterday and that yesterday started with Sushruta from the Vedic times and slowly passed to Greeks, Romans and finally the Christian era.

It is beyond a book of the size to describe the history in detail. It will, however, serve the purpose if the back ground is given in a chronological order so that we know our ancestors on whose thinking modern ophthalmology has been built. Even in building this chronological order, space permits the inclusion of only those names whose concepts and contributions were specifically substantive. The following ophthalmic chronology is full of these limitations:

A.	Indian ophthalmologySushruta	1000 BC or earlier	Devised first cataract operation in history Described pterygium operation Described 76 eye diseases
B.	Egyptian ophthalmology Hammurabi	2000 BC	Described varieties of ophthalmia including trachoma
C.	Greek ophthalmology		
	Hippocrate	450 BC	Gave the Hippocratic oath for medical ethics
	Plato	400 BC	Theories of vision
	Aristotle	350 BC	Difference between distant and near vision

Contd.

Contd.

D. Roman ophthalmology

Celsus	AD 50	First original writings available to date prescribed eye drops
Galen	AD 150	Described lens as organ of vision
		Described seven coats of eye
		Recognised seven cranial nerves
		Performed paracentesis

E. Dark periods Ophthalmology in oblivion

F. Renaissance period of Middle ages

1.	Leonardo da Vinci	15th century	Studied ocular anatomy
			Recognised retina as organ of vision
			Described pupillary reaction to light
2.	George Bartische (German)	1583	Wrote the first textbook of ophthalmology

G. Modern Ophthalmology

1.	J. Daviel	1747	First extraction of cataract
2.	I.G. Zinn	1720-1759	Described zonule of Zinn of lens
			Described vascular circle of Zinn round optic nerve head
3.	JR Tenon	1724-1816	Demonstrated Tenon's capsule
4.	J Descemet	1732-1810	Identified Descemet's membrane of cornea
5.	Thomas young	1773-1829	Theory of colour vision
			Theory of accommodation
			Described astigmatism
			Mapped normal field of vision
6.	William Mackenzie	1791-1868	Treatise on glaucoma
			Described sympathetic ophthalmia
7.	F Schlemm	1795-1858	Described Schlemm's canal
8.	J. Muller	1801-1858	Described M. fibres in retina
			Described M. muscle of ciliary body
			Described M. muscle fibres of levator palpebrae superioris
			Described M. muscle of orbit
9.	Loui Braille	1809-1852	Devised writing for the blind, Braille system
10.	C. Ruete	1810-1867	Invented indirect ophthalmoscope
11.	W. Bowman	1816-1892	Originated iridectomy operation
			Introduced retinoscopy
			Defined Bowman's membrane
12.	F.C. Donders	1818-1889	Pioneered optics and refraction
			Described blind spot
13.	C.C. Crede	1857	Silver nitrate prophylaxis for ophthalmia neonatorum
14.	Helmholtz	1851	Developed direct ophthalmoscope
15.	Dieffenbach	1839	First operation for squint
16.	Von Graefe	1828-1870	Used iridectomy for glaucoma
			Described Graefe's sign for Grave's disease
			Designed knife for cataract operation
17.	J. Hutchinson	1838-1913	Described Hutchinson's triad in congenital syphilis
18.	J.F. Horner	1831-1913	Described Horner's syndrome
19.	Snellen	1862	Devised Snellen's charts for distant and near vision record
20.	Holmgren	1866	Discovered electro retinogram
			Holmgren's test for colour vision
21.	DeWecker	1832-1867	Initiated filtering operation for glaucoma
			Designed DeWecker's iris scissors

Contd.

Contd.

22.	E. Fuchs	1851-1889	Masterpice book on ophthalmology in German
23.	Col. Smith (Madras, India)	1903	Practised intracapsular cataract extraction by tumbling
24.	Schiotz	1905	Devised the impression tonometer
25.	Zirm	1863-1906	Performed first keratoplasty operation
26.	Lagrange	1906	Originated sclerectomy for glaucoma
27.	Elliot (Madras, India)	1909	Developed comeoscleral trephining for glaucoma
28.	Gullstrand	1911	Designed a slit lamp
29.	Barraquer (Sr)	1921	Described the eriseiphake for cataract operation
30.	Mathuradas Pahwa (India)	1920	Pioneered rural eye camps
31.	Von Lint	1914	Facial block for akinesia at outer canthus
32.	O'Brien	1929	Facial block at mandibular neck
33.	Elschnig	1865-1928	Retrobulbar anaesthesia
34.	Filatov	1875-1956	Pioneered use of cadaver eyes for corneal transplantation
35.	Ida Mann	1925-1937	Two classic Treatise on Development of Eye Ball and Developmental Anomalies
36.	Goldmann	1938	Developed gonioscopy on slit lamp Devised gonio lens and contact lens for fundu examination Developed applanation tonometry Designed dome projection perimeter
37.	Charles L. Schepens	1945	Developed binocular indirect ophthalmoscope
38.	G. Karpe	1945	Developed clinical electroretinography
39.	Dalios	1948	Contact lenses introduced
40.	Dhanda, RP	1951	First ERG in India recorded
41.	Franceschetti (Switzerland)	1940-1950	Designed newer instruments and developed modern techniques of corneal grafting
42.	Castroviejo, R.	1940-1970	Developed corneal surgery, Designed instruments
43.	Meyerschwikerath (Germany)	1954	Developed photocoagulation techniques

H. Drugs that revolutionized therapy

i.	Antibiotics	1945	Started with penicillin followed by newer generation after generation of broad-spectrum antibiotics
ii.	Steroids	1950	
iii.	Diamox	1954	
iv.	Chymotrypsin	1958	

I. Newer Diagnostic Aids

i.	Applanation tonometry	1955
ii.	Clinical electroretinography	1945
iii.	Ultrasonography	1956
iv.	Optical coherence Tomography	1990

J. Newer procedure

i.	Photocoagulation	1954	
ii.	Phacoemulsification	1966	
iii.	Cryoextraction cataract	1961	
iv.	Corneal grafting	1960	First regular corneal service and Eye Bank in India.
v.	Keratoprosthesis	1951	
vi.	Intra-ocular lens implant	Late fifties	
vii.	Vitreous surgery	1971	
viii.	Pars Plana intra-ocular surgery	Late seventies	
ix.	Radial keratotomy (FyodoroV)	Late seventies	

Many institutions have created a place in history like Filatov's institute in Odessa, Moorfields Hospital in London and Egmore Hospital in Madras. India. Before all these, was the Ophthalmological School in Vienna, Austria, which was the world's first University Eye Clinic, no institution can boast of so many pioneers in ophthalmology who have been on its staff, have taught there or have attracted students from all over the world. It is stimulating to read the list of so many pioneers from one institution.

1.	G.J. Beer (First Director)	For Beer's triangular cataract knife
2.	A. Arlt	Arlt's line of cicatrisatin in Trachoma
3.	T. Benedict	For Benedict's syndrome
4.	DeWecker	DeWecker's iris scissors
5.	F. Dimmer	For description of corneal dystrophy
6.	A. Elschnig	For Elschnig intracapsular forceps
7.	E. Fuchs	Of Fuchs' dystrophy and his wonderful book of ophthalmology
8.	Von Graefe	For Graefe's knife and many other things
9.	K. Hruby	For Hruby's preset lens for fundoscopy
10.	F. Jager	Of Jager's near vision charts
11.	H. Knapps	Knapps roller forceps
12.	W. Mackenzie	For Glaucoma iridectomy
13.	J. Muller	First book on Medical Ophthalmology
14.	K. Stellwag	For Stellwag's sign in thyrotoxicosis
15.	J. Schnabel	Cavernous optic atrophy
16.	M. Salzmann	Salzmann's corneal dystrophy
17.	H. Sattler	For Sattler's veil in contact lens use
18.	E. Zirm	For first keratoplasty

The history of ophthalmology will remain incomplete without recognition of the first ever lens extraction which was performed in the middle of the eighteenth century by a French surgeon, J. Daviel published in 1753 in French and translated into English in 1914 and published in 1947.

Lebensohn, JE. The bicentennial of cataract extraction, *Am. J. Ophth.* 30:922-923,1947.

BIOGRAPHICAL NOTE

Jacques Daviel (1696-1762) was born in La Barre, Normandy. Shortly after completing his medical studies at Hotel Dieu in Paris he volunteered for medical duty during the plague at Toulon and was cited for his ability. After two years he married the daughter of an eye surgeon. In 1747, he successfully performed the first deliberate cataract extraction in history. By the end of 1756, Daviel has done 434 cataract extractions of which 384 were successful. Among his distinguished patients was King Ferdin VII of Spain. Daviel died in 1762.

2

Evolution of Sense of Vision
Development of Eye Ball

Light sense is the essence of all life on earth whether vegetative or biological and the presence of special and specific pigments in the photo-receptors is the basic requirement for light sense because pigment absorbs light which leads to its synthesis and utilization. It is common knowledge that plants need sunlight for proper growth. There are flowers which tend to follow the direction of light from sunrise to sunset.

Biologically the evolution of light sense which is the same as the sense of vision, has been recorded ever since pre-historic times. The pigment producing the protoplasmic cell responsive to light is the most primitive visual organ. Further development and differentiation of cells resulted in the more complex and functionally efficient eyes of invertebrates and the vertebrates. This anatomical evolution was simultaneously associated with complex evolution leading to binocularity, stereopsis, colour vision, etc. in the most developed organism, the man. All organs of light sense in all species are basically epithelial in development. They may be facets on the surface epithelium or sub-epithelial in the form of a vesicular eye. Even the eye developed from the neuro-epithelium as in mammals is basically epithelial in character because the

neuro-epithelium is also the specialized derivative from the ectoderm.

The Evolution of the Eye can best be described in two groups
1. In invertebrates
2. In vertebrates.

THE EYE IN INVERTEBRATES

Amoeba is a typical example of the most primitive unicellular organism which reacts as a whole to light.

A multi-cellular organism may have two types of eyes:
1. The simple eye
2. The compound eye

Simple eye: It is a group of light sensitive cells acting without any discriminating functional association. The simple eye may be epithelial facets on the surface epithelium, the typical example being the vesicular eye of snail. It is interesting that spiders have multiple groups of simple eyes acting independent of each other.

Compound eye: It is composed of sensory cells arranged in different functioning groups. These eyes have a lens and pigment cells. Typical examples are arthropodes like insects, crabs, scorpions etc.

EYE IN VERTEBRATES

The evolution of vertebrates in order of antiquity are:
1. Pre-fish fossils
2. Fish and amphibians
3. Reptiles
4. Avians (birds)
5. Mammals like monkey and man.

The special features of the vertebrate eye are that they develop from the neural ectoderm and are hence called cerebral eyes. They are complex eyes well developed with special features in different species.

It is interesting to note that even early species like amphibians and reptiles have well-developed functions like foveal functions and accommodation. The evolutionary change from amphibians to reptiles to man has been rather small. The special character of the vertebrate eyes is the inverted retina that is the visual cells point outwards, their nutrition being largely from the choroidal circulation and they are nearer the pigment layers. The light in all vertebrate retina reaches the visual cells, the rods and cones. The second special character of vertebrate eyes is the transmission of impulses to the brain through relays or neurons. There are commonly three neurons from each eye, the first neuron, the percipient, the second, the association neuron and the third conductive neuron.

The eyes of fish are adapted to vision in water and therefore the first essential requirement is the covering over the cornea of a transparent nictitating membrane. The cornea being immersed in water and with aqueous behind has no refractive power. Most refraction is therefore carried on by the lens. The lens in fish is situated very near the cornea and accommodation is brought about by pulling the lens back by a ligamentous structure. The eyes are large in size with a flat cornea and hypermetropic character when in the air.

Amphibians differ from the fishes in that they have no gills and respiration is carried on by lungs. In evolution the amphibians have moved from total under water life to breathing from the air when on land. A good example is a frog. The eyes in amphibians are more round with a convex cornea as against the flat cornea of fishes. The lens is placed away from the cornea and the accommodation is brought about by a change in the shape of the lens as in man. Amphibians have lacrimal glands which are absent in fishes. The retina as in fishes, is avascular.

Reptiles also have an avascular retina but have good accommodation brought about by changing the shape of the lens. Snakes in this group have no lacrimal glands and hence no lacrimal fluid. The cornea is however protected by an oily secretion.

Birds eyes are more like reptiles but with a higher degree of specialization. Birds have the highest degree of visual acuity even more than in man, the superiority of man however being the higher degree of cerebral association of vision sense. Interestingly, where man has 200,000 cones per sq. mm in foveal area, the birds have 400,000 cones per sq. mm and the hawk with the highest degree of visual acuity has one million cones per sq. mm. Birds have a high degree of binocularity. The size of the eyes is larger than the brain but the eyes are less mobile, this deficiency being compensated by a greater excursion of the movement of the head.

Mammals

There are three groups of mammals:
1. *Oviparous* which lay eggs.
2. *Marsupials,* where the infant is born immature, the remaining part of which develops outside the mother, a typical example being the kangaroo.
3. *Placentals* where the infant is born mature. It is evident that the eyes of placentals are

most highly developed among the mammals, the highest being the eyes of man which in terms of vision however in second to birds but has the highest quality of discriminating functions like colour sense, fusion and stereopsis and bilateral representation in the brain.

Situation of the eye balls: Eye balls are wider apart in animals which do not need convergence and accommodation but more importantly need a larger field of vision. The most forward placed eyes are in man and hence the binocular capability.

Nictitating membrane: The plica seminularis in the human eye is considered the vestigial remnant of the nictitating membrane. When fully developed, it is a protective membrane for the cornea, under-water as in fish, underground as in frogs and snakes and while flying as in birds. A variant of the nictitating membrane in reptiles burrowing underground is a tough membrane and is called brille (the spectacle).

Lacrimal gland: It is typically absent in snakes.

Pupil: The common shapes of pupil are a slit pupil or a round pupil. The slit pupil is a peculiarity of fish and amphibians.

Lens: The special features are in snakes, fishes, sharks and other amphibians, in which the lens is pulled back or pushed forwards for accommodation rather than become thicker or thinner as in human beings.

Extra-ocular muscles: A special feature in carnivorous animals and some reptiles is a muscle called the retractor bulbi which pulls the eye back in time of emergencies.

Retinal vascularity: Direct blood supply through the retinal arteries is a feature of man, mammals and reptiles while many other species have no retinal vessels and nourishment comes only from choroidal circulation specially in birds. There is a special vascular membrane in some birds extending from the disc into the vitreous which is called pecten.

Tapetum: It is a membrane that is either fibrous or cellular situated between the retina and the choroid. It reflects light and therefore the eyes of the species with tapetum shine at night. It is present in a large number of animals being cellular in carnivorous and fibrous in unguates (animals with hoofs).

The macula, although anatomically present in all animals, is functionally highly developed in man and monkey to the extent that one-third of the optic nerve fibres are from the macula alone.

Chiasmal crossing: It is a characteristic of vertebrates. In mammals, it is partly crossed and partly uncrossed. The higher the species the more are the crossed fibres. This anatomical fact gives the binocular representation of each eye on both sides of the brain.

The pineal gland is homologus of a vestigial pineal eye in most species. Some remnants of which are noted in frogs and is called a pineal eye.

The superior corpora quadrigemina along with lateral geniculate body are important relay centres and do the function of visual cortex in invertebrates and are therefore called optic lobes as against corpora quadrigemina in man. As we get nearer the mammalian stage, corpora quadrigemina become functionless, so that ultimately in man 90% of fibres that reach the cerebral cortex are relayed in the lateral geniculate body.

DEVELOPMENT OF EYE BALL

The general plan of development of an organ consists of an initial stage of (a) *embryogenesis* when the primary layers of embryo are segregated (b) *organogenesis* when the segregated layers develop into identifiable organs and (c) *differentiation* when these organs develop their characteristic feature, structural and functional.

The process of embryogenesis includes the initial development of a fertilized ovum when the germ layers are differentiated and specific cell groups destined to form different organs are separated. For the development of the eye ball, this stage ends with the appearance of optic primordium just before 2.6 mm stage at the third week after fertilization. It can be identified as the future eye ball at a very early stage of development of the embryo.

All the three germinal layers contribute in its development, the *neuroectoderm* forms the visual apparatus, the *surface ectoderm* helps develop the important elements of the dioptric system and the *mesoderm* contributes to the development of vascular and supportive connective tissue elements and the adnexa.

At the anterior end of the neural tube, the optic pits, one on either side, make their appearance as early as the 3 mm stage. They grow to form the primary optic vesicles and remain attached to the neural tube (future fore-brain) by the optic stalk. The invagination of the optic vesicle anteriorly by the surface ectoderm to form the lens and formation of embryonic or foetal fissure on the under surface lead to the convertion of the optic vesicle to the optic cup. This is the stage of organogenesis occurring during 5-6 weeks after fertilization. Later on further development and differentiation take place.

The optic vesicle forms as a spherical pouch from the optic pit. As it increases in size, its distal part comes in apposition to the overlying surface ectoderm which indents and ultimately invaginates into the optic vesicle. A similar indentation (without invagination of surface ectoderm) takes place on lower medial aspect of the optic vesicle, the foetal fissure. Eventually the single walled optic vesicle becomes converted into a double walled secondary optic vesicle also called optic cup. The original cavity of the primary optic vesicle is reduced to a potential space between the two layers of the secondary optic cup. The foetal fissure on the lower aspect

gives entry to the surrounding mesoderm into the optic cup. The foetal fissure starts forming at 4.5-5 mm stage and is closed by 13-15 mm stage. By this time the lens vesicle has also separated from the surface ectoderm and lies at the anterior opening of the optic cup.

These two invaginations are a very important stage in the development of the eye ball. If these do not occur, the complete future development is arrested at this stage resulting into microphthalmos with cyst where the primary optic vesicle persist as the cyst. The formation of the foetal fissure is also important for enabling the nerve fibres to enter the optic stalk to constitute the optic nerve (Figs. 2.1 and 2.2).

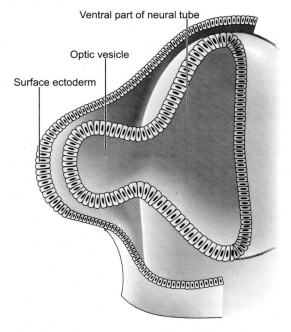

Fig. 2.1: Development of eye—Primary optic vesicle stage

The optic cup also called the secondary optic vesicle is a double-walled structure. The invagination to form the foetal fissure extends into the optic stalk. The posterior or the proximal end of the fissure exists even after the rest of the fissure has closed, as the entrance point of the central artery of the retina into the optic nerve.

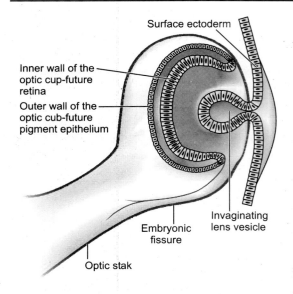

Fig. 2.2: Development of eye ball—Secondary optic vesicle

The optic cup is now surrounded by the mesoderm on all sides with a layer of surface ectoderm anteriorly. The mesodermal elements also occupy the cavity of the cup behind the lens vesicle as the hyaloid system of vessels. The outer wall of the optic cup differentiates into the pigment epithelial layer of the retina while the inner wall of the optic cup develops to differentiate into the different layers of retina except the rods and cones which are formed the last as ciliary projections from the basement layers of the inner wall of neuroectodermal cells.

The anterior edge of the cup develops to project forward in front of the lens vesicle and forms the double-layered iris epithelium and iris muscle (only muscle developed from neuro-ectoderm) and the folded posterior part, the ciliary epithelium of the ciliary processes.

The pigment appears in the outer wall of the optic cup and gradually extends forwards into the ciliary and iris parts, to continue into the inner layer of the neuroepithelium of iris but stops short at the root of iris so that the inner layer of ciliary epithelium remains without pigments.

The cells of the inner wall of the optic cup multiply fast to form a multi-celled layer. These cells are called *neuroblasts*. They proliferate nearer the cavity of the cup and in further development migrate inwards to the acellular marginal zone thus becoming divided into two layers, inner and outer neuroblastic layers with a narrow acellular zone called the transient *fibre layer of Chievitz*. The neuroblastic layers further differentiate into the different layers of adult retina.

Differentiation in the macular area is early and rapid up to the third month of intra-uterine life. Later however it lags behind the rest of the retina until about the eight month. In the last month of intra-uterine life the macular area again starts developing and differentiating which continues to 4 months after birth.

Differentiation into individual layers of the retina is in the reverse direction of the sensory light stimulus, that is, the ganglion cells are differentiated first while the rods and cones come last.

Cilio-iridic neuro-ectoderm: Soon after the foetal fissure has closed and the lens vesicle has separated from the surface ectoderm, the anterior rim of the optic cup starts rapidly growing forwards. Radial folds appear which are the future ciliary professes. The growing edge advances in front of the lens vesicle to form the neuroectodermal epithelium of iris (60-65mm stage). Over this the mesoderm develops to form the iris stroma and its vasculature. Each of the primitive ciliary process is invaded by meso-dermal tissue to form its core. The pigmentation process of this part of neuro-epithelium is already described.

Muscles of iris: The anterior layer of the neuroectoderm of the iris becomes differentiated to form the sphincter pupillae which is more defined and functionally active. It becomes identifiable at about the 65 mm stage. As the growth of the iris proceeds, fine myofibrils make their appearance in the anterior layer of the neuroepithelium near the pupillary margin where pigmentation has not occurred. This forms a mass of muscle fibrils which is invaded by fine capillaries and connective tissue at six months' stage as the iris stroma develops from the anterior mesoderm. The invading mesoderm divides the muscles fibres into the individual bundles and separates them from the parent epithelium. The muscle, although called a sphincter, is not a continuous circular bundle of muscle fibres but is arranged as distinct separate muscle units round the pupillary aperture. This is the basis for part of the pupillary margin responding to light stimulus even after a complete iridectomy.

The dilator muscle makes its appearance well after the sphincter has well developed. It remains ill defined and is identifiable as only fine myofibrils in the cytoplasm of the anterior epithelial cells in the peripheral part at about 6 months' stage. The dilator muscle which is functionally much less active, remains an integral part of the epithelium and is therefore not easily identified.

Optic nerve: The optic stalk which connects the optic vesicle to the forebrain shares in the process of invagination of the vesicle into a cup. The foetal fissure invagination extends into the stalk and as already described, its posterior extremity remains patent as the point of entrance of the central artery of retina. The optic stalk is open to both cavities, proximally to that of the forebrain and distally to optic vesicle and has a wide lumen. As development proceeds, it becomes longer with progressively diminishing lumen.

The nerve fibres start growing from the ganglion cells (15 mm stage). The fibres reach the future optic disc area and turn at right angles to enter the optic stalk. Since this occurs all around the rim, a small mass of glial cells in the centre are cut off as a cone-shaped papilla in front of the disc, *Bergmeister's papilla* which atrophies when the main hyaloid artery disappears before birth. The degree of atrophy of the papilla determines the depth of the physiological cup.

The lumen of the optic stalk is nearly filled up with the nerve fibres, axons of ganglion cells, by 25 mm stage. Cells derived from the primitive epithelium of the optic stalk form the supporting glial framework of the optic nerve.

From the Surface Ectoderm Develop

1. Epithelium of the cornea.
2. Epithelium of conjunctiva, lacrimal gland.
3. Epithelium of lids and its derivatives, cilia, tarsal glands and the ciliary and conjunctival glands.
4. Epithelial lining of lacrimal apparatus.
5. Lens.

From Neuro Ectoderm Develop

1. Retina with pigment epithelium.
2. Epithelium of ciliary processes and iris.
3. Pigment epithelium on the posterior surface of iris.
4. Sphincter and dilator pupillae muscles.
5. Optic nerve (Neuroglial and nervous elements only).

From Mesoderm Develop

1. Blood vessels of eye ball and orbit.
2. The sclera.
3. Ciliary muscles.
4. Substantia propria of cornea and its endothelium.
5. Stroma and anterior endothelium of the iris.
6. The extrinsic muscles of the eye.
7. Bony walls of orbit.
8. Connective tissue, muscles and vasculature of lids.

SURFACE ECTODERM

Lens

There is a single cell layer of surface ectoderm overlying the optic vesicle. As the optic vesicle grows and approaches the surface ectodermal layer, there is a thickening in the single cell layer, the lens plate, at 4.5 mm stage.

The lens plate begins to show a depression, lens pit, and at the same time starts invaginating the optic vesicle. The process continues till 7 mm stage when the lens pit has become a lens vesicle lined by a single cell layer, and the stalk attaching it to the surface ectoderm disappears separating the vesicle and reestablishing a continuity of the overlying surface ectoderm. This is the first stage of lens development, that of formation of lens vesicle from surface ectoderm. The surface ectodermal layer that has become continuous again is the future corneal and conjunctival epithelium (Fig. 2.3).

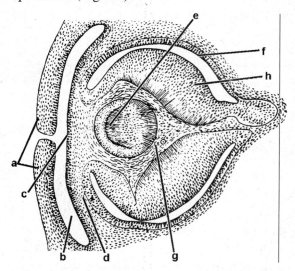

Fig. 2.3: Development of eye ball (a) Lid fold; (b) Conjunctival sac; (c) Corneal epithelium; (d) Anterior mesoderm–to be differentiated into corneal stroma and mesoderm of the iris; (e) Developing lens, primary lens fibres from posterior epithelium form; (f) Pigment epithelial layer of retina–outer neuro-ectodermal layer of secondary of optic cup; (g) Developing vitreous; (h) Inner neuro-ectodermal layer differentiating into retinal cell layers.

The lens vesicle, a hollow sphere, after the 10 mm stage, enters the second stage of development. The anterior wall of the vesicle is formed by the peripheral cell of the lens plate which remain unchanged and as single cell layer of cubical cells all through life under the anterior capsule. The cells of the posterior wall start differentiating, first central then peripheral, into elongated columnar cells stretching from posterior to anterior so as to encroach into the cavity of the vesicle and, on reaching the anterior wall they completely obliterate the cavity, about 18 mm stage. These constitute primary lens fibres which form the embryonic nucleus. During this process the posterior cells have exhausted themselves and henceforth the posterior capsule is devoid of cellular elements. It is the equatorial area of the cubical cells which go on forming the lens fibres throughout life. These secondary fibres grow in a peculiar but regular fashion. The anterior end of each passes to the anterior pole of lens under the anterior cubical epithelium and the posterior end backwards to the posterior pole under the posterior capsule. Layer upon layer of fibres form from the equatorial cells, each fresh layer pushing the previous layer towards the centre of the lens thus surrounding the embryonic nucleus of primary fibres. The increase in equatorial diameter makes the primitive spherical lens to a biconvex-shaped structure of the adult.

The primary fibres run from the posterior to the anterior pole without interruption but the secondary fibres are not long enough to reach from one end to another and therefore they unite to form sutures. During a transient stage, they form an anterior vertical and posterior horizontal lines which, towards third month, branch into a tri-radiate form resembling Y, erect anteriorly and inverted posteriorly. In successive layers, the suture lines become more complex progressively as the layers of secondary fibres are laid down.

The lens capsule develops as a thickening of the fine basement layer of the surface ectodermal cells and becomes evident about 8-10 mm stage.

A fully developed lens by adult sage shows the following zones on slit lamp

1. **The embryonic nucleus** is the optically clear central area formed by primary lens fibres from posterior epithelium and visible in the centre of the adult nucleus.
2. **The foetal nucleus** which surrounds the embryonic nucleus is formed from secondary lens fibres laid down during 3rd–8th month of foetal life and contains the Y sutures.
3. **The adult nucleus** is formed after puberty in adult life.
4. **Cortex** is formed by secondary fibres which lie between the nuclei and the subcapsular epithelium anteriorly and the capsule posteriorly.

VITREOUS

Development of vitreous can be divided into three stages:

1. Primary
2. Secondary
3. Tertiary.

Primary

As the lens vesicle separates from surface ectoderm and lies at the anterior opening of the optic cup which is deepening, the cavity of the cup is bridged by protoplasmic threads connected posteriorly to the neuro-epithelium and anteriorly to the lens epithelium, and this forms the primary vitreous.

Around the 10 mm stage, the mesodermal vascularised elements enter through the foetal fissure and invade the vitreous chamber. These merge with the ectodermal protoplasmic elements. The hyaloid artery proliferates and separates the lens from primary vitreous which is homogenous in the beginning but soon becomes fibrillar entangling the hyaloid capillaries. Near the equator of the lens the fibrillar pattern starts assuming a fan-like arrangement.

Secondary or Definitive Vitreous

This stage lasts from the 13 to 70 mm stage. A finer but denser layer of vitreous makes its appearance near the surface of retina with the fibrils parallel to the surface of retina. There are no capillaries. Thicker fibrils are seen at the anterior part. The vitreous is attached to the internal limiting membrane of the retina. It also has connections to the posterior capsule of the lens in the form of a ring called *hyaloido-capsular ligament* as well as to the region of optic disc.

Atrophy of the hyaloid capillaries and growth of secondary vitreous which now fills large part of vitreous cavity leads to localization of primary vitreous along with hyaloid remnants to the centre of the vitreous cavity known as Cloquet' canal when the vascular elements have atrophied. The hyaloid artery or its remnant, when they persist, occupy the canal.

Tertiary Vitreous or Zonule

At 170 mm stage well-formed fibrils are seen extending between the ciliary processes and lens, forming the tertiary vitreous.

As the vascular coat of lens atrophies and disappears and the eye grows in size, there fibrils become longer and stronger and well defined eventually becoming grouped as anterior and posterior bundles. This also causes atrophy of the most anterior and peripheral part of secondary vitreous so that its connection with internal limiting membrane is retained only upto ora serrata leaving the tertiary vitreous in front attached to the ciliary body and lens, *the zonule*.

MESODERMAL STRUCTURES OF THE EYE

It is the para axial mesoderm which contributes the vascular and stromal elements to the eye ball in its development.

The mesoderm surrounds the developing optic vesicle and optic cup. After separation of lens vesicle, it insinuates between the surface and neuro-ectoderm and also into the cavity of the optic cup. The anterior mesoderm forms the iris stroma and corneal substantia propria. The middle portion of this mesodermal mass atrophies giving rise to the space recognised as anterior chamber. Similarly, the conjunctival vessels and connective tissue is formed under the epithelial layer of surface ectoderm which is the future conjunctival epithelium.

The sclera and choroid develop from the mesoderm surrounding the optic cup. The condensation of mesoderm to form the sclera begins about 20 mm stage, first at the limbus and then gradually extending backwards. At the end of 5 months the condensation has reached the posterior pole of the eye ball. Further condensation and differentiation into collagen and elastic fibres make the sclera thicker. Tenon's capsule is also the result of peripheral condensation enveloping the formed sclera.

The development of choroid is nearly complete by the fifth month. The chorio-capillaries form the first layer of vessels. Venous channels form on the outer side in the third month. The arterial plexus makes its appearance between the chorio-capillaries and the venous plexus in 4th month. The choroid as a whole is well differentiated by the seventh month.

The hyaloid artery enters the optic cup through the foetal fissure and contributes to the formation of the posterior vascular sheath of lens. It also provides vascularisation to the interior of growing eye ball during 40-60 mm stage. At 60 mm stage, the hyaloid system starts to atrophy. The main trunk loses its connection with its branches in the primary vitreous and the part embedded in the optic nerve is then called the trunk of the central artery of retina. At about the forth month two solid buds appear on the disc. These represent the upper and lower branches of the central artery. These soon grow and become canalised. More budding and ramifications occur and at about the eighth month the retinal vasculature reaches the periphery. Venous channels develop simultaneously and accompany the arterial tree.

LIDS AND LACRIMAL PASSAGES

They are formed both from the surface ectoderm and mesoderm. The single layer of surface ectoderm overlying the growing optic cup forms the corneal and conjunctival epithelium. After the sixth week, two folds appear in the surface ectoderm to form the upper and lower lids. These grow and unite together in front of optic cup in the ninth week. They remain united throughout the development, as if to protect the developing eye ball.

During the period of union, lacrimal gland and naso-lacrimal passages are formed from the epithelium of surface ectoderm. The upper and outer surface ectodermal buds grow towards the outer and upper orbital angle where it differentiates to form lacrimal gland. Mesodermal structures are formed later from the paraxial mesoderm. The development of two canaliculi, lacrimal sac and the naso-lacrimal duct takes place from epithelial down-growths. These are solid in the beginning but canalise just before birth. A delayed canalisation results in blockage of naso-lacrimal passages and is the basis of congenital or infantile dacryocystitis.

While lid folds remain untied, changes are taking place at the future lid margins and in the lid folds.

Around the fourth month, eyelashes and the glands of lid appear. Mesodermal ingrowths develop vasculature and tarsal plates. The orbicularis oculi develops along with other facial muscles. The lid folds remain united till the eighth month of intra-uterine life when keratinisation at the site of union of the two folds separates the lids.

It is good to remember at least the approximate age of the embryo and foetus when different stages of development of eye ball take place. This is important to understand pathogenesis of developmental anomalies and is also of significance in clinical diagnosis of congenital defects.

CHRONOLOGY OF DEVELOPMENT OF THE EYE BALL

A. **Embryonic period**

It extends from the beginning of the fourth to end of the eighth week of gestation. It is a very important period in the development of eye ball. Number of important events take place.

1. Appearance of optic pits	2.6 mm	25 days
2. Optic vesicle forms	3.2 mm	28 days
3. Lens plate appears	4.2 mm	
4. Invagination and formation of lens vesicle	5.0 mm	5 weeks
5. Embryonic fissure forms giving access to vascularised mesoderm	6.0 mm	
6. Retinal differentiation starts. The lens vesicle is detached	8-9 mm	
7. Embryonic fissure starts closing and lens vesicle is filled by fibres from the posterior epithelium	11-12 mm	
8. Embryonic fissure completely closed, ganglion cells of retina differentiated with their axons entering the optic stalk (future optic nerve)	13-14 mm	
9. Rudimentary lids appear	15-16 mm	
10. Retinal layers well differentiated. Iris mesoderm is identifiable and scleral condensation starts	17-18 mm	
11. Chiasmal crossing of optic nerve fibres	20-21 mm	
12. Mesodermal corneal stroma appears along with beginning of anterior chamber identification	22-30 mm	8th week

5 to 30 mm growth is equal to 5 to 8 weeks of gestation

B. **Foetal Period**

At the end of eighth week of gestation, the embryo has developed into an identifiable foetus and so the intra-uterine period extending from the beginning of third month to birth is called the foetal period. During this period of about 31 weeks, the growth of the foetus is rapid and fairly constant, approximately 10 mm per week. A simple formula for age and mm length relationship after 8 weeks of embryonic life is:

Length of foetus = (Age in weeks–5) × 10.

Stages of development of the eye ball during foetal period are summarized below:

1. Individual layers of the retina become identifiable and the secondary vitreous is fully developed. The lid folds unite to close the palpebral fissure. *Diameter of eye ball is 1 mm*	30-40 mm	9 weeks
2. Ciliary body formed with differentiation of its muscles and appearance of lens zonule	40-50 mm	10 weeks
3. Macular area can be recognised	50-60 mm	11 weeks
4. Rudimentary rods and cones appear. Sphincter pupillae muscle differentiates from the iris neuroepithelium. The limbal area is demarcated	60-70 mm	12 weeks
5. Hyaloid system and the posterior vascular sheath of lens atrophy. Ciliary processes are well formed. Eye lashes and glands appear in lids. *Diameter of the eye ball is 7 mm*	75-110 mm	16 weeks

Contd.

Contd.

6.	Choroidal layers well recognised. Melanoblasts appear. The iris is fully developed and scleral condensation is well advanced.	110-150 mm	20 weeks
7.	Dilator muscle of the iris makes its appearance. Descemet's membrane of cornea can be identified. Nuclei of rods and cones are differentiated.	150-200 mm	26 weeks
8.	Pupillary membrane and Bergmeister's papilla atrophy starts. Myelination of nerve fibres reaches chiasma. *Diameter of eye ball is 14 mm*	200-230 mm	28 weeks
9.	Retinal vasculature is well developed, Myelination extends into the optic nerve, Lids separate	230-265 mm	31 weeks
10.	Mesoderm in angle of anterior chamber has atrophied up to trabecular meshwork. Myelination has reached up to lamina cribrosa and except the macular area, retina is completely developed. *Diameter of the eye ball is 16 mm.*	265-300 mm	35 weeks

THE EYE BALL AT BIRTH

The eye ball at birth is 16 mm in diameter and hence hypermetropic. The cornea is relatively large in size. The sclera is thin and bluish in colour. The anterior chamber is rather shallow and the pupil small. The uveal tract has scarce pigments. The lens is rounder. The cones are short. The fovea is not properly developed structurally and functionally also. It continues to develop till 4-6 weeks after birth and hence the frequent consequence of nystagmus in bilateral ocular lesions of congenital origin or lesions developing in both eyes soon after birth. The infant starts fixing objects by 6 weeks. He follows objects with both eyes by six months of age and develops full range of binocular vision by age of 6 years. The eye ball as a whole is developed to full normal adult size by the age of 10 years.

3

Anatomy of the Eye Ball

The eye ball is the most highly specialised sense organ serving the most vital function of providing sight to living creatures. It is not generally under stood that the eye ball only serves the purpose of condensing and directing the rays of light on a sensitive retina from which impulses are transmitted to the occipital lobe of the brain. The eye ball, therefore, acts mainly as a peripheral receptor and all the images formed on the retina are actually appreciated, interpreted, evaluated and analysed at the higher centres only.

The shell of the eye ball is formed by the sclera and cornea on the outer side, the retina on the inner side and the choroid in between the two. The interior of the eye ball is divided into anterior segment and posterior segment, the dividing line being the lens. The anterior segment is divided by the iris-lens diaphragm into anterior and posterior chambers containing the aqueous humour. The posterior segment is filled by jelly-like vitreous.

The Adult Eye Ball

The eye ball is not quite spherical in structure although it is nearly so. It has the following statistics in an emmetropic normal eye:

a.	Anterio-posterior length	24 mm appx.
b.	Horizontal diameter	23.5 mm appx.
c.	Vertical diameter	23.0 mm appx.
d.	Volume of eye ball	7.0 cc
e.	Weight of the eye ball	6.8 gms
f.	Circumference of eye ball	72 mm
g.	Radius of curvature of posterior 5/6th (scleral shell)	12 mm
h.	Radius of curvature of anterior 1/6th (cornea)	8 mm

The eye ball is situated slightly higher in the orbital cavity with a cushion of orbital fat for support below. Posteriorly it is fixed by the optic nerve, anteriorly supported by the lids, inferiorly by the hammock of the suspensory ligaments attached to the orbit through the medial and lateral check ligaments. The movements are controlled by the four recti and two oblique muscles. Tenon's capsule enveloping the sclera provides a smooth surface like the synovial sheath of joint.

Surface Anatomy of the Eye Ball

Most of the measurements needed for intra-ocular surgery are done on the outer surface of the sclera. These measurements are usually in relation to the limbus which forms the junction between the cornea and sclera. One should be particularly conversant with the surface representation of the ciliary zone, the pars plana, the ora serrata and the equator of the eye ball.

Newer advances in the techniques of intra-ocular surgery through the pars plana have made the subject still more important (Figs 3.1A and 3.1B).

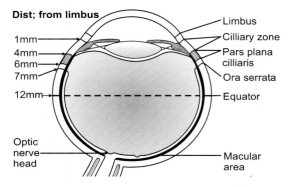

Fig. 3.1A: Eye ball external

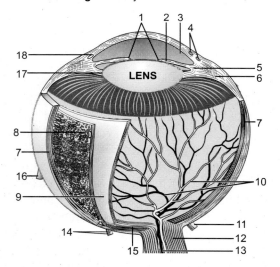

Fig. 3.1B: Inside of eye ball (1) Pupil (2) Iris (3) Anterior chamber (4) Episcleral veins (5) Posterior chamber (6) Ciliary body (7) Sclera (8) Choroid (9) Retina (10) Retinal vasculature (11) Short posterior ciliary vessels (12) Optic nerve (13) Central reitnal artery and vein (14) Long posterior ciliary vessels (15) Macula (16) Vortex vein (17) Suspensory ligament of lens (Zonule) (18) Canal of schlemm

The whole of the ciliary zone from limbus to 7 mm all around was considered a danger zone. This is not considered true now. The actual ciliary zone which represents the corona of the ciliary processes inside is only a strip 2.5 mm wide all round called pars plicata. Entry into the eye for a pars plana surgery at a point 3.5 mm to 5.5 mm will avoid the ciliary zone anteriorly. Posterior to this safety zone, is 1 mm zone of ora serrata, where the vitreous base and retina are adherent to the choroid. The ora serrata can be identified as a narrow dark girdle behind the illuminated pars plana by transillumination through the pupil. It is also to be noted that the ora serrata is slightly more anterior on the nasal side than the temporal side.

The four recti muscles are attached to the sclera, the medial rectus being nearest to limbus 5.5 mm, the inferior rectus 6.5 mm, the lateral rectus 6.9 mm and superior rectus being farthest, 7.7 mm from the limbus. Because of this, the superior rectus muscle should be the first to be cut in enucleation and then the medial rectus, inferior rectus and lastly the lateral rectus.

The equator is situated approximately 13 mm from the limbus. The vortex veins (vena vorticosae), four is number, two above and two below on either side of the superior and inferior recti, pierce the sclera obliquely from before backwards appearing on the surface about 6-7 mm behind the equator.

Both the oblique muscles are attached on the sclera behind the equator on the temporal side. The superior oblique is inserted in the upper and outer quadrant. The inferior oblique is inserted just above the horizontal meridian with the posterior end being about 2 mm from the macula.

The optic nerve which is 1.5 mm thick and surrounded by its meningeas pierces the sclera about 3.5 mm medially from the posterior pole corresponding to the macula.

Identification of the enucleated eye ball, whether it is a right eye or left, can be done by the following points:

a. Determining the upper limbus by slight scleral encroachment.

b. Measuring the attachment of the four recti muscles from the limbus, the superior rectus being farthest and the medial rectus nearest to limbus.

c. The vortex veins, two each, above the below, behind the equator.

d. The insertion of superior oblique in the upper and outer quadrant behind the equator.

e. The direction of the optic nerve stump in relation to the posterior pole, the optic nerve is attached medial to the posterior pole.

When the eye is examined, with the cornea in front and the encroached limbus above, if the optic nerve is to the right of the posterior pole, it is the right eye, if it is on the left side, it is the left eye.

NERVE SUPPLY OF THE EYE BALL AND ITS ADNEXA

Oculomotor Nerves

The third, fourth and sixth cranial nerves are the principal motor supply of the extrinsic and intrinsic muscles of the eye and therefore control ocular movements, pupillary contraction and accommodation. The nuclei of these nerves are situated in the floor of aqueduct of Sylvius and upper part of the floor of the 4th ventricle. These oculomotor nuclei in turn have extensive association communications with the higher visual centres through the pyramidal tract, the medial longitudinal bundle and possibly other tracts not yet understood.

Third Oculomotor Nerve

The third nerve nucleus is a composite nucleus for both sides with specific representation of the various muscles supplied by this nerve. The levator palpabrae superioris and the superior rectus nuclei are farther away from the mid-line and medial rectus nuclei are very close to each other and the two portions representing medial recti are connected with each other centrally and this part is called Perlias nucleus responsible for convergence.

Anteriorly is a paired Edinger Westphal nucleus supplying parasympathetic fibres to the sphincter muscles of the pupil and the circular muscle of the ciliary body and thus responsible for accommodation and contraction of the pupil.

The two third nerves starting from the nucleus, leave the brain substance in the groove between the pons below and cerebral punduncle above. The posterior cerebellar arteries are in close association with the roots of the third nerve. The nerve, after leaving the brain substance passes between the posterior cerebral and superior cerebellar arteries and then lies in the lateral wall of cavernous sinus anteriorly. Here it is closely related to the sixth cranial nerve medially. The fourth nerve and 1st and 2nd divisions of fifth nerve are posteriorly to the third nerve.

The third nerve after dividing into two divisions passes through the central part of the superior orbital fissure within the annulus of Zinn. The nerve supplies the superior rectus, medial rectus, inferior oblique and levator palpabrae superioris. The nerve fibres to the medial and inferior recti are on the inner surface of the muscle belly, while the nerve supply to the superior rectus is between this muscle and levator palpabrae superioris. The parasympathetic nerve fibres to the sphincter muscle of iris and ciliary muscle accompany the branch to the inferior oblique muscle from which they separate and reach the ciliary ganglion to form synaptic connections (Figs 3.2A and 3.2B).

Fourth Trochlear Nerve

The fibres from the nucleus of the 4th nerve in the mid brain decussate to the opposite side before leaving on the dorsal aspect of the brain stem at the upper border of the pons and hence it is closely

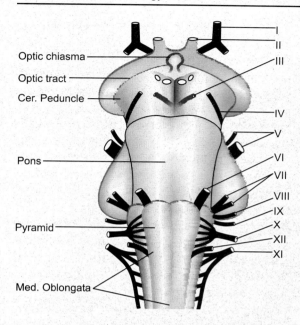

Optic chiasma

Optic tract

Cer. Peduncle

Pons

Pyramid

Med. Oblongata

I
II
III
IV
V
VI
VII
VIII
IX
X
XII
XI

Fig. 3.2A: Cranial nerves (I to XII) at their exit from the base of the brain

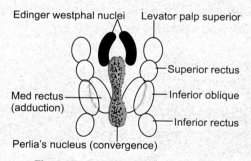

Edinger westphal nuclei   Levator palp superior

Med rectus (adduction)

Perlia's nucleus (convergence)

Superior rectus

Inferior oblique

Inferior rectus

Fig. 3.2B: Oculomotor (III) nerve nuclei

related to the posterior cerebral and superior cerebellar arteries. This nerve has the longest intracranial course during which it lies in the lateral wall of the cavernous sinus behind the 3rd nerve and enters the orbit through the upper part of the superior orbital fissure above the annulus of Zinn. It supplies the superior oblique muscle on the upper surface and hence may escape the effect of retrobulbar injection which may paralyse all the movements of the eye except intorsion.

Sixth Abducent Nerve

The 6th or the abducent nerve starts from its nucleus in the pons. The nerve leaves the brain substance in the groove between the pons above and the medulla below. In its intra-cranial course it crosses over the apex of the petrous portion of temporal bone under the petro-sphenoidal ligament. It lies within the cavernous sinus between the internal carotid artery on the medial side and nerves in the wall of the cavernous sinus on the lateral side. It enters the orbit through the central part of the superior orbital fissure within the annulus of Zinn and supplies the lateral rectus muscle.

Facial Nerve

It is the motor nerve. The fibres starting from the nucleus in the pons, circle the sixth nerve nucleus emerging at lower border of pons lateral to the sixth nerve. It leaves the intra-cranial cavity along with the 8th nerve through the internal auditary meatus. During its course, it lies in the wall of the middle ear and after emerging through the stylo-mastoid foramen turns forward to lie over the neck of the condyloid process of mandible from which it fans into five branches, the upper three supplying the orbicularis oculi and the frontal part of occipito-frontalis muscle. The secretary fibres to the lacrimal gland in part of their course accompany the facial nerve before joining the greater superficial petrosal nerve.

Trigeminal Nerve (Fig. 3.3)

The fifth cranial or the trigeminal nerve which is the principal sensory nerve of the eye ball and face, has a long nucleus extending from the pons to the 2nd cervical segment. The sensory supply of the upper part of the face is represented in the lowest part of the nucleus of the fifth nerve. It has three divisions namely, ophthalmic, maxillary and mandibular. The first (ophthalmic) division, is the sensory supplier to the skin of lids, conjunctiva, cornea, iris and ciliary body through its three branches, i.e. the lacrimal, frontal and nasociliary nerves which enter the orbit through the superior orbital fissure.

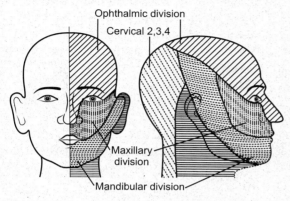

Fig. 3.3: Diagram showing the sensory nerve supply of the face, forehead and occipital region. (Note that the first division (ophthalmic) of trigeminal nerve carries sensation from the forehead, upper lid and the side of the nose up to the tip. Also note that cervical segments 2.3 and 4 are responsible for sensation from occipital region of the scalp and the upper part of neck which explains the referred occipital ache due to ocular conditions.

Autonomic Nerve Supply

The sympathetic and para-sympathetic nerves control important structures and functions of the eye.

The para-sympathetic supply from the nuclei in the midbrain comes along the 3rd (oculomotor) nerve reaching the orbit through the central part of the superior orbital fissure. The supply is relayed through the ciliary ganglion to the iris and ciliary body and through the spheno-palatine ganglion to the lacrimal gland (Fig. 3.4).

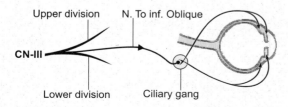

Fig. 3.4: Para-sympathetic supply of the eye ball

The sympathetic supply to the eye ball and adenexa is through the cervical sympathetic and then through the superior cervical ganglion. The fibres are carried along the plexus around the internal carotid artery. The sympathetic supply to the eye ball is principally along the ophthalmic artery while some fibres enter the orbit through the superior orbital fissure along with the naso-ciliary branch. The supply to the iris and ciliary body is through the ciliary ganglion (without synaptic connections) along the long ciliary nerves while the supply to the Muller's muscle in the lid is along the naso-ciliary nerve (Fig. 3.5).

The lacrimal gland receives the sympathetic fibres along with the lacrimal vessels.

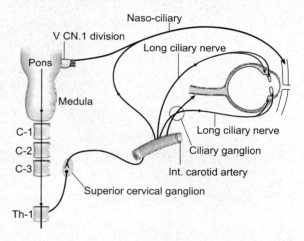

Fig. 3.5: Sympathetic supply of Eye ball

Blood Supply of Eye Ball

Blood supply to the eye ball is essential for nutrition to its tissues and their functions. Tissues, like the uveal tract, have a rich blood supply while the sclera is relatively avascular with scanty blood vessels. It is interesting that the optically most important structures, the cornea, the lens and the vitreous are avascular and receive their nutrition indirectly from the surrounding vascular structures. The avascularity of the cornea, lens and vitreous is responsible for their transparency which allows free passage of light to reach the retina, an essential factor for good visual acuity.

The blood supply to the eye ball and most of its adenexa is principally received from the ophthalmic artery and its branches. The only other source of arterial supply is through a few branches of facial artery and the external carotid artery supplying the lids (Fig. 3.6).

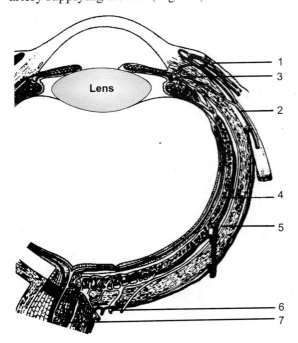

Fig. 3.6: Blood supply of eye ball. (1) Posterior conjunctival artery; (2) Anterior ciliary artery as it gives a perforating branch and then anastomoses with posterior conjunctival vessels; (3) Circular iridis major; (4) Choroidal plexus; (5) Long posterior ciliary artery; (6) Short posterior ciliary arteries forming choroidal plexus; (7) Central artery of retina

Ophthalmic Artery

It is a branch of the internal carotid artery and enters the orbit with the optic nerve through the bony optic canal. In the canal, it first lies under the optic nerve to the medial side and then on its lateral side. In the posterior part of the orbit, it lies between the optic nerve on inner side and

the ciliary ganglion and lateral rectus on the outer side. It then crosses over the optic nerve to reach the medial wall of the orbit.

The ophthalmic artery, during its course gives off following branches as it courses from behind forwards:
1. Central retinal artery
2. Posterior ciliary arteries
3. Lacrimal artery
4. Muscular arteries
5. Supra-orbital artery
6. Ethmoidal artery
7. Medial palpebral artery
8. Terminal nasal and frontal arteries

Central Retinal Artery

It branches off from the ophthalmic artery near the optic foramen and runs along the optic nerve near its lower and medial surface. It then pierces the meningeal coverings of the optic nerve and before it enters the nerve substance, it gives off a small branch, the post-central artery, which provides blood supply to the orbital portion of the optic nerve.

The central retinal artery traverses forward and enters the eye ball in the centre of optic disc with the artery on the medial and vein on the lateral side. Here it divides into upper and lower divisions each of which divide into temporal and nasal branches as they cross over the optic disc margin. The branches of central retinal artery lie in the nerve fibre layer of retina. They have a special feature in that they are all end arteries and do not anastomoses with each other. In a majority of places, the artery crosses in front of the vein. At the crossing, they have a common outer sheath. Another special feature of central retinal artery at the optic disc and the retinal layers is its non-pulsating character. This is due to the sudden change from the high intra-arterial pressure in the ophthalmic artery to the low intraocular pressure to which the central artery is exposed.

The central retinal artery supplies blood and thus nutrition and oxygen to the retina upto the inner nuclear layer while the outer layers including layer of rods and cones and pigment epithelium receive blood supply from choriocapillaries. The twigs from the temporal branches of the central retinal artery terminate round the macular area which also receives its nutrition from chorio-capillaries. Anteriorly the terminal branches do not reach the ora serrata and therefore the peripheral retina has a relatively poor blood supply.

Posterior Ciliary Arteries

There are groups of posterior ciliary arteries; the long and short posterior ciliary arteries. Two branches take off from the ophthalmic artery below the optic nerve. They divide and subdivide into 15 to 20 branches which pierce the sclera round the optic nerve and enter the posterior choroid and are called the *short posterior ciliary arteries*. These arteries branch and anastomose to form the choroidal net work. The two *long posterior ciliary arteries* are branches of the ophthalmic artery and pierce the sclera obliquely in horizontal meridian on either side of the optic nerve and traverse forward between the sclera and choroid to enter the ciliary body where they divide and anastomose with each other to form the circulus iridis major near the root of the iris. They also anastomose with the perforating branches of anterior ciliary arteries and together supply the ciliary body and anterior choroid.

Lacrimal Artery

After branching off from the ophthalmic artery it runs along the lateral rectus and supplies the lacrimal gland and contributes to the blood supply of conjunctiva and eye lids through its palpebral and zygomatic branches.

Muscular Arteries

These are lateral and medial branches. The lateral supplies the lateral and superior recti, superior oblique and levator palpebrae. The medial branch supplies the medial, inferior rectus and inferior oblique.

Supra-orbital Artery

It courses along the superior rectus and accompanies the supra-orbital nerve through the supra-orbital notch or foramen. It contributes to the blood supply of the upper lid and scalp over the frontal bone.

Ethmoidal Artery

It branches off from the ophthalmic artery during its course in the medial part of the orbit and passes into the nasal cavity along with the ethmoidal nerves to supply the ethmoidal air cells and nasal mucosa.

Medial Palpebral Artery

It takes off from the ophthalmic artery in anterior part of the orbit and anastomoses with corresponding branches of the lacrimal artery to form the palpebral arcades.

Terminal Nasal and Frontal Artery

They supply the skin and muscles of the forehead, the root of the nose and the lacrimal sac.

Anterior Ciliary Artery

These arteries which arise from the muscular branches are seven in number, two each from the arteries to the superior, inferior and medial recti and one from the artery to external rectus. These arteries give off the anterior conjunctival branches which anastomose with the posterior conjunctival vessels round the limbus. The arteries pierce the sclera about 3-5 mm from the limbus and anastomose with the long posterior ciliary arteries to form the circulus iridis major at the root of the iris. A recurrent branch takes off before this anastomosis which joins the choroidal plexus and supplies the anterior choroid.

The facial artery: supplies blood through its anterior facial branch running from below upwards from the mandibular border to the lateral side of the nose and becomes the angular artery and courses along the angular vein near the inner side of the eye. The angular artery can be seen on the lateral side of the nose lying under the skin where it curves from the medial to lateral side above the medial palpebral ligament to joint the frontal artery which contributes to the formation of arterial arcades of the lid. It is an important vessel in the surgery of the lacrimal sac. It should be identified and a voided during the operative procedure to avoid brisk bleeding if it is inadvertently cut.

External carotid artery: It gives a superficial temporal branch coursing from behind the angle of the mandible towards the lateral orbital margin to anastomose with the lacrimal artery and contributes to form the arterial arcade of lids.

Venous Drainage of Eye

The venous drainage from inside the eye is principally through the two superior and two inferior vena verticosae, draining respectively into the superior and inferior ophthalmic veins. The extra ocular venous drainage from the deeper structure drains posteriorly into the ophthalmic veins and anteriorly into the angular vein. The superior and inferior ophthalmic vein passing through the orbital fissure drain into the cavernous sinus.

Cavernous Sinus

This is an important structure for ophthalmologist from point of view of ocular features resulting from pathology in the cavernous sinus.

The two cavernous sinuses are large venous channels, one on either side of the body of the sphenoid bone in the middle cranial fossa. Each cavernous sinus receives venous blood anteriorly from the inferior and superior ophthalmic veins, and in turn drains posteriorly via the inferior and superior petrosal sinuses into the internal jugular vein. The two cavernous sinuses communicate with each other through a narrow venous channel called the *sinus intercavernosus*. It also communicates with the pterygoid plexus of veins in the pterygo-palatine fossa through emissary veins (Fig. 3.7).

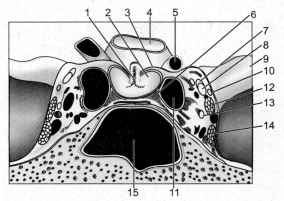

Fig. 3.7: Anatomy of cavernous sinus and its contents. (1) Infundibulum; (2) Pituitary gland; (3) Diaphragmatic sella; (4) Optic chiasma; (5) Internal carotid artery as it comes out of cavernous sinus; (6) Sinus inter-cavernosus; (7) and (8) Two divisions of oculo-motor nerve, (9) Lesser wing of sphenoid, (10) Trochlear nerve, (11) Internal carotid artery in cavernous sinus, (12) Trigeminal nerve-ophthalmic division, (13) Abducent nerve; (14) Trigeminal nerve-maxillary division, (15) Sphenoid sinus

The internal carotid artery enters the cavernous sinus from below and leaves the cavernous sinus through its root. A communication between the internal carotid artery and cavernous sinus following injury, atherosclerosis or aneurysm of the artery results in carotico-cavernous fistula with serious ocular manifestations.

The sixth cranial nerve passes through the cavernous sinus between the internal carotid artery and the lateral wall of the sinus and is therefore the first cranial nerve to be affected in sinus thrombosis.

The lateral wall of the cavernous sinus contains the fallowing structures in order from before backwards.

1. Upper division of the third neve
2. Lower division of the third nerve
3. Fourth cranial nerve
4. First division of the fifth nerve (ophthalmic)
5. Second division of the fifth neve (Maxillary).

LYMPHATIC DRAINAGE OF THE EYE BALL

The inside of the eye ball has no lymphatic spaces or lymphatic vessels. The only circulating fluid inside the eye is the aqueous humour which fills the anterior and posterior chambers. This fluid drains anteriorly into the anterior ciliary veins via the angle of the anterior chamber and the canal of Schlemm. Posteriorly some amount of fluid drains out from behind the lens via the Cloquet's canal into the lymphatics around the optic nerve. A small quantity of aqueous also drians from the angle of anterior chamber into the supra choroidal space and then via the lymphatics surrounding the vortex veins.

True lymphatic channels are however present in the tissues of the adnexa of the eye ball and the orbit. There are three main groups of lymph glands into which these lymphatics drain:

1. The submandibular lymph glands
2. The pre-auricular lymph glands
3. The deep cervical lymph glands.

From the inner half of the lids and conjunctiva, the medial orbital space and the lacrimal drianage area, the lymphatics go along the anterior facial vein and drain into the sub-mandibular lymph glands. Similarly, lymphatics from the outer conjunctiva, lids and orbit drain into the pre-auricular lymph gland. The lymphatics from the deeper part of orbit drain posteriorly mostly via the inferior orbital fissure along the pterygoid plexus of veins and then into the deep cervical lymph glands.

Vision and Visual Functions

The sense of sight is not only the most important of all the senses in body, but is also important for the social, economical and psychological development of the individual. It is surprising how different the reactions are of individuals with different grades of visual acquity. A myopic may have only 50 to 60% of the normal vision and yet he may live through his span of life without ever going to the ophthalmologist. He is not only content with the distance vision he has, but is happier in old age seeing that his contemporaries of the same age are so dependent on near glasses for reading and writing while he does not need them. It is not uncommon to come across patients with one eye normal while the other eye is myopic, hypermetropic or amblyopic and yet not realising that they have been seeing only with one eye. A routine examination of school children is often the first pointer to a defect in vision.

To be able to qualitatively record vision, it is necessary to have methods giving comparable observations, not only in literates and illiterates but also in children and sometimes in infants.

It is well known fact that light rays do not form a point focus on the macular area because of spherical and chromatic aberrations in the refractive media. The focus of light rays on the other hand forms a circle of diffusion and the smallest circle is called the circle of least diffusion. This establishes that more than one rod or cells are stimulated by each of the different components of the objects seen. For critical and discriminate appreciation of the size and shape of the object, the circle of least diffusion must stimulate at least 4 cones at a time, the total diameter of which is 0.04 mm in macular area, and this forms the basis of vision charts. The largely accepted Snellen's charts (Fig. 4.1) of vision for distance are so made that the outline of each letter is divisible into 20 squares and the two ends of each of the twenty squares subtend an angle of 1 min. at different distances depending on the size of the letters. For example, each component of the top letter of the Snellen's chart subtends an angle of 1 min. at 60 meters, while the letters in the line indicating normal visual acuity (6/6) subtend the same angle at a distance of 6 meters.

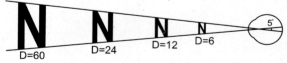

Fig. 4.1: Principle of Snellen's chart

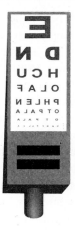

Fig. 4.2: Vision record drum

Six meters is accepted from the practical point of view because most rays from a distance of 6 meters and more are as good as parallel rays. Depending on the number of lines the patient can read, distance vision is recorded as 6/60 to 6/6 with Snellen's chart illuminated either externally or internally with uniform standard illumination. Some charts have letters for recording visual acuity up to 6/5 and 6/4. If a person misses or incorrectly reads some letters of a line, the record is qualified as 'partial'. Further more vision should be recorded for each eye separately as well as binocularly. It is to be noted that the binocular vision (both eyes open) is always one line more than the uniocular vision provided both eyes have equal visual acuity.

The macular part of the retina is most sensitive part and maximum visual acuity is derived form this area. Retinal sensitivity gradually diminishes from the centre to the periphery, so much so that the peripheral retina has only 10% of the central sensation. It is an every day experience that a person with gross localised foveal lesion with whole of the remaining retina normal will not have visual acuity more than 6/60 or 6/36 partial. On the other hand with gross pathological lesions in the peripheral retina but an unaffected macular area, the patient may have 6/6 vision although this will be tubular in character because of the loss of peripheral field.

The standards of visual acuity graded by the World Health Organization are now internationally accepted both from the economic point of view as well as from the point of view of vision as a criteria of disability for recruitment and compensation. If vision with both eyes open is 3/60 or less (with correction if necessary), it is total blindness because a person with that poor a visual acuity cannot independently move about except in very familiar surroundings. If vision, with both eyes open, and with correction if necessary, is more than 3/60 but 6/60 or less, it is considered as economic blindness, because such a person by virtue of his visual handicap cannot earn his living independently. Vision better than 6/60 but 6/18 or less (with both eyes open and with correction) is considered a visual handicap because such a person is visually challenged and may be unfit for service or jobs requiring better visual acuity. Similarly the field of vision reduced to 20 degrees or less is economic blindness even though visual acuity may be good.

In the grades of vision like 6/60, 6/36, ... 6/9, 6/6 the constant number 6 in the numerator indicating the distance from which the patient is reading and the denominator indicates the distance in meters from which the patient should be able to read that line. The vision record in some charts is noted differently but on the same principles. Countries not following the metric system denote it in feet as 20/200 to 20/20. Similarly in some countries, the notation is in decimal, for example 6/6 is 1.0 and 6/60 is 0.1. Another criteria for denoting vision which is particularly important for recording visual improvement or deterioration is on the percentage basis. The percentages however cannot be on the basis of Snellen's criteria but on a more clinically oriented basis. A satisfactory percentage equivalent of vision recorded in Snellen's chart could be as follows:

Percent equivalent of vision:

PR 4+ to 2/60	PR to HM	0.0%
1/60 to 2/60	3/200 to 6/200	5.0%
3/60 to 5/60	10/200 to 15/200	10.0%
6/60	20/200	20.0%
6/36	20/120	40.0%
6/24	20/80	50.0%
6/18	20/60	60.0%
6/12	20/40	80.0%
6/9	20/30	90.0%
6/6	20/20	100.0%

This percentage equivalent of vision is very important to assess percent of visual improvement or otherwise after treatment, medical or surgical.

Different types of vision charts are in use. Charts for literate people are made in different languages maintaining the principle that the maximum thickness of every component of the letter should form the same angle at the same distance as described above. Three types of charts are used for illiterate people. The Landolts 'C' charts are accepted as standard for testing visual acuity for various professions in preference to others. The 'E' charts are also identical and can be used under the same guide lines as 'C' charts. The dot charts showing a different number of dots of different sizes are also convenient. Charts with pictures of different objects are specially meant for pre school children. Multi-coloured balls can be used from different distances for the toddlers. Optokinetic drums are used for infants where it is questionable whether the child has vision or is blind, a problem raised by many parents.

COLOUR VISION AND COLOUR BLINDNESS

Colour vision is a special acquisition in human beings. Although this has been a universally known fact, the physiological understanding of colour vision has remained a subject of controversial theories. The hypothesis put forward by Thomas Young and later supported by Helmholtz were the only concepts that carried conviction. In the confusion that has persisted for many decades the most universally accepted concept at present is the trichromatic theory of colour vision which states that there are three types of cones with three types of pigments for red, green and blue colours and that there are possibly three sets of nerve fibres carrying the colour sense to the brain. The pigments responsible for colour vision are present only in cones and therefore colour vision is the specific function of only the cone cells in the retina. Colour sense being a function of the cones, is therefore most efficiently appreciated in day light. With gradually increasing illumination, the colours become visible in a particular order, the earliest being blue followed by green, yellow and red. Similarly from day light to dark the colour red becomes invisible first and blue the last. Complementary colours are any two spectral colour which when mixed, produce white. The common combinations of complementary colours are red and green, orange and blue, yellow and green. On this basis individuals with normal colour sense are called *trichromats*. Individuals who have no colour sense or a sense of only white, are called *archromats*. *Dichromats* are individuals who can perceive only two of the three primary complementary combinations, usually green and blue or red and blue. The first, *protanopes* are green blind and use green and blue to match to white. *Deuteranopes* are green blind and use red and blue to match for white. *Tritanopes* are blue blind, this is rare in incidence. They use red and green to match for white.

Colour blindness, better known as colour vision defect is, in most cases a congenital and genetically mediated visual defect. Acquired colour blindness is rare and is secondary to pathologies which disturb the chemistry of the retinal cells. The common acquired conditions which cause relative colour defects are choroidal atrophy, extensive macular degeneration, malignant myopia, retinal detachment, vascular retinopathies, glaucoma, optic atrophy, papillo-edema and toxic amplyopia. In most of these conditions visual loss is the prime consideration and the colour defect is consequential.

On an average 2 per cent of population has some form of colour defect of a primary hereditary nature. These colour defectives usually remain undetected except when they opt for certain technical jobs and are then picked up during a routine examination. The professions where colour vision is of particular importance are driving, defence services, flying, professions needing accurate colour matching like the textile industry and the diamond industry.

The Common Method of Testing Colour Vision

1. Colour plates of Ishihara
2. Edridge Green lantern
3. Holmgren wool matching
4. Anomaloscope

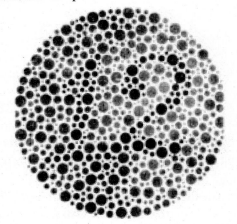

Fig. 4.3: Plate from Ishihara colour vision book

Primary congenital colour blindness is not a reversible pathology, and no treatment is therefore indicated. In acquired colour blindness, treatment is for the causative pathology and not for colour detect.

Field of vision is the peripheral extent to which the eyes can see while fixed on an object straight in front. As against this, the field of fixation is the peripheral extent to which the eye can appreciate the objects by turning the eye maximally in that direction. It is obvious that the field of fixation will be larger than the field of vision.

The field of vision has been described by Traquair as an island of vision in a sea of blindness, and the island is depicted as sloping from the maximal height to the sea level the slope being unequal representing the unequal field in different directions. Near the top of the island is a dark crater which represents the blind spot in the field of vision.

The extent of the field of vision depends on the anatomical configuration of the face. Nature has provided variations depending on the needs of living creatures. Eyes which are more laterally placed as in certain animals, have a greater field of vision but poor binocularity. Eyes which are placed further forwards have a smaller field of vision but better binocularity. The field of vision is contoured by the bony surroundings of the eye ball. For example, in man the field is larger on the temporal side where the eye ball is an front of the level of zygomatico-temporal bony arch, while it is restricted nasally by the bridge of nose and superiorly by the over-hanging supra orbital bony arch.

The extent of the field of vision is different for white as compared to colours, the order being white, yellow, blue, red and green being the smallest. It also varies with the size of the object used. Visual field for a particular object size at a particular distance is called the isoptre for that size and distance. It naturally varies both for the size of the object and the distance from which the object is shown. The method of recording field of vision (perimetry) and the field defects in common clinical conditions are given in the chapter on the examination of the eye.

ACCOMMODATION

Accommodation means the capacity to focus objects at different distances in quick succession. Although it is present in most animals, its relation to convergence and binocularity is developed at its best in human being. Accommodation is a function of each eye separately and both eyes together.

Accommodation in the human eye is brought about by two distinct components, the physiological component in the ciliary body and the physical component in the lens. The physiological part which initiates accommodation is the action of the muscle in the ciliary body. As the circular muscle fibres contract, the zonular fibres of the lens attached to the ciliary processes are relaxed leaving the physical part of the function to take place in the lens.

The anterior capsule of the lens can change its position and shape. The posterior capsule is supported by the hyaloid fossa of the vitreous and is therefore not free to shift. In the anterior capsule, the central part is the thinnest and the anterior surface of the lens therefore protrudes forwards only in the pupillary area, thereby making the lens more convex in the axial part and thus increasing the power of the lens.

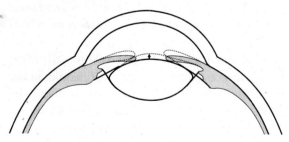

Fig. 4.4: "Lens in accommodative state. Anterior surface more convex and iris pushed forward"

There is another view that instead of relaxing the zonular fibres, the contraction of the ciliary muscle pulls the zonular fibres backwards and thereby physically brings about a change in the shape of the lens. This change in the lens is possibly further augmented by the contraction of longitudinal muscle fibres of the ciliary body, the contraction of which pulls the choroid and vitreous forwards causing pressure on the lens from behind.

It is possible, that both the parasympathetic nerve supply to the circular muscle fibres of the ciliary body and the sympathetic nerve supply to the longitudinal muscle fibres of the ciliary body innervate the accommodative action of the ciliary body (Fig. 4.5).

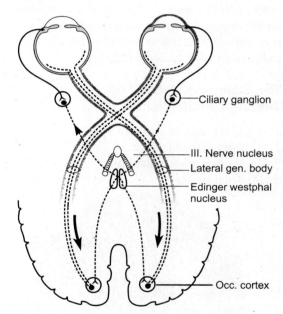

Fig. 4.5: Accommodation reflex, nerve pathway

The accommodation reflex is mediated through the occipital cortex. Blurred vision activates a desire to see clear and this stimulus from the retina is carried along the visual fibres to the occipital cortex from where it is relayed to the Edinger-Westphal nucleus of the 3rd nerve in the mid brain. From there efferent impulses are carried along the parasympathetic fibres in the 3rd nerve and then via the ciliary ganglion in the orbit to the circular muscle fibres of the ciliary body.

The sympathetic innervation of the ciliary muscle is along the sympathetic fibres entering the orbit and supplying the meridional and longitudinal fibres of the ciliary muscle.

Physiologically, accommodation is maximum in childhood and gradually becomes weaker as the age advances. A child has an accommodation power of about 14 diopters which is reduced to 3.5 to 4 diopters by the age of 45 years. It is further reduced to one diopter by the age of 60 years.

To see an object at infinity which for all practical purposes is at 6 meters or more, no accommodation is required. It is evident that hypermetropes use accommodation even for seeing distant objects and therefore higher accommodation for near while myopes use no accommodation for distance and less accommodation for near objects. Myopes however have to use all their accommodation within a limited range of distance between their far and near point which are closer to each other than in emmetropes and hypermetropes. Anomalies of accommodation can therefore cause symptoms not only in hypermetropes but also in myopes.

Measurements of Accommodation

Accommodation is expressed in diopters inversely proportional to the distance in meters. So that seeing an object at 1 meter distance will need an accommodation of 1 diopter and an object at 1/2 meter will need an accommodation of 2 diopters. Accommodation can therefore be measured for a particular distance, and this is called *relative accommodation*. The accommodation which can be enhanced against concave lenses is called *positive accommodation* and the one which can be relaxed against a convex lens is called a *negative accommodation*. It is important for comfortable working that the positive and negative parts should be equal. The total available accommodation in an individual is called *amplitude of accommodation* which is the difference between the dioptric distance of far point and the dioptric distance of near point.

Clinically, for comfortable near work, it is important that all available accommodation should not be used but at least 1/3rd to 1/4th accommodation should remain unused and in reserve. An emmetropic eye needs no accommodation for distance and therefore the amplitude of accommodation is the nearest distance in centimeters at which the individual can see the object clearly, 100 divided by the distance gives the amplitude of accommodation in diopters.

Accommodation is an active physiological process and any disturbance can cause symptoms of asthenopia. It becomes clinically evident when the near point recedes beyond a comfortable working distance. A person requires about 3 diopters of accommodation for near work at a comfortable distance of 1/3 meter while the accommodation power at the age of 45 years is reduced to about 3.5 to 4 diopters. Keeping in reserve of 1/4th to 1/3rd accommodation, the available accommodation at this stage will be less than 3 diopters and hence the need to augment it by convex lenses, the condition called *presbyopia*. This gradual weakening of accommodation is partly due to weakening of the ciliary muscles but largely brought about by the reduced plasticity of the lens. The central part of the lens hardens to form the nucleus and therefore the lens is not as amenable to change its shape as it could do in younger age.

Accommodation is closely related to convergence for all near work. When a person exerts accommodation for near, the eyes simultaneously converge so that the focus of the image falls on the macular area of both eyes. The correlation between accommodation and convergence is brought about by a fusional reflex which is co-ordinated at the occipital cortex of the brain. This correlation is described as AC/A ratio, which is accommodative-convergene and accommodation ratio. It is not only important for the physiological function of the eye but also has an important bearing on conditions like accommodative squint and its treatment. Normal AC/A ratio is 3:1 to 5:1.

Convergence

Convergence is an essential requirement for near work. When looking at a near object, the two eyes are moved inwards by the coordinated action of two medial recti muscles. The meeting point of two visual axes from two eyes forms an angle which is measured in meter angles. The angle formed at 1 meter is 1 meter angle and like accommodation, will be inversely proportional to distance. Clinically, convergence is measured in prism diopters.

For doing near work comfortably and without symptoms, the eyes should not only be able to converge adequately but also maintain the convergence. Any deficiency in convergence or ill-sustained convergence will have to be compensated. If possible by extra effort. This

extra effort for any length of time will cause symptoms of eye strain. If convergence is so weak that it cannot be compensated by extra effort, the result will be loss of binocularity which may result in exophoria or exotropia for near.

Convergence is a binocular action which is controlled by a centre in the mid brain. The nucleus of convergence is called Perlia's nucleus, which is situated in the median line close to that part of third nerve which controls the action of the two medial recti.

The pathway of convergence reflex is not fully understood. The afferent stimulus either starts from the retina with a desire to see a near object clearly or from the sensory nerve endings in medial recti muscles; the former travel along the optic nerve and optic tract upto the lateral geniculate body and then accompany the pupillary fibres to the third nerve nucleus to reach the nucleus of Perlia. The possible origin of afferent stimulus from the medial recti partly goes as afferent fibres along part of the third nerve and

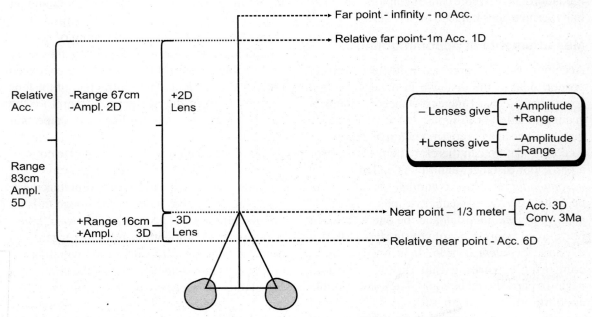

Fig. 4.6: Accommodation and convergence range

these are then probably mediated along the mesencephalic fibres of fifth nerve to reach the mid brain and Perlia's nucleus (Fig. 4.7).

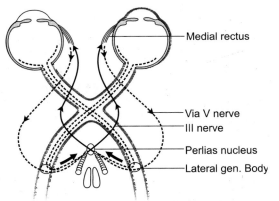

Fig. 4.7: Convergence reflex—Nerve pathways

The efferent fibres of the convergence reflex pathways, after decussation, reach the medial recti along the lower division of the 3rd nerve.

Convergence is an essential physiological function and its deficiency can cause ocular symptoms. It is therefore a good practice to test for convergence in routine out-patients examination.

Accommodation-Convergence/ Accommodation Ratio (AC/A ratio)

When a person accommodates to see a near object clearly, this effort also causes the response of convergence of both eyes. The convergence response to accommodation may be anything from being deficient to excessive. Excessive convergence is inhibited by fusional convergence from higher centres and the patient does not develop squint. The ratio of accommodative-convergence in prism dioptres and accommodation in dioptres is called AC/A ratio. The importance of AC/A ratio is significant in accommodative squint with good binocular vision.

Physiology of the Pupil

Pupillary reaction has a close inter-relationship with accommodation and convergence. Just as the pupil reacts to light stimulus, it also reflexly reacts to accommodation and convergence. Like accommodation and convergence, the efferent pupillary pathways are also mediated through the third nerve.

The afferent pathway starts with the stimulation of the retina by light. This stimulus is carried along the visuo-motor fibres in optic nerve and the optic chiasma. These pupillary fibres leave the optic tract just before the lateral geniculate body and pass along the superior colliculus to the third neve nucleus from where the efferent fibres travel along the third nerve and reach the ciliary ganglion via the nerve to inferior oblique muscle. From the ciliary ganglion the pupillary fibres travel along the ciliary nerves and reach the sphincter pupillae muscle.

The pupillary fibres partially decussate both in the chiasma and at the third nerve nucleus in the mid brain. This explains the direct and consensual reaction of pupil to light even though only one eye is stimulated.

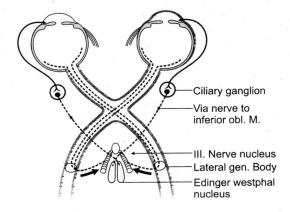

Fig. 4.8: Pupillary reflex—nerve pathways

5

History Taking and
Ocular Symptomatology

Machines and laboratories have made the diagnosis of diseases easier and simpler. It has, however, suppressed the ingenuity of clinicians and made them depend on the diagnosis to be made, not in clinics but in laboratories. This may be commensurate with the scientific advances of today but it has taken away the pleasure and pride of diagnosing the problems of a patient on the basis of personal experience and critical evaluation of clinical findings. It is not sarcasm but serious and respectful amusement to be told that the physicians in the pre-investigative era often made a correct diagnosis on clinical evaluation alone. They would look under the bed of the patient to get an indication of what he had eaten. They would keep their fingers on the pulse of the patient for minutes together with a meditative expression. And all this was a part of clinical acumen. The best clinician is one who is armed with scientific knowledge, practices medicine using clinical judgement. True, that the present diagnostic facilities available should be used to confirm the diagnosis but one should stretch his clinical knowledge and experience to the maximum before depending on investigative procedures. It will certainly give the patient a feeling that the doctor has examined him carefully and minutely and it will enhance the status of the clinician in the eyes of the patient.

The medical man, by accepting technical advancements totally, forgets, the art of healing by compassion and understanding which are important. Observations and perceptions must take precedence over investigative and technical advancements.

The first clinical step is to listen to the patient talk about his complaints. Patient with endless stories may sometimes exhaust the patience of a doctor and a tactful approach is needed to cut a long story short. Most patients, however, will be precise and a note of the history of the patient and a few cross questions will go a long way in the making a diagnosis. Patients should be asked more than once "what else"? It will be very embarrassing to the clinician if a diagnosis is made after a short and hurried history and at the end of it all, patient comes up with further symptoms needing further examination. Often, half the diagnosis will have been made by the time the dialogue between the doctor and the patient, is through.

The Terminology of symptoms used by a patient of what are called complaints of the patient or the patient's problems pertaining to his eyes or his body, depend varyingly on the language and the regional areas but should pose no difficulty as one gets used to them soon enough. However, a symptom may mean one thing for one patient and a different thing for another. One should understand the patient for proper interpretation of his complaints. It is good practice that the patient should first be made to speak of his present complaints and should then be asked to narrate the past history, family history, personal history and more important, any history of previous treatment and/or surgery.

VISUAL SYMPTOMS

The variety of visual symptoms complained of are:
  i. Defective vision
 ii. Defective near vision
iii. Black spots in front of the eye
 iv. Night blindness
  v. Double vision
 vi. Flashes in the eyes
vii. Distorted shape of objects
viii. Running of letters

Transient obscuration of vision or visual blackouts may be due to:
  i. Bullous keratopathy when vision is obscured early in the morning and becomes clear later in the day.
 ii. Spasm of accommodation due to any cause results in transient myopia and the diminution of distant vision. Accommodation inertia or weakness causes diminution or difficulty in near vision.
iii. In the early stages of congestive glaucoma, vision is obscured in the rising phase and becomes normal when the intra-ocular tension becomes normal.
 iv. Retinal arterial spasm in systemic hypertension
  v. Migrainous amaurosis in prodromal stage of an attack.

 vi. Amaurosis fugax
vii. Cerebral angiospasm
viii. Vaso-vagal attacks with temporary visual blackouts.

Defective Vision Distance and Near

The two normal age groups where the patient complains of defective vision are school going children and older persons. Both these groups complain of defective vision in majority, for distance although some may complain of defective near and distant vision both. The third age group of 43–45 age for the first time complain of defective vision for near work only.

In the younger age group, myopia is the commonest cause. It is detected either in routine school examination or because the child complains that he can not see the writing on the black broad from the back bench in school. It is not unusual that the parents are the first to note the defect because the child holds the book or slate too close.

In the older age group, defective vision may be due to any of the following cause:
  i. Hypermetropic or myopic shift in the refractive status of the eye.
 ii. Lenticular changes like nuclear sclerosis and senile incipient cataract.
iii. Symptomless open angle glaucoma.
 iv. Vascular retinopathies.
  v. Senile degenerative changes in retina or optic nerve.
 vi. Degenerative conditions like myopic degeneration and retinal detachments.

Defective Vision for Near Alone

Presbyopic symptoms usually start between the age of 42-45 years; earlier in the hypermetropes and later in myopes. The earliest symptom in presbyopia is difficulty in reading or threading a needle in evenings or in dim light or that the patient has to hold the object farther away to be able to see clearly.

Black Spots in Front of the Eyes

It is important to elicit from the patient whether the spots he sees are floaters or are fixed. The patient should be able to explain whether the black spots he sees follow the movement of the eye or are freely moving independent of eye movement.

Floaters are always in the vitreous. The most common vitreous floaters are fine thready or web-like opacities commonly seen when looking at the sky or looking against a lighted background like a white ceiling. These fine vitreous opacties are common in most people in grown up age and are due to the breakdown of the fibrillar net work of vitreous. These, in healthy eyes are called *muscae volitantes*. Some patients become too conscious of them and they have to be persuaded to overlook them as they are harmless. It is a good proverb to tell to an understanding patient that "many see them but only fools look at them".

Vitreous opacities of different shapes and sizes are commonly present in myopia and are due to vitreous degeneration. Black solid vitreous floaters are more likely to be from the degenerative areas of retina. A large single vitreous floater may come from a retinal tear. It is, therefore, very important that the peripheral fundus should be critically examined for any such areas like chorio-retinitis, cystic retinal degeneration or retinal holes. Round single floaters may, in tropical countries, be parasitic in origin.

Fixed black areas (scotoma) in the field of vision are mostly chorio-retinal in origin and represent positive scotoma. They always follow the movement of the eye and remain stationary with the eye. In macular lesion with central scotoma, a dark area is seen on every object the eye tries to focus on.

Night Blindness (Nyctalopia)

Night vision is the retinal rod function and anything that disturbs the rod layer of the retina can cause symptoms of defective night vision. Some patients in the early stage of presbyopia may present symptoms as if connected with night vision. A clearer history should be elicited and a good question to ask is whether the patients knocks against things in the dark.

Common causes of defective night vision are:

i. Congenital night blindness—an incurable condition.

ii. Oguchi's disease—a hereditary condition in certain racial groups.

iii. Retinitis pigmentosa more appropriately called primary pigmentary degeneration of retina, is a hereditary progressive disease for which there is hardly any effective treatment to date. Early and irreversible extinction of ERG is diagnostic.

iv. Vitamin A deficiency. Common in children of poorer communities in poor and developing countries. The blood level of vitamin-A must come down to 20 IU/100 cc of plasma to cause night blindness. This is a reversible condition with the administration of vitamin A.

v. Nyctalopia as a symptom of early cataract formation is a misnomer. The patient's history indicates that he sees better in bright light than in the shade or inside the room.

Diplopia or Double Vision

It is a binocular condition. It is a very disturbing symptom and may sometimes even cause giddiness. The most common cause of diplopia is ocular palsies, when diplopia is maximum in the direction of action of the affected muscle. Although in most cases, restriction of movement is evident, diplopia may sometimes persist even after the movements have clinically recovered. Transient diplopia may also occur in myasthenia gravis due to temporary muscle weakness.

Diplopia may follow squint surgery. Diplopia can also be caused by displacement of one eye ball by an orbital lesion. This can be simulated by mechanical displacement of one eye ball with the finger through the lid.

A near object is seen as double when held closer than the near point and convergence breaks down. Physiological diplopia is present for near vision when focussing on a distant object or for distance when focussing on a near object. Binocular diplopia can be readily overcome the disturbing symptoms caused by diplopia or adopt head postures.

Uniocular diplopia or polyopia is truly not diplopia. The patient may sometimes see one moon as more than one moon in case of early incipient cataract because different clear parts of the lens may act as different pupils at night. A subluxated lens may also cause a relative degree of uniocular diplopia, one image being through the phakic area and the other through the aphakic area of the pupil. Congenital polycoria or more than one surgical coloboma in the iris, rarely if ever, causes a feeling of diplopia.

Flashes in Front of Eyes (Photopsae)

Flashes may be complained of as sparks of light seen even with closed eyes. Flashes originate in the retina. They are suggestive of a retinal pathology in some stage of activity or a healed lesion adjoining an active area. They may be caused by arterial spasm. They are often seen by high myopes and may indicate an impending retinal detachment. Sudden onset of flashes of light is also due to posterior vitreous detachment, due to traction of detached vitreous on retina.

Flashes are distinct from entoptic phenomenon. The latter are also retinal in origin but are present in normal healthy eyes.

Halos may be complained of in different forms in the following conditions:
  i. Mucous discharge on cornea.
 ii. Corneal oedema.
iii. Early lens opacities

 iv. Early chronic simple glaucoma. Coloured halos in the form of rings a round lights
  v. Halos during migraine which are coloured wavy lines, appearing during the prodromal aura preceding the migrainous attack
 vi. Halos of cerebral origin are usually functional but sometimes organic similar to migrainous halos.

Distortion of Objects

This may be complained of in different forms:
  i. Difference in size and shape of objects seen with both eyes open in aniseikonia.
 ii. Words of a line seen at different levels due to the prismatic effect of glasses.
iii. Objects look farther away and smaller in overcorrected myopia and closer and magnified in overcorrected hypermetropia.
 iv. Metamorphopsia is a condition where objects appear distorted. It is usually the result of displacement of rods and cones in the retina as in retinal detachment or exudates in the retina.
  v. Macropsia, when the objects appear larger with the affected eye. This is due to crowding of rods and cones. This may also be complained of in spasm of accommodation, miosis and aniseikonia.
 vi. Micropsia, when the object appears smaller. This happens when the rods and cones are spread apart as in oedema of retina. Objects may appear smaller in paralysis of accommodation. The patient sometimes complains of objects looking smaller when full myopic correction is prescribed for the first time in grown up life.
vii. Chromatopsia which means coloured vision. There may be different types like erythropsia meaning red vision in case of a haemorrhage in the vitreous or when a large amount of light passes into the eye as in a dilated pupil, broad iridectomy and aphakia.

Xanthopsia is yellow vision as seen in jaundice and carbon monoxide poisoning.

Cyanopsia is blue vision felt soon after cataract extraction.

Other colour disturbances like green, violet and black vision are sometimes complained of following the ingestion of certain drugs like digitalis or after smoking hashish.

The prejudice or distaste for glasses; particularly among girls, is a common reason for not taking cognisance of visual defect because in any case if they are myopic they are able to read and write without difficulty. One should also keep in mind malingering as a cause of visual symptoms in adolescents and adults. A brisk pupillary reaction is a satisfactory guide to attract the possibility of a functional visual complaint.

SYMPTOMS OF EYE STRAIN

Among the common symptoms due to eye strain are:
   i Headache
  ii. Tiredness at the end of the day
 iii. Heaviness following work, movies and driving
  iv. Recurrent redness of eyes
   v. Feeling of irritation
  vi. Lacrimation
 vii. Recurrent stye and chalazion.

Pain in the eyes as a symptom of eye strain is vaguely stated and vaguely understood. It is probably a part of tiredness of eyes. True pain is usually due to ocular inflammation.

Headache

Headache is among the most common symptoms of eye patients. It is so much attributed to the eye that a physician or surgeon would like an ocular cause to be first excluded before further investigations. Patients themselves often first consult the ophthalmologist for headache.

The exact site of headache has not been clearly defined except in conditions where local tissue cause is evident. The intracranial site of headache is probably the meaninges of brain where congestion of venous sinuses causes stretching of the dura which causes headache. The scalp is another site from where headache commonly originates.

The character of the headache, the site of the headache, the timing of the headache may vary with the causative condition. Association of other clinical symptoms with headache is characteristic of ceratin conditions. In every case of headache, therefore, the following pointed questions may be asked and answers noted:
   i. Site of the headache—frontal, temporal, occipital or all over.
  ii. Related to near work or follows after movies, or watching moving objects.
 iii. Constant or intermittent
  iv. On one side or both sides
   v. The type of headache—dull, severe, throbbing
  vi. At what time of the day is it most intense
 vii. Any associated halo before or at the time of the headache
viii. Whether associated with visual disturbances
  ix. Any nausea or vomiting at the time of the headache
   x. History of recurrent attacks of cold or flu
  xi. Condition of teeth.

There are different groups of causes of a headache:
   i. Ocular causes
  ii. Sinus causes due to inflammation in the paranasal sinuses (vacuum-headache)
 iii. Intracranial causes due to raised intracranial tension
  iv. Systemic causes like hypertension
   v. Vasomotor causes like migraine
  vi. Neuralgic headache like trigeminal neuralgia
 vii. Functional headache like neurasthenia, hysteria and malingering.

Ocular headache: The causes of an ocular headache are:

i. Errors of refraction.

ii. Muscle imbalance and convergence deficiency

iii. Aniseikonia

iv. Raised intra-ocular tension.

v. Inflammation in and around the eyes.

The modalities of headache due to errors to refraction or muscle imbalance are not clearly understood. It is likely to be a reflex headache where the afferent stimulus arises either in the extraocular muscles or iris and ciliary muscles. It is transmitted along the fifth nerve and is reflexly located in some part of the scalp, the sensory supply of which is either by the fifth nerve or closely linked with it. This explains the headache located in the occipital area which has sensory supply from the second cervical segment upto which level the lower end of sensory nucleus of the fifth nerve extends.

Headache due to raised intraocular tension as well as inflammations in and around the eye, is evidently due to irritation of the fifth nerve endings. The referred pain is, therefore, in the area of sensory supply of the fifth nerve.

Quite often headache, often called pain is referred to the temporal region. This is also reflex in nature except when there is a local organic disease like temporal arteritis or when it is referred from the teeth or the sinuses.

A feeling or tiredness at the end of the day or a feeling of heaviness after near work is largely accommodative in origin due to ciliary muscle strain. Similarly the symptoms aggravated after a movie or driving, are muscular in origin and are worse in persons with muscle imbalance.

Symptoms of irritation like redness and lacrimation due to eye strain are reflex in origin. It is difficult to explain precisely the relationship between the errors of refraction and recurrent styes and chalazia. They are likely to be due to vascular congestion and staphylococcal infection co-related in some way.

Frequent Change of Glasses

i. Change of presbyopic glasses for near vision every 2-3 years after the age of 45 years, is a physiological change because of gradually weakening accommodation and the hardening of the lens as age advances. Rapidly increasing presbyopia is considered to be a manifestation of early glaucoma.

ii. Incorrect prescription of glasses often prescribed by optometrists who may be theoretically trained in the subject but do not take into consideration the physiological factors of the eye and the body. To be a good refractionist, even an ophthalmologist needs a few years of concentration and experience in this aspect of ophthalmology. The reputation of an ophthalmologist in his early career will depend on the percentage of prescribed glasses that are not comfortable and patients who come back for re-examination. Every change in glasses means extra cost to the patient, the responsibility for which is often the person's who prescribed the glasses.

iii. Glasses which are not fitted and centered properly often need to be adjusted even though the prescription may have been correct.

iv. Axial myopia is progressive condition till the body grows, in females till about the age of 16 years and in males about 20 years. Myopic glasses, therefore, need to be changed from time to time till the refractive state of eye stabilises. The change is usually needed not earlier than two years except when the first prescription is under-corrected and the change in the first two years may be more frequent. Unlike simple myopia, malignant or pathological myopia, however continues to progress even in later life and a change is needed whenever indicated. Axial hypermetropia, on the other hand, tends to decrease as the child grows but stabilises at a much earlier age than myopia.

v. Changes in the refractive index of the lens as in older age needs change in glasses although only for a temporary phase till vision cannot be further improved due to gross lens changes.

vi. Active disease like a change in corneal curvature or irregularity in corneal surface as in keratoconus and trachomatous cornea will often need frequent change of glasses.

vii. Prescription of high cylindrical error incorporated for the first time in grown up age is often not tolerated even though the prescription is correctly based on retinoscopic findings. The patient complains of intolerable slanting of ground or tilting of objects when walking or going downstairs. If the patient cannot get adjusted, glasses need to be changed by reducing the cylinder and proportionately adding to the spherical component.

viii. Glasses may not be suitable because the quality of the lenses may not be good or the lenses may not be properly centered or the frame too light or too loose. It is the responsibility of the optician to satisfy the patient on these points.

Ocular Neuralgia

Neuralgic pain is not an uncommon symptom in eye patients. The most common neuralgia is supra-orbital neuralgia which may be due to sinusitis or peripheral neuritis. The patient usually points to the origin of neuralgia from the supraorbital notch and describes its extension towards the forehead. In cases of unilateral neuralgia of this type, pressure at the supraorbital nerve area elicitis tenderness if this is the cause of neuralgia. Comparison on the two sides will always be helpful. Examination of the nose and X-ray sinuses is indicated in such cases.

Trigeminal neuralgia of the ophthalmic division of the trigeminal nerve is not uncommon. It is nearly always unilateral. The patient clearly defines the area of neuralgic pain. The characteristic recurrent nature of sudden onset and sudden relief in elderly patients are typical clinical features. Pathology of causative ganglionitis of the trigeminal ganglion will need to be investigated and treated by a neuro physician and/or a neurosurgeon.

Post-herpetic neuralgia following herpes zoster infection of the ophthalmic division of the fifth nerve may simulate supraorbital or trigeminal neuralgia.

Pain of neuralgic nature may also be due to intraocular or orbital inflammations or may be referred to around the eye from teeth and sinuses.

SYMPTOMS OF OCULAR INFLAMMATIONS AND IRRITATION

Among the common symptoms are:

i. Redness of the eye
ii. Lacrimation or watering
iii. Discharge
iv. Feeling of a foreign body
v. Burning of the eyes
vi. Itching
vii. Falling off of eye lashes
viii. Crusts at the lid margins
ix. Swelling of lids
x. Photophobia
xi. Pain
xii. Frothy collection at the outer canthus
xiii. Cosmetic symptoms.

Redness of the eye is in most cases due to conjunctival or ciliary congestion. Reactionary conjunctival congestion is common when an eye with allergic conjunctivitis is rubbed. Conjunctival congestion may also be an extension from the inflammations of lid, lacrimal sac and the orbit.

Localised redness may be due to subconjunctival haemorrhage, a congenital capillary naevus or a localised inflammation like phlyctenular conjunctivitis or episcleritis. The subject has been discussed in detail in the chapter on conjunctiva.

Lacrimation is due to reflex irritation either due to external or internal inflammation or may be psychic in nature. Lacrimation should be differentiated from epiphora which is due to obstruction in the naso-lacrimal channels. Whatever the cause of irritation, the reflex acts via the sensory nerve endings through the trigeminal nucleus and along the secretory nerve fibres reaching the lacrimal gland.

Discharge may be anything from sticking of the lids in the morning to a profuse mucopurulent secretion. Discharge from the conjunctiva is always indicative of inflammatory reaction.

Foreign body sensation is a gritty feeling as the lids move over the eye ball. Apart from the foreign body in the conjunctival sac or a corneal ulceration, a foreign body feeling is a common symptom caused by conjunctival follicles or conjunctival concreations. In acute conjunctivitis, dilated capillaries in the palpebral conjunctiva may make the conjunctival surface rough which causes a feeling of a gritty sensation in the eye.

Burning in the eyes is characteristically a symptom of angular conjunctivitis. Burning may, however, be vaguely complained of in many conjunctival conditions.

Itching is a characteristic clinical feature of allergic conjunctivitis like spring catarrh. Like burning it may also be vaguely complained of in other external conditions of the eye.

Falling off eye lashes: It should be remembered that the life span of an eye lash is about 10 weeks and lashes which have lived their span, fall off during rubbing or washing. New lashes grow in their places. Unusual falling off of lashes may be associated with many conditions like:

  i. Blepharitis
  ii. Aviaminosis and malnutrition
  iii. Leprosy
  iv. Syndromes like Vogt-Koyangi-Harada's disease
  v. Myxoedema.

Whitish deposits at the lid margins are commonly seen in squamous or ulcerative blepharitis. Dandruff and lice infestation at the roots of eye lashes also cause a white deposit at the lid margin.

Swelling: Lid swelling usually limits itself upto the orbital margins because the skin is adherent to the orbital margin.

Bagginess of the lids is common in older age and is due to herniation of orbital fat. Inflammatory swelling may be due to any of the following causes:

  i. Stye
  ii. Inflammed chalazion
  iii. Purulent conjunctivitis
  iv. Lid abscess
  v. Acute dacryocystitis
  vi. Pan-ophthalmitis and end-ophthalmitis
  vii. Orbital cellulitis

Passive oedema of lids may be due to:

  i. Thrombosis of cavernous sinus
  ii. Exophthalmic ophthalmoplegia
  iii. Acute nephritis
  iv. Myxoedema.

Pain: Pain is symptom which is complained of and is interpreted variedly by different patients in different ocular conditions. It has already been emphasised that pain inside the eye ball is typically due to iridocyclitis and deep scleritis. However, gross inflammations like endophthalmitis, panophthalmitis and orbital cellulitis cause generalised pain in and around the eye. Localised pain is typical of a stye, or acute dacryocystitis. A painful blind eye in absolute glaucoma or pain in acute congestive glaucoma are well known clinical complaints. Pain referred to the eye from surrounding may be complained of as pain in the eye but is due to causes in neighbouring structure. The pain of an acute prolapse of the eye can be excruciating.

Photophobia is a common complaint whenever there is irritation of superficial nerve endings like severe conjunctivitis and corneal epithelialitis. Photophobia is a prominent symptom of phlyctenular ophthalmia and intraocular inflammation like iritis. Photophobia in case of central lens opacity is due to marked diminution of vision as soon as patient goes into bright light.

The collection of a frothy secretion along the inner border of the lid margin and more commonly at the outer canthus is due to excessive Meibomian secretion or Meibomianitis.

Cosmetic symptoms: Though few, they are important from patient's point of view and when present they are prominently complained of.

Squint and white spots on the eye are among the common cosmetic complaints. By white spots, patient usually means corneal opacities. Sometimes Bitot's spot as white patches are mentioned by the patient as white spots.

A fairly common symptomless complaint is the yellowish plaque on either side of the cornea which may be a localised lipid deposit or pinguecula. An early pterygium or a limbal epithelioma may start as a localised raised area in the inter marginal zone on either side of the cornea.

A frequent complaint is the dark discolouration of the lower lid skin, commonly bilateral and frequently seen in women. It may be due to loss of orbital fat. It is sometimes related to menstrual period. It may, therefore, be a manifestation of endocrinal disturbances.

6

Examination of the Eye

Just taking a patient's history in detail not only guides the clinician towards diagnosis but also helps the patient develop confidence in the doctor. A complete and routine examination will not only satisfy the patient but also help the ophthalmologist reach a diagnosis. Further more, it will save the clinician from the embarrassment of having to go back to the patient for some more examination after having apparently completed it. As in all systems of medicine, ophthalmology is no exception to the practice of a total approach to the patient instead of examining just those parts which are related to the symptoms of the patient. It is, therefore, always good practice that the clinical examinations should be completed in well determined stages, so that no findings are missed and some findings may even be incidentally discovered which are unrelated to the patient's symptoms. It is only after a complete clinical examination that further investigative procedures of the eye and systemic examinations, if necessary in other disciplines of medicine, should follow.

Clinical examination should appropriately start as the patient enters the clinic, noting his expression, gait, degree of visual handicap if any, head posture, proptosis, squint etc. An acromegalic face, a tabetic gait, the blank expression of a blind person, the head posture of a paralytic squint, closing one eye to overcome diplopia, screwing the eyes in myopia, folds in forehead to lift the upper lid in ptosis, are some of the findings of distant inspection which go more than half way in making a diagnosis.

An outline of the clinical examination of the eye and a list of investigation is given below:

i. *History taking:* This should include the present complaints followed by the background history, personal history and family history as already discussed.

ii. *Record of visual acquity:* It is only natural that vision record should be the first step because the patient is an eye patient.

iii. *Examination of anterior segment:*

   a. Near inspection: A look at the patient's face to note any squint, nystagmus, tumour swelling, ptosis etc. before the examination with illumination is started, is always desirable.

   b. Examination with focal illumination and magnification (oblique-illumination examination).

   c. Cover test and power of convergence.

d. Eye movements in all cardinal directions, uniocular and binocular.

e. Test for regurgitation, if any, by pressure on lacrimal sac area.

f. Tonometry (Schiotz and Applanation). Intraocular tension record must be routinely done in all patients above the age of 35 years whatever symptoms they come with and also in younger age patients where symptoms and clinical findings so demand.

g. Syringing of naso-lacrimal passages when indicated.

h. Fluorescein and rose Bengal staining tests whenever necessary.

i. Keratoscopy with Placido's disc, if needed.

j. Slit lamp examination for confirmation of findings under focal illumination and more detailed study. This also helps in detecting something which may not have been noted under focal illumination.

iv. *Dark room examination*

a. To determine the refractive state of eye by retinoscopy or plain mirror examination and post-mydriatic (PMT)/post-cycloplegic test.

b. Direct ophthalmoscopy to examine media and fundus.

c. Indirect ophthalmoscopy, if necessary, to examine the peripheral fundus.

d. Slit-lamp examination under mydriasis, for:
   - examination of lens
   - examination of posterior fundus with Hruby lens
   - examination of posterior fundus with Goldmann lens.

e. Fluorescein angiography-scopy wherever indicated.

v. *Special methods of eye examination.* These are required when specifically indicated on the basis of clinical findings and

for confirmation of the diagnosis and evaluation of prognosis.

a. Macular function tests

b. Colour vision tests

c. Visual field studies.
   - Perimetry on Lister's perimeter, projection perimeter and Goldmann's perimeter.
   - Scotometry on Bjerrum's screen and Goldmann's perimeter.

d. Diplopia charting.

e. Keratometry and contact lens trial.

f. Hess screen examination

g. Synoptophore examination in cases of muscle imbalance and squint.

h. Glaucoma provocative tests.

i. Gonioscopy

k. Pachometry

l. Ophthalmo dynamometry

m. Therapeutic tests with prostigmine and vitamin A

n. Photography, anterior segment and fundus.

vi. *Special investigative procedures.* The advanced procedures which are now available to the ophthalmologists are listed below, but should be advised only after careful assessment of their necessity for diagnosis, prognosis and treatment.

a. Radiological investigations

b. Fluorescein angiography

c. Tonography

d. Ultrasonic investigations (echography)

e. Electro-physiological investigations

vii. *General systemic examination*

viii. *Reference to other disciplines of medicine.*

RECORDING OF VISION

Visual acuity is recorded on the basis of the patient's reading of various charts already described. Vision without correction and with correction if any, should be recorded separately.

If a person cannot read or identify the top figure, his vision is less than 6/60. The vision of such person is recorded as 5/60, 4/60 or 3/60 depending on at what distance from the chart he can read or identify the top letter or figure. If the vision is poorer than 3/60, patient is asked to count figures and vision recorded as finger counting (F.C.) at the distance at which he can correctly count fingers. If a person cannot even count fingers, he is asked to identify the hand movement and is so recorded. If he cannot identify the movement of fingers, the vision is tested by throwing a light beam on the eye. If he can appreciate the difference between dark and light, it is recorded as light perception (PL). Light is then directed from four principal sides and patient is asked to indicate the direction from which the light is coming. Depending on the number of directions he correctly answers, it is recorded as PR 4+, 3+, 2+ or 1+. If a person has no perception of light, he is recorded as PL absent or no PL.

Near chart: The near vision charts are based on Jager's principle of sizes of printer's letter. Near vision is therefore recorded as J1, J2, J3, etc.

EXAMINATION OF ANTERIOR SEGMENT

This is the first step in the examination of every patient whatever the symptoms he comes with. The anterior segment examination includes examination under good illumination and adequate magnification.

EXAMINATION WITH GOOD ILLUMINATION AND MAGNIFICATION (OBLIQUE OR FOCAL ILLUMINATION)

The requirements for this examination are a good focussing light, or a pen torch and uniocular or binocular magnifying loupe. The following routine is a good procedure.

Near Inspection

The patient should be asked to look at the examiner with the light focussed on his eyes. Any squint or nystagmus, if present, is noted. Any other gross abnormality; anatomical or pathological, should become evident if this examination is done with some concentration.

Examination of Lids and Conjunctiva

i. The position, density and direction of eye lashes should be noted. Normally, the direction of upper eye lashes is downwards, forwards and upwards.

ii. The position of the lid margins should be carefully examined. Normally, the acute angled posterior border of lid margin rests on the eye ball and the lacrimal puncta are in apposition to the conjunctiva fold near the caruncle. Any inturning (entropion or evertion (ectropion) should be looked for.

iii. Examination of palpebral conjunctiva. The lower palpebral conjunctiva can easily be examined by pulling the lower lids downwards and away from the eye ball. Any abnormality of the lower palpebral conjunctiva and depth of lower fornix should be assessed.

To examine the upper palpebral conjunctiva, the upper lid should be everted. Eversion can be easily done by using the thumb and index finger of the left hand for the right eye and the right hand for the left eye. The patient is asked to look down with both eyes and the margin of upper lid is made to override the upper margin of lower lid. Using the tip of the index finger as a fulcrum, the thumb rolls and everts the lid over the index finger which is now withdrawn and the everted lid is held in position by the thumb exposing the conjunctival surface of the upper tarsus. The procedure is very simple but needs some practice. It has the advantage of preventing cross infection if the same hand is used for both eyes.

Another method of everting the upper lid is to pull down the upper lid by holding the eye lashes and using the tip of a pencil or the tip of the middle finger as a fulcrum to roll and evert the upper lid. The procedure is unpleasant at least from one point of view, in that quite a few lashes come out and not many patients will appreciate it, at least not the women.

Eversion of the lids by the first method is difficult when patient is non co-operative and cannot look down, when the eyes are deep set, and in eyes where the tarsal plate is excised as in some entropion operations. In these cases, the second method is more applicable.

Double eversion of lid is needed to examine the conjunctiva of the upper fornix. This is best done with the help of a Desmarres lid retractor. The retractor is engaged on the skin surface of the lid above the upper border of the tarsal plate. Holding the lid margin against the retractor it is turned to show the upper tarsal surface as well as upper fornix conjunctiva as illustrated in (Fig. 6.1).

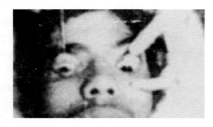

Fig. 6.1: Evertion of lid, (RE—Double evertion with lid retractor showing fornix conjunctiva; LE—Simple evertion showing only palpebral conjunctiva)

The normal appearance of healthy palpebral conjunctiva is indicated by its translucency through which the Meibomian ducts underneath are visible along with the normal pattern of vasculature with the conjunctival vessels running parallel and dividing and redividing into branches.

In tropical climatic conditions, the palpebral conjunctiva may not always presents this healthy appearance because of some degree of hyper-

trophy caused by chronic irritation or mild inflammation even though there may be no evidence of a trachoma or no history of any gross conjunctivitis.

The bulbar conjunctiva is easy to examine by pulling the lids apart and asking the patient to turn his eyes in different directions. Normal bulbar conjunctiva is nearly transparent so that the anterior sclera shows through and it is relatively avascular except the main blood vessels running from fornix to limbus. Another vascular pattern that is visible near the limbus in 30% of normal eyes is that of aqueous veins which have a bilamellar column with blood and aqueous flowing side by side, as they travel to join the anterior ciliary veins.

The bulbar conjunctiva is freely movable over the sclera except about 2–3 mm round the limbus. Conjunctival movement can be elicited by moving the lid margin against the sclera with a finger. The conjunctival vessels are seen moving with the movement of the bulbar conjunctiva. The direction of blood flow in conjunctival vessels is from the fornix to the limbus. This can be demonstrated by pressing a vessel with a glass rod and noting the flow on release of pressure.

Sclera: This is the dull white opaque outer coat of the eye ball which can be seen under the bulbar conjunctiva only for a distance of about 10-12 mm from the limbus all round. The sclera in infants is thinner and therefore bluish in colour due to the dark uveal lining underneath.

The sclera is relatively avascular and only large conjunctival vessels are seen against it. However, when there is congestion of the sclera itself, a localised pinkish discolouration is indicative of inflammation.

Cornea: This is the transparent and optically most important structure which needs to be examined by various methods. The points to be noted include the size, shape, transparency and curvature.

The cornea is nearly circular except along the upper limbus. The size is half a millimeter less along its vertical extent than its horizontal extent. The normal cornea is perfectly transparent with uniform anterior curvature except for a sight flattening near the limbus.

The examination of the cornea at this initial stage is best done with a focussed light or a narrow beam. A simple magnification like a monocular or binocular loupe is often necessary specially to see a foreign body or keratic precipitates. A thin beam of light moved across the cornea from one side to the other may show a very faint corneal nebula which may otherwise not be visible with focal illumination.

The continuity of the corneal epithelium can best be determined by fluorescein staining which may show fine abrasions otherwise invisible. It is important to emphasize that fluorescein strips should be used in preference to fluorescein solution, as the latter may be the source of bacterial contamination.

Corneal sensation should be tested whenever clinical conditions indicate its importance. This test can be done with a pointed wisp of cotton. The patient is asked to look slightly upwards and the point of the wisp touched on the cornea as near the centre as possible. A brisk reflex closure of the eye indicates good normal sensation. Aesthesiometers have been designed to quantify the corneal sensation, but clinical purpose is adequately served by this simple test.

Cosmetically and functionally, the normal brightness of the cornea and the surrounding conjunctiva are important. This brightness is maintained by a normal tear film comprised of various biochemical constituents. The dryness of cornea and conjunctiva are therefore always indicative of the pathological state of these structures.

Detailed anterior segment examination is very important in non-cooperative children or when the lids are markedly swollen. A wire lid retractor may be needed to expose the cornea. One should not hesitate to take the help of sedatives or general anaesthesia if necessary, the latter, infact, should be very helpful in making a detailed and complete examination in a child.

Slit lamp examination to see the details of corneal structure, keratometry to measure the different meridia of curvature and pachometry to measure the thickness of the cornea are specialized methods of examining this vital structure.

Limbus: One should not lose sight of the corneo-scleral junction called the limbus. Its physiological and pathological importance has been described in appropriate places. Clinically, one should not its clear cut outline. In normal eyes, blood vessels from the conjunctival side end at the limbus except in the upper part where a few loops of blood vessels may extend into the corneal tissue usually not beyond 1/2 to 1 millimeter. In endemically trachomatous areas however, limbus along its upper border is rarely well defined and clear cut. The cloudiness encroaches across the limbus into the cornea in most trachomatous eyes. A row of brownish pits, seen along the upper limbus, are an everlasting evidence of past trachoma healing or healed. A thin ring of opacity just inside the limbus in one sector or all around called arcus juveniles or arcus senilis when present is of very little pathological significance and as such, never encroaches further into the cornea and never affects vision.

Anterior Chamber: While examining the anterior chamber, the points to be noted are its depth, contents and the angle.

Depth of anterior chamber: A very important clinical observation is the depth of the anterior chamber. It cannot be measured except with the sophisticated technique of pachometry II. Clinical assessment is therefore based on experience. One must know what a normal anterior chamber looks like.

The shallowness of anterior chamber may be graded as, rather shallow, distinctly shallow, very shallow and absent anterior chamber. The physiological variations have a wide range. The anterior chamber maybe distinctly shallow even though the eye may otherwise be normal.

The presence or absence of the anterior chamber in eyes with total and dense corneal opacities, can be noted with the help of scleral scatter of light by throwing a narrow beam of light at one side of limbus. If the anterior chamber is present, the light shows through on the opposite limbus. If the anterior chamber is absent, no light scatter is seen. This can be done in a dark room with any point of light, but better done with the slit lamp.

Contents of the anterior chamber: Normal aqueous is transparent with no cellular or particulate material. The anterior chamber is, therefore optically empty with no reflection or defraction of light passing through it. The anterior chamber may appear hazy as seen through a clear cornea, either due to pus cells or due to red blood cells. The transparency of the anterior chamber is best determined on a slit lamp to observe presence of aqueous flare, if any. The details of this method are given in the section on slit lamp examination.

Angle of anterior chamber: Examination of the angle is important for the diagnosis of certain conditions. As the angle is hidden behind the anterior rim of sclera, it is not visible by oblique illumination. It can only be seen with the help of a gonio-prism or a reflecting gonio-mirror. The best method of examination of the angle is by a gonio-lens used with a slit lamp. The procedure is called gonioscopy and is described in the section on slit-lamp examination.

An open angle is necessary for unobstructed passage of the aqueous into the canal of Schlemn and thence into the aqueous veins and general circulation. A narrow or a closed angle will obviously impede this circulation and may cause raised intraocular tension. Common conditions where the angle may be narrow or closed are:

i. Physiological narrowing with no persistent or transient rise of intraocular pressure above the normal variation.
ii. Narrow or closed angle glaucoma.
iii. Peripheral anterior synechiae as in chronic iridocyclitis or iris bombe.
iv. Following cataract or glaucoma surgery.
v. Ciliary cysts or tumours causing localised narrowing.

Examination of the Iris

The iris diaphragm is normally opaque to light and controls the size of the pupil and thus the amount of light entering the eye. It acts like the diaphragm of the camera. The pupil represents the aperture of the camera. Just as the smaller aperture gives a finer definition of the picture, a smaller pupil improves the definition of the object seen.

The colour of the iris has wide physiological variations not only in different races but also in the same race. The colour of the iris in two eyes may not be identical. There may also be a difference of colour of the iris diaphragm on either side of the collarette.

A dark coloured iris or a light coloured iris is of very little clinical importance except that a light brown or a blue iris has its racial characteristic in Caucasian races and colder countries while a darker iris is peculiar to tropical and Asiatic races. Partial discoloration of one eye or gross difference of colour of two eyes is sometimes of pathological significance and the condition is called *heterochromia*.

Magnification with a loupe or slit lamp may be necessary to examine a lesion in detail or locate a foreign body on the iris. Gonioscopy helps examinations of the root of iris.

A retro-illumination test is very helpful in determining whether a black spot is a pigment or a hole in the iris. The translucency of iris is also positive in an albinotic iris when fundus glow can be seen through the iris diaphragm.

In an Examination of the Iris, the following points should be noted

i. **Iris pattern:** The dividing line of the collarette at the junction of the inner one-third and outer two-third of the iris diaphragm is to be noted. The position of the collarette is an important point of differential diagnosis between a congenital coloboma of the iris and a sector iridectomy coloboma. Uneven iris pattern is obscured when the iris is oedematous as in inflammation. The iris pattern is also disturbed in areas of iris atrophy either primary or secondary.

ii. **Iris vessels:** Although a vascular tissue, the iris blood vessels are not visible on the surface. Presence of visible vessels, therefore, is always pathological. They are commonly seen in:

a. Diabetic rubeosis of the iris
b. Thrombosis of the central retinal vein
c. Thrombotic glaucoma
d. Tumours of iris.

Examination of Pupil

The examination of the pupil is a MUST during an anterior segment examination. Examination of the pupil is done with a source of light both for inspection as well as for testing the pupillary reactions with the patient looking at a distance and also while looking at a near object. The important points to note are:

i. Size of the pupil
ii. Shape of the pupil
iii. Site of the pupil
iv. Pupillary area
v. Pupillary reactions
vi. Symmetry of the pupil between the eyes.

i. **Size of the pupil:** The pupil is unstable in different lights and different functioning states. A normal pupil may have a diameter as large as 4-5 mm or as small as 2 mm. The size of pupil should however be specifically noted because it may have a close relationship to further examination of the eye. The normal pupil is smaller in light, in convergence and in hypermetropic eyes. It is smaller in infants and in senility. It is also small in addicts of opium or its derivatives. The pupil is relatively larger in size in the dark, when looking at distance and in myopic eyes. There is a transient mydriasis in fear, shock and deep anaesthesia.

ii. **Shape of the pupil:** The normal pupil in most cases, is round in shape but not always so. Small degree of variations is not uncommon in otherwise normal eyes. This is best recorded as 'unround pupil'. Ectropion of the iris pigment epithelium at few points gives the appearance of a crenated margin which is otherwise perfectly normal. Any gross irregularity may become manifest only after mydriasis as in mild iridocyclitis with early posterior synechia.

iii. **Site of the pupil:** A normal pupil is almost always in the centre of the iris diaphragm and the centre of the pupil remains central though the margins change position as in dilatation and constriction. The pupil may falsely appear eccentric when the corneal out-line is disturbed. Rarely, the pupil may be slightly eccentric in otherwise perfectly normal eyes.

iv. **Pupillary area:** In normal eyes the pupil is occupied by the central part of anterior surface of the lens and the pupillary margin gently rests on this surface. It glides on the lens surface during dilatation and contraction and thus makes the pupillary area correspondingly larger or smaller. The colour of the pupillary area is dark in younger age and becomes greyish in older age. It is jet black in aphakic eyes. The change in old age is not necessarily due to cataractous changes in the lens. A greyish discolouration of the pupil is often due to change in refractive index of the lens with age but otherwise a perfectly transparent lens.

v. **Pupillary reactions:** This is a vital part of the examination of the anterior segment and should be carefully done for dependable interpretations. The pupillary reactions are indicative not only of the intraocular conditions but are a dependable guide to many intracranial pathologies and therefore an ophthalmologist, a physician or for that matter even a surgeon should be familiar with correct method of testing pupillary reactions. It is important to repeat that the pupillary reflex pathway starts from the retina at the peripheral end, accompanies the optic nerve and the optic tract upto the lateral geniculate body where they leave the optic tract and reach the third nerve nucleus. The efferent fibres for the reflex are carried along the third nerve in the lower division and thence along the nerve to the inferior oblique to reach the sphincter muscle of the iris. The different pupillary reaction to be tested are:

1. Light reflex (Fig. 6.2)
   a. Direct
   b. Indirect or consensual
2. Pupillary reaction to accommodation and convergence (near reflex).

Direct light reflex: This is tested with the patient looking at a distance. Light is thrown on the eye slightly obliquely so that the patient's concentration on the distant object is not disturbed. The light should be maintained on the eye for a few seconds. A normal pupil contracts as soon as light falls on the eye. It remains contracted or shows hippus movement of small contraction and dilatation alternatingly with the light still maintained. Each pupil should be tested separately with the other eye properly covered. During the examination, the patient should avoid looking at the source of light as this adds the accommodation reaction of the pupil

Reactions to Direct Light may be:
  i. Absence of reaction

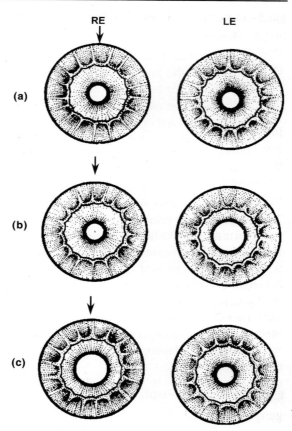

Fig. 6.2: Pupillary light reflex—Light on right eye (a) Pupil contracts in both eyes—Direct reaction in RE and consensual in LE present (b) RE pupil contracts, LE no reaction—direct reaction in RE present and consensual in LE absent (c) RE pupil no reaction, LE pupil contracts—direct reaction in RE absent and consensual in LE present

  ii. Sluggish reaction
  iii. Ill-sustained reaction.

When reaction to direct light is absent, the pupil is large in size and remains immobile. This is noted as 'dilated fixed pupil'.

If the pupil reacts to light but the movement is slow and it is called 'sluggish reaction'. When the pupil contracts to the desired size but tends to dilate even though the light is maintained, it is called ill-sustained reaction'.

Consensual light reflex: The pupillary fibres from each eye are connected to both third nerve nuclei in the mid-brain and therefore light stimulus from one eye causes contraction of the pupil in both eyes. A consensual light reaction or indirect pupillary reaction is one where the pupil contracts due to light thrown on the opposite eye.

To elicit this reaction, the patient is asked to look at a distant object. The eye to be observed for consensual reaction is very lightly illuminated, just enough to be able to observe the pupil. A bright light is now thrown on the other eye. The consensual pupil reaction is then noted in the dimly lighted eye.

Near light reflex: A normal pupil reacts both to accommodation and convergence. The accommodation reflex initiates in the retina and is carried along the visual pathways to the cortical centre and from there down to the third nerve nucleus. The convergence reflex starts either in the retina or in the sensory nerve endings in the medial recti and reaches the third nerve nucleus via the association fibres in higher centres. The efferent path follows the same course as that of the light reflex in the third nerve and reaches the sphincter pupillae, the former via the accessory ganglion and the latter via the ciliary ganglion.

Near reflex is tested by asking the patient to look at a distant object and illuminating the eyes moderately with light. The patient is then asked to look at a near object and pupillary contraction is noted. One may find that a pupil not reacting to direct light may briskly contract to near reflex.

Interpretations of Pupillary Reactions

a. When the pathology is on the afferent side, in the retina, optic nerve or the optic tract, there is absence of light reflex on the same side as well as consensual reaction on the opposite side. The other eye responds to direct light reflex as well as causes consensual reflex on the affected side.

b. When the lesion is on the efferent side, for example, the right third nerve, the right pupil is immobile to direct as well as consensual

reflex. At the same time, the left pupil reacts both to direct and consensual stimulation.

c. Just as the near reflex may be present when the light reflex is absent, similarly near reflex may be absent although light reflex may be normal. This is typically seen in paralysis of accommodation.

Some specific anomalous pupillary reactions are:

i. *Adie's tonic pupil* when there is delayed pupillary reaction.

ii. *Argyll-Robertson pupil:* When light reflex is absent but accommodation reflex is present.

iii. *Hutchinson's pupil* due to pressure on the third nerve at the base of the brain as in meningeal haemorrhage. On light stimulation there is dilatation of the pupil on the side of the lesion and consensual contraction on the opposite side.

iv. *Wernick's hemianopic pupil* is associated with hemianopia. When light is thrown from the side of the hemianopic field, there is no pupillary contraction. If light is thrown from the intact field area, the pupil reacts normally.

v. *Marcus-Gunn sign* as in retro-bulber neuritis when the pupil contracts to direct light initially but dilates immediately thereafter.

vi. *A paradoxical pupillary* reaction is sometimes noted when instead of contraction, the pupil dilates on light stimulation. This is due to central inhibition to light stimulation.

Examination of the Lens

When the lens is cataractous, different types of central lens opacities can be seen in the pupillary area.

A clinical picture of these lens opacities as seen by oblique illumination is described in the appropriate chapter. Examination of the detailed morphology of lens changes and examination of the peripheral part of the lens will require dilatation of the pupil and examination with an ophthalmoscope and slit lamp.

OTHER EXAMINATIONS

Cover test and test for convergence power. Convergence deficiency, and muscle imbalance are important causes of eye strain: next only to errors of refraction. This examination should therefore be done as a routine in every case of eye strain.

Cover Test is described in detail in the chapter on Squint and Orthoptics: The Convergence test is done by holding an object or a pencil of light in front of the eyes about one-third meter away and the patient is asked to look at it.

The object or light is gradually moved closer to the eyes while the patient keeps looking at it. One of the two eyes deviates out as soon as convergence breaks down. The distance of the object from the eyes at this point is noted. With good convergence, the patient may be able to maintain binocular convergence even at as close as 3-4 inches. Farther the distance at which convergence breaks, the weaker is the convergence. Convergence can also be measured on the synoptophore which gives quantitative assessment.

Maddox rod and Maddox wing test: Binocularity of vision and muscle balance can be dependably measured for distance by the Maddox rod test on a tangent scale and for near by the Maddox wing. These require very simple equipment and the test can be quickly and routinely done in the clinic. A further reference to this is made in the chapter on squint.

Eye movement in all cardinal directions should be tested in each eye separately. Binocular movements should also be tested to detect faults in conjugate movements and to discover paresis of extraocular muscles. This is also important to diagnose overaction or under action of contra-lateral and ipsilateral synergists or antagonists. The description will be found in the section on paralytic squint.

The above non-invasive procedures of examinations of the anterior segment have taken many pages to describe but will not take as many minutes to complete routine examination covering all points mentioned.

Peep into nasal cavity: It is always a good practice to end the examination of the anterior segment with a peep into the nose. An ophthalmologist is quite capable of detecting gross infection in the nose which maybe the cause of recurrent conjunctival congestion, a hypertrophied turbinate or a markedly derivated septum which may be blocking the naso-lacrimal duct opening or an atrophic rhinitis which may be a part of dry eye syndrome. A peep into the nose can, therefore, be very rewarding in determining the line of treatment.

Tenderness at the supra-orbital notch: It is also good practice to elicit tenderness at the supra-orbital notch whenever symptoms like neuralgia in the area supplied by the supra-orbital nerve or vacuum headache in the morning is complained of, especially when it is unilateral. A comparison of two sides will always be helpful. In bilateral cases, feeling of difference between the lateral orbital margin and supra-orbital notch area will often confirm tenderness over the notch area.

Palpation of lymph nodes: Whenever indicated, one should make it a point to palpate for enlargement of the lymph nodes. One should specifically palpate the submandibular and pre-auricular areas for secondary involvement due to an inflammation or a neoplastic growth in and around the eye ball. Palpation of deep cervical glands is done by pushing the fingers under the sternomastoid muscle.

The palpation of anterior and posterior triangle of the neck is also indicated when ever a tuberculous diathesis is considered as a possible etiological factor.

Lacrimal passage patency test: Pressure against the nasal bone from below upwards over the lacrimal sac area will indicate whether there is any regurgitation of fluid through the upper or lower or both punca. As the sac area is pressed, the lower lid is pulled down to bring the lower punctum in view and at the same time, one should look at the upper punctum. If there is any obstruction in the naso-lacrimal duct preventing the fluid from passing into the nasal cavity, the fluid regurgitates on pressure through the canaliculi and puncta. One should note whether the regurgitated fluid is watery and clear, mucoid, mucopurulent or purulent and sometimes sanguinous (bloody).

In all cases where there is epiphora, a lacrimal syringing with normal saline should be done. This helps in differentiating between physiological obstruction and organic obstruction. It also helps deciding whether obstruction is in the naso-lacrimal duct, at the canalicular opening in the sac or in the canaliculus. In small children, syringing is better done under general anaesthesia. In infants, it is possible to do it by holding the child steady. It may be advisable to add a drop of fluorescein to normal saline to note the colour of fluid passing down the same side nostril or by swabbing the throat of children for coloured fluid which may pass into the throat.

Tonometry: It is a good practice to record tension in all patients aged 35 and above whatever symptoms they come with. This is one simple procedure which helps detect early or suspect cases of glaucoma. Tension upto 20-21 mm of mercury is within normal limits. Patients with tension 22-25 mmHg should be considered as glaucoma suspects and be further investigated. A tension 26 mmHg and above should be considered glaucomatous unless proved otherwise by various confirmatory investigations. Importance should be given to diurnal variations of tensions as well as difference of tension in two eyes. The subject will be discussed in detail in the chapter on glaucoma.

The simplest but an unreliable method of assessing intraocular tension is the digital method. The patient is asked to look down. The tips of the index fingers are placed 1 cm apart on the upper lid. One finger is kept stationary and the other gives a pressure on the eye through the lid. The thrust is felt by the stationary finger. The harder the eye, the greater the pressure needed to elicit the thrust. The method needs experience to be dependable to some degree. It can at best detect fairly well developed ocular hypertension. It is relatively more dependable when one eye is normal and other eye has comparatively raised or very low tension.

Schoitz tonometry is the simplest procedure of tension record practised in most eye clinics. There are however serious objections to the accuracy of this method. The most important variable element is the scleral rigidity factor. This scleral rigidity factor can, to some extent, be taken care of by doing differential Schoitz tonometry. Tension is recorded with 5.0, 7.5 and 10.0 gm weights and the average of these three readings is corrected for scleral rigidity factor from a graph (Fig. 6.3, Plate 1).

An impression tonometer designed by Maklakov, USSR has the advantage that it leaves a permanent impression of tension record on the case file for ready comparison during follow-up.

Applanation tonometry is considered much more dependable and should be the preferred method if the equipment is available. This procedure excludes the scleral rigidity factor and the record is therefore more acceptable and reliable.

Non contact tonometers are available and are considered dependable.

Staining tests: Fluorescein and Rose Bengal are among the common dyes used. Fluorescein is particularly suitable for corneal staining. It is important in corneal ulcers to define their outline. It stains an epithelial defect, which may not otherwise be clinically visible as for example a small abrasion. It should always be done in all cases of foreign body feeling. It is important to emphasize that a fluorescein strip should be used instead of a stock solution of fluorescein since the latter is fraught with the danger of introducing infection.

Rose Bengal can also be used to stain filamentary and punctate lesions of the cornea and devitalized keratinized epithelial cells. It stains the devitalized or keratinized cells of the conjunctiva and the cornea bright pink in colour.

Keratoscopy: This identifies the regularity or otherwise of anterior corneal curvature. It is an important test in trachomatous eyes where an irregular corneal surface gives irregular retinoscopy readings due to irregular astigmatism and vision cannot be improved with glasses even though the cornea on focal illumination appears clear. The test also indicates contact lens trial for improvement of vision in cases of corneal astigmatism. Keratoscopy is also important for diagnosing early keratoconus.

Keratoscopy can be done with a Placido's disc either a reflecting type or a self-illuminating type. A similar but miniature device can be mounted on a direct ophthalmoscope.

Slit-lamp examination: Biomicroscopy with the slit-lamp is part of routine examination and should be available to ophthalmologists in larger numbers than in the past.

Slit Lamp in Anterior Segment Examination Helps

1. To observe under magnification and higher illumination the lesions on corneal and conjunctival surface.
2. To localise whether a corneal lesion is in anterior stromal layers, posterior stromal layers or at the endothelial layer level.
3. Detect aqueous flare and keratic precipitates.

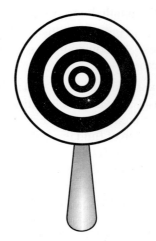

Fig. 6.4: Keratoscopy—Placido's Disc

4. Detailed examination of lens opacities.
5. Measuring tear film break up time.
6. Recording intraocular tension by applanation tonometry.

The detailed procedure to be done with the slit lamp for examination of the eye or gonioscopy and pachometry are give in the section on slit lamp biomicroscopy.

DARK ROOM EXAMINATION

Retinoscopy

Retinoscopy is the first dark room procedure in a majority of eye patients coming to the clinic or hospital because defective vision and symptoms of eye strain are common. The procedure has been described in detail in the chapter or retinoscopy and errors of refraction.

Ophthalmoscopy—Direct and Indirect

To Helmholtz goes the credit of devising the ophthalmoscope in 1850 and opening the interior of the eye to ophthalmologist. After initial scepticism, the fear of injuring the eye by light, soon disappeared. The original crude ophthalmoscope of Helmholtz was improved upon in quick succession and the reflecting ophthalmoscope came into being. In the following ten years everybody started using the ophthalmoscope and diseases like retinoblastoma, retinitis pigmentosa, papilloedema, thrombosis central retinal vein, occlusion of artery and cupping of the disc became clinically identified. The concept of indirect ophthalmoscopy with a small concave reflecting mirror was also introduced about the same time. However, the present generation of self-illuminating ophthalmoscope, both direct and indirect, are a great advancement over the old reflecting ophthalmoscope. Ophthalmoscope for ophthalmologist is like a stethoscope for a physician and the indirect ophthalmoscope must always be on hand for examination of those parts which the direct ophthalmoscope cannot reach.

Direct ophthalmoscopy: Direct ophthalmoscopy permits detailed examination of all refractive media. With the direct ophthalmoscope one can know whether the opacity is in the anterior part of the lens or the posterior part of the lens, whether opacity is in the anterior vitreous, mid-vitreous or the posterior vitreous. Against retro-illumination with the direct ophthalmoscope, even corneal vascularization can be seen.

Direct ophthalmoscope is ideally suited for the examination of posterior fundus which includes disc, retinal vessels, macular area and fundus background upto or little beyond the equator. In addition, fluorescein angioscopy is possible with those direct ophthalmoscopes which have a cobalt filter incorporated in them. Most of the newer models of direct ophthalmoscopes have a red-free filter for discrimination of haemorrhagic lesions and blood vessels, a central star to test the type of macular fixation and a grid to measure the degree of eccentricity. The slit light in the ophthalmoscope is to determine the level of the lesion in relation to the retinal surface as between a macular hole and a macular cyst. Some ophthalmoscopes have an additional half circle light mechanism for examination of the macular area which avoids pupillary contraction caused by macular stimulation. The ophthalmoscope may be powered by dry

batteries, chargeable batteries or from the mains through a transformer.

The optics of the direct ophthalmoscope is based on the principle that the observer is very close to the patient's eye and the light of the ophthalmoscope is reflected back from patient's fundus. The emergent rays from retina of patient are divergent from hypermetropic eye and convergent from myopic eye. This emergent light is caught by the observer's eye and can be focussed on his retina either by the observer's accommodation or by incorporating the convex or concave lenses in the viewing aperture of the ophthalmoscope. In either case, the light is caught by the observer's eye before it forms focus.

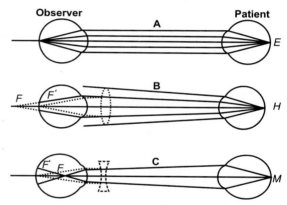

Fig. 6.5: Optical principle of direct ophthalmoscopy (A) Emmetropic eye—retina of the patient and the observer are at conjugate focus to each other. The fundus details of the patient's eye can be seen with 0 lens in the ophthalmoscope aperture (B) The light rays out of a hypermetropic eye are divergent and will need a convex lens in the ophthalmoscope aperture to bring them to a focus on the observer's retina (C) The light rays out of a myopic eye are convergent and will need a concave lens in the ophthalmoscope aperture to bring them to a focus on the observer's retina.

The fundus image seen with the direct ophthalmoscope is magnified 14–16 times, less in hypermetropic eyes and more in myopic eyes.

The method of direct ophthalmoscopy. The basic requirements of direct ophthalmoscopy are:
1. The observer has to be as close to the patient as possible.

2. The patient is asked to direct his attention to a distant object.

3. The observer should relax his accommodation. This can best be done by keeping the other eye open and mentally feeling that he is looking at a distant object, not always quite easy to do.

It is advisable to do direct ophthalmoscopy with a dilated pupil. Even a general physician can use a drug like phenylephrine which quickly dilates pupil, does not affect accommodation and the action passes off within one and a half to two hours.

The difficulty of direct ophthalmoscopy with an undilated pupil is two fold, the first is the corneal reflex, which corresponds to the centre of the pupil. Secondly, the brisk pupillary contraction as soon as ophthalmoscope light is directed towards the macular area. The patient's own pupillary reflex, his own accommodation and convergence make it still more difficult.

Most direct ophthalmoscopes have an additional half circle smaller aperture and a rheostat for using lesser intensities of light. This obviates the difficulties to a certain extent.

With a dilated pupil, all these difficulties are overcome and examination of fundus is comfortably completed in detail upto as far in the periphery as the equator or even a little anterior to it.

For satisfactory examination of fundus details, two things are necessary. The media should be clear and gross error of refraction, if any, of the observer and the patient, should be neutralised by an appropriate lens in the ophthalmoscope. It is, therefore, important that one should enquire if a patient is using glasses and if so find out the power of glasses used. This is particularly important in myopic eyes, the emergent rays from which are forming a focus in front of the observer's retina somewhere in his vitreous and the observer's own accommodation cannot help unlike in divergent rays of hypermetropic eyes and parallel rays of emmetropic eyes. It is for this reason that to examine a myopic fundus, one needs a more myopic lens than the degree of myopia because it has to provide for the observer's own unavoidable accommodation also. It is always advisable that ophthalmoscopy follows retinoscopy so that amount of refractive error is known and adjusted in the ophthalmoscope. It is equally satisfactory to see the fundus details of a highly myopic eye through the patient's own glasses. Keeping all the above points in view, direct ophthalmoscopy should follow clear and well defined steps.

Steps of Direct Ophthalmoscopy
(Fig. 6.6, Plate 1)

1. Ophthalmoscopy is done with the right eye when examining the patient's right eye, and with the left eye when examining the patient's left eye. Both should be done from the temporal side and not across the face and nose of the patient. To this, there is one exception. To see the extreme temporal periphery, one can see more of the fundus when looked into from the opposite side, i.e. across the nose.

2. Ophthalmoscopy should be started at a distance of 1/3 meter (distant direct ophthalmoscopy). From this distance, any gross opacities in the media can be seen against the red glow of the fundus. The observer then approaches the patient with + 10.0. Diopter lens in the aperture, the opacities in the media, if present, become more defined and they can be studied in further detail by changing the power of the convex lens in the aperture, either on the higher or on the lower side. The opacities in vitreous can also be defined and their location whether in anterior vitreous or in posterior vitreous can be determined.

3. With the media examined, the examiner should get closure to the patient and at the same time the lens power in the aperture is rapidly reduced. With the patient looking straight ahead and the observer seeing from temporal side, the first structure of the fundus seen is the optic disc and the retinal vessels on and around the disc.

4. With patient looking straight ahead, the observer turns the direction of light towards the macular area and looks for the foveal reflex and any changes at and around the macula.

5. It is then necessary to scan the fundus background upto as far a periphery as possible. With the patient still looking straight ahead one can observe the posterior fundus upto 3 to 4 disc. diameter all round the disc by changing the direction of the ophthalmoscope light. The patient is now asked to look into the eight cardinal directions one after the other in clockwise direction when examining the right eye, and anti-clockwise when examining the left eye. By doing this, it is possible to see the mid peripheral fundus upto or a little beyond the equator. Any structure normal or abnormal can be focussed by changing the power of the lens if necessary. In high myopic eyes, one has to get too close to the eye to see the fundus details. To avoid this, it is preferable that a highly myopic fundus should be seen through the patient's own spectacles or through a similar lens in a trial frame. This will allow examination from the usual distance and give a larger field of illumination.

6. One should also note the power of the lens in the aperture with which the particular area of the fundus or particular lesion is best seen.

7. Any further step of ophthalmoscopy like finding the type of fixation or measuring the distance of a lesion from the disc or foveal area and assessing the elevation or depression of a fundus lesion in relation to retinal level can now be done.

It is good to bear in mind that a prolonged fundus examination titres both the observer and the patient apart from the symptoms of lacrimation due to photophobia. A few seconds of rest at intervals will, therefore, be appreciated by the patient.

The examination of fundus in small children is best done under short general anaesthesia, open masks inhalation anaesthesia or IV catalar. A wire speculum and a conjunctival forceps should be at hand during this procedure.

Direct Ophthalmoscopy Permits the Following Observations

A. Media

1. Corneal vascularization and keratic precipitates by retro illuminations with +20 Diopter lens in the aperture.

2. Any posterior synechia and pigments on the lens with +14 to +16 Diopter lens in the aperture.

3. Anterior part of lens with +12 diopter and posterior part of lens with +8 Dioptres.

4. Anterior vitreous with +6 dioptres, middle vitreous with +4 diopter and posterior with 0.0 to +2 dioptres.

The power of the lens needed in the aperture is in relation to the distance from ophthalmoscope of the tissue under examination so that the same power of the lens is needed to focus the lens and the anterior vitreous whether the eye is hypermetropic, emmetropic or myopic. The refractive state of the eye however affects the power of the lens needed when examining the posterior vitreous and fundus of eye. It is, therefore, possible with ophthalmoscope to make a rough estimate of the refractive state of the eye. It should however be kept in mind that a less convex lens in needed to focus a hypermetropic fundus and a more concave lens for a myopic, than the actual error of refraction.

B. Fundus

1. *Disc:* The size, shape and colour are noted. The central part of the disc should be particularly viewed for the presence of normal or abnormal cupping and for

the relation of the artery and vein to each other. The artery enters the eye ball in the centre of the disc on the medial side of the vein. Many normal eyes show venous pulsation while the artery seen with the ophthalmoscope is normally non-pulsating. This is because of the relation of intraocular pressure which is slightly higher than the ophthalmic venous pressure but is appreciably lower than the ophthalmic artery pressure.

2. *Disc margin* should be carefully focussed and note made whether they are well defined or fluffy or markedly blurred. In case of blurring of the disc margin, the elevation when significant, can be fairly dependably measured by increasing the dioptric power of the lens in the aperture. Note is also made of the vessels as they cross the disc margin. Any sheathing if present, is noted.

3. *Blood vessels:* Blood vessels need to be examined in great detail. One should be able to differentiate between an artery and the vein as seen with the ophthalmoscope. Arteries are lighter in colour, narrower in calibre and have a prominent linear reflex along their course. Veins are darker in colour, broader in diameter and the light linear reflex is less conspicuous.

   One should examine the blood vessels from the centre of the disc upto the periphery. Their character or course whether straight or tortuous, should be noted. Their branching pattern should be seen. Any sheathing along their course should be looked for.

   Special attention is necessary to the arterio-venous crossing. In the majority of places, the artery crosses in front of the vein but it may be vice-a-versa. At least two to three arterio-venous crossings should be studied about 2–3 disc dia-

meters away from the disc margin. Although there is a common sheath between artery and vein at crossing, their lumen is unaffected in the normal condition of the blood vessels.

4. *Macular area:* Being functionally the most important part of the retina, it should be carefully examined in detail. If size of the pupil is small, one may not be able to examine this area. There should be no hesitation in dilating the pupil.

   The best method of examining the macular area is to ask the patient to keep looking straight and for the observer to change the direction of the ophthalmoscope light slightly temporal from the disc. During examination of an undilated eye it is a bad practice to ask the patient to look into the light. This may bring the macular area in the line with the visual axis of the observer but it causes marked photophobia to the patient and makes the pupil small due to accommodation and convergence reflex.

   The macular area is identified by a small star like reflex which represents the fovea centralis. If the star is absent or dull, as may be in some normal eyes also, the macular area is identified by being the area free from the retinal capillaries. One sees a few fine blood vessels converging from above and below but ending at the outline of the macular area.

5. *Fundus background.* It includes the examination of the posterior as well as mid peripheral fundus. Any abnormal findings during fundus examination should be recorded and better still sketched on paper for comparison during follow up.

It is to be kept in mind that an emmetropic eye, the posterior fundus is best seen with –0.5 to –1.0 Diopter lens, the peripheral fundus can best to be focussed with +1.0 to 2.0 diopter or even more. For the same reason, a less minus lens in myopic eyes and higher plus lens in hypermetropic eyes is needed to focus the peripheral fundus as compared to lenses needed for focussing the disc, macula and the area around (Fig. 6.7, Plate 1).

Indirect Ophthalmoscopy

It is called indirect because fundus is seen as an image in the air between the observer and the convex lens used in this procedure. The optical principle of indirect ophthalmoscopy is to make the eye highly myopic by interposing a high power convex lens which is held at its focal distance from the retina of the eye under examination. The bright light from indirect ophthalmoscope is reflected back from the patient's retina which is then refracted by the hand held convex lens. The image formed in air between the lens and the observer is real and inverted. The convex lens is held by the observer in front of the patient's eye and the distance between the eye under examination and the lens will depend on the power of the lens used. Commonly a lens of 16–18 diopters is used so that it can be conveniently held with the hand and at the focal distance from the retina. A +13.0 diopter lens recommended earlier was inconvenient because of its longer focal length. The retinal image in air is magnified 4–5 times with +16 to +18 diopter convex lens. The higher the power of lens used, the smaller its focal length, the closer it has to be held from the eye, the lesser the field of illumination but greater is the magnification. High power convex lenses are available upto 30 dioptres. These high power lenses are particularly useful for reaching further into the periphery than with a 16–18 diopter convex lens. They are also particularly useful where pupil cannot be widely dilated.

There are two types of indirect ophthalmoscopes available, binocular and monocular. Special optical devices have been introduced to permit indirect ophthalmoscopy even through a

less dilated pupil and they are known as small pupil ophthalmoscopes. The binocular indirect ophthalmoscope has the advantage that one hand of the observer is free for indentation before or during operation. The second advantage is that the binocularity adds to the view, stereopsis and depth of focus. The monocular indirect ophthalmoscope is preferred by some because it is considered less cumbersome but then indentation has to be done by the assistant. It has been said that binocular ophthalmoscope gives a headache while the monocular gives a handache.

It is important to emphasize that indirect ophthalmoscopy needs good practice before one acquires ease in this method. One has to get used to looking at the aerial image and not at the eye of the patient and he has to orient himself to the inverted character of the image (Fig. 6.8).

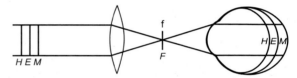

Fig. 6.8: Indirect ophthalmoscopy optical Principle. The high power convex lens used in indirect ophthalmoscopy is held at such a distance from the patient's eye that the focus of the lens coincides with the anterior focus of the eye ball, and the size of the image seen will be the same irrespective of whether the patient's eye is emmetropic, hypermetropic or myopic. If, however, the position of the lens is changed, the size of the image will increase or decrease depending on whether the lens is moved towards or away from the patient's eye and whether the eye is myopic or hypermetropic

Because of the inverted image in the indirect ophthalmoscopy, what we see above is of the lower retina and what we see below is of the upper retina. Similarly, what we see on the nasal side is of the temporal retina and vice versa. With the patient looking straight in front, the macular area is seen on the nasal side of the disc. All these have to be kept in mind when recording the findings of indirect ophthalmoscopy (Fig. 6.9 and 6.10, Plate 1).

Direct Versus Indirect Ophthalmoscopy

Both the procedures have their advantages and disadvantages

Direct Ophthalmoscopy	*Indirect Ophthalmoscopy*
1. More useful for examination of posterior fundus	1. Specially valuable for peripheral fundoscopy
2. Magnification is 14 to 16 times	2. Magnification is 4 to 5 times
3. Fundus image is erect	3. Fundus image is inverted
4. Illumination is less bright 3-5 watts	4. Illumination is very bright 25-30 watts
5. Field of illumination is smaller	5. Field of illumination is larger
6. Fundus examination is possible upto a little beyond the equator only	6. Fundus can be seen further into the periphery even upto ora serata with special aids.
7. Examiner too close to the patient	7. Examiner is 1/3 to 1/2 meter away from the patient
8. Detailed examination of media is a distinct advantage	8. Only gross details of media possible
9. Rough assessment of refractive status of the eye is possible	9. Assessment of refractive status not possible
10. Swelling of the disc or elevation of retinal lesions can measured in dioptres	10. Dioptric measurement not possible

Biomicroscopy

Slit lamp examination is now an essential part of clinical examination of the eye. It is as important for examination of the anterior segment of the eye as ophthalmoscopy for the posterior segment. The optical principle of the slit lamp examination is based on the passage of a slit of light through the cornea, anterior chamber and the lens and in doing so the tissues in its path reflect certain amount of light and the path appears as if a microscpic section of the tissue is presented to the observer's eye.

The original concept of a slit lamp was based on the need to examine different layers of the cornea and hence the original name of this equipment was corneal microscope. Further developments however have made it a multipurpose equipments which provides outstanding facilities not only to examine the cornea, the anterior chamber, the lens but also to be used with accessories, for gonioscopy, fundoscopy and examining the extreme periphery of retina. The examination of various tissues of the eye on slit lamp is now called Bio-microscopy.

The credit goes to Gullstrand who made the first corneal microscope and demonstrated its use in 1911. Vogt improved the illumination system and developed the modern slit salmp techniques. The gonioscopy technique was successfully done first by Salzmann by using a contact lens. A mirrored contact lens to facilitate examination of the anterior chamber angle and the posterior segment was designed by Goldmann in 1938.

Once its utility and importance was realised, many started manufacturing their models of slit lamps, prominent amongst them being Hamblin of London, Haag-streit of Switzerland and Carl Zeiss of West Germany. The last few years have seen further sophistication and the Japanese and Americans have added their newer models. The attempts by Indian firms to manufacture a slit lamp have succeeded to a fairly satisfactory extent. The Haag-Streit slit lamp 900 has the advantage of simplicity, convenience of use and ease of manipulation with one hand, leaving the other hand of the observer free to lift up the upper lid or gently pull down the lower lid of the patient if and when required (Fig. 6.11A and Fig. 6.11B, Plate 2).

It is important to mention that a slit lamp does not replace routine inspection and examination

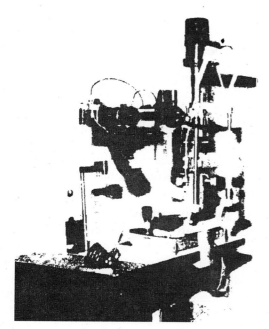

Fig. 6.11A: Haag-Streit Slit Lamp with accessories for applanation tonometry. Pachometry and photography

for the slit lamp in addition to attachments for tonometry, angle visualisation, fundus examination and depth measuring devices.

In cases of a corneal opacity, with good illuminations and magnifying aids, one can determine the surface extent, density and vascularization in the opacity but not the depth at which it lies in the cornea. A nebular opacity may be deep in the posterior stroma while a dense leucoma may be absolutely superficial. This can be determined only on slit lamp.

Similarly, in a case of early cataract, ordinary good illumination and magnification reveals a layer of opacity in the lens. The same on a slit lamp reveals where exactly the opacity is.

It is only after visualizing the angle of anterior chamber by the slit lamp gonioscopy in case of a primary glaucoma, that a correct surgical procedure can be planned.

Biomicroscopy is also important to study the progress of disease because it gives the correct picture of whether a lesion is receding by therapy or is progressing in spite of it.

Before proceeding to examine a patient on the slit lamp, the following adjustments should be done. These are common to all the procedure of slit lamp examination.

1. The height of the instrument should be comfortable for both, the observer and patient. This is done by adjusting the slit lamp height and height of the rotating stool for the patient and position of observer so that all three can be aligned for comfortable examination.
2. The chin rest should be adjusted so that the patient's eyes are level with a marker on the side of the head rest and the forehead of the patient is firmly pressed against the headband.
3. Any large refractive error of the observer should be incorporated in the eye pieces of the binocular microscope.
4. The inter-pupillary distance of the observer is to be adjusted in the binocular microscope.
5. Loosen the fixing screws of the microscope and the illumination arm so that the angle

of the anterior or posterior segment of the eye, but it certainly stimulates and trains for greater accuracy of observation with a loupe or ophthalmoscope. This is particularly so in the case of anterior segment examination.

To be able to carry out a critical examination on a slit lamp, it is absolutely necessary to be completely familiar with all the controls of the equipment to the extent that with a flick of the fingers, the observer should be able to change over from one type of illumination to another, increase or decrease the magnification, change the width and length of the light beam or insert a particular colour filter. Practice of using a slit lamp is the first requisite. It is important to be able to see normal and abnormal structures and pathological lesions, with the accessories which are now available with most models of slit lamps.

In earlier days, one had to make elaborate drawings of slit lamp findings to clinically present the observations. Today, we have anterior segment as well as slit photography attachments between them and their position can be adjusted depending on the requirements for a particular procedure. For routine slit lamp examination, the microscope is best kept stationary in the centre while the illuminations arm should be mobile to swing from the right to left side at different angles and inclinations.

Other adjustments vary according to the requirements of a particular procedure and should be made accordingly. These are usually necessary for procedures carried out with accessory attachments such as applanation tonometer, preset lens for fundus examination or a contact lens for fundus and gonioscopy examination.

The different methods of ocular examination that can be done on a slit lamp are grouped as follows:

A. Those possible with a slit lamp alone.
B. Those which need accessory equipment.
A. The examination with a slit lamp alone consists of using different types of illumination and changing the width of the light beam. They are:
1. **Direct illumination:**
   a. Broad beam
   b. Narrow beam—slit of light
   c. Small circular beam.

Examination with a broad beam: In all biomicroscopes, the illumination can be adjusted to obtain an extremely narrow beam of light and get an optical section. This is the most commonly used method of examination and most useful too. With adequate magnification, an optical section helps determine the depth of the lesion. This is of great significance in the localisation of lesions in the cornea, lens and anterior vitreous. By varying the angle between the microscope and the illumination arm, the slit beam gives a narrower or wider optical section for observation.

By moving the slit of light across the cornea from the right to the left or vice versa, lesion can be observed in succeeding optical sections like serial sections under a microscope. The graded slow movement of the focussed slit is extremely useful in determining the change in the depth of a lesion in its different parts. For example, a corneal opacity may be partly superficial being only in the epithelial and subepithelial zones, extend into the stroma in an adjoining area and at the same time involve the endothelial and Descement's zone also. Similarly, the crystalline lens can be studied under full mydriasis to localise the extent and depth of opacities or determine different types of lens opacities.

Examination with narrow beam: This is useful for gross inspection under bright illumination and high magnification. This does not give a sectional view but if the angle between the microscope and illumination is kept wide enough, an illuminated parallelogram is visualised. By varying the length and width of the light beam, the sides of the parallelogram can be varied to illuminate the pathological lesion. This is particularly useful to study the anterior and posterior surface of the cornea.

Examination with a small circular beam: This is sometimes called a conical beam. It is obtained by reducing the length of the beam to the smallest and opening the slit wide. It is useful for observing anterior chamber. The normal anterior chamber described as 'optically empty' appears as a dark zone behind the cornea because normal aqueous does not contain any particulate matter and therefore there is no reflection of light from it. In inflammations of the ciliary body and iris, aqueous becomes plasmoid due to fibrinous and cellular elements. These cause reflection of light and show themselves as floating matter in the aqueous called 'aqueous flare'. Gross turbidity of aqueous can be visualised readily in a broad or narrow beam but in early cases a small circular beam is necessary. Instead of recording it as an aqueous flare present or absent it is often useful to grade the density of visible matter and record it as aqueous flare one plus, two plus etc.

2. **Indirect illumination:** Although this is being described separately, it is done at the same time as examination with direct illumination. Indirect illumination is most often combined with narrow beam examination under direct illumination. The light is focussed on an adjoining area instead of on the lesion directly. When indirect illumination is practised, a medium width of the beam should be focussed on an area adjacent to the lesion which is seen in far greater detail than under direct illumination. Such lesions include small neovascularisation or haemorrhage on the iris. A combination of indirect and retro-illuminations can be used to examine very fine lesions of the cornea such as early dystrophic changes, fine pigmentation on the endothelial layer, ghost vessels etc.

3. **Retro-illumination:** Most of the light that enters the eye is refracted and then absorbed by the pigmented layers in the eye ball. Part of the light is reflected back and acquires the red colour, 'the fundus glow'. This phenomenon is made use of in examining transparent structures against the red fundus glow. The best example is the appearance of the vitreous, lens or corneal opacities against fundus glow in a fully dilated pupil. The denser the lesion, the darker the appearance against this red glow.

4. **Oscillating beam:** This is a combination of different illuminations, direct, indirect and retro-illumination. It becomes second nature to a person who has acquired good practice on slit lamp. When a lesion is being focussed under direct illuminations and the adjacent area is seen under indirect illumination and at the same time, a corneal lesion can be examined under retro-illumination. Thus alternating the direct, indirect and retro-illumination

methods, one or more lesions at the same or different levels in the anterior segment, can be examined.

5. **Scleral scatter:** When a beam of light is focussed on the limbal region, the opposite limbal zone is illuminated in addition to the adjacent area of the cornea. This is due to the light passing through by internal reflection. The procedure is particularly important because it determines the presence or absence of the anterior chamber, or in other words, the presence or absence of anterior synechiae when the whole cornea is opaque and the deeper structures cannot be examined by direct or indirect illumination. The beam of light can be focussed on different sectors of the limbus, observing the diametrically opposite limbus which gets lit up if the iris is not adherent and light can pass through an intact anterior chamber with no opaque obstruction in its path. If however, there is an obstruction and light cannot pass across, the opposite limbal sclera remains unilluminated indicating anterior synechiae.

6. **Zone of specular reflection:** It is based on the principle that if an object is observed along the line of reflected rays, finer irregularities in texture become visible, which remain otherwise invisible on direct or indirect illumination. The method is useful in examining corneal endothelium, individual cells of which form surface irregularities, inspite of the curvature of the surface as a whole being regular. Each of those irregularities acts either as a concave or convex mirror and in a zone of specular reflection show up in a mosaic pattern representing the endothelial cells individually.

The procedure consists of adjusting the slit lamp microscope and the illumination arm, one or either side, at an equal angle to the normal straight ahead direction. The broad light beam of medium length is focussed on the cornea and the same is observed through microscope which is set on the opposite side along the path of reflected light. A bright image of the source of light is seen and in it is seen as a golden mosaic pattern which is the endothelium seen in specular reflection.

It is important to understand that the zone of specular reflection shows a small endothelial area at a particular time. No diagnostic definitive opinion can be passed on visualisation of one area alone. Secondly, specular reflection can be observed only if the stroma and epithelium are transparent. Any endothelial pathology, advanced enough to cause secondary changes in the corneal stroma and epithelium will make observation of endothelium under a zone of specular reflection impossible. An examination of the corneal endothelium under a zone of specular reflection is rarely practised by ophthalmologists. Even cornea specialists resort to using a specular microscope, a separate equipment, available to study cell morphology of the endothelium and determine the endothelial cell count per square mm. This is a very dependable method to study corneal endothelium.

The slit lamp methods just described can be appropriately used in the examination of different structures and tissues of the anterior segment of the eye ball, amongst which the cornea and the lens are the most important. In addition, this will obviously include examination of the anterior chamber, iris and the pupil.

Slit Lamp Examination of the Cornea

The anterior surface of cornea is examined by focal illuminations with a broad beam. This is a better alternative to oblique illumination because it provides better illuminations and higher magnification.

The different layers of the cornea can be examined with a narrow slit illumination which determines the depth of a corneal lesion, level of vascularisation and condition of endothelial and epithelial surfaces. An important observation is any unevenness in the thickness of the cornea or any localised thinning. Epithelial bullae are best seen on a slit lamp. Stromal oedema indicated by increase in the thickness of the cornea can be quantitatively evaluated by a slit lamp. Folds in Descemets membrane and deposits on the endothelial surface of the cornea are seen along the posterior edge of the slit illumination.

It is therefore evident that a slit lamp which was originally called a corneal microscope gives a variety of information about corneal pathology and is a dependable guide not for conservative treatment but also for planning a surgical procedure like a lamellar or penetrating corneal grafting (Fig. 6.12A).

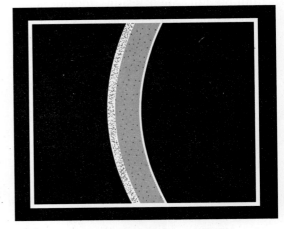

Fig. 6.12A: Cornea on the slit lamp

Examination of the Anterior Chamber, Iris and Pupil

The aqueous flare produced by cells in the anterior chamber is an extremely important observation to diagnose anterior uveal inflammations. Peripheral synechiae following operative procedures like cataract extraction or corneal grafting are best detected and studied on a slit lamp. Rubeosis iris, evidence of posterior synechia, presence of a persistent pupillary membrane remnant are important clinical findings with a slit lamp examinations.

Pupillary reaction when doubtful can be confirmed on the slit lamp by changing the illumination from zero to brightest and noting the movement of pupillary margin through the binocular microscope.

Examination of Lens with Slit Lamp

It is possible to study lens at different depths from the anterior to the posterior capsule. The oblique beam passing through the lens shows the anterior capsule, the anterior cortex, outline of the nucleus when formed, the posterior cortex and posterior capsule of the lens. The sutures of the lens in the nuclear area can be visualised in the transparent lens. One can even see the hyloido-capsular ligament attached to the posterior capsule, moving with slightest movement of the eye which is called the assension phenomenon (Fig. 6.12B).

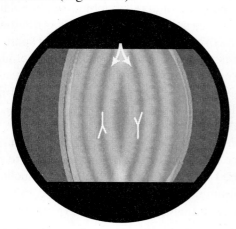

Fig. 6.12B: Normal lens seen on slit lamp (Note: Posterior surface more convex than anterior, differentiation of cortical zones: Outlines of foetal nucleus (arrow); anterior and posterior Y sutures, and cleft of embryonic nucleus in the centre).

Opacities in lens can be clearly seen in different shapes and forms. Their morphology can be studied by moving the beam across the dilated pupil and noting the location of the opacity and its level of depth in the lens. Nuclear sclerosis and nuclear cataract are seen with a distinct biconvex outline in the centre of the lens. Retro-illumination differentiates between nuclear sclerosis and nuclear cataract. In the former, the fundus glow is well seen and the outline is distinctly visible. In the latter, a dark central opacity shows against the fundus glow of retro-illumination. Physiological changes in the posterior capsule and pathological posterior capsular opacities can be very clearly studied by focussing the slit lamp beam.

SLIT LAMP PROCEDURES (WITH ACCESSORIES)

In addition to the different methods of examination with slit lamp, a number of other procedures can be carried out with suitable extra attachments. These are:
1. Applanation tonometry
2. Gonioscopy
3. Fundus examination
    i. with pre-set lens
    ii. with Goldmann contact lens
4. Depth measurement of
    i. cornea
    ii. anterior chamber
    iii. lens
5. Slit lamp photography

Applanation Tonometry

This has become a common procedure. A significant advantage of applanation over routine Schiotz tonometry is that the scleral rigidity factor is excluded and therefore the intra-ocular pressure recorded by applanation is more realistic. Another advantage is that applanation tonometry is carried out on the slit lamp with the patient in a sitting position and becomes a routine procedure. In the sitting position, the gravity factor of Schiotz tonometry is also obviated. Repeated measurements with a Schiotz tonometer induce a massage effect to show a decrease in intraocular tension with each reading. This is also obviated with applanation.

Applanation tonometry is based on measuring the force required to flatten the corneal surface in a known and constant area. The exact measurement of the flattened area is made with the microscope under a magnification of ten times. It is important to mention that viewing is uniocular, either with the right or left eye piece of the microscope. The tonometer is mounted either on the guide plate provided (in older models) or above the binocular microscope (in newer models of slit lamp). The cornea is anaesthetized with 4% xylocaine drops. A fluorescein strip is placed in the lower fornix and a cobalt blue filter is interposed in the path of the light of the slit lamp.

The prism is mounted in the ring at the end of the tonometer arm. The diameter of the flat surface of prism is 7.0 mm and has a rounded edge to prevent corneal injury. By advancing the slit lamp, the prism is brought in contact with the cornea. At this stage, two small half rings of fluorescein are seen at a distance apart as shown in the illustration in the illustration (Fig. 6.13).

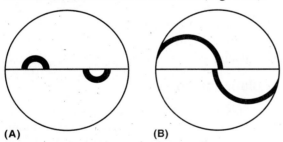

(A)   **(B)**

Fig. 6.13: Fluorescein rings as seen in Applanation tonometery (A) Before (B) At final measurement

The pressure on the cornea through the prism surface is now gradually increased by turning the knob on the recording drum till the inner ends of both half rings just touch each other which indicates flattening of the known area of the cornea. The value obtained on the recording drum when multiplied by ten, gives the intraocular pressure in mmHg.

Gonioscopy

The visualisation of the angle of the anterior chamber forms an integral part of the study in a case of primary glaucoma. This has become very easy and becomes a routine procedure with a single mirror or a three mirror Goldmann contact lens.

It is based on the principle of the periscope in a submarine. The reflected image of the angle of the anterior chamber is seen in the mirror on the opposite side when the contact lens is in perfect optical contact with the cornea. To achieve this, an optically perfect medium is necessary. Methyl cellulose in 2% strength fulfills this requirement. Goldmann contact lenses have 7.4 mm radius of corneal curvature and 12 mm diameter. Xylocaine 4% drops are instilled for surface anaesthesia. This should be effective so that pain or irritative symptoms are alleviated. The cornea side of the contact lens is filled with 2% methyl cellulose. Holding the lids apart, the lens is placed on the cornea. Methyl cellulose prevents air bubbles and if there is one, it an be easily displaced by a slight pressure and tilt of the lens if necessary (Fig. 6.14A and B).

A narrow slit beam is focussed and the opposite side angle is visualised in the mirror. Since the beam of light can be turned to any desired angle and also tilted upto 20° by inclining the illumination arm of the microscope, the angle of the anterior chamber all round can be

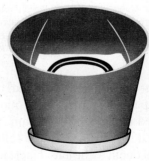

Fig. 6.14A: Goldmann gonioscope lens

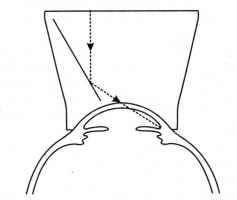

Fig. 6.14B: Gonioscopy—the angle of anterior chamber seen as a reflected image in the Gonio lens

examined within a few minutes. A single mirror contact lens needs to be rotated during this procedure while a three mirror contact lens is held steady without rotation and the angle observed in any one of the mirrors, remembering that it is the angle of the opposite side.

Fundus Examination

There are two devices available for fundus examination on the slit lamp—the preset lens and the contact lens.

1. Posterior fundus examination with preset lens—Hruby's lens. The shank of the pre set lens of –58.0 diopres is inserted in the slot on the guide plate under the chin rest which couples it to the microscope to follow its movements. The illumination is inclined by 10° and kept in the central position. The short mirror is used with a medium length of beam. The concave side of the lens is towards the patient's eye. The lens is centered as close to the patient's eye as possible with the pencil of light passing through the centre of the lens. Mydriasis is the only requisite for the procedure which can be undertaken following routine biomicroscopy. By focussing, central vitreous and central fundus can be seen with a slit beam. The mid-peripheral region can also be seen if the light is focussed through the periphery of the lens.

2. Goldmann three mirror contact lens. This lens used is conjunction with a good slit lamp, has proved to be a valuable diagnostic aid in ophthalmic practice and research. It enables binocular stereoscopic observation of an area of the fundus (already examined by direct and/or indirect ophthalmoscopy) which needs detailed observation. A contact lens has a distinct advantage over the preset lens because of the absence of two refracting separations (glass to air and air to cornea in use of preset lens). This is obviated by the Goldmann lens being in direct contact with the cornea.

The requirements for fundus examination with a three-mirror contact lens are:
1. Widely dilated pupil
2. Anaesthesized anterior surface of the eye ball.

The lens is inserted with methyl cellulose 2% as already described for gonioscopy. A fixation lamp helps to direct the patient's direction of gaze. A bright narrow beam of light is focussed under 10X or 16X magnification. The stereoscopic view is improved by increasing the angle between the micro scope and illumination. The three mirrors are at different angles leaving the central part of the lens without a mirror. The posterior fundus and vitreous are observed through this central mirrorless part of the lens. The steepest mirror is used for observing fundus beyond 30° while the least inclined mirror is used mainly for examination of the vitreous, extreme fundus periphery and gonioscopy. The third mirror with inclination of medium grade is used for examination of fundus near and just posterior to ora serrata.

A 90D aspheric lens used with slit lamp biomicroscopy is an important adjunct to get a magnified 3D image of posterior pole. This is an ideal method to examine macula specially in small pupil.

Sterilization of contact lenses: The contact lenses used as accessories with a slit lamp are cleaned by washing in cold water to remove methyl cellulose and lacrimal fluid etc. Their sterilisation is done by keeping them in 5% formalin solution for 20 minutes which is washed off with distilled water. The lenses are dried clean and stored.

Depth Measuring Device

Depth measuring or pachometry is an accessory for Haag-Streit slit lamp. The design of the pachometer was first developed by Jaeger in 1952. It is a simple method for measuring the actual thickness of the transparent media of the eye ball. It is of importance in many clinical conditions of the cornea, particularly those where stromal swelling is one of the important clinical manifestations. A record of the actual thickness of the cornea in millimeter fractions helps assess the progress of the disease and the effectiveness of therapy.

Two different attachments are available. Pachometer-I measures upto 1.2 mm and is suitable for measuring corneal thickness. Pachometer-II measures upto 6 mm and is used for measuring depth of the anterior chamber and the anterio-posterior axis of the lens in mm.

The principle of a pachometer is to split the optical section in upper and lower halves and then focus them so as to coincide the measuring points, described later.

Each of the attachments consists of a fixation base, measuring device, a split image eye piece and a corrective table. The fixation base and split image eye piece are common for both attachments. The measuring device is separate and has to be interchanged if after measurement of corneal thickness, the depth of anterior chamber or lens is to be measured. The measuring device has a diaphragm with a vertical slit which reduces the light to a smaller pencil for better depth of focus. It also ensures the correct angle of 40°

between the microscope and illumination which is necessary.

A split image eye piece replaces the right eye piece of the microscope, +2.5 dioptre is added to the normal setting of the observer on the right eye piece for pachometer-I and +6.0D for Pachometer-II. The junctional line in the split image eye piece should be perfectly horizontal and made so by rotating the eye piece in its socket and observing correct horizontal position through the eye piece. The illumination arm is moved from the left side till the light passes through the vertical slit of the diaphragm on measuring device and falls on cornea. It is observed uniocularly through the right eye piece and appears in two halves, upper and lower, separated by a horizontal line. These slit images are focussed and the scale is moved from 0 to a point when the slit images meet one above the other and the measuring points coincide.

Measuring Points

1. For corneal thickness, the endothelium and epithelium are the measuring points (Fig. 6.15).

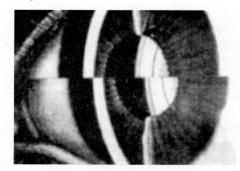

Fig. 6.15: Measurement of corneal thickness

2. To measure the depth of the anterior chamber, the measuring points are the epithelium of the cornea and anterior surface of the lens in the centre of the pupil. The corneal thickness is first determined and then deducted to get the corrected depth of the anterior chamber.

3. For measurement of the lens, the measuring points are the anterior and posterior poles of the lens.

Once the slit images are coincided as described above, the value in millimeters is read off on the scale. Three readings are take and the mean value determined. The corrective value from the appropriate table is added to the mean measured value to obtain the final result in millimeters or fraction of mm for cornea.

Slit Lamp Photography

These photographic attachments are available for anterior segment as well as slit photography. The importance of photographic records does not need to be emphasized. In medical profession, it is enhanced from the academic as well as the research point of view.

Special Methods of Eye Examination

One or more of these procedures are required on the basis of interpretations of the findings of anterior segment and dark room examinations. Not all these procedures given below, can be a part of routine ophthalmic examination. Some are simple procedures which are a part of regular clinical ophthalmology while others need special equipment and are to be done by ophthalmologists trained specially.

With scientific developments, both academic and technological, many newer investigative procedures are now available providing more precise information and guidelines. It is now possible to study the anatomy of the internal eye by ultrasonics even where opaque media do not permit use of a ophthalmoscope. It is now possible to assess functioning state of the retina much more dependably by electro-physiological studies, a subject which was only in its experimental stages before 1950. Nuclear medicine has so advanced that its clinical application in diagnosis and therapy has become an important armamentarium in medical science. It is important to emphasize that these procedures which are available at institutional levels should not be advised purely on academic grounds or for confirmation of well made clinical diagnosis. These costly procedures should be reserved for situations where they will make an appreciable difference in diagnosis, prognosis and treatment.

A detailed description of some and a short description of others is given below:

Macular Function: The macular area is responsible for 90% of visual acuity. If macular area is punched out or destroyed by pathology, visual acuity from the whole of the remaining retina will be 6/60 or at the most 6/36 partial. The macular function test is, therefore, very important particularly when haziness or opacities in media obstruct direct view of the macula. The common tests are:

1. Two point discrimination test: A card with two round holes near each other, is placed in front of the eye to be tested and the card is illuminated from behind. An eye, with normal macular function should be able to identify light coming from two separate holes.

2. Macular dazzle test. This can be useful in eyes which have subnormal vision and the macular appearance has to be differentiated for physiological or pathological state. Best visual acuity with correction, if necessary is recorded before the test. The eye is exposed to bright halogen ophthalmoscope light at a close range and the patient is asked to look into the light. The dazzling maintained for 30 seconds. After dazzling, time interval taken for vision to return to the predazzle level is recorded. If time taken is 45 seconds or more, it indicates disturbed macular function.

Hadinger brushes in synoptophore and laser interferometry are also used as macular function tests.

3. Electro-retinography can also be helpful in evaluating macular function in eyes with hazy media. The suitable procedures are photopic

ERG, chromatic ERG and determining flicker fusion frequency by ERG.

Colour Vision Test: There are many methods of assessing colour vision. The simplest and most handy are Ishihara's Charts which can fairly dependably detect partial or total colour blindness.

The Edridge lantern test is more sophisticated when higher degrees of colour vision discrimination needs to be tested. Chromato-electro-retinography can also be done with different colour stimuli. Based on the old coloured wool test, Fransworth has developed a 100 hue test.

FIELD OF VISION STUDIES

These are indicated not only in ocular conditions like glaucoma, optic neuritis, papilloedema and optic atrophy but also in neurologic conditions affecting the visual pathways.

There are various methods and with developments of technology, visual field studies have reached a high precision. The methods practised are:

1. Confrontation test.
2. Perimetry on Lister's perimeter, with targets or projection perimeter with illuminated spots.
3. Scotometry or Bjerrum's screen.
4. Differential perimetry on Goldmann's perimeter.
5. Amsler grid. Field defects can present themselves in various forms.
6. Automated perimeters available have added significantly to understand field defects to an extent hereto not possible.

There can be localised defects in the field not necessarily extending to the periphery. These localised islands of field defects within the extent of peripheral field are called scotoma. A scotoma may be negative or positive; absolute or relative. A scotoma which does not enter the consciousness of patient is called a negative scotoma while if the patient sees and appreciates the scotoma, it is called a positive scotoma. A typical *negative scotoma* is blind spot in the field of vision which is present in all normal eyes. This physiological scotoma represents the optic disc area where there are no retinal cells. Similarly, scotoma caused by glaucoma and lesions affecting the retinal elements are also negative scotoma, example being ring scotoma of retinitis pigmentosa.

Positive scotoma is caused by gross lesions like opacities in the lens, vitreous, patches of deep choroiditis, early stages of active macular pathology and retinal detachment.

An *absolute scotoma* is one, the size and shape of which remains the same for white and different colours and also for different sizes of objects. Blind spot and healed lesions of chorio-retinitis are typical examples of absolute scotoma. *Relative scotoma*, is one where the size of the scotoma varies for white light and colours—the largest field being of white and next in order, blue, yellow, green and red. Lesions affecting the conducting elements, nerve fiber layer of retina and optic nerve, cause more field loss for blue colour while lesions affecting cellular layers of retina, rods, and cones, cause greater defect for red.

Field defects are an important diagnostic criteria. The field defects depend on the site of the lesion which may be any where from the optic disc to the cerebral cortex. The various sites of lesion and the field defects produced are described in the chapter on neuro-ophthalmology.

Method of Recording Field of Vision

Of the different methods listed, perimetry and scotometry are the ones described because these are practised by most ophthalmologists.

Sophisticated equipment like the Goldmann perimeter and automated field recorders carry their own instructions to be followed. The confrontation method for roughly detecting any gross defect like hemianopia is mostly adopted by the physicians and is described in the chapter on neuro-ophthalmology (Fig. 6.16, Plate 2).

Perimetry

The equipment used are either a Lister's perimeter with a movable target and the arc illuminated by lights at each end or a projection perimeter where a projected light spot is moved along the arc from an in built source of illumination.

Perimetry can record the peripheral extent of the field of vision alround. It can demarcate blind spot. It can detect gross field detects like hemianopia or a large absolute scotoma within the field of vision.

The perimeter has a half circle arc with a radius of 1/3 meter or 330 mm painted dark on the inner surface. The arc has a fixation point or a fixation light in its centre on which the patient fixes his eye. The target or a projected light spot can be moved in the middle of the arc along its whole extent. This movement can be manually controlled. The perimeter has a disc at the back of the arc on which the standard perimetry chart can be fixed.

Method: Perimetry is done in a dark room. The patient is seated infront of the arc of the perimeter with the chin resting in the chin rest of the perimeter and his eye is to be examined on level with the point of the fixation point or the fixation light. The other eye of the patient is occluded by an occluder with an elastic head band. The patient is explained that he has to keep looking at the fixation spot and should not try to look at the moving target or the light spot by turning the eye. The target is then moved from the periphery to the centre of the arc, that is, from the blind to the seeing area. As soon as the patient sees the target coming into his peripheral field, he should immediately knock to indicate the same and instantly the target should stop moving. This should be repeated to confirm that the patient knocks at the same or about the same site to indicate visibility of target. At this point, a mark is made on the chart with a spike that is provided. The target is then moved further towards the centre of the arc and the patient is asked to indicate if he continues to see the target all along or if there is an area where he does not see the target. The linear length of this unseeing area can also be recorded at the point the patient stops seeing the target and at the point where he restarts seeing it. This procedure is repeated every 15° of the 360° of the circle for each eye separately.

The size of the target commonly used is 3 mm which subtends an angle of 0.5° at the patient's eye. Smaller targets can be used for a more critical study. Coloured targets can also be used in for colours fields.

After the recording is completed, the points of mark on the chart are joined bylines to indicate the peripheral extent of the field. Deficiency in the field as compared to the normal on the chart is shaded to make it clearly evident.

It is important to bear in mind that perimetry needs co-operation and some degree of intelligence on the part of the patient or else its interpretation is vitiated. It may often be observed that the peripheral extent of the field may be beyond the normal drawn on the chart in some sector. It will usually be inside the normal on the opposite sector. This is due to either the patient keeping his face turned in the vertical or horizontal direction or his eyes may not be level with the fixation point or the chart may not be properly centered or its holder. Bony variations in the orbital margins and the bridge of the nose can also cause variations in the peripheral extent of field.

The normal peripheral field of vision extend from 90°–110° on the temporal side, 60°–70° downwards, 50°–60° upwards, 45°–50° down and in and 50°–55° up and in. This contour is due to the outline of the bony orbit and height of nose.

Scotometry: Scotoma is a field defect somewhere within the peripheral boundaries of field of vision. As such, it is always surrounded by the intact part of the field. The types of scotoma have already been described.

Scotometry is done on a Bjerrum's screen which is within the means of an average practitioner. Bjerrum's screen findings are fairly dependable for clinical evaluation. More sophisticated equipment like the Goldmann's perimeter provides facilities for scotometry with great analytical details which is not absolutely necessary in routine practice. Bjerrum's screen is available in two sizes, one meter square and 2 meter square. The screen is made of black woolen felt cloth. It has roller at the upper and lower edges which help to keep it spread out during examination. The screen has circular markings all-around the central fixation every 5° upto 30°. It also has radial markings starting at the fixation point upto the outer circle and are spaced every 15°.

The equipment of Bjerrum's screen also includes a set of targets in white, blue and red in different sizes from 1 mm to 20 mm diameter. When doing scotometry, these targets can be fixed into a black painted pointer rod.

Field studies on Bjerrums screen cover only the central 26° of the central field of vision. It is therefore evident that outline of the central field is circular unlike the outer extent of the peripheral field recorded on a perimeter. This is considered adequate because this is the part of field of vision which is functionally more important as the retinal sensitivity continues to decrease towards the periphery.

The screen is lighted both from the upper and lower side with a diffuse illumination of covered fluorescent tubes in such a way that the light does not fall on the patient but the screen is uniformly illuminated.

Method of Scotometry on Bjerrum's Screen

The patient is seated at a distance of one meter in front of a one meter square screen and at 2 meters in front of a 2 meter square screen in such a way that the eye is level with the fixation point and the patient is asked, as in perimetry, to keep looking at the fixation point and not try to look at the object coming from the periphery. One eye is examined at a time with other eye occluded. The examiner holds the pointer rod with the target at its end and stands by the side of the screen. He should preferably wear arm length gloves of a dark colour so that the attention of the patient is not diverted.

Bjerrum's screen studies include demarcating the blind spot and detecting the size, shape and location of a scotoma if any, within the 26° of central field. The size of the targets used are generally 10 mm for the blind spot and 1 mm for scotometry. A large sized target is preferred for blind spot because it is an absolute scotoma and the size of target will not make any difference in size of the scotoma.

The blind spot is charted first as it is easy to do. When charting the blind spot the target is moved from the blind area to the sighted area because every eye has a blind spot and it is easy for the patient to observe as soon as the target becomes visible. The blind spot is situated on temporal side of the fixation point and normally extends from 12°–18° from fixation point in the horizontal extent and about 3° above and 5° below the horizontal line in vertical extent. The centre of blind spot is slightly below the horizontal meridian. The extent of the blind spot is marked on the screen and is then transcribed on the scotometry chart.

To detect any scotoma in central field, the target is moved along one of the meridional lines and the patient is asked to indicate if he ceases to see the target at any point during its movement from periphery to the fixation point. A pin is planted where the target disappears and where it reappears. The procedure is repeated on every 15° radial markings covering all the 360°. Scotomatous areas if any, are transcribed on the scotometry chart corresponding to the location on the screen, based on the distance in degrees from fixation point both with reference to circular and radial markings.

Visual field studies are important and every eye clinic should possess these two simple equipments. Field defects, if any, will help the ophthalmologist not only for supporting his clinical diagnosis but also enable him to provide complete report to the Neurosurgeon or Neuro Physician.

Patients with central scotoma may not see the fixation point on Bjerrum's screen and therefore may not be able to fix the eye. In such a situation, a white circle is drawn round the fixation point with a chalk. The circle should be larger than the central scotoma so that the patient can see the outline of the circle. The patient is now instructed to look approximately in the centre of white circle so that he can maintain fixation.

Diplopia charting: Binocular diplopia is usually associated with neurological or orthoptic conditions. The diplopia charting helps in identifying muscle palsies and also provides a follow-up record. Clinically, diplopia charting is done with the help of a linear light source like a lighted candle. The patient wearing red and green goggles (red in front of the right eye) is asked to indicate the distance between two images and the level of the two images and also whether the red image is on the right side of the green image or on the left side of it. He is also asked whether both the images are parallel or one is obliquely placed in relation to the other. The method is described in detail in the section on paralytic squint.

Hess screen test: This test is also based on the principle of diplopia chart. It is of special importance to study the relative actions of synergists and antagonists among the paralysed muscles. It provides a dependable record of the rate of recovery, if any, during the follow-up period. This test is described along with diplopia charting in the section of paralytic squint.

Keratometry: Keratometry determines the radius of curvature of the anterior surface of the cornea and is, therefore, a useful procedure in studying corneal astigmation. It also gives dipotric equivalent of radius of curvature of cornea.

Keratometry is clinically indicated to determine the base curve on which a contact lens is to be made and fitted (Fig. 6.17, Plate 2).

Glaucoma provocative tests: The principle is to find out whether intraocular tension is raised by a provocative test. Pro-glaucomatous eyes show a higher positive response as compared to the normal eyes. The test is, therefore, important in cases of glaucoma suspects.

Various provocative tests have been developed from time to time: The two commonly used are the dark-room or mydriatic test for narrow angle cases and water drinking test for open angle cases. Topical instillations of steroids have been used as a provocation to the rise of intraocular tension but it takes at least three weeks before a positive or negative result can be interpreted. It is not advisable to have to use local steroids since it can cause untowards effects. The detailed procedure for carrying out these test is given in the chapter on Glaucoma.

Schirmer's test and tear film break-up time (TFBT): Schirmer's test is a quantitative test for measuring amount of lacrimal secretion and therefore is of value in dry eye syndromes.

Tear film break-up determination is a very useful test for faulty tear film composition, a condition which is often overlooked. The test should therefore be done in all cases of vague symptoms of burning and irritation of eyes for which no local cause is found. Both these tests are described in detail in chapter on the Cornea.

Ophthalmo-dynamometry: This is an important procedure to determine the pressure in the central retinal artery, a branch of ophthalmic artery and the test, therefore, is indirectly useful in vascular conditions affecting retina. It is also a useful guide to neuro-physician and cardio-vascular clinician in diseases like carotid artery syndrome and pulseless disease.

Therapeutic tests: Common ones are prostigmin test and the Vitamin-A therapeutic test.

Prostigmin test is specially indicated in transient and intermittent symptoms of ocular palsies in Myasthenia gravis.

A therapeutic dosage of Vitamin-A is a good method to differentiate between functional cause of night blindness and organic cause. Single dose of 100,000 units of vitamin-A given intramuscularly will restore night vision and also scotopic ERG if night blindness is due to Vitamin-A deficiency.

Synoptophore examination: It is a subject by itself and an important part of ophthalmology. Diagnostic examination on synoptophore helps quantitative evaluation of muscle imbalance, degree of convergence and accommodation, AC/A ratio, grade of binocularity and degree of suppression.

Photography: Modern ophthalmology and academic interest of the clinicians require photography for more than one purpose.

Anterior segment photography, Colour and black and white photography is useful for:
1. Pre-operative and post-operative record of clinical conditions like corneal opacity treated by keratoplasty and squint treated by muscle surgery.
2. Permanent record for filing or publishing a paper on anterior segment conditions of clinical interest.
3. Recording operative procedures for demonstration.
4. Movie films for academic demonstrations and for pubic education in community ophthalmology.

Posterior Segment Photography is useful for:
1. Colour photographs of fundus lesion.
2. Black and white photography for fluorescein angiography.

Radiological Investigations

Radiological investigations are fairly frequently required in clinical ophthalmology. The radiological investigations which are primarily requested for by an ophthalmologist are listed below:
1. X-ray pictures of orbit
2. X-ray pictures of optic foramen and orbital fissures
3. X-ray skull
4. Localisation of intra-ocular foreign body
5. Orbital venography.

Radiographs of orbit, orbital fissures and the optic foramen. It is important that the X-ray pictures of these structures should show both sides for comparison. Among the important conditions are retro-bulbar mass causing proptosis, enlargement of superior orbital fissure due to extension of an intracranial lesion into the orbit or enlargement of optic foramen due to extension of a retinoblastoma along the optic nerve. Fractures of the apex or the floor of the orbit, contra-coupe or otherwise, can often be shown in a carefully taken X-ray plate (Fig. 6.18).

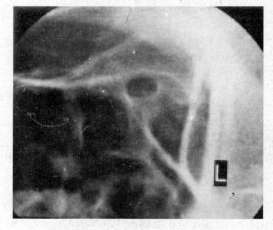

Fig. 6.18: X-ray—normal optic formen

Radiograph of skull: An ophthalmologist often requires lateral view of skull, particularly for pituitary fossa, to show its size, shape, volume and the clinoid processes, anterior and posterior. A shadow of a suprasellar cyst or growth is sometimes seen. An X-ray of the skull should always be asked for in cases of macular lesions due to congenital toxoplasmosis because the same infection in cerebral tissues may show spots of calcification. Calcification may also be seen in aneurysm of the internal carotid artery or its branches at the base of the skull and meningioma of greater wing of sphenoid. In case of hydrocephalus, congenital or acquired. X-ray of skull is very important to study the skull vault for separation of sutures, silver or copper beaten appearance of skull bones and vascular markings of the bones (Fig. 6.19).

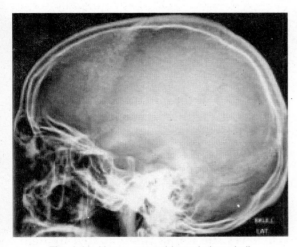

Fig. 6.19: X-ray—normal lateral view skull

Location of a radio opaque intra-ocular foreign body: With the increasing incidence of intraocular foreign bodies due to rapid and sophisticated industrialisation, this facility should be available to all ophthalmologists. Not all foreign bodies are, however, radio opaque. Metallic foreign bodies like iron, copper, brass, lead etc. are radio opaque. Among the glass foreign bodies, only lead glass is opaque. The procedure of localisation is described in the chapter on injuries.

Dacryocystography: A radio opaque dye is injected through one of the puncta and an X-ray picture of the lacrimal sac is taken. Care should be taken that the radio opaque fluid does not spill on the skin or conjunctival sac which might obscure the actual sac shadow.

Dacryocystography shows the size and shape of lacrimal sac: It indicates the direction and track of any fistula either into the nose or towards the surface. It is a good guide to decide whether a dacryocystorhinostomy is feasible in a particular case. The procedure is of great importance to investigate the condition of the lacrimal sac following recurrence of epiphora and regurgitation after dacryocystectomy or dacryocystorhinostomy operation.

Orbital venography: A radio opaque dye is injected in the angular, frontal or supraorbital vein. While injecting the dye, a head band is tightened round the forehead and both the facial veins are compressed with the fingers. Orbital venography is particularly indicated in reducible and pulsating exophthalmos.

Fluorescein Angiography

This is an extremely helpful procedure to study retinal circulation and has helped not only in diagnosis of retinal conditions but has also helped in understanding the pathogenesis of many of these conditions not well understood before. It provides a permanent record helpful in follow up studies of a case under treatment. In retina

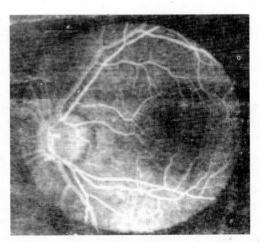

Fig. 6.20: Normal fluorescein angiogram showing arterial phase (Dye is still more concentrated in arteries than in veins. No leakage of dye any where)

clinics, it has become a common procedure which can be undertaken with hardly any risk to patients.

Fluorescein angiography is done on a fundus camera which takes successive pictures of different phases of fluorescein either passing through the vessels or accumulating in tissues because of leakage. As the retinal picture is seen and photographed through a cobalt blue filter, fluorescein appears white. This photography is done with a black and white film. Fluorescein administered intra-venously is used either as a 10% 10 cc solution or 20% 5 cc solution. The newer trend is to use 3 cc of 25% solution.

Fluorescein angiography records arterial phase and the venous phase. It also shows finer neovascularisation and micro-aneurysms which may otherwise not be seen. Leakage from choroidal vessels perfusing into the retina can also be seen in angiography pictures. The observations help in localizing the lesions needing active treatment by light or laser coagulation.

Fluorescein angiography is particularly helpful in:
  i. Diabetic retinopathy
  ii. Central serous retinopathy
  iii. Papilloedema
  iv. Haemangioma—choroidal, retinal and other tumours
  v. Cystoid macular oedema
  vi. Disciform degeneration macula and other macular lesions
  vii. Many other vascular and non-vascular conditions.

Tonography: It is an investigative procedure, more of an academic importance than of clinical utility. Tonography studies indicate aqueous out flow facility from anterior chamber. It is particularly helpful in differentiating hyper-secretion glaucoma from glaucoma due to obstruction in the drainage channels.

The recording is done on an electronic tono-meter with a recorder. The readings are noted during a four minute continuous pressure of the tonometer on the eye. These are reproduced on a graph paper. The readings are referred to standard tables to get the corrected C value for aqueous outflow facility. The normal C values are 0.20 or more as per earlier calibrations and 0.30 as per present calibrations. Value of C less than 0.12 indicates glaucoma while in between the normal and 0.12 is to be treated as glaucoma suspects. It is more informative if C value is co-related to original pressure (PO). If Po/c is less than 100, it is normal, If it is more than 100, it is suggestive of glaucoma.

Like any other part of the body, any physical tissue activity results in developing an action potential, for example, an electro-cardiogram from the heart muscle and an electro-myogram from skeletal muscles. Similarly, a cellular activity also results in the production of electrical potentials like an electro-encephalogram from the brain cells and electro-retinogram from the retina. Measurements of these electrical potentials is a fairly dependable guide of the functioning capacity of these tissues and cellular elements.

Electroretinogram (ERG)

Whenever the retina is stimulated by light, three changes take places:
  i. Physical change in the form of shortening of the cones.
  ii. Chemical change in the form of bleaching of retinal pigments.
  iii. Electrical change in the form of action potential.

An ERG is the record of electrical potential produced at the level of retina when the latter is stimulated with a flash of light. Granit was the first to analyse the components of an ERG using microelectrodes in animal experiments. It has been established that the inner layers of the retina are electrically negative as compared to the outer layers of retina which are electrically positive. When retina is stimulated by light, certain electrical waves are produced which result in the record of an ERG (Fig. 6.21).

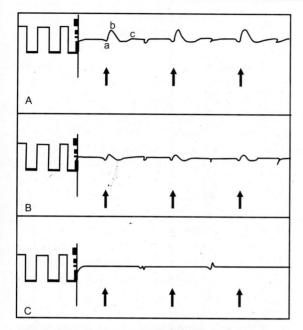

Fig. 6.21: Electroretinography (ERG) (A) Normal ERG with average b-potential of 0.3 mV. (B) Subnormal ERG b potential less than 0.2 mV. (C) An extinguished ERG with no electrical potential recorded. (Note that each ERG curve has a small negative a-wave, main positive b-wave and a slow recovery phase, the c-wave)

An ERG is called a scotopic ERG when the light stimulation is given after dark adaptation and it is called photopic ERG when a bright light stimulus is given after moderate light adaptation of the eye. The exact site where the different components of ERG are produced has been a matter of investigation for a long time. It is generally agreed that the ERG is produced at the outer nuclear layer and level of bipolar cells of retina. It has been suggested that the 'C' wave in addition to being retinal in original, may also have a part of the potential produced due to pupillary muscle activity. From clinical point of view however, an ERG is a composite response of retina as a whole. It cannot indicate any localising site of retinal lesion. Special methods can however be adopted by which function of the individual retinal elements maybe studied. For example, instead of white light, coloured lights

are used and the response is called *chromato-electro-retinogram* which indicates functioning status of cone cells of the retina. Similarly, quick stimuli in succession may be given and a point determined at which the number of stimuli per second result in a continuous response instead of separate response to each stimulus and this is called flicker ERG (Foveal ERG) and the rate of stimuli which leads to fusion of responses is called *flicker fusion frequency* (FFF). Both these special tests are indicated for cone function of retina and hence the macular function.

An ERG is recorded using two indifferent electrodes, the +ve on the cornea and the –ve on the forehead or the temple. The one on the cornea is fitted to a contact lens and the other on the forehead is stuck on the skin. The +ve electrode on the cornea represents the +ve outer layers of the retina which are in close apposition to the sclera, which in turn, is anteriorly continuous to the cornea, white the -ve inner layers have a continuity via the nerve fibres of the optic nerve through its contact with the bony optic canal and then to the frontal bone. These electrodes are connected to an oscillograph. Each light stimulus results in the production of the electrical potential which is recorded by the amplifier.

An ERG is measured as the height of the 'b' wave. A normal 'b' wave varies between 0.2 to 0.35 millivolts. 'b' potential less than 0.20 mV is a subnormal ERG and more than 0.45 millivolts is a super-normal ERG. If there is no electrical response and ERG is a flat line, it is called extinguished ERG.

The clinical use of an ERG has become more and more since Karpe's pioneering work which brought ERG from experimental research into clinical application. The first ERG in India was recorded in 1951 by R.P. Dhanda. More recently ERG is used as a dependable guide for evaluation of the functions of retina when media are hazy and do not permit fundoscopy.

The important subjects where ERG has proved of significant clinical application are:

1. *Night blindness:* due to Vitamin-A deficiency. By the time the child develops night blindness, ERG is usually extinguished, but unlike congenital night blindness, it is reversible with the improvement of the vitamin-A level. Research studies based on ERG records and biochemical studies have indicated that minimum threshold level of Vitamin-A in plasma is around 20 IU/100 cc as against an average of 100-200 IU/100 cc in normal human beings. ERG studies in Vitamin-A deficiency have also indicated that clinical manifestations of malnutrition like xerosis of conjunctiva and kerato-malacia are not pure Vitamin-A deficiency syndromes in which an ERG is not necessarily extinguished.

2. *Retinal detachment:* An ERG being a composite response of the retina as whole, it is affected in proportion to the extent and duration of retina detachment and is a sub-normal response. It is a fairly dependable guide for evaluating pre-operatively prognosis of retinal detachment surgery, the same being poor if ERG is extinguished or markedly sub-normal.

3. *Retinitis pigmentosa:* Scotopic ERG is extinguished at a very early stage of the disease, even before the retinal changes have become clinically evident. It is an important diagnostic feature for differential diagnosis between primary retinitis pigmentosa and secondary pigmentary degeneration due to disseminated or diffuse choroiditis. As the disease is incurable, ERG also is irreversibly extinguished.

4. *Siderosis retinae:* A subnormal ERG is prognostically important to indicate that the eye is likely to end in blindness even if the intraocular foreign body is successfully removed.

5. *Retinal pathology* like vascular retinopathy: Diabetic and hypertensive retinopathies have been observed to have influence on the height of 'b' wave in ERG. The initial irritative phase of these pathologies have supernormal response which becomes sub-normal when degenerative process has advanced.

6. *Malingering:* ERG is precise procedure at our disposal to prove malingering in patients where subjective vision is poor but fundus picture is normal. An objective record of ERG, if normal, will prove normal functioning of the retina. Uniocular feigned blindness is not distinguishable from unilocular amblyopia because in both ERG is normal. Chromato-electro retinography can similarly be helpful in proving or disproving the existence of colour blindness.

It is interesting to note that an ERG may be normal or near normal in gross fundus pathologies where the retinal cellular elements may not be affected. The ERG may be as good as normal in optic atrophy. It may also be near normal in eyes blinded due to glaucomatous changes in the optic disc.

Correlation between ERG and visually evoked response (VER) in the occipital cortex has proved useful in localizing pathology in the visual pathways where the retina is unaffected. The records are made simultaneously for ERG and VER. If the patient cannot see and ERG is normal, a faulty VER indicates a conduction defect in visual pathways. VER may also be affected in amblyopic eyes where ERG and fundus are normal.

Electro-oculogram (EOG)

An EOG is a record of corneo-fundal potentials. It is indicative of the functioning of the outer layers of the retina and the integrity of choroidal blood supply. Cornea is treated as +ve pole and the skin under either of the two canthi as negative pole. The eye under standard illumination is made to move in and out in a horizontal plane at a regular frequency in a fixed range. This evokes an electrical response which is called an electro-oculogram (EOG). A normal response is approximately 6 millivolts.

An EOG can help in the localization of the site of the lesion which the ERG cannot. For example, an EOG may be abnormal when the outer layers of the retina are involved in which case ERG may be normal. Like ERG, EOG is recorded in light adapted and dark adapted eyes. The record in a dark adapted eye appears in the form of dark trough and in light adapted eyes, as a light peak. The clinical application of EOG has been studied in following conditions.
1. Retinitis pigmentosa and night blindness
2. Disseminated choroiditis
3. Retinal detachment
4. Chloroquine retinopathy.

Ocular Electro-Myography

It is a record of action potential produced in the muscle fibres of the extra-ocular muscles of the eye. It is useful investigation not only for diagnosis of muscular functional abnormalities but is also a dependable record in the follow up of treatment. The record is made by introducing a bipolar electrode into the belly of the muscle to be investigated and the eye moved to activate that muscle. The action potential is recorded in an amplifier. Electro-myography is important in neuro-muscular lesions like myasthenia gravis, muscle degenerations like myopathies, muscle palsies due to peripheral neuritis and exophthalmic ophthalmoplegia. It is also useful in investigating muscle palsies due to central innervational disturbances.

Radio-active Isotope Uptake Test

The uptake of radioactive element like P32 by tissues is recorded by electronic radioactivity detectors. The radioactive element gets heavily concentrated in malignant neoplasm. This test was used to determine malignancy in a growth particularly when a biopsy is not possible. There

are however better scanning procedures now available which give more dependable information.

ULTRASONOGRAPHY OF THE EYE AND ORBIT

Ultrasonography was first developed to locate submarines in the first World War. It was only after 1955 that its use in medicine was investigated. It is now extensively used in ophthalmology, neurology and cardiology and has therefore an importance in diagnosis and therapy.

Ultrasonography is a non-invasive, painless and safe procedure with no radiational hazard. It is a dependable guide to study intraocular anatomy and pathology. It helps in accurate measurement of the eye ball in situ. It can record position of the retina, presence or absence of lens and other intraocular pathologies even in eyes where opaque media do not permit examination of inner eye. It is as useful for study of soft tissues as the study of bones with X-rays. Ultra sound can resolve objects of even 0.1 mm size.

Ultra sound is a high frequency of sonic energy that is above the human audible range. This energy is produced by electrically stimulated quartz or lithium sulphate crystals. Each crystal has a specific frequency and produces ultrasonic waves of a specific wave length. The differential reflection of these waves from the objects in the beam pathway is also received by the crystals and converted for visual display on the cathode ray oscilloscope.

In this procedure ultrasonic waves are directed along the visual axis. Some of these waves are obstructed and reflected back by the cornea, the lens and pathological lesions in the posterior segment of the eye ball. These reflected waves are called ECHOES which are seen on a screen or photographically recorded. The recorded tracing is called an echogram.

There are two types of scans commonly used for display of ultrasonic energy, namely the A and B-scans.

A-Scan

This is uni-dimensional time amplitude trace received along the beam path. The distance between the echoes provides an indirect measurement of tissues such as axial length of the globe or lens thickness. The height of the echo represents the strength of the tissue which reflects it. On the A-scan echo spikes are produced by the anterior and posterior cornea, anterior and posterior lens surface and sclera (Fig. 6.22A to C).

B-Scan

This is two dimensional trace where the echoes are displayed as brightness dots instead of spikes and a cut section of the eye as such, is obtained.

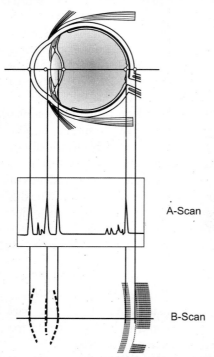

Fig. 6.22A: Ultrasonography of normal eye recorded on A-scan equipment. The spikes indicate, from before backwards echoes from cornea, anterior surface of lens, posterior surface of lens and posterior coats of eye ball; Recorded on B-scan ultrasonogram showing an outline of eye ball with echoes from various structures. The blank space in posterior wall in the optic nerve

The location, size and configuration of the structures and the relationship of the abnormalities to other ocular structures are readily apparent. The normal eye has a smooth rounded contour, the reflecting surface being produced by the cornea, lens and sclera.

Ultrasonography may be performed by one of the following methods

a. Contact method: The transducer probe which is hand held and wet with distilled water is placed over the closed eyelid of a patient. It can also be used directly over cornea after a suitable anaesthetic solution is used. Either A or B scan alone or combined A and B scans can be done in the commercially available models.

   The equipment can be used with ease in children, un-cooperative adults and mentally retarded. It is also a quick method of studying the inside of eye ball. This method of scanning is quite satisfactory for detecting most intraocular pathologies, but is of limited value for orbit.

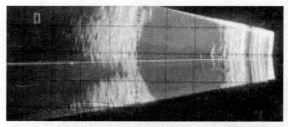

Fig. 6.22B: Echogram of normal eye ball recorded on A and B Scan ultrasonograph. Upper echogram showing eye ball outline by A-scan and lower echogram on B-scan

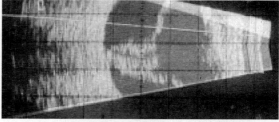

Fig. 6.22C: Combined A and B scan ultrasonogram showing total detachment of retina

b. Immersion method. This is a more sophisticated method. The eye to be examined is kept open. A plastic drape fixed to the orbital rim serves as a water bath. The transducer probe is placed just beneath the surface of the water, but not in direct contact with the globe. The transducer is operated manually and the entire cross section of the globe can be constructed on the screen using linear, sector or compound scans. It is ideal for study of both intraorbital and intraocular pathologies.

Uses of Ultrasonography in Ocular Pathology

Variations in the shape and size of the globe can be demonstrated by ultrasonography e.g. enlarged globes with increased axial length as in high myopes, buphthalmos, shrunken and distorted shape of posterior wall due to staphylomata or scleral buckle. Clinical conditions for which ultrasonography is useful:

1. Depth of the anterior chamber.
2. Dislocations of the lens (anterior or posterior)
3. Cataractous lens changes
4. Changes like iris bombe
5. Cysts and tumour of the iris
6. Vitreous haemorrhage, asteroids or inflammatory debris
7. Membranes in the vitreous
8. Retinal detachment or its attachment can be traced to the optic nerve head on one hand and ora serrata on the other.
9. Long standing retinal detachments are seen as thickened membranes in a typical funnel shaped pattern.
10. Choroidal detachments appear typically convex in shape, showing an attachment further anterior to the ora and no attachment to the optic neve head posteriorly.
11. Solid tumours of the eye produce a compact collection of echoes adjacent to the globe wall.
12. Localization of intraocular foreign bodies in the presence of unclear media and is probably the only method of locating nonmetallic intraocular foreign bodies.
13. Evaluation of proptosis. Soft tissue lesions behind the globe can be easily detected and differentiated into cystic, solid, angiomatous or infiltrative lesion.
14. Biometry when axial length of the globe can be accurately measured with an A-scan. It is highly valuable in calculating power of the intraocular lens to be implanted after cataract extraction.

Ultrasonography is an important investigative procedure in the present era of advanced ophthalmology and should be taken advantage of when necessary and where such facility is available. Its high rate of accuracy both in ocular and orbital pathology, and its safety make ultrasonography an invaluable diagnostic technique.

Computerised Tomography (CT Scan) is helpful in locating intraocular foreign bodies and growths but has the disadvantage that it is radiational investigation and therefore avoided as far as possible. Moreover, CT scan is relatively non-specific for tissue characterisation.

Magnetic Resonance Imaging (MRI) is a non-radiational and more dependable method of diagnostic modality particularly for orbital pathology.

Optical Coherence Tomography

It is a non-invasive, non-contact imaging technique first developed by collaborative group at MIT Boston USA in 1990 reported in 1991 and demonstrated in vivo in 1995.

It gives cross sectional image measuring depth resolved reflectance of tissue by employing low coherence inferometry. The equipment set up essentially consists of an inferometer with a low coherence, broad band light source. OCT provides cross sectional images of posterior sequent as well as high resolution and high definition images of surface anatomy of fundus.

It is a vital investigative modality (Fig. 6.23, Plate 2).

Slit lamp OCT evolved over the last decade specifically improves anterior segment imaging with non-contact and high resolution technique essential for cross sectional image of anterior segment particularly in refractive surgery, corneal transplant surgery and glaucoma procedures, preintra- and post-operatively.

In addition to ocular examination and investigations, reference may some times be necessary to other disciplines of medicine for the following purposes:

 i. Laboratory tests, routine and special as indicated by clinical examination.

 ii. ENT and dental examination because of its neighbourly status to orbit and the eyes, causing referred symptoms, acting as focus of infection or extension of a pathology into the orbit.

 iii. Neurological examination because of the close relationship and communications between the intra-cranial cavity and its contents and the orbit. Fundus picture and ocular palsies are often the result of intra-cranial lesions. A reference for a neurological examination by the ophthalmologist is therefore as often required as the reference by a neurophysician or neurosurgeon to ophthalmologist.

 iv. Reference to cardio-vascular physician or a physician in other disciplines of medicine may sometimes be necessary not only in diagnosis of ocular conditions but also their help in treatment of ocular pathology due to systemic diseases.

 v. *Allergy Test:* Sensitivity to allergens, exogenous or endogenous has become an important aspect in etiology of many ocular conditions. Allergy test to detect the specific allergens, wherever possible, will help effective therapeutic measures.

General Systemic Examination

Whether a student of ophthalmology or a practising ophthalmologist, one cannot take stand that because he has taken to ophthalmology, he ceases to be a general physician. An examinee in ophthalmology may be given a case of systemic problem like hemiplegia, intracranial space occupying lesions, systemic hypertension, thyrotoxicosis with ocular manifestation and expected not only to examine the eyes but also other systems. A practising ophthalmologist may have to depend on his own knowledge to make systemic examination related to the case before him. A general knowledge of the procedure for systemic examination, therefore, needs to be refreshed both for the student of ophthalmology and practising ophthalmologist. It is important that the knowledge of anatomy and physiology which he acquired as a student should continue to stay with him to a good residual extent to enable him to complete clinical examination and detect abnormalities in the system. In addition, requirements for general clinical examination like a thermometer, a stethoscope, a blood pressure instrument and a neurological examination tray should always be at hand.

It is however not possible to make this section, a section of clinical medicine. Sequence of clinical approach is indicated with particular emphasis on those aspects where systemic findings have an important bearing on ocular diagnosis.

The systemic examination consists of interrogation of the patient and physical examination. Enough has been written earlier regarding history taking and its importance in diagnosis. The same is applicable to questioning the patient for his non-ocular symptoms with particular emphasis during interrogation on intelligence, memory, co-operation, speech and expression.

Physical Examination

Physical examination includes inspection, palpation, percussion and auscultation.

Inspection: Inspection includes a look at the patient from head to foot. One can note the appearance of illness, the state of nutrition, the condition of face and hands which contain guidelines for clinical evaluation. Inspection will show any gross abnormalities which maybe evident from a distance. Pointed inspection should be extended to other systems guided by probable ocular diagnosis.

Palpation: Palpation for enlarged lymph glands in neck, axilla and inguinal regions and palpation of abdomen and for oedema of extremities and on the thyroid gland in neck will often be an important addition to ocular examination.

Percussion: To maintain correct methodology of percussion one should continue to do it whenever there is occasion to do so in ophthalmic practice. The size of the heart in cases of hypertension, any fluid in the pleural spaces in tuberculosis and ascites in the abdomen may demand percussion of these areas.

Auscultation: This is important in cases with ocular manifestation due to cardiovascular disease to detect any abnormality in the cardiovascular and respiratory systems.

Recording blood pressure: This should be as dependably done by an ophthalmologist as by a physician. The record of blood pressure should be based on atleast three readings of systolic and diastolic pressure. One should be conscious of the silent zone in some cases between 150-180 mmHg and therefore should raise the manometer level to 200 or more to avoid false recording of lower than real systolic pressure.

Neurological Examination

An examination of neurological system has particular significance because many ocular conditions are closely related directly or indirectly to the lesions of nervous system.

Knowledge of at least gross anatomy is necessary to complete a routine neurological examination..., important among these are:

1. The surface areas and deeper structures of the brain.
2. The location of tracts in the spinal cord.
3. The segmental sensory and motor anatomy of the body.
4. The neuro-anatomy of various tendon reflexes.

The location of functional areas on the lateral and medial surface of the cerebral hemisphere is given in the illustrations 6.24 and 6.25. The location of tracts in the spinal cord is detailed in the illustration (Fig. 6.26).

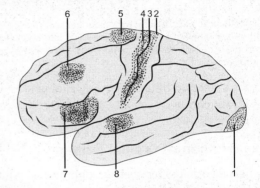

Fig. 6.24: Lateral surface of cerebral hemisphere (1) Occipital visual cortex striate area (2) Sensory cortical area (3) Central sulcus (4) Motor cortical area represented upside down, head and neck being lowest (5) Centre of conjugate ocular movement (6) Visio-psychic centre (7) Broca's area for speech (8) Auditory area

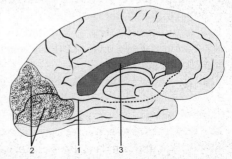

Fig. 6.25: Medial surface of cerebral hemisphere (1) Calcarine fissure (2) Visual cortex (3) Corpus callosum

Neurological examination includes:
1. Determination of intelligence
2. Type of speech

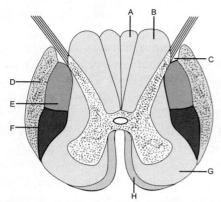

Fig. 6.26: Tracts in spinal cord: (A) Column of GOLL (B) Column of Burdach (C) Dorso-lateral fasciculus (D) Cerebellar tracts (E) Lateral pyramidal tracts (crossed) (F) Lateral spinothalamic. Tract of Gower (G) Intersegmental tract (H) Anterior cerebro-spinal tract (Pyramidal tract uncrossed)

3. Examination of the twelve cranial nerves
4. Examination of sensory and motor systems of the body.

Examination of Cranial Nerves

Important cranial nerves from ophthalmic point of view are II to VII which need to be particularly examined.

   I. **The olfactory nerve** is tested by asking the patient to smell oil of clove with each nostril separately.

  II. **The optic nerve** is tested by recording visual acuity and fields of vision.

 III. **The oculo-motor** nerve is tested by the movements of eye ball, pupillary reaction and accommodation.

  IV. **The trochlear nerve** is tested by the movements of eye related to the superior oblique muscle.

   V. **The trigeminal nerve** is largely a sensory but partly a motor nerve. The sensory area of the face is tested for each of the divisions, ophthalmic, maxillary and mandibular, separately. Sensation is tested with a pin touched on identical points on either side in the corresponding areas.

The sense of taste of the anterior two-third of the tongue is mediated via the fifth nerve. To test this, the patient is asked to protrude his tongue and keep it protruded. The tongue is dried and then powdered salt or sugar is gently rubbed on each half of the tongue by turn. The patient is asked to indicate whether it is salt or sugar by raising one or two fingers respectively.

The motor function of the trigeminal nerve is tested by asking the patient to clench his teeth and feeling the masseter muscle on either side.

  VI. **The abducent nerve** is tested by amplitude of the action of the external rectus muscle.

 VII. **The facial nerve is motor nerve:** There is more than one tests to determine its integrity.

   1. The patient is asked to forcibly close his eyes against a pull on the upper lid. Each side is tested separately. Inability or partial ability to close the lids will indicate weakness off VII nerve.

   2. The patient is asked to raise his brows and frown. The folds in the forehead skin will be absent on the side of paralysis.

   3. The patient is asked to show his teeth. Angle of the mouth will not move out on the side of VII nerve paralysis, if any.

   4. The patient is asked to blow his checks. Escape of air occurs from the side of paralysis of VII nerve.

Whether the facial paralysis is upper motor or lower motor neuron type, can be distinguished by the second test noted above because the frontalis belly of occipito-frontalis muscle escapes in the upper motor neuron type paralysis but is affected in lower motor neuron lesions.

Motor and sensory function may be necessary to be tested when an ophthalmic pathology is associated or is due to a systemic/neurological diseases.

Eye Lid and its Diseases

Function of the lids is not only protective but they help in the lubrication of the exposed part of the eye ball, conjunctiva and the sensitive corneal surface, in the passage of the lacrimal fluid from the lateral to the medial part of the conjunctival sac and help in the drainage of the lacrimal secretion by its pumping action on lacrimal sac.

Development

The lids are developed from mesoderm and ectoderm. The skin and conjunctiva are from surface ectoderm and the intervening structures from the mesoderm. During development, the two lid borders are at first fused together with the eye ball developing under their protective cover. The lids however have separated before birth, but some remnants of developmental adhesions may persist resulting in a condition called *ankyloblepheron*.

The lids may present special racial features. A small fold of skin covering the medial canthus is sometimes present in new born children which disappears as the base of the nose grows. The fold may however persist and is characteristic of races like the Chinese or Japanese and is called epicanthus. The two lids join at an acute angle on lateral side and a rounded angle on the medial side. The lateral angle is at a slightly higher level than the medial angle. This slant is increased in the Mongolian races. The inter-palpebral fissure which at the widest part is on an average 15 mm with wide variations in different individuals. The conjunctiva and cornea remain exposed in the inter marginal zone except during blinking.

The upper lid is wider and the lower narrower. The upper lid covers 1/4th to 1/3rd of upper cornea with the eye ball looking straight. The upper lid is more active with a larger excursion of movements.

STRUCTURES OF LID

These from before backwards, are:
1. The skin
2. Sub-cutaneous tissues
3. The palpebral part of orbicularis oculi, interspersed with aponeurotic fibres of levator palpebrae superioris.
4. Tarsal plate.
5. Palpebral conjunctiva.

The skin: The skin of the lid is one of the two places in the body which do not have sub-cutaneous fat. Because of this, lids have horizontal folds, the main folds being accentuated by the attachment of few fibers of the levator palpebrae superiors muscle (Fig. 7.1).

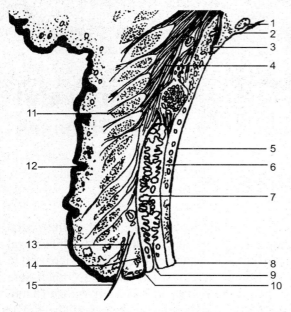

Fig. 7.1: Eye lid—Gross anatomy (1) Krause's accessory lacrimal gland (2) Loose fornix conjunctiva (3) Muller's muscle of lid, deeper extension from levator palpebrae superioris (4) Levator palpabrae superioris (5) Palpebral conjunctiva adherent to the subjacent tarsal plate (6) Tarsal plate (7) Racemose type Meibomian gland (8) Sharp-angled posterior border of lid margin (9) Opening of Meibomian duct (10) Grey line of muco-cutaneous junction in the middle of lid margin (11) Orbicularis oculi muscle bundles (12) Eye lid skin (13) Hair follicle of eye lash (14) Glands of Zeiss and Moll (15) Rounded anterior border of lid margin.

The margin of the lid is an important anatomical structure. A line can clearly be seen between the anterior cutaneous and posterior mucous part. A row of eye lashes come out of the cutaneous anterior part and there is a row of openings of meibomian ducts in the mucous posterior part of the lid margin. The junction between the cutaneous and mucous part is called the grey line of the lid. The direction of the normal eye lashes is downwards forward and upwards in the upper lid and downwards, forwards and

backwards in the lower lid. The eye lashes have hair follicles in the sub-cutaneous part of the lid margin. There are small glandular structures in the sub-cutaneous tissue of the lid called the sebaceous glands of "Zeiss" the sweat gland of "Moll". The ducts of Zeiss glands usually open into the hair follicle at the root of an eye lash.

The orbicularis oculi muscle: The fibres of the orbilaris oculi muscle form a sheet in front of the tarsal plate in both the lids. They fuse together on the lateral side into a fibrous band called the lateral palpebral raphae which is attached to the orbital margin. This gives it the anatomical continuity and helps in simultaneous action of both the lids. Medially the orbicularis oculi has a bony attachment just in front of the anterior lacrimal crest. The fibres of orbicularis oculi muscle are traversed by anterior extension of the aponeurosis of levator palpebrae superioris some of which are attached to the tarsal plate and few fibres into the skin of the lid. The vascular arcade of the lids are situated deep to the muscle sheet in front of the tarsus.

Tarsal plate: It is a firm fibrous structure which maintains the shape of the lids, its regular margin and smooth conjunctival surface. The upper tarsus is wider than the lower tarsus. The marginal border is straight and the free border is convex. The tarsal plates are attached laterally to the lateral palpebral ligament and medially to the medial palpebral ligament. The meibomian glands are situated in parallel rows in vertical direction within the tarsal plate. The ducts of the meibomian glands open into the mucous part of the lid margin. To the upper border of the upper tarsus is attached the fibres of levator palpebrae superioris.

Palpebral conjunctiva: It covers the inner surface of the tarsal plate. Muller's muscle of lid and its attachment to the superior fornix conjunctiva have already been described.

Septum orbital: It is a thin fibrous sheet extending from the orbital margin to the tarsal plate. It forms a compartmental partition between the orbital fat behind and the tissues of the lid in front. Above, it is attached all along to the orbital margin. On the medial side it is attached to the medial palpebral ligament infront of the lacrimal sac and posterior lacrimal crest behind the sac except for the trochlea at the superior oblique. It is from here that in older age when the septum becomes weak, the herniation of fat can take place. The septum is pierced by levator palpebrae superioris muscle, to the sheath of which, a reflection from the septum gets attached. It is an important structure to be taken note of when performing operation for ptosis. If this membranous sheath is cut during surgery. The orbital fat herniates forward and makes anatomical approach to surgery very difficult.

Lateral palpebral ligament: This attaches the lateral ends of the upper and lower tarsus to the orbital margin at the Whitnall tubercle below the zyomatico-temporal suture. To the lateral palpebral ligament is also attached the lateral raphae of the orbicularis oculi muscle and the check ligament from the lateral rectus muscle. The outer margin of the levator palpebrae superioris above and the inferior rectus and inferior oblique below also have a thin extension to the ligament.

Medial palpebral ligament: This is more important of the two, both anatomically and functionally. The ligament divides into upper and lower divisions laterally, each being attached to the medial ends of the two tarsal plates. Medially, the ligament divides into anterior and posterior divisions. The anterior part crosses over the lacrimal sac and is attached to the anterior lacrimal crest. The deep or the posterior part is attached to the posterior lacrimal crest behind the sac. The medial extension of the orbicularis oculi muscle is also attached to the upper border

of the medial palpebral ligament which in turn is continuous with the orbital periosteum.

The muscles of the forehead are also functionally associated with the elevation of the lid. The frontalis portion of the occipito frontalis muscle is attached to the periosteum and helps raising the upper lid to some degree particularly in cases of weakness of the levator palpebrae superioris as in ptosis.

Nerve and Blood Supply of the Structures of Lid

The skin of the lid is supplied by the sensory division of the trigeminal nerve. The facial nerve supplies the orbicularis oculi muscle. The upper division of the third oculomotor nerve supplies the levator palpebrae superioris. The Muller's muscle of lid is supplied by sympathetic fibres.

The main blood supply of the lid is from the vascular arcades, two in the upper lid and one in the low lid as illustrated (Fig. 7.2).

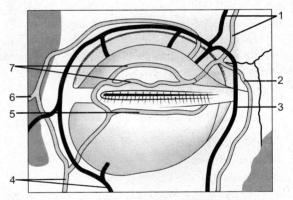

Fig. 7.2: Blood supply of lids (Note the important angular artery and the vein and the vascular arcades of upper and lower lids): (1) Supra-orbital artery and vein (2) Angular artery (3) Angular vein (4) Inferior orbital artery and vein (5) Arterial arcade of lower lid (6) Superficial temporal branches of external carotid artery (7) Superior and inferior arterial arcades of upper lid.

Lymphatics from the outer half of lids drain into the pre-auricular glands and the medial half along the anterior facial vein into the submandibular glands.

General Pathology

From the pathological point of view, the thickness of the lid is divisible in three anatomical layers.

1. Skin and the sub-cutaneous tissue including the orbicularis oculi, the terminal part of the levator palpebrae superioris and the anterior cutaneous part of the lid margin.
2. Tarsal plate with the Meibomian glands embedded within it along with the tarsal part of the lid margin behind the grey line.
3. Palpebral conjunctiva including the posterior conjunctival border of the lid margin.

Being devoid of sub-cutaneous fat and the deep fascia, oedema, sub-cutaneous haemorrhage and inflammatory reaction cause marked thickening of the lids.

Sub-cutaneous haemorrhage in the lids (black eye) may be local haemorrhage, an extension from behind the eye ball or an extension from fracture of base of skull. Sub-cutaneous chemosis following trauma or an enucleation of the eye can extend to the opposite side. The bleeding or chemosis seeps under the skin of the bridge of the nose to the opposite sub-cutaneous tissues. The continuity of the sheet of blood over the bridge of the nose is not visible because the skin there, is thicker than the lid skin.

Causes of Lid Oedema are:

1. Allergic due to:
   - Insect bite
   - Urticaria
   - Drugs and cosmetics
   - Angio-neurotic oedema
2. Inflammatory
   - Stye
   - Lid abscess
   - Acute dacryocystitis
   - Panophthalmitis
   - Orbital cellulitis
3. Passive oedema:
   - Renal failure
   - Cardiac failure
   - Thrombosis of cavernous sinus
   - Arterio-venous fistula in the cavernous sinus.
4. Solid oedema due to obstruction of lymphatic drainage following extensive surgery in the area of lymphatic drainage.

Oedema of the lids can be so severe as to completely obscure the eye ball. One may have to use a retractor to examine the cornea and the eye ball.

An allergic oedema is characterised by sudden onset, absence of inflammatory signs and recurrence. Oedema due to drug allergy is very common, particularly due to atropine, penicillin, sulfonamides and use of cosmetics. The skin of lid develops redness, eczematous condition with superficial excoriations and thickening of the epidermis giving an appearance of weeping eczema.

Angio-neurotic oedema, more common in females, appearing in the morning hours, recurrent in nature is sometimes related to menstruation.

Inflammatory oedema is characterised by redness, tenderness and pain. Sometimes a point of suppuration may become visible. Solid oedema characterised by absence of pitting on pressure, is due to obstruction to the lymphatic drainage of the lid area. It may be mild or severe (Figs 7.3A, Fig. 7.3B, Plate 2 and 7.4).

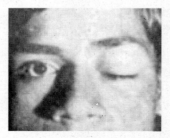

Fig. 7.3A: Left eye—Insect Bite, Allergic swelling

The treatment of oedema depends on the cause. Allergic oedema should be treated with cold compresses while inflammatory oedema with hot fermentation. Anti-histaminic and

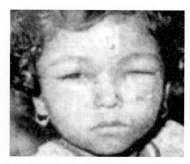

Fig. 7.4: Multiple infected boils on face (Note reactive oedema of lids more left side)

antibiotics may be added to the treatment in severe cases.

VASCULAR LESIONS OF LID

Among the common lesions of the lids are:
• Telangiectases
• Capillary haemangioma
• Cavernous haemangioma
• Haemorrhage in the lids.

Telangiectases is localised dilatation of the superficial cutaneous blood vessels and when present, is clinically more evident in fair skinned persons. It sometimes becomes clinically very evident after irradiation for the malignant lesions of the lids.

Capillary haemangioma is congenital in origin. It may be localised to the skin surface alone or may extend and involve palpebral or even bulbar conjunctiva.

Clinically the capillary angioma is a raised lesion, reddish brown in colour, usually uniocular and limited to the trigeminal nerve supply area of the face. It may be localised to the skin of the lid or may involve a large part of the skin of the face on one side including the upper lip on that side, giving it a markedly thickened appearance.

A large capillary haemangioma involving the lids may be associated with similar neovascularisation in the angle of anterior chamber causing a rise of intraocular tension. This syndrome consisting of haemangioma and Buphthalmos (infantile glaucoma) is called the *Sturge-Weber's syndrome* (Fig. 7.5A and 7.5B, Plate 2).

Cavernous haemangioma: These are saccular venous spaces usually situated deeper than the epidermis. A caverous angioma is a bunch of such wide channels that these are visible from a distance. They have large feeding vessels which may be many. They are reducible on pressure and become more prominent on bending down. Cavernous angioma is usually not limited to the lid only but may extend on the temporal area and forehead. If the lesion has extended to the orbit; it will cause reducible proptosis of the eye ball.

Treatment: Small congenital capillary angioma has a definite tendency to regress as the child grows. There should, therefore, be no hurry for surgical treatment. If treatment is necessary for cosmetic reasons, cryo therapy can help most of these cases. The larger one can be excised with skin grafting of the raw area.

Cavernous angioma however needs treatment much earlier. The lines of treatment that have been practised are:
1. Injection of sclerosing fluid in the cavernous space which may help shrinkage of the mass.
2. X-rays or radium are more effective but disadvantage of extensive irradiation is the radiation cataract in the eye, radiation burns in the retina and malignant change in the irradiated area.
3. Systemic steroids in large doses by mouth has helped in some cases by inhibiting the proliferating endothelial cells.
4. Radical surgery is necessary in locally defined masses which will also need tying the feeding vessels.

Allergic dermatitis of skin: This allergic condition of the skin of the lid is becoming more common due to the extensive use of cosmetics and dyes and the system developing allergy to various drugs.

The common agents are:
- Cosmetics
- Hair dyes
- Plastic spectacle frames
- Synthetic clothes

Medicines like atropine, sulfonamide, penicillin (Fig. 7.3B).

In addition, the skin of the lid may develop allergic manifestations as a part of eczematous condition of the body.

The clinical picture is fairly easy to identify. In all such cases, a careful history is important to find out the cause if any. Clinical manifestations are:
1. Oedema of the lids
2. Thickening and scaling of the lids.
3. Excoriation of skin like in weeping eczema.

Depending on whether the allergy is to a local agent or is systemic in nature, the condition may be unilateral or bilateral.

Treatment is largely preventive by excluding the causative allergen whether used locally or ingested or injected. Local treatment should be to keep the skin dry and give anti-histaminic by oral administration. A steroid used locally gives fairly quick relief.

INFLAMMATIONS OF THE LIDS

Lids undergo inflammatory reaction as elsewhere in the body. Because of the absence of sub-cutaneous fat, the tissue reaction is highly exaggerated so that even with a small localised infection, the whole lids gets oedematous and swollen.

Lid Abscess

The infection may be local infection and exogenous, extension from nearby structures like lacrimal passages, sinuses or orbit or due to systemic infection (Fig. 7.6).

The clinical picture is easy to identify: All the signs of inflammation are present. There is

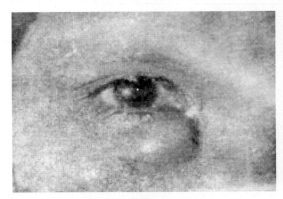

Fig. 7.6: Lid abscess

acute tenderness on the area of origin. The abscess usually points out through the surface of the skin. In more serious and necrotic inflammatory lesions there may be sloughing.

Treatment: Antibiotic therapy is helpful in most cases if started early. If, however, an abscess is pointing, it should be promptly incised by a horizontal incision in the skin of the lid.

In case of sloughing abscess, eye should be protected pending control of active inflammation. At a later stage, reconstructive plastic surgery may be needed to save the cornea from damage.

Inflammation of Lid Margin (Blepharitis)

It has been emphasized that lid margin has a surface which is anteriorly cutaneous and posteriorly mucous, demarcated by the junctional grey line. Situated as it is, the lid margin may be involved by inflammation of skin and also by inflammation of conjunctiva.

The inflammations of lid margin proper are clinically differentiated as:
1. Simple squamous blepharitis
2. Ulcerative blepharitis.

Squamous blepharitis: The patient complains of collection of dandruff like flakes at the roots of eye lashes, itching and falling off of eye lashes.

On examination, lid margins may appear congested. Scales/flakes are usually present at roots of eye lashes. In chronic and recurrent cases, lid margins are thickened, with tendency to ectropion.

Ulcerative blepharitis: Patient complains of redness and collection of discharge on the lid margin. The lid margins are swollen. There is collection of discharge with matting of eye lashes. In severe cases, pustules breakdown and leave ulcers on the lid margins. Inflammation may extend to Meibomian and Zeiss glands with the result that there may be recurrent styes and chalazia. Healing by cicatrisation results in rounding up of the acute angled posterior border of lid margin affecting its capillary action leading to epiphora. Lid margins may becomes sinuous and there may be irregular growth of the eyelashes (Trichiasis). Sometimes, in severe cases ectropion of the lid may result and all the eye lashes may have disappeared (madarosis).

Aetiology of Blepharitis

The causes of blepharitis may be varied:
1. Unlean personal habits, using dirty linen frequently to clean the eyes thus transmitting infection.
2. Refractive errors and muscle imbalance have been considered an important cause though not adequately explained.
3. Extension from surrounding areas like chronic conjunctivitis and recurrent dermatitis or chronic dacryocystitis.
4. Systemic causes like septic foci in the body.
5. Allergic causes either exogenous or endogenous.
6. Deficiency of vitamin-B complex (Riboflavian factor) as a part of the syndrome of angular stomatitis and angular conjunctivitis.
7. Rarely specific diseases like syphilis, tuberculosis, leprosy, parasitic and mycotic infections may cause blepharitis.

Treatment: Squamous blepharitis is fairly easy to treat although recurrences are difficult to avoid.
1. Improvement of personal hygiene.

2. Removal of scaly crust collection on lid margins which should be done every day. Their removal can be facilitated by rubbing the lid margins with a wet cotton swab soaked in 10% warm soda-bicarb solution.
3. An antibiotic ointment to be rubbed in the lid margins twice a day.
4. Treatment of the adjoining skin and conjunctival conditions, if any.
5. Oral therapy with Vitamin B-complex.
6. Examination for error of refraction or muscle imbalance and corrective treatment, if required.
7. Exclude allergic factor if evidently detected.

In pustular blepharitis, the lid margins need to be cleaned more energetically and repeatedly. The pustules should be opened if necessary. Cilia with an infected root may be pulled out. In severe cases oral antibiotics may be given.

Recurrence can be avoided by:
1. Massaging the lid margins and expressing the contents of Meibomian ducts.
2. Eradicating the source of septic infection in the lacrimal passages, nose, teeth and throat.
3. A course of auto-vaccine of the material from the inflammed lid margins.
4. In cases which do not readily respond to treatment, think of the possibility of specific causes like tuberculosis, syphilis, leprosy, myotic and parasitic infections and adequate treatment of necessary.

Surgical repair is needed where the lids have grossly deformed or there is destruction of the tissues during the healing process.

Inflammation of The Zeiss Glands (Stye)—Hordeolum Externum

The ducts of Zeiss glands open into the hair follicles and through them communicate with the surface of the lid margin.

A stye is an acute inflammation which is localised and sudden in onset. The patient complains of local pain, tenderness and swelling.

Pain may sometimes be severe and throbbing in character.

On examination, the condition may vary from a localised congested area near the lid margin to a swelling of the whole lid and rarely abscess formation.

An on-coming stye can often be diagnosed by a careful palpation along the lid margin and detecting the point of tenderness even before a loaclised swelling has become evident. Palpation along the lid margin will also help in making the diagnosis when the local lesion is overshadowed by the lid swelling.

The fate of a stye may be spontaneous resolution in the first 48 to 72 hours or it may reach a stage of suppuration and may point at the lid margin near the root of an eye lash, seen as a yellowish white point, where it may spontaneously rupture and ultimately resolve.

The recurrence of stye is a common feature: They sometimes appear in succession one after the other. Recurrence maybe in the same eye or sometimes in each eye by turn.

Aetiology: No exact cause is known except that the staphylococcus is the most common causative organism. The contributory factors may be unhygienic personal habits, errors of refraction, a septic focus or poor general health.

Treatment: An early stye can be aborted by:
1. Repeated fomentation alone.
2. In a well established case, fomentation can be combined with local antibiotics, particularly in cases where it affects the routine work antibiotics.
3. Normally, it is best to avoid incising a style because they all respond to treatment. Pulling out of the eye lash at the pointing yellow spot may help let out the pus.

For preventing recurrence of a stye, error of refraction, if any, should be corrected. An antibiotic ointment at bed time should be rubbed at the root of the eye lashes in the lid margin and general health should be improved. Administration of vitamin-A has been suggested.

Chalazion

It is also called Meibomian cyst or a tarsal cyst. This is a chronic inflammatory condition of Meibomian glands. Though not a true retention cyst, the lesion is circumscribed and comprised of a fibrous wall lined by granulation tissue on the inner surface and the remaining space filled with thick pultaceous material.

The etiology of chalazion is obscure: It may be an endogenous infection which excites a local infective process leading to blockage of the Meibomian ducts and collection of secretion. The chronic infective process leads to granulation tissue formation from which fibrous layers are laid down all around converting into a cystic swelling. Other causes attributed are Vitamin-A deficiency and chronic inflammations of the lid margins.

Symptoms are mostly cosmetic except when it gets inflammed: A swelling is visible through the lid surface which is hard is consistency. It is circumscribed and fixed in the tarsal plate. Lid skin is freely movable over it. There is no sign of active inflammation. On everting the lid the palpebral conjunctiva corresponding to chalazion area is distinctly identifiable as purplish or reddish in colour (Fig. 7.7 and 7.8).

There may be more than one chalazia in the same lid or in the either lid or in either eye.

A chalazion may undergo a spontaneous resolution and disappear but most chalazia persist for a long time. A chalazion may sometimes rupture though the tarsal plate and the palpebral conjunctiva. If the rupture opening is small, the granulation tissue protrudes out, proliferates and gives rise to a granuloma with a pedicle. This granulomatous condition often causes irritation, watering and discharge due to secondary infection. A chalazion is rarely known to undergo a malignant change of carcinomatous nature. A

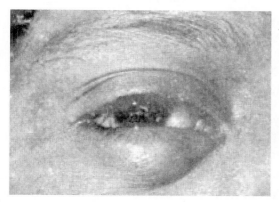

Fig. 7.7: Big chalazion—Right lower lid
(Seen through skin)

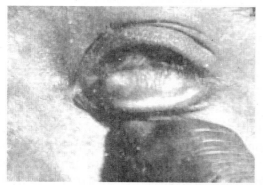

Fig.7.8: Big Chalazion—Right lower lid seen through
conjunctiva

Meibomian carcinoma should always be though of, if a chalazion repeatedly occurs in the same place in spite of adequate opening and curettage of the cyst cavity.

Treatment: A chalazion is better treated surgically in every case. A clean incision is better than spontaneous rupture.

The small surgical process is simple but should be properly undertaken and always from the conjunctival surface. The anaesthesia includes local instillation in the eye and infiltration under the skin corresponding to the chalazion site. The lid is everted and held either with a chalazion clamp or between the thumb and index finger by the surgeon. A vertical incision parallel to Meibomian ducts is made through the purplish area of the tarsal conjunctiva. If the incision is in the proper place, the contents of the chalazion immediately pour out. A small chalazion scoop is introduced through the opening and the wall of the cystic space is thoroughly curetted all round and all its contents are expressed out. If the chalazion is large a strip of incised edges of the opening should be excised with scissors so that the opening does not close and the healing by granulation takes place from inside. In large chalazia, the wall of the cavity should be cauterized with 5% carbolic acid or 10% silver nitrate to prevent recurrence.

In recurrent case, a biopsy should be done of a piece excised from the opening for histological evidence of carcinomatous change if any.

Some surgeons would prefer to enucleate the cyst cavity in entirety through a horizontal incision in the lid skin, to forestall any change of malignancy. The procedure is not difficult but is not necessary except in cases of recurrent chalazia.

Hordeolum Internum

This is a condition of acute inflammation of Meibomian gland which may therefore be termed acute Meibomian adenitis. It may be a primary infection starting as an acute process or a pre-existing chalazion may get secondarily infected.

Clinically there is an inflammatory lesion localized in nature and showing sign of acute inflammation like pain and tenderness. The corresponding area on the conjunctival surface is angry looking. Sometimes a pus point may appear on the opening of Meibomian duct at the lid margin.

Treatment should be conservative with fomentations and antibiotics. Only when signs of active inflammation disappear, surgery should be undertaken to remove the lesion.

Chronic Tarsitis

The tarsal plate being a compact fibrous tissue and relatively avascular, is not the usual seat of active inflammation. The tarsal plate is however grossly affected in trachomatous pathology with repeated secondary infections (described elsewhere). Syphilitic tarsitis leads to a typical clinical picture. The third condition of significance in the tarsal plate is the chronic inflammation of Meibomian glands; a condition called meibomianitis.

Syphilitic tarsitis, although rare, selectively affects the tarsal plate in its tertiary stage. The wooden hard character of the tarsal plate is characteristic of syphilitic tarsitis, seen in no other condition. As a result, the lid droops down causing some degree of ptosis.

Meibomianitis: It is a chronic inflammatory condition of Meibomian glands and is often associated with chronic conjunctivitis and squamous blepharitis.

The typical clinical feature is collection of frothy white secretion along lid margin and the outer canthus. The material is the excessive Meibomian secretion churned up by lid movements and is therefore frothy in nature.

Symptoms are often cosmetic due to the collection of white frothy secretion and irritation in the eye due to chronic conjunctivitis. Sometimes there may be recurrent chalazia.

A tarsal massage by holding the lid between thumb and the index finger is done. The lid margin should be cleaned with 10% soda bi-carb solution and an antibiotic ointment applied twice a day.

SYSTEMIC CONDITIONS AFFECTING THE LIDS

Lids are affected functionally, morphologically in many systemic and metabolic diseases. Lid features are however rarely of diagnostic significance except in few conditions like thyrotoxicosis or where there is a paralytic effect. It is, therefore, not necessary to give a long list of such systemic conditions. A few conditions, however, are described in brief which are important from the diagnostic point or which need treatment of the lid proper.

Xanthelasma: The term indicates presence of xanthoma cells which are histiocytes and excite a local tissue reaction. This is a lipid metabolic condition. In case of xanthelasma, blood cholesterol should be estimated and diabetes excluded.

Clinically, xanthelasma is seen as muddy yellowish plaques raised above the skin surface. They are more frequently seen above and below the inner angle of the eye but may be present in other parts also.

Treatment is necessary only for cosmetic reasons: They can be simply excised. Less satisfactory methods are cryo application, irradiation or light coagulation.

Myxoedema: This is due to hypothyroidism which causes typical solid oedema of lids.

The clinical features of myxoedema are more important for diagnosis.

Lupus erythematosis: This is a collagen disease probably based on the auto-immune reaction. Clinical appearance of the lesion involving both sides of the face and both lower lids has a typical and characteristic butterfly appearance. The healing process may lead to cicatricial ectropion of the lower lid.

Deficiency of vitamin-A: It causes characteristic changes like hypertrichosis of eye lashes, keratinization (hyperkeratosis) and pigmentation of skin.

Deficiency of riboflavin: Causes excoriation of the lid margin and the outer canthus.

Deficiency of nicotinic acid: Causes typical skin changes or pellagra like dryness, thickening and pigmentation.

Deficiency of vitamin C (Scurvy): Can cause haemorrhage under the skin of the lids.

Protein and calorie deficiency: Causes Kwashiorkor disease with oedema and chemosis of lids.

ATROPHY AND PIGMENTATIONS OF THE LID

Senile Atrophy

Characteristic of old age, clinical features develop after the 5th or 6th decade. The laxity of skin exaggerates the lid folds and furrows and can cause ectropion of the lower lid due to atrophy of the subcutaneous tissue and atony of orbicularis oculi muscle. The herniation of fat, particularly through the lower lid is due to loss of elasticity in the orbital fascia or the septum orbitale.

Blephero-chalasis

The condition shows overhanging of skin of upper lid over the upper lid margin due to laxity. It may be present at any age. No exact cause is known but there may be a hereditary factor.

Clinically it is more of cosmetic importance because it narrows the interpalpebral aperture, giving a sleepy and ptotic appearance to the face. The extra fold of skin can be excised with two horizontal incisions enclosing an elliptical area of skin, broader in the centre and narrow in the periphery (Fig. 7.9) for cosmetic improvement.

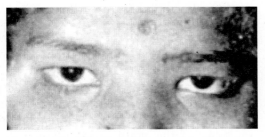

Fig. 7.9: Blepharo-chalasis congenital—Both eyes (Note the skin overhanging the upper lid margin)

Pigmentation of the Skin

A common complaint is the pigmentation of the lids, more often the lower lid and commonly complained of by women. Pigmentation is sometimes transitory during menstrual period. No cause is known but it is probably due to vasomotor disturbances.

Pigmentation of lids can also become evident following loss of weight and loss of orbital fat thereby the skin is no longer stretched and therefore appears darker. Pigmentation in women during pregnancy and menopause is probably due to the disturbance of ovarian hormones.

A transient pigmentation of the lid following ecchymosis of the lid is a very common feature and is due to the blood pigment under the skin. Pigmentary disturbances as in Vogt-Koyanagi. Harada's disease have been mentioned. Patches of leucoderma are not an ophthalmic problem.

EYE LASHES, EYE-BROWS AND ITS DISEASES

Eye lashes act as a filter for the dust and foreign particles. Much more significant is the cosmetic importance of eye lashes, their number, length and direction. Eye-brows have largely cosmetic importance. These are evident from the various dyes and cosmetics used for the eye-brows and how frequently bushy eyebrows are shaped to a fine outline.

It is important to know that the average life of an eye lash is ten weeks and they keep on falling and regrowing one by one without causing a cosmetic blemish. The fall of eye lashes is often noticed when one rubs the eyes and finds one or two eye lashes on the hand. The eye lashes may fall into the conjunctival sac and may be carried by lacrimal secretion into either puncta, the pointed end going in and the bulbous peeping out of the punctum, resulting in epiphora.

Among the common disorders of the eye lashes are:
- Hypertrichosis
- Madarosis
- Alopecia
- Poliosis
- Trichiasis

Hypertrichosis is abnormal length of eye lashes and increase in their number. When the arrangement of eye lashes at the lid margin is irregular or they form more than the normal rows; it is called *distichiasis*. No cause is known. Some hereditary or endocrine factor may probably have something to do with the anomaly.

Long and dry eye lashes are however a common feature of vitamin-A deficiency, particularly in children.

Madarosis is partial or complete loss of eye lashes due to local lid pathology. among the common causes are:
- Ulcerative blepharitis
- Trachoma
- Mycotic infections
- Chemical burns
- Loss of lid tissue by trauma
- Malnutrition

Alopecia or loss of hair usually affects the eye lashes, eye brows or even the scalp. This may be hereditary or due to local or constitutional diseases. Among the common causes are:
1. Leprosy
2. Syphilis
3. Myxodema
4. Psoriasis
5. Vogt Koyanagi's syndrome
6. Horner's syndrome
7. Acid burns of face
8. Irradiation.

Treatment of etiological factor, if evident, may in some cases be followed by normal growth of eye lashes.

Trichiasis: The term trichiasis means inturning of the eye lashes with the result that they may start rubbing on the cornea. The misdirection of the individual eye lashes is usually due to direction of the hair follicles having been distorted by local pathology. The whole row of eye lashes may also be turned inside when the tarsal border of the lid margins turns in as in Entropion.

Trichiasis is due to a cicatricial pathology of the lid margin. The common conditions are:
- Trachoma
- Ulcerative blepharitis
- Acid and alkali burns
- Badly done entropion operation.

Trichiasis is a serious complication because the eye lashes rub on the cornea and cause irritation and corneal epithelial abrasion. Constant irritation by many eye lashes as in entropion also induces corneal vascularization.

Treatment: Trichiasis should always be treated to save the cornea from permanent damage.

A few inturned individual eye lashes are best treated by destroying the hair follicles with electrolysis or cryopexy. This can be done for quite a number of inturned cilia. If, however, there is a bunch of eye lashes in one area, many points of electrolysis, near each other may cause local cicatrisation and therefore is not desirable.

There are quite a few surgical procedures that have been developed to deal with the whole row of eye lashes turned inside or a large bunch in one area. These surgical procedures are:
1. Mucous graft at the grey line of the lid margin. The graft may be along the whole lid margin or limited to a small part against the bunch of inturned eye lashes. The mucous flap is from the inside of lip or cheek.
2. Out turning of the tarsal border by deep incision along the tarsal sulcus on the conjunctival surface and suturing the cut edge of the main tarsal plate to the marginal tarsus, turned at right angle.
3. Regular entropion operation through the skin and removing the wedge of tarsal thickness and resuturing is so that the lid margin turns out.

Whatever the corrective surgery adopted, it is important that the causative pathology should be adequately treated to prevent recurrence.

ANOMALIES OF LID POSITION, LID MOVEMENTS AND INTER-PALPEBRAL FISSURE

A lid with normal anatomy, normal muscular function and normal nerve supply has features of its own, any disturbance of which, specially if in the upper id, readily attracts the attention of an observer. These normal features are:

1. Upper lid margin (when looking straight) covers the upper 2.0–3.0 mm of cornea.
2. Two horizontal folds are constantly present in the skin of the lid.
3. When the eye looks down, the upper lid follows it by downward movement of the lid margin.
4. When the eye looks up, the upper lid proportionately moves up.
5. When the eyes are gently closed, the eyeballs move up. This is called the Bell's phenomenon.

Among the conditions that deserve to be described as anomalous conditions of the lids are:

1. Ptosis
2. Lid retraction
3. Lid lag
4. Lagophthalmos
5. Blepherophimosis
6. Epicanthus
7. Symblepheron
8. Ankyloblepheron
9. Entropion
10. Ectropion

Ptosis (Blepheroptosis)

The term ptosis means drooping of the upper lid. Ptosis of congenital origin is a fairly common condition. In trachomatous regions a mechanical drooping of the upper lid (Tylosis) is also not uncommon.

The clinical effects of ptosis are:

1. Cosmetic disfiguring.
2. Visual defect due to the lid covering the pupil
3. Exaggerated folds in the forehead caused by the effort to raise the lid with help of the frontalis part of occipito-frontalis muscle.
4. Postural attitude of elevating the chin to get better vision.
5. Development of amblyopia in uniocular ptosis.

Degree of ptosis: It is important from the surgical point of view to measure degree of ptosis present because this is one of the factors which will indicate the amount of resection of the levator palpebrae muscle needed. This is best done by holding a scale in the vertical direction supported on the upper orbital margin. The patient is asked to look down, look straight and then look up. The movement of the upper lid margin from one position to the other is noted, measured in millimeters and recorded.

Types of ptosis: Ptosis may be classified in the following types, each of which is a clinical entity and etiologically different:

1. Pseudoptosis
2. Congenital ptosis
3. Tylosis (Mechanical ptosis)
4. Paralytic ptosis
5. Cicatricial ptosis (e.g. due to injury)
6. Myogenic ptosis (e.g. Myasthenia gravis)
7. Ptosis in Marcus-Gunn phenomenon.

Pseudoptosis: This is a condition where the lid appears ptotic although there is no abnormality in the anatomy or the nerve supply of the lid. Pseudoptosis is commonly observed when the lid has lost the support of the eye ball as in:

1. After enucleation
2. Phthisis or atrophic bulbi
3. Anophthalmos
4. Displacement of eye or microphthalmos
5. Loss of orbital fat in old age
6. Fracture of the floor of the orbit
7. Duane's retraction syndrome
8. Blepherochalasis.

Tylosis: This is a mechanical drooping of lid because of increase in weight. Common causes are:

1. Trachoma
2. Tumours of the lid
3. Swelling or haemorrhage in the lid.

Paralytic ptosis: This is due to paralysis of the levator palpebare superioris which could be caused by the lesion anywhere from the nerve endings in the muscle to the third nerve nucleus in the midbrain. Lesions of the sympathetic supply to the Muller's muscle of the lid as in Horner's syndrome, can also cause ptosis (Fig. 7.10).

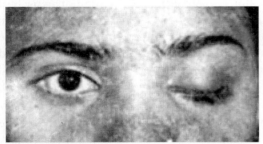

Fig. 7.10: Total ptosis, paralysis of levator palpabrae superioris muscle

Marcus-Gunn phenomenon is a clinical condition usually unilateral where one eye has ptosis. On opening the mouth, the ptotic lid is retracted. Similarly, on moving the jaw side to side, the lid alternatively moves up and down. The upward movement i.e. the retraction part being when the jaw is moved towards the opposite side and downward when the jaw is moved to the same side. This is due to abnormal connections between the third, fifth and seventh nerves either at the nuclear or peripheral level (Fig. 7.11A and 7.11B).

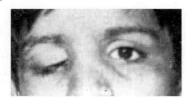

Fig. 7.11A: Marcus—Gunn phenomenon (right ptosis with internal squint)

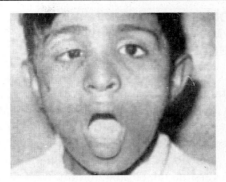

Fig. 7.11B: On opening the jaw, right upper lid is retracted

Myasthenic ptosis: This is transient and intermittent ptosis appearing in the later part of the day following fatigue.

Myasthenia is due to deficiency of acetyl choline at the myo-neural junction. It is usually bilateral. Common in old age, its diagnosis is confirmed by injection of prostigmin (0.5 mgm). I.M. when ptosis quickly disappears, though temporarily. There may be evidence of myasthenia in other parts of body. An electromyogram of the levator palpebrae superioris shows low electrical potential during tiredness and myasthenic phase.

Cicatricial ptosis: This condition is because lid is prevented from moving by cicatricial lesions like osteomyelitis of orbital margin and extensive symblepharon (Fig. 7.12).

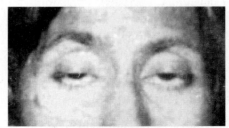

Fig. 7.12: Congenital ptosis—Both eyes

Congenital ptosis: This is the most common type of ptosis and is due to defective development of the levator palpebrae superioris muscle. It is usually present from birth but noticed by the parents sometime later (Fig. 7.13A and 7.13B).

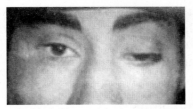

Fig. 7.13A: Congenital ptosis left eye with superior rectus paralysis (Looking straight—Left upper lid ptotic, left eye hypotropic)

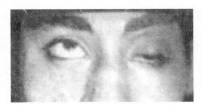

Fig. 7.13B: Looking up—Left eye no upward movement of eye

Congenital ptosis is not uncommonly associated with poor functioning of the superior rectus muscle. This combined anomaly is explained on the basis of the development of the levator palpebrae and superior rectus muscle from common mesoderm and lack of differentiation which should normally result in separation of the two muscle.

Clinical examination of a case of ptosis should includes:

1. Inspection to note the presence, diminution or absence of skin folds in the upper lid.
2. Degree of ptosis measured as described eralier.
3. Eye movements particularly in the upward direction. The latter is done by pulling the ptotic lid up and then noticing whether on being asked to look up, the eye moves up or not.
4. Residual power in the levator palpebrae if any. The action of the frontalis muscle should first be neutralized by firm compression above the superior orbital margin so that the action of the frontalis muscle cannot be transmitted to the lid.

The patient is then asked to follow the movement of a finger which is moved from below upwards. The amount of elevation of lid margin if present, will indicate the amount of residual power in the muscle. A congenital ptosis usually has some residual power, while in paralytic ptosis, the lid may remain completely immobile. The amount of residual power present will be a guide to the amount of levator muscle resection needed.

5. To check if there is any diplopia, lift the upper lid and ask the patient to follow the finger in different directions and note if he gets diplopia in any part of the field of vision, particularly so in paralytic muscle involvement.
6. Record of vision in each eye, retinoscopy and fundus examination, to exclude amblyopia and any evidence the effects of intracranial lesions on the optic disc.

Treatment of ptosis: Surgery is the only procedure which can correct the position of ptotic lids. Some mechanical devices have been developed by incorporating them in a spectacle frame or in a haptic contact lens which can mechanically keep the lid raised. These devices are inconvenient and so they are very rarely used.

Before planning surgery for ptosis, one must differentiate between congenital and paralytic ptosis because in the former, surgery can be undertaken at any time, the earlier the better. In paralytic ptosis, the surgical correction should be postponed till at lest 9 months to a year, the time being allowed for regeneration of the nerve fibers. Also one must ensure the absence of diplopia because diplopia persisting after surgical correction of the lid will be worse than the lid anomaly. It is also important to determine before operation if the levator muscle has any residual power or the power is totally absent as explained above.

Surgery for ptosis is principally of two types. First is the shortening by resection of levator palpebrae superioris muscle, thereby enhancing its action which is like strengthening the weaker muscle. The second is the sling operation for mechanically elevating the upper lid.

Of these procedures, the resection of the levator muscle is the most appropriate procedure, provided there is some residual power in the muscle. Levator resection is done either externally through the skin or internally through the fornix conjunctiva. The amount of resection is proportional to the degree of ptosis and anything from 10 to 20 mm of resection is required in most cases.

The second procedure to mechanically sling and elevate the lid margin is to anchor the lid to the anterior attachment of the frontalis muscle. The slings can be provided by using the fascia lata strips, strips of sclera or less satisfactorily, silk suture material. Another procedure is to use the superior rectus muscle for elevating the lid. A strip of this muscle is detached from its insertion and the end is attached to anterior surface of the tarsal plate so that when the eye moves up, the lid is also elevated.

Lid Retraction

The lid is considered to be retracted if the sclera above the cornea at the 12 O' clock position is exposed. Lid retraction may be present in the following conditions:

1. Congenitally present in normal eyes giving an unpleasant cosmetic appearance.
2. During voluntary effort when staring or showing expression.
3. When the eye is proptosed.
4. True lid retraction as in thyrotoxicosis and thyrotropic exophthalmos.
5. Cicatricial retraction due to scars pulling the lid up.
6. Conditions like high myopia and Parkinsonism can also give the appearance of lid retraction.

In cases of mild retraction, confusion should be avoided when the opposite eye looks relatively

ptotic. It may be necessary to decide whether one eye has ptosis or other eye has lid retraction. This can usually be determined by careful history or examination of the case for either of the conditions.

Lagophthalmos

This is a condition where the lid does not adequately cover the eyeball. It may vary from eyes remaining slightly open during sleep to inability to close the lid even by efforts.

Mild degrees of lagophthalmos are compensated by Bell's phenomenon so that during sleep or when the eye is voluntarily closed, the eye ball moves up and there is no irritation or damage to the cornea. In severe degrees, however, cornea undergoes pathological changes due to its unprotected exposure (Fig. 7.14).

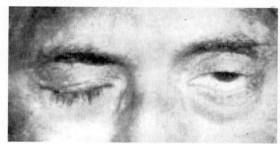

Fig. 7.14: Lagophthalmos—Left facial nerve paralysis, inability to close LE

Lagophthalmos may be present in:

1. A physiological state where some persons are known to sleep with their eyes half open. This causes no symptoms except that some foreign matter may enter the eye during sleep.
2. Proptosis or exophthalmos of a severe degree so that the lids cannot be closed over the eye balls. These cases are likely to develop exposure keratitis and even further damage unless some protective measures are taken.
3. Cicatricial lagophthalmos caused by scars following tissue loss due to trauma, inflammation, ulceration etc.

4. Paralysis of the seventh cranial nerve where the eyes cannot be closed even by effort.

Treatment, It is Directed Towards Protection of Cornea

As a temporary measure, in a condition like nerve paralysis, a central tarsorrhaphy will protect cornea till nerve regeneration restores the orbicularis function.

In permanent lagophthalmos of mild degree, a lateral tarsorrhaphy at the outer canthus may narrow the interpalpebral aperture and protect cornea.

In severe degrees of lagophthalmos, strips of temporalis maybe invaginated in both lids to help replace the function of orbicularis oculi muscle.

Plastic surgery is needed in severe degrees of tissue loss in lids.

Blepherophimosis

The condition indicates that the interpalpebral aperture is distinctly smaller than normal. It includes partial ptosis of the upper lid, slight elevation of the lower lid margin and a shorter canthus to canthus length.

Most cases are primary and congenital. It may be associated with epicanthus.

Secondary blepherophimosis may be caused by adhesion of lid margin at the canthi following ulcerative conditions. Marked thickening of lids and symblepharon in the inner and outer conjunctival fornices may also give an appearance of blepherophimosis.

Treatment of the condition is entirely plastic surgical repair, done mostly at the outer canthus.

Ankyloblepheron

This is a condition where there are adhesions between the upper and lower lid margins. Congenitally, one or more tags of skin maybe present extending from one lid margin to the other. Firm cictricial adhesions may cause fusion of the lid margins at places or along the whole

length in conditions like ulcerative blepharitis, diphtheric conjunctivitis, acid burns and specific ulcerative conditions due to systemic diseases. The treatment includes separating the lid margins and preventing their re-adhesion by mucous grafts.

Symblepheron

It is a condition where there are adhesions between lid margin and cornea or the lid margin to bulbar conjunctiva. The term symblepheron also includes adhesions between the palpebral conjunctiva and the cornea, bulbar conjunctiva and the cornea and between the palpebral and bulbar conjunctiva. The treatment includes separation of adhesions, covering the raw area with mucous graft and prevention of re-adhesion during the healing process. Causes of symblepheron have been discussed in the chapter on conjunctiva.

Entropion

Entropion is the inturning of the lid margin which may be due to lid margin pathology or as a part of the inturning of tarsal plate causing inturning of the lid as a whole. Entropion should also be differentiated from trichiasis. In the latter, it is the inturning of the eye lashes alone while in entropion, the inturning of the eye lashes is due to the inturning of the lid margins. Trachomatous entropion may however be associated with trichiasis. Entropion maybe spastic, cicatricial or senile.

Spastic Entropion

It is commonly due to spasm of the orbicualris oculi muscle caused by chronic irritation. Bandaging of the eye in some cases makes it worse. Spastic entropion in most cases affects the lower lid alone. The condition is usually reversed to normal when the cause of spasm is treated. In persistent cases, an injection of 1/2 to

1 cc of absolute alcohol in the orbicualris muscle in the lower lid gives a lasting effect.

Senile Entropion

This is much more common and usually affect elderly patients. It is due to diminution of orbital fat. It is the lower lid which is mostly affected. The in-turning leads to in-turning of all the eye lashes thereby also causing irritation and congestion of the bulbar conjunctiva. This conjunctival congestion further aggravates the spasm and the vicious cycle continues, one helping the other. Like spastic entropion, it is precipitated by post-operative bandaging.

The patient should be advised to pull the lid down frequently during the day. A narrow strip of adhesive with one end stuck near the lid margin and the other on the check to keep the lid margin in a normal position is helpful. At the same time, conjunctival congestion should be treated with astringent and decongestive drops. In persistent cases, excision of skin-muscle tissue of an elliptical shape of 3.0 mm breadth in the centre and the skin edges sutured cures the condition.

Cicatricial Entropion

This is far more common in trachomatous countries. Entropion used to be an everyday problem for eye surgeons. With the advent of sulphas, antibiotics and improvement in personal and environmental hygiene, the incidence of trachomatous entropion has markedly reduced. In endemic areas however there are pockets of population where the incidence continues to be high.

Cicatricial entropion can also be due to trauma, chemical burns, purulent and memb-ranous conjunctivitis.

Trachomatous entropion in most cases involves the upper lid. The inturning of the lid margin is the result of persistent and recurrent secondary infection in trachomatous eyes. The resulting cicatrisation involves the tarsal plate particularly near the margin causing distortion and inturning of lid.

Treatment is surgical correction. There are various surgical procedures for correcting a cicatricial entropion. All aim at altering the shape of the tarsal plate so that the lid margin is brought into its normal position and eye lashes are restored to their normal direction. A common procedure is the excision of a wedge shaped thickness of tarsal plate all along its length from the skin side and then suturing the cut edges and bringing them together.

Ectropion may be Senile, Spastic, Paralytic or Cicatricial

Ectropion is the out-turning of the lid margins. The effects of ectropion are:

1. Epiphora due to loss of capillary action to retain the lacrimal secretion within the conjunctival sac, because the sharp angled posterior border of the lid margin is no longer resting on the eye ball.
2. Exposure of conjunctiva and cornea adds to epiphora due to excessive lacrimation.
3. Constant exposure and irritation of the conjunctiva leading to keratinization and xerosis of the exposed conjunctival surface. **Senile ectropion** is quite common in elderly patients and affects mostly the lower lid. It is due to the loss of tone in the orbicularis oculi muscle. Senile ectropion usually first starts on the nasal side causing eversion of the lower punctum and later the whole lid may sag down. It all cases of epiphora in elderly people with no obstruction in naso-lacrimal passages, one should look for the position of the lower punctum and note whether it is in apposition with the conjunctival surface near the caruncle or is everted.

Spastic ectropion: It is the opposite of spastic entropion. In prominent eyes, a spasm of orbicularis muscle causes ectropion instead of entropion.

Paralytic ectropion: It is caused by paralysis of the facial nerve and like senile ectropion it affects the lower lid.

Cicatricial ectropion: This is due to scars in the skin of the lids; either local or extending from the cheek or the orbital margin. Any ulcerative or neoplastic lesion which causes a pull on the lid skin can also cause cicatricial ectropion. It may affect either the upper or lower lid or sometimes both the lids as in chemical burns.

Treatment: Early senile ectropion limited to the punctum area can some times be effectively corrected by a few diathermy points applied to the conjunctiva behind the punctum and along the canaliculus. Most cases of senile and spastic ectropion however need some surgical procedures like V-Y operation in which the lid margin is shortened in length and suturing of cut edges pulls the lid inside. Paralytic ectropion, if permanent, can be corrected by the Kuhnt-Szymanowski operation.

Cicatricial ectropion, however, needs varied surgeries of reconstructive and plastic nature depending on type and extent of the cicatricial lesion.

Functional Disorders of the Lid

Spasmodic and clonic tics of the eye lids, when present are psychological and cosmetic embarrassment. The condition is often unilateral. It may be limited to lids but more frequently it is associated with spasmodic retraction of the angle of the mouth on the same side.

The condition is due to irritation somewhere in the course of the facial nerve. If the condition is limited to the lids, the cause may be in the peripheral nerve endings. If the face is also involved, the cause should be looked for behind the angle of jaw, in the middle ear or higher up. In most cases, however, no cause can be detected. The condition in a majority of cases is transient but may sometimes last for weeks or months.

Treatment, in the absence of any detected cause, is non-specific. If mild and transient, no treatment is necessary. If persisting, the condition can be relieved by an injection of absolute alcohol at the site where the facial nerve crosses the neck of the condyloid process of the mandible. It is advisable that about 3 cc of xylocaine should be injected at the site 10-15 minutes before alcohol injection. This will not only make the injection of alcohol painless but also work as a test dose for the effectiveness of alcohol injection. The treatment is effective for quite a few weeks and twitching may not return even afterwards. Alcohol injection can be repeated.

The resulting lagophthalmos due to the facial palsy caused by the treatment is usually not a matter of concern because the Bell's phenomenon will protect the cornea. A small lateral tarsorrhaphy may sometimes be needed.

TUMOURS OF LID

The lid tissues consist of the skin, the glands, the muscles, the tarsus, the nerves, the blood vessels and the palpebral conjunctiva. Therefore, there can be variety of tumours of the lid and these are not uncommon. The list of these tumours can, therefore, be very long and will include tumours of the skin, lymphatics, blood vessels, nervous tissue, connective tissue and in addition, pigmented and developmental tumours. There may be primary malignant tumours and secondary metastasis from elsewhere.

The common neoplastic growths of the lids are:

Benign
1. Dermoid
2. Naevus
3. Haemangioma
4. Neurofibroma

5. Sebaceous cyst
6. Meibomian cyst
7. Granuloma
8. Warts

Malignant
1. Basal cell carcinoma (Locally malignant)
2. Squamous cell carcinoma
3. Adenocarcinoma
4. Malignant melanoma
5. Xeroderma pigmentosa
6. Secondary metastasis

Although clinical diagnosis of tumour is evident in most cases, histological diagnosis can only be confirmed by biopsy of the tissue.

Dermoid: It is present from birth and can grow to a fairly large size. It is typically found at the outer orbital margin but may be elsewhere also. It is cystic in nature. The tumour mass is usually fixed to the bone underneath at the zygomatico-temporal suture. The skin overlying the growth is freely movable.

The treatment is surgical excision. Care should be taken that it is removed intact. The attachment at the bony suture should be cauterized.

Naevus: A congenital naevus or a pigmented patch is commonly seen at the muco-cutanoues junction of the lid. Multiple pigmented naevi from small to large size may be seen on the skin of the lid and sometimes palpebral conjunctiva. Pigmentation or melanosis can also be in the form of a diffuse patch on the lid skin (Fig. 7.15).

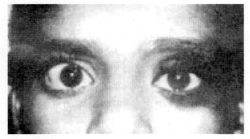

Fig. 7.15: Congenital melanosis of skin around left eye involving left lids

Haemangioma: A capillary and cavernous haemangioma have already been described.

Neurofibroma: These are pedunculated multiple growths of varying sizes from the skin of the lid. They may be present on the face as a part of generalised neurofibromatosis (Von- Rechling Hausen's disease).

Sebaceous cyst: Clinically looks like a dermoid but is differentiated by the fact that it is freely movable over the underlying structures and there is usually a pigmented point on the skin where the skin is adherent to the underlying cyst. Unlike a dermoid, it can be present anywhere and is commonly seen at the inner part of the upper eye lid.

Warts: These may be small or large and pigmented or unpigmented. They are limited to the skin only (Fig. 7.16).

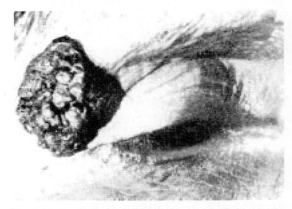

Fig. 7.16: Large pigmented wart outer angle RE upper lid.

Malignant Tumours

Basal cell carcinoma (rodent ulcer). The characteristic features are the chronic ulcerative condition of the skin with everted edges. Commonly starting in the lower lid near the inner canthus but may extend to involve larger areas of skin of the lower and upper lids.

Basal cell carcinoma does not metastatise to other parts of the body but is locally malignant.

It may involve the deeper structures and even the underlying bone. The histological picture is characteristic with columns of basal cell of skin growing into the deeper tissue. There are no cell nests which is an important histological differentiation from epithelioma (squamous cell carcinoma).

Squamous cell carcinoma: It may start as a small lesion but may rapidly grow into an ulcerative condition with ill-defined and undermined edges. The disease may extend to involve the surrounding and deeper structures and may even extend into the orbit. There is an enlargement of lymph nodes draining the area because squamous cell carcinoma metasatises through the lymphatic system.

Histologically the columns of epithelial cells growing down divide at the ends and destroy the basement membrane. The cornification of the embedded squamous cells may lead to formation of cell nests or pearls which are a characteristic feature of squamous cell carcinoma.

Treatment: Both basal cell carcinoma and squamous cell carcinoma are radiosensitive.

However, complete excision at the earliest is the preferred line of treatment, not only because it can be easily accomplished but also because radiation hazards to the face and eyes may cause undesirable effects. Moreover, radiation, should be considered for the enlarged lymph nodes rather than the primary growth. The gap caused by the surgical excision is covered by a skin graft. A careful watch should however be kept for any recurrence at the dissected edges.

In advanced cases with a large amount of tissue destruction, radiation is an important therapy in addition to the extensive surgery that is needed. In these cases, more complicated repair is required.

Adenocarcinoma and malignant melanoma are highly malignant growths causing early metastasis. Early diagnosis with histological confirmation is the only chance of effective treatment.

Xeroderma pigmentosa is described elsewhere.

Secondary metastasis in the lid from the primary elsewhere is extremely uncommon.

8

Conjunctiva and its Diseases

The conjunctiva is a thin translucent, vascular membrane covering the anterior part of the sclera and lining the inner surface of both lids. The conjunctiva is exposed to dust, wind, environmental and radiation heat. Therefore, suffers from ill effects of environments which are severe in tropical climates. The conjunctival diseases are more common and more severe in the tropics.

The conjunctiva also reacts to diseases of the skin. It reacts to the inflammations of the cornea and the intra-ocular structures. The conjunctival sac being continuous with the nasal cavity and sinuses through the lacrimal passages, inflammation in these areas often extends to the conjunctiva. The conjunctiva is particularly sensitive to allergic reactions both endogenous and exogenous. It often reacts to septic foci in the body.

Development

The epithelial layer of the conjunctiva develops from the surface ectoderm while sub-epithelial tissues and the blood vessels are mesodermal in origin.

Anatomy

The conjunctiva extends from the margins of both lids, covers the inner surface of lids, is reflected across the fornices to cover anterior part of the scleral surface and ends at the corneo-scleral junction. The term "conjunctival sac" is a misnomer because it encloses a space only when the lids are closed and the lid margins are apposed to each other. Otherwise, a larger part of the bulbar conjunctiva is exposed lo the exterior (Fig. 8.1).

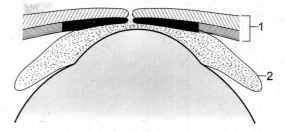

Fig. 8.1: Conjunctival Sac : An outline when the lid margins are apposed. (1) lids (2) conjunctival sac

Anatomically the entire conjunctival lining can be divided into three portions:
1. The palpebral conjunctiva
2. The fornix conjunctiva
3. The bulbar conjunctiva.

Palpebral conjunctiva: The palpebral conjunctiva starts from the mucocutaneous junction (the grey line) at the lid margin. It covers inner tarsal surface of the lids and continues as fornix conjunctiva. The palpebral conjunctiva is adherent to the tarsus and cannot be easily dissected. The marginal conjunctiva is pierced by the openings of the Meibomian ducts, and at its medial end by superior and inferior lacrimal puncta. The tarsal conjunctiva is so thin that the ducts of the Meibomian glands can be seen through normal tarsal conjunctiva.

The fornix conjunctiva is a loose but thicker membrane and covers superior, inferior, medial and the lateral fornices. The subconjunctival tissue of the fornices has fibrous connective tissue extensions to the levator palpebrae superioris and superior rectus muscles in the upper fornix and inferior rectus in lower fornix. The lateral and the superior fornices are deeper than the medial and inferior fornices, respectively.

The bulbar conjunctiva is continuation of the fornix conjunctiva and covers anterior portion of the scleral surface. It is loosely attached to the underlying tissue, but 3 mm round the limbus, the bulbar conjunctiva is firmly adherent to the Tenon's capsule and episclera underneath.

Medially the bulbar conjunctiva forms a vertical fold called the *Plica semilunaris*. This semilunar fold is the vestigeal third lid, counterpart of the nictitating membrane in the lower animals, specially those living in water or hibernating underground.

At medial canthus, there is a small nodular structure in the conjunctiva called *caruncle* which has the structure of the skin like the squamous epithelium, hair follicles and sweat glands.

Histologically, character of the conjunctival epithelium is different at different sites. It is a transitional epithelium at the lid margin changing from the squamous epithelium of the cutaneous part to cylindrical and cubical cells of the palpebral conjunctiva. The epithelial cells of the rest of the conjunctiva i.e. bulbar and forniccs are largely columnar. Near the limbus, the epithelium becomes stratified and heaped up into 7-8 cell layers.

The goblet cells which provide a very important constituent of the corneal tear film are found in the epithelial layers of the conjunctiva. They are larger in number in the fornix and plica-semilunaris and fewer in the bulbar conjunctiva. These are unicellular glands providing mucous part of tri-lamellar corneal film. A few other glandular structures, the accessory lacrimal glands (glands of Krause and Wolfring) are also found in the upper and outer bulbar and fornix conjunctiva.

The sub-epithelial tissue of the conjunctiva, substantia-propria, is comprised of the connective tissue, blood vessels, lymphatics and the nerves.

Blood supply: The arterial supply of the conjunctiva is mainly from the arterial arcades of lids (described in blood supply of the lids). The branches from the arcades supply the tarsal conjunctiva and the fornix conjunctiva and then continue as posterior conjunctival vessels to supply large part of the bulbar conjunctiva. The conjunctiva around the limbus is supplied by the anterior conjunctival branches of the anterior ciliary vessels which anastomose with the posterior conjunctival branches. This anastomotic network round the limbus is involved in the circum-corneal congestion.

The conjunctival veins accompany the corresponding arteries. Those from palpebral, fornix and posterior conjunctiva drain ultimately in the ophthalmic veins. The venous plexus round the limbus drains into the veins of the recti muscles. A special feature of the veins around the limbus is that they also carry aqueous and such veins are called aqueous veins. With careful examination and adequate magnification, aqueous veins are seen in most eyes. Their characteristic feature is that the blood and aqueous run without mixing and appear as if the fluid column is laminated.

Normal Conjunctiva

A normal conjunctiva has a shining bright surface.

It is kept moist by a thin tear film (Tri-lamellar) described later on. It is important to emphasize clinical features of healthy palpebral conjunctiva.

A normal palpebral conjunctiva has the following features:

1. The racemose pattern of Meibomian ducts is visible through its translucency.
2. The normal vascular pattern is parallel rows of blood vessels branching and re-branching as they traverse from the fornix towards the lid margins on the everted lids (Fig. 8.2A and Fig. 8.2B, Plate 3).

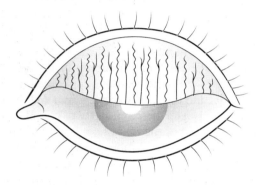

Fig. 8.2A: Everted lid showing healthy translucent palpebral conjuctiva showing Meibomian ducts and normal pattern of blood vessels

If conjunctiva is thickened due to inflammation or chronic irritation, the Meibomian ducts are no longer visible. Similarly, if the vascular pattern is disturbed or there is irregular capillary anastomosis, it is a positive indication of inflammation, past or present. Subconjunctival cicatrisation also disturbs the visibility of the meibomian ducts and the normal vascular pattern.

A normal conjunctival sac is usually not sterile. Common non-pathogens in the conjunctival sac are bacillus xerosis of the diphtheroid group and staphylococcus albus. Because of the communication of conjunctival sac with the nasal cavity through the naso-lacrimal passages, pneumococci may also be present.

PATHOLOGICAL CONSIDERATIONS

Being subjected to environmental and physical pollutions, the conjunctiva suffers from various pathological processes.

Trauma

When traumatised, conjunctiva heals rapidly and completely if not disturbed by infection. Any gaps in the conjunctival surface which cannot be bridged over, cause sub-epithelial tissue reaction which forms a granuloma.

Haemorrhage

Bulbar and fornix conjunctiva being loose tissues, the blood vessels are likely to bleed either due to trauma, inflammations or stress and strain. The haemorrhage may be small and localised or it may spread under a large part of the bulbar conjunctiva. A subconjunctival haemorrhage may also be an extension of an orbital haemorrhage or from inside the skull as in a fracture of the anterior cranial fossa.

Inflammation

An inflammatory reaction in the conjunctiva follows usual response to inflammation of any vascular tissue. When the inflammation is acute, there is exudation which may first be only mucous secretion and later mucopurulent when a large number of pus cells from the dilated vessels are added. The exudates may sometimes be sanguinous when mixed with blood from the engorged vessels. Severe inflammatory reaction, as in streptococcal and diphtheric infection, may form a membrane. There are two types of membranes formed.

A true membrane permeates the epithelial lining and a pseudomembrane is a coagulation of exudates lying over the epithelial surface.

In chronic inflammations of conjunctiva, epithelial hyperplasia and keratinisation of superficial epithelial layers may cause dryness of the conjunctiva and diminished sensation. This is particularly evident in bulbar conjunctiva. In the palpebral conjunctiva, formation of follicles is a common feature of virus infections. A follicle is an aggregation of lymphocytes and plasma cells in the adenoid layer of conjunctiva. Follicle formation is often associated with formation of papillae which comprise of convoluted capillaries and is a manifestation of a vascular tissue reaction.

Chronic inflammatory reactions and heavy vascularisation may lead to cicatrisation which may be in superficial layers or may involve the subconjunctival tissue. Extensive cicatrisation may cause obliteration of the ducts of the secreting glands causing secondary xerosis and dryness of the eye. A severe degree of sub-conjunctival cicatrisation may result in shallowing of the fornices and formation of symblepharon.

Chemosis

Conjunctival chemosis is a swelling of the conjunctiva due to collection of fluid in its tissues. It is commonly due to a local or a systemic allergy or it may be due to obstruction to the outflow of lymphatic fluid. If swelling is due to collection of blood, it is called ecchymosis.

Degeneration

The degeneration of conjunctiva usually follows chronic inflammation or constant exposure and irritation. Among the few specific degenerative changes are fatty and amyloid degenerations. Degeneration has also been attributed to be the cause of pterygium.

Neoplasms

Among neoplastic lesions of conjunctiva, which are not many, a *pigmented naevus* is usually a congenital lesion. A *capillary angioma* may extend from the skin to the conjunctiva. *Squamous cell epithelioma* which may either arise from the limbus or extend from the conjunctiva to the limbus and cornea is only locally malignant and does not cause metastases. A *malignant melanoma*, however, is a rare but highly malignant lesion.

A malignant condition of conjunctiva is *xeroderma pigmentosa* commonly associated with similar lesions particularly facial skin and other tissues with pigment cells.

A cyst in the conjunctiva may be congenital, or acquired. Parasitic cysts are particularly more often seen in tropical countries.

Conjunctival Response to Allergy

The conjunctiva is the easiest victim of exogenous allergy and also suffers from effects of endogenous allergy as often as the other tissue of the eye.

DISEASES OF CONJUNCTIVA

Conjunctival diseases are a very common ailment in tropical and developing countries. Some are mild while others may be as serious as to distort the lids and involve the cornea. The reason for the high incidence of conjunctival diseases in developing countries is the rigors of heat and dust in a tropical climate, poor personal hygiene and poor sanitation further complicated by mal-nutrition. Many conjunctival diseases are communicable. Communication of disease in poorer countries is due to over crowded living conditions, heavy fly incidence and poor personal hygiene. Conjunctival diseases are therefore an every day problem to be dealt with by the general medical practitioner and ophthalmologist alike. Inflammations of the conjunctiva comprise the largest group of conditions among the conjunctival diseases.

Inflammations of Conjunctiva

Inflammation of the conjunctiva, if grouped etiologically, is more academic than clinical. In the case of conjunctiva, one has to depend more on clinical manifestations than on laboratory investigations, the latter being needed mainly to confirm the diagnosis or change the line of treatment already adopted. Economy is also an important consideration for depending on clinical evaluation, because most conjunctival diseases predominantly affect poorer communities.

Conjunctival inflammations from clinical point of view are grouped as follows:

Acute conjunctival inflammations
a. Epidemic conjunctivitis.
b. Muco-purulent conjunctivitis.
c. Purulent conjunctivitis including ophthalmia neonatorum.
d. Membranous conjunctivitis.

Chronic conjunctival inflammations
a. Chronic catarrhal conjunctivitis.
b. Chronic follicular conjunctivitis.
c. Trachoma.
d. Angular conjunctivitis.

Allergic inflammations of conjunctiva
a. Phlyctenular Ophthalmia.
b. Spring Catarrh.
c. Allergy to drugs and cosmetics.

Specific inflammations
a. Tuberculosis.
b. Leprosy.
c. Syphilis.
d. Parinaud's disease.

EPIDEMIC CONJUNCTIVITIS

Acute epidemic conjunctivitis is different from seasonal muco-purulent conjunctivitis or epidemic keralo-conjunctivitis. Acute epidemic conjunctivitis has been introduced into Indian subcontinent and nearby countries decades ago, the first epidemic was in 1975 affecting crowded urban populations. Since then, it has been regularly appearing in the rainy season and has extended even to rural areas. The disease affects all age groups and both sexes. The cause of acute conjunctivitis is adeno-viral infection. Secondary bacterial infection, when present, is only of a milder degree.

The disease is highly contagious and communicable. The causative agent can be in the nose and throat. It can possibly be airborne. Common places of getting the contagion are crowded places and cinema houses.

Clinically, the onset is sudden and acute. It may start in one eye and the other eye is usually affected within 2-3 days. The symptoms start with an acute feeling of foreign body sensation. Within the next 12-24 hours, watering and photophobia cause severe inconvenience.

On examination, there is a moderate degree of swelling on lids and the conjunctiva is markedly congested, more severely in the fornices. A characteristic feature of the disease is petechial subconjunctival haemorrhages under the bulbar conjunctiva. Discharge is usually absent, and when present, it is scanty. The lids do not stick overnight. The cornea remains unaffected. There is no deterioration of vision.

The disease is self-limiting and in most cases, cures itself in 7-8 days. Recurrence within the same epidemic is very unlikely. Prognosis therefore is usually good. There are no serious complications. Some patients complain of transient disturbance in near vision after the acute part is over, may be the virus affects the nerve supply of accommodation.

Being a highly contagious disease, prophylaxis is less effective. One should avoid visiting crowded places, keep at a distance from an affected person and adopt careful means of personal and domestic prophylaxis.

Treatment is largely palliative. Decongestant drops provide maximum relief from symptoms. Simple antibiotic drops are used only empirically to control secondary bacterial infection when present. The drops should be used every two hours during all waking hours. A simple antibiotic ointment at bed time is helpful.

ACUTE MUCOPURULENT CONJUNCTIVITIS

The synonyms of this condition are, acute bacterial conjunctivitis and seasonal conjunctivitis. The condition is distinctly more common in children living in insanitary environments and in a state of nutritional deficiency. It has a distinct seasonal relationship with two seasonal peaks, one in April-May and other in August-September in north India. The seasonal incidence of the disease is also closely related to fly incidence which is highest before and after the rainy season.

Etiology

The identification of causative bacteria has indicated different organisms in different climatic and geographical areas. First three among the causative organisms are gram negative Koch Week's bacillus, gram positive pneumococcus and micrococcus catarrhalis. Staphylococcus aureus, streptococcus and influenza bacillus are sometimes significantly detected.

Clinical Features

Clinically the onset is sudden and both eyes are affected. The symptoms may be from very mild to very severe.

In mild cases, the patient may only complain of sticky lids on waking up in the morning. On examination, there may be matting of eye lashes and congestion of fornix and palpebral conjunctiva.

In a well developed acute case, the symptoms of a foreign body feeling, mucopurulent discharge, photophobia, lacrimation and redness of the eye are present. On examination, collection of discharge is seen at the inner angle and lid margins. Conjunctival congestion is maximum in the fornices and becomes less and less towards the limbus. A collar of non-congested conjunctiva round the limbus is quite evident at times. There may be petechial haemorrhages in the bulbar or fornix conjunctiva, more common in pneumococcal infection.

In severe degrees of conjunctivitis, lid margins may be oedematous. There may be chemosis of the conjunctiva and extensive discharge.

It is necessary to evert the lids particularly to look for a membrane formation on the palpebral conjunctiva and any involvement of the cornea. It may sometimes be difficult to separate the swollen lids and examine cornea which is important to do to detect early corneal complications particularly common in severe cases. It may, therefore, be necessary in children to examine the eyes under some type of short general anaesthesia.

Clinical diagnosis of conjunctivitis is fairly easy. Any laboratory investigations are largely of academic interest. It may however be essential where corneal complications are present. A conjunctival smear examination and culture from conjunctival discharge reveal causative organism. Slit lamp examination will show some degree of oedema in the corneal epithelium although the transparency is unaffected.

Prognosis

Prognosis of acute bacterial conjunctivitis is usually good. The disease is self-limiting. Moreover, common causative organisms cannot penetrate intact corneal epithelium. Any abrasion of the odematous epithelium, may, however allow bacteria to get a foothold and cause an infected corneal ulcer with it consequences.

Prophylaxis

Prophylaxis is extremely important and the condition is by and large preventable with attention to personal hygiene, environmental sanitation and improvement in nutrition. Parents should be told that working mothers should not dope the children with opiates, because under sedation, swarms of flies sit on the infected eyes which the child is too dull to ward off. These flies from the infected eyes are a common mode of transmission of infection to others. Personal prophylaxis should also include washing and cleaning the eyes daily and in epidemic months, to apply an antibiotic ointment at bed lime. Family prophylaxis should be observed by not using common kajal and surma rods for all children in the house and mothers should not use their saree ends to wipe the faces of children.

Treatment

Treatment of acute bacterial conjunctivitis has become simpler with the advent of antibiotics. Common antibiotics act against both, gram positive and gram negative organisms and are therefore effective against most causative organisms. The frequency of the eye drops instillations depends on severity of the condition. In moderate to severe cases, eye drops may be repeated every 2 hours for one or two days and then the frequency reduced gradually. Before the drops are instilled, the eyes should be cleaned with boiled cotton swabs to remove any discharge. An antibiotic ointment must be applied at bed lime.

Silver nitrate, 1% solution as eye drops, once a day in the mornings still continues to be the favourite treatment and is very effective too. It may be added to the antibiotic treatment. Silver nitrate coagulates the oedematous epithelial cells in which the causative bacteria are maximally concentrated. These cells are peeled off by the movements of the lids and thus the infection is mechanically removed. Excessive lacrimation caused by silver nitrate further helps removal of these cells and bacteria. Moreover, silver nitrate has some bactericidal effect as well.

In acute cases, symptoms can be relieved by repeated hot fomentation and decongestant drops.

It is important to categorically emphasize that one should not give in to the temptation of using steroids in bacterial conjunctivitis. Steroids do help quick relief of symptoms but they can do something worse and this has been emphasized elsewhere in this text.

Recurrence or non-response to routine therapy invites investigations to trace source of recurrent infection. The most common place to look for is the lacrimal passages. Some of these cases will readily respond to repeated syringing of the lacrimal passages with an antibiotic solution in addition to the local therapy.

PURULENT CONJUNCTIVITIS AND OPHTHALMIA NEONATORUM

Gonococcus used to be the most important cause of acute purulent conjunctivitis. Conjunctivitis due to other organisms is rarely so severe. The common manifestation of gonorrheal conjunctivitis is ophthalmia neonatorum which is fortunately very rare now, thanks to penicillin which is so effective against gonococcus. The infection in ophthalmia neonatorum is from maternal passages. Infection in grown-up children and adults is however transmitted from genitals through hands and towels etc.

Ophthalmia Neonatorum

Gonococcal conjunctivitis in the new born was, till the middle of the twentieth century, a very serious cause of corneal blindness in children. Other organisms can sometimes cause a clinical picture of purulent conjunctivitis but it is good to consider and treat all cases of purulent conjunctivitis in new born as ophthalmia neonatorum due to gonococcus unless proved otherwise. In most cases, infection sets in during labour when the eyes of the infant are opened after the presentation of the head and it is at this moment that the infection is introduced in the conjunctival sac.

Clinical evidence of conjunctivitis usually starts 24-48 hours after birth. There is profuse discharge. Lids are inflamed and swollen. The infant may have temperature. In all cases of purulent conjunctivitis in infants, the cornea should be examined regularly for any corneal complication because gonococcus can invade even a healthy, intact corneal epithelium. If necessary lids should be separated with wire lid retractors to examine the cornea.

Complications

Corneal complications in pre-antibiotic days were a very frequent occurrence. Corneal ulcers developed, which quickly perforated and infection entered the inside of the eye. Fortunately, not only is the disease much less common but complications are also uncommon because effective therapy is available.

Prophylaxis

Prophylaxis of ophthalmia neonatorum was a matter of very great significance in the first half of the twentieth century and before. An advance was made when silver nitrate 1% solution as eye drops instilled immediately the infant is born, was adopted. The credit for this goes to Crede dating back to 1857. Silver nitrate has now been replaced by penicillin solution 5000 units/cc as prophylactic drops. Prophylaxis has further improved with the availability of better maternity services and qualified midwives even in the remotest areas of developing countries.

If the history of infection in the maternal passages is known before labour, effective treatment should be given locally and systemically to cure the infection in the mother before delivery.

Ophthalmia neonatorum was a notifiable disease but is no longer necessarily so because it has been eradicated by effective prophylaxis in most countries even through gonorrhoea as a venereal disease has persisted.

Treatment: Once ophthalmia neonatorum has set in, treatment should be energetically carried out. The pent-up discharge in the conjunctival sac should be let out by frequent separation of the lids. Penicillin solution 50,000 units per c.c. should be instilled in the conjunctival sac every 15 minutes to begin with and the frequency gradually reduced as the condition improves. An antibiotic ointment should be applied 2-3 times a day. Atropine 0.5 per cent solution should be instilled once a day. If any corneal involvement is detected, a subconjunctival injection of penicillin should be added to therapy. Chemical cauterisation of the corneal ulcer may be considered if it tends to extend. Penicillin should also be administered systemically.

Treatment of gonococcal conjunctivitis in adults is on the same lines and can be carried out more easily. Corneal complications are less common and easily manageable. The treatment of gonorrhoea in genitals, if present, should be simultaneously carried out.

It is important that even in the presence of corneal complications, eyes should not be bandaged.

ACUTE MEMBRANOUS CONJUNCTIVITIS

This is a type of conjunctivitis where there is formation of a membrane, usually on the palpebral conjunctiva, in addition to the usual features of acute conjunctivitis. There are two types of membranes. One is where the epithelium has necrosed and is replaced by membrane formation. This is a true membrane and can be caused by any virulent organisms like streptococcus and cannot be peeled. The other type of membrane is a coagulum of the superficial epithelial cells. This is called a pseudo membrane because it can readily be peeled off leaving behind only few punctate bleeding points. Pseudomembrane is caused by C. diphtheria.

In most cases of diphtheric conjunctivitis, a primary infection is usually present in the throat. It is rather uncommon in incidence and affects children in young age.

Symptoms

They are moderately severe. There is swelling of lids, congestion of conjunctiva and severe lacrimation.

On examination, a membrane on the palpebral conjunctiva is noted when the upper lid is everted. It bleeds when an attempt is made to displace the membrane with a swab. Lymph nodes may be enlarged in the pre-parotid region. In all cases of membranous conjunctivitis, a careful examination of the throat should be made to look for diphtheric patches.

Diagnosis

It can be confirmed by a smear examination of the conjunctival membrane and a throat swab which should be further confirmed by culture studies if needed.

Corneal complications are not uncommon because C. diphtheria also can invade an intact corneal epithelium. Prognosis of diphtheric conjunctivitis therefore improves if specific therapy is started at the earliest. If treatment is delayed, conjunctival adhesions may form. Systemic complications may also develop. Rarely, paralysis of accommodation following diphtheric infection may affect near vision.

Treatment: All cases of membranous conjunctivitis should be treated as diphtheric conjunctivitis until proved otherwise. Specific treatment should therefore start immediately.

1. The patient should be isolated to prevent transmission of the disease to others.
2. If uniocular, the other eye should have repeated penicillin 10,000 units per c.c. solution as prophylactic eye drops.
3. The affected eye should be locally treated with anti-diphtheric serum and penicillin, eye drops alternating with each other every 2 hours.
4. Atropine 1% eye drops in the affected eye once a day even if the cornea is not involved.

5. A bland ointment should be applied in both eyes at night.
6. Silver nitrate should not be used.
7. Systemically. Injection of heavy dose of anti-diphtheric serum in consultation with Paediatrician should be given.
8. Penicillin 50,000 units should be given by intramuscular route twice a day in addition to the anti-serum.
9. The eye should not be bandaged to avoid formation of adhesions and symblepharon.

CHRONIC INFLAMMATIONS— CHRONIC CATARRHAL CONJUNCTIVITIS

This is not a specific etiological entity. It comprises conjunctival reaction to many causes, for which the patient often consults the ophthalmologist. This group comprises various conditions which lead to conjunctival congestion with mild symptoms of conjunctival catarrh.

The groups of causes which can lead to a chronic conjunctival congestion are:

1. Exposure to tropical winds and sun.
2. Occupational irritants like gases, smoke and industrial dust.
3. Mild bacterial infection.
4. Chronic inflammation in the surrounding tissues e.g. chronic sinusitis.
5. Chronic infection in the lacrimal sac.
6. Septic focus in the teeth, tonsils etc.
7. Use of irritant drugs.
8. Introduction of foreign matter in conjunctival sac e.g. by malingerers.
9. Tear film anomalies.
10. Personal habits like smoking and alcohol consumption.
11. Allergic reactions, endogenous or exogenous.
12. Errors of refraction.

Red eye is a fairly common complaint in tropical environments: The complaints vary depending on profession and modalities of living. The patient may complain of redness of the eyes, burning, tiredness of eyes and sometimes a feeling of irritation. Some patients have no symptoms but complain that to others they appear as if drunk. The patient may complain of stringy discharge, feeling of dryness, itching etc. [Pointed questions should be asked to exclude dry eye conditions].

The signs will depend on the causative factor: In chronic mild bacterial infection, the palpebral conjunctiva is thickened and the meibomian ducts are no longer visible through it. The palpebral conjunctival vessels do not appear in parallel rows but are seen in an irregular pattern. When congestion is due to environmental factors, it is largely limited to bulbar conjunctiva of the intermarginal area, other parts of bulbar and palpebral conjunctiva being normal. When due to a local irritant, congestion is usually limited to lower fornix. Congestion is mostly limited to inner canthus when source of infection is in lacrimal passage or in nose. In long standing chronic congestion, one may find epithelial papillary hypertrophy in upper fornix.

Etiological diagnosis is difficult to establish in most cases: These patients have already used numerous local therapies, antibiotics, steroids, decongestants etc. A conjunctival smear is usually negative. It is a very rewarding habit, that in all such cases, one should peep into the nasal cavity on either side and a source of infection may be detected. Tear film break-up lime, if found defective may indicate correct approach to treatment where nothing else has worked. Syringing of lacrimal passages may reveal a partial obstruction or a physiological block.

Treatment is largely empirical and palliative: If the cause can be detected it should be excluded and adequately treated. Use of protective goggles when outdoor may help. Protective measures in industry are necessary for eyes. The most useful eye drops are decongestants and astringents. Steroids are avoided.

CHRONIC FOLLICULAR CONJUNCTIVITIS

It is a group of etiological conditions where a common feature is the presence of non-trachomatous follicles in the conjunctiva, mostly in palpebral and fornix conjunctiva. The conditions which fall under this group are:
1. Folliculosis.
2. Primary Follicular conjunctivitis.
3. Follicular conjunctivitis secondary to causative agents.

Conjunctival Folliculosis

It is a simple lymphatic hyperplasia of adenoid tissue of the conjunctiva. It commonly affects children and young adults.

Clinically, there is formation of follicles of the size of a pin-head, translucent and arranged in rows. It is most frequently seen in lower fornix conjunctiva. The condition is often associated with hypertrophy of the tonsils and adenoids.

Symptoms are mild irritation and photophobia. The absence of inflammation, cicatrisation and absence of corneal involvement distinguish it from follicular conjunctivitis and trachoma.

Treatment is only palliative. Astringent drops are helpful. Removing the adenoids may sometimes reverse the condition.

Primary Follicular Conjunctivitis

Most clinical forms of chronic follicular conjunctivitis are due to a virus although identity of the virus has not been fully established. Virus of epidemic kerato-conjunctivitis and adeno-virus are among the common ones known to cause follicular conjunctivitis. A common feature of different types of chronic follicular conjunctivitis is associated lymph-adenopathy affecting the pre-parotid and the sub-mandibular glands.

Clinically the condition may sometimes present itself as a subacute condition but otherwise it is mostly chronic in nature. The symptoms are relatively mild and include watering, with a small amount of mucous discharge. The conjunctiva is moderately congested in fornices. Numerous yellowish, round, flat dots are seen in palpebral and fornix conjunctiva. There is no cicatrisation even after the condition has lasted for a long time. The condition usually lasts from a few days to a few weeks and disappears without leaving behind any after-effects of inflammation.

Differential diagnosis is from the conditions where follicle formation is a part of clinical entity particularly trachoma. Trachoma is associated with follicles at the upper limbus, pannus in the cornea and cicatrisation in the late stages. All these are absent in follicular conjunctivitis.

Follicular Conjunctivitis Secondary to Toxic Agents

Amongst the causative agents are local eye drops like miotics, eserine, pilocarpinc and DFP. The follicles are not associated with any inflammatory reaction and usually disappear with the cessation of drug therapy. The same is true in case of cosmetics.

TRACHOMA

Trachoma is a truly tropical disease because it is so closely linked to tropical factors like dusty, dry and windy climate and factors promoting transmission of disease like fly incidence, poor personal hygiene and defective environmental sanitation. Being endemic in many parts of the world and having been investigated extensively, there are many synonyms of the disease like granular conjunctivitis, chronic follicular conjunctivitis, Egyptian ophthalmia, military ophthalmia etc. Names like 'Rohe' in Punjab, 'kukre' in UP and Rajasthan, 'khil' in Gujarat, 'Dane' in Central India are well known regional terminologies in local dialects.

The clinical part of the disease has been known for centuries and the earliest records are from China, India and Egypt. Its etiology however, was not really understood till the beginning of 20th century when evidence of a virus as an etiological factor was first suggested on a histological basis. Isolation and culture of the trachoma virus however, became possible only in 1957. Since then there have been differing opinions whether the causative organism is a true virus. The large-sized virus has been suggested to be something between a true virus and bacteria.

Epidemiology

Trachoma has been known to spare no region and no race but is endemic in areas where the environmental factors are favourable to the spread of trachoma. Its first home was Egypt from where it spread to large parts of the world through invading armies and travellers. The armies of Napoleon carried it to Europe and the Muslim invaders to the east. The most endemic areas are northern India, Pakistan, Afghanistan, near and middle east countries. Its incidence is significantly high in southern Russia and China. The morbidity of trachoma and its clinical picture have however undergone a drastic change not only because of national and international programmes of eradication but also because of ready availability of effective drugs. These observations are supported by the available data that a hospital which used to do upto 500 operations of entropion and trichiasis in a year now does less than 50 such operations in the same period. The ravages of past trachoma, however, are still seen and will continue to be seen so as long as these victims of trachoma of earlier years continue to need treatment.

The incidence of trachoma in India is maximum in the dry belts of the northern region because of climatic factors. It was reported on the basis of a national survey conducted in India from 1956-1959 that 50–75% of population in northern states has or had trachoma. The heaviest incidence was in the States of Punjab, Haryana, Uttar Pradesh and Rajasthan. It is interesting to know that the incidence of trachoma is very low indeed in the southern and eastern states of India where the climate is humid and the rainfall heavy.

Aetiology

Trachoma for long was known to be due to bacterial infection. The reason for this was the presence of bacteria as a secondary infection in most cases of trachoma. Noguchi (1928) described the morphology of what he called bacillus granulosis found in trachomatous eyes. His observations were not supported by reports from other laboratories.

It is now established that trachoma is caused by a virus of Chlamydia group belonging to psittacosis-Lymphogranuloma-Trachoma (PLT) family of atypical viruses. The specific trachoma organism is a small non-motile, gram negative, obligate intracellular parasite. The organism grows in the cytoplasm of the host-cells forming micro-colonies or 'inclusion bodies'. The causative trachoma virus is called trachoma-inclusion conjunctivitis agent, the TRIC agent.

The first evidence of the virus as an etiological agent was the finding of elementary bodies with inclusions and the causative virus was called Halberstaedter Prowazek Korpurchen (1907) after names of the authors who reported their findings. The isolation of the causative virus proper, however, became possible after successful cultivation of the virus in egg yolk by Teng (1957). Although trachoma virus has been isolated, cultured and identified, the strains of the causative virus vary from country to country and

region to region and therefore the culture study reports in one laboratory may not be entirely applicable to another laboratory.

To summarise, it is now established that trachoma is a virus disease, that the virus is a large sized virus, that it belongs to psittacosis group and that it can be grown on egg yolk and passaged again and again.

Infection by other organisms commonly found is only secondarily imposed but this secondary bacterial infection influences the consequences of trachoma in a significant way.

Pathology of Trachoma

Trachoma is a chronic inflammatory process and primarily involves epithelial and sub-epithelial layers of conjunctiva and remains localised to eye only. In the early stages, there is epithelial hyperplasia of palpebral conjunctiva. The evidence of virus in epithelial cells is proved by presence of intracellular inclusion and elementary bodies, easily stained by Giemsa stain and identified under microscope. As the inflammation spreads to the deeper layers, there is lymphocytic infiltration in sub-epithelial tissues, increased vascularisation and formation of follicles and papillae. The natural process of healing is initiated by cicatrisation and is directly proportional to the severity of secondary bacterial infection. The cicatrisation of subconjunctival tissues in the fornices leads to shallowing of fornices and symblepharon. Cicatrisation of the bulbar conjunctiva can result in dryness and keralinisation of conjunctival surface. At the limbus, cicatrised follicles are seen as Herbert's pits. Scarring in corneal tissues may cause varying degree of corneal opacities. There is evidence that trachomatous pathology may infiltrate into the angle of the anterior chamber and cause a secondary rise of intra-ocular tension, which may be further exaggerated by occlusion of aqueous veins due to cicatrisation under bulbar conjunctiva.

Once trachomatous pathology has established itself, it is rare for conjunctiva to return to complete normalcy. Evidence of past trachoma can be seen for years after the disease has completely healed and patient has no symptoms. The typical features of past evidence of trachoma are Herbert's pits at limbus, cicatrisation in the palpebral conjunctiva obscuring its translucency and resulting in an altered pattern of the vascular arrangement of vessels in the upper palpebral conjunctiva. Ghost vessels in the upper cornea may also be seen.

Clinical Features of Trachoma

It mostly affects both sexes but features are more severe in females because of hazards of domestic life and poor personal hygiene like cooking in smoke, the customary veil in certain communities and habit of using the saree end to clean the eye each time. The incubation period is 5–12 days.

The clinical features of trachoma follow a set pattern starting with subacute inflammation and ending with cicatrisation and its consequences. Trachoma is therefore described in a series of clinical stages. The earliest clinical classification was by McCallam from his experience in Egypt. The present and internationally accepted classification is based on WHO classification dividing the clinical stages into:

Trachoma 0	Trachoma dubium or doubtful trachoma
Trachoma I	With active infiltration and conjunctival inflammation
Trachoma II-A	With follicles and early pannus
Trachoma II-B	With follicles, papillary hyperplasia and progressive pannus
Trachoma III-A	With early cicatrisation and regressive pannus
Trachoma III-B	With advanced cicatrisation and hypertrophy of the tarsus
Trachoma IV	Quiet healed trachoma
Trachoma IV-S	With sequelae, complications and degenerative changes
Trachoma IV-R	Recurrence after healed trachoma.

Trachoma-I: This is a stage of infiltration. The clinical features are that of subacute conjunctivitis with watering, photophobia and conjunctival congestion. The specific features of trachoma are not yet manifest. It is therefore not easy to clinically diagnose trachoma at this stage. It is however a good rule that any conjunctivitis in endemic areas which does not readily respond to routine treatment of conjunctivitis in 7–10 days or recurs again and again should be provisionally considered as trachoma unless proved otherwise. Specific and definite diagnosis is however possible by examination of conjunctival smear for inclusion bodies.

Trachoma-II: This is stage of follicles and papillae. The follicles are yellowish dots, the size of a pin-head commonly seen in the upper palpebral conjunctiva. Less commonly these may be present in lower palpebral conjunctiva also. Each follicle is usually surrounded by a capillary loop. At places the dilated capillaries form reddish areas called the papillae. The palpebral conjunctiva is oedematous so that the pattern of meibomian ducts is not seen through it. Similar follicles may also be seen along the upper limbus. Blood vessels from the upper limbus grow into the upper cornea and form a typical progressive trachomatous pannus, the characteristics of which are that the blood vessels run parallel to each other from above downwards and end in a more or less horizontal line corresponding to the contact of the upper lid margin to the cornea. Trachoma- II has been divided in to II-A and II-B. The former being milder and the latter with papillary hypertrophy and intense infiltration. In the progressive stage there may be spots of infiltration in advance of the pannus line. A slit lamp examination may show pattern of the blood vessels more clearly and may also reveal some follicles in other parts of the cornea.

The symptoms in this stage are watering, a feeling of sand particles in the eye and redness. There may be some degree of photophobia. Discharge may be present along with lacrimation depending on the degree of secondary infection which is a common accompaniment in this stage (Figs 8.3, 8.4 and 8.5).

Trachoma-III: This is the stage of cicatrisation. The earliest cicatrisation is seen in the upper palpebral conjunctiva. Cicatrisation commonly starts near the sub-tarsal sulcus and is seen as fine linear bands of fibrosis. These may acquire

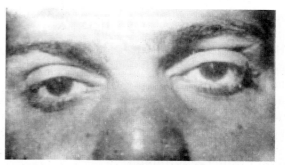

Fig. 8.5: Typical appearance of trachomatous lids, thickened and with slight mechanical ptosis

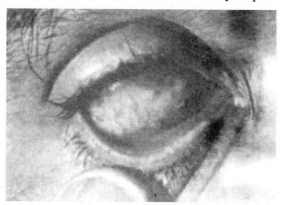

Fig. 8.3: Marked thickening and trachoma follicles in lower bulbar conjunction— Rarely seen

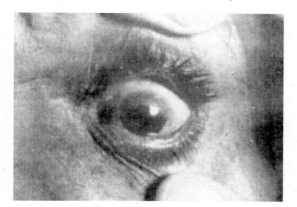

Fig. 8.4: Healed trachomatous pannus with scarring upper cornea

different shapes and sizes. In between the lines of cicatrisation, the palpebral conjunctiva is thickened, congested and hypertrophied. Few follicles may still be seen. Cicatrisation at the upper limbus is seen as Herbert's pits which appear like brownish dots which are depressed in the centre. Pannus is in the regressive stage. Cicatrisation in the fornices and bulbar conjunctiva has not yet become clinically evident. The difference between Trachoma III-A and III-B is based on the relative proportion between the degree of cicatrisation and area of active disease. If there are more active areas and less cicatrisation, it is Trachoma III-A. If there is more cicatrisation tarsal hypertrophy and less active areas, it is Trachoma III-B.

The symptoms of Trachoma III stage are less severe but chronic in nature and their severity depends on the degree of active disease present. There may be diminution of vision due to involvement of the cornea.

Trachoma-IV: This is a non-infective stage of healed trachoma. In the absence of gross secondary bacterial infection and with appropriate treatment in the active stage, trachomatous pathology may end up as healed trachoma stage IV. The eyes are quiet. The palpebral conjunctiva is not congested but remains thickened so that the Meibomian ducts are not seen through it. The normal vascular pattern is absent and irregularly formed new blood vessels are seen. Herbert's pits are seen at the upper limbus. Sometimes Herbert 'spits are present at the lower limbus also'. The trachomatous pannus has regressed but ghost blood vessels in the upper cornea can be seen against retro-illumination of a slit lamp. There are no symptoms but vision may be diminished due to corneal astigmatism.

Trachoma Complicated (Trachoma-IV-S)

This is the stage of sequelae and complications. The incidence and severity of complications is directly proportional to the degree of secondary infection. Complications may be as a result of changes in the lid margin, the tarsal plate, the bulbar conjunctiva and the cornea. The following may be listed as the sequelae and complications of trachoma:

1. **Trichiasis** is due to cicatrisation involving hair follicles of the lashes distorting the direction so that the lashes are in-turned, rub on the cornea and aggravate symptoms.

2. **Entropion** is in-turning of lid margin. This is due to disease infiltrating the tarsal plate. The tarsus gets thickened. Due to cicatrisation, there is increased convexity of the anterior surface and in-turning of the upper lid margin due to inversion of the tarsus. The eye lashes, consequently also get inturned, rub and irritate the bulbar conjunctival and corneal surface.

3. **Shallowing of fornices and symblepharon.** In trachomatous populations, the fornices are often shallow, due to cicatrisation in the subconjunctival tissues of the loose fornix conjunctiva.

4. **Corneal haze and astigmatism.** These are due to changes in the upper cornea which gets flattened due to cicatrisation. This introduces astigmatism which sometimes may be of a high order. Localised keratectasia (Keratocele), may sometimes be seen which is due to thinning of the cornea in the upper part.

5. **Conjunctival xerosis and tear film breakup anomaly.** Conjunctival xerosis is due to keratinisation of the conjunctival epithelium. The lid movements help collection of this keratinised material on the bulbar conjunctiva in the inter-marginal zone on either side of cornea. Tear film anomaly is due to fine cicatrisation in the subconjunctival tissues blocking or strangulating the ducts of the mucous glands or destroying goblet cells.

6. **Corneal vascularisation.** Severe vascularisation of whole corneal surface is common with a severe degree of trichiasis and entropion.

7. **Exposure keratitis.** This is commonly due to shortening of the upper lid as a result of cicatrisation. The exposure of the lower cornea can also result from over correction of entropion or a faulty procedure causing a notch in the upper lid margin.

8. **Trachomatous ptosis.** There is a small degree of ptosis in the infiltrative stage of Trachoma-II and Trachoma-III when the lid becomes thicker. Trachoma pathology may involve the levator palpebrae superior muscle through the upper fornix or the lid may become heavier due to thickening. It is in trachomatous ptosis, that the pannus and corneal haze may be more prominent in the lower than the usual upper corneal involvement.

9. **Trachomatous dacryocystitis and dacryoadenitis.** Trachomatous pathology may extend into the lacrimal sac and the ducts of the lacrimal gland to cause consequent inflammation. The lacrimal sac and the gland may actually serve as hideouts for the virus. This lingering infection may be a source of recurrence and exacerbations from time to time. Trachomatous

pathology may involve the sac epithelial lining, block the nasolacrimal duct and result in dacryocystitis.

10. **Corneal ulcer and opacities.** In addition to the corneal involvement noted above, trachomatous follicles in the cornea may get secondarily infected and cause an infected corneal ulcer. Such an infected corneal ulcer undergoes exactly the same course as any other infected ulcer. In the absence of adequate and effective therapy, all the sequelae and consequences of an infected corneal ulcer with or without perforation may occur in these cases. It is this complication which is commonly responsible for the high incidence of corneal blindness in trachomatous eyes.

Degenerative Changes

Being a chronic inflammatory process, the palpebral conjunctiva and the underlying tarsal plate undergo degenerative changes. The commonest degenerative change is calcific degeneration. Concretions form in the palpebral conjunctiva. These may be few isolated or in groups. So long as they are covered by epithelium, they cause no symptoms but as they migrate and point above the surface, they cause a foreign body feeling in the eyes. These concretions are inspissated material from the epithelium and conjunctival glandular tissue. They may be present in any chronic inflammatory conditions not necessarily specifically in trachoma. Further more, the tarsal plate may be markedly thickened, fibrosed and distorted due to hyaline and calcareous degeneration.

Although trachoma has been categorised and described in different stages, clear cut bordering between one stage and other is not always evident. From the therapeutic point of view, however, the most important consideration is whether trachoma is in a stage of active inflammation because then it needs anti-trachoma therapy, local, systemic or both.

Relapse or Recurrence of Trachoma (Trachoma-R)

It is doubtful whether trachoma, even though a virus disease ever confers any lasting immunity. Healing by fibrosis reduces the chance of recurrence. However, a relapse of trachoma infection has been reported after long intervals. The common sites where the trachoma virus may remain a source of re-infection is possibly Ihe lacrimal gland or sac. Vaginal passages have been known to harbour trachoma infection which may also be responsible for reinfection.

Diagnosis of Trachoma

It is curious that in trachomatous areas, trachoma is often diagnosed even when there is no trachomatous pathology. On the other hand, in areas with low incidence, it is rarely thought of even if it is present. Clinical diagnosis of trachoma should always be possible if one kept in mind Ihe basic criteria.

The three most important clinical criteria for diagnosing active trachoma are follicles in the palpebral conjunctiva, follicles at the upper limbus and active pannus in the upper cornea. The process of healing is indicated by cicatrisation under palpebral conjunctiva and Herbert's pits at the upper limbus. It is true that evidence of past trachoma can always be diagnosed with certainty even years after pathology. The criteria are thickening and cicatrisation of palpebral conjunctiva and Herbert's pits at upper limbus. Laboratory investigations are of academic importance only and rarely need to be done in clinical practice to prove or disprove trachoma.

Prognosis of trachoma is largely dependent on the degree of secondary infection. If secondary infection can be entirely avoided, which is not always possible in the type of patients who are the commonest victims, the disease can go through its usual stages, complete the circle in 2–3 months time and completely heal without any harmful effects but leaving behind some mild evidence of past trachoma. Prognosis, however, becomes worse with higher incidence and severity of secondary bacterial infection. It is for this reason that in endemic areas, trachoma is considered to be directly or indirectly responsible for the high incidence of corneal blindness in children.

Prophylaxis and Treatment

Prophylaxis

Trachoma is a truely preventable disease. The World Health Organization, the UNICEF and the governments of various countries have co-ordinated national and international trachoma programmes and have, to a large extent succeeded in eradicating the disease or at least diluting its harmful effects. The introduction of sulpha drugs and broad spectrum antibiotics has made the task easy.

In India, a national trachoma eradication programme was carried out with co-ordination of WHO, UNICEF, ICMR and the Ministry of Health, Government of India in 1956-59 all over the country. The programme was extended in selective areas for a few more years and later continued by the State Government under their own health projects. The result of these efforts has been rewarding.

Truly effective prophylaxis of trachoma involved efforts at all levels. The WHO recommended schedule used to be use of Achromycin drops or an ointment 5 days in each of the months from May to August in the eyes of all pre-school children. WHO programmes in different countries also provided guidelines to prevent transport of infection from one region to the other.

Treatment: In pre-sulpha era, numerous medications have been used for trachoma. There is a long list of these drugs which include zinc sulphate, chaulmoogra oil, mercurochrome, fresh infusion of abrus pricatorius (Ratti), Oxycyanide of mercury, hydrargy perchlor, copper sulphate and silver nitrate. The application of carbon dioxide snow, radium and X-rays were all tried because nothing better was then available. Of all these agents, silver nitrate alone has stood the test of time. Earlier destructive application of 6% solution of silver nitrate was reduced to a sensible use of 2% application once a day.

Active Trachoma Needs Active Treatment and the Following Routine is Recommended

1. Sulphacetamide solution 20% eye drops four times a day for 2-3 months.
2. Long acting sulpha oral drugs for 10 days in a month, 2-3 such courses.
3. Silver nitrate continues to hold ground. This is particularly indicated in trachoma-II where follicles and papillae need to be locally treated. Silver nitrate is used as 2% solution painted with a cotton stick swab on the everted palpebral conjunctiva once a day in the mornings only. Its mode of action has already been described.
4. An antibiotic ointment at bed time is needed when there is collection of discharge in the conjunctival sac overnight.

With appropriate treatment, it is now possible to convert active trachoma to healed trachoma. The earlier it is started, the quicker and more effective are the results. It is reasonable to expect that with the proper treatment, trachoma can be controlled though it is not correct to use the word 'cured' because some evidence of past trachoma remains for long years and recrudescence is not uncommon. The treatment of sequelae and complication is largely surgical, often combined with anti-trachoma therapy.

CHRONIC ANGULAR CONJUNCTIVITIS

The term angular conjunctivitis is partly a misnomer because the prominent clinical manifestations are more on the lid margins than at the angles of the eye. The cause of angular conjunctivitis is diplobacillus of Morax-Axenfeld which is a gram negative organism. Secondary staphylococcal infection may be associated. The clinical features of angular conjunctivitis have also been reported to be associated with riboflavin deficiency in the form of a syndrome, angular conjunctivitis and angular stomatitis, common in the rice eating population of south India.

The symptoms of angular conjunctivitis are characteristically burning of the eyes and a thready secretion.

On examination, the lid margins appear congested and reddened along the mucous border. The congestion may also be present in inter-marginal area of the bulbar conjunctiva. There may be excoriation of skin and even a fissure may even be seen at the outer canthus. Diagnosis is mostly based on clinical examination but it can be confirmed by examination of a conjunctival smear for the causative organism.

Prognosis of angular conjunctivitis is good although it takes time to get cured. The disease, in most cases, follows a benign course. Diplobacillus has rarely been known to cause corneal ulcer.

Treatment of the diplobacillary angular conjunctivitis was zinc sulphate 0.5% eye drops, repeated four to five times a day and zinc oxide ointment 5% applied at bed time. This is the cheapest drug used in ophthalmology. Broad spectrum antibiotic solutions are also effective particularly to combat the staphylococcal infection activated by the diplobacillus. Vitamin-B complex with an added dose of riboflavin is indicated in cases of deficiency syndrome.

PHLYCTENULAR CONJUNCTIVITIS

It is part of a more composite syndrome and is described under various names—phlyctenulosis, phlyctenular kerato-conjunctivitis, phlyctenular ophthalmia, eczematous conjunctivitis and scrofulous conjunctivitis.

Phlyctenular conjunctivitis affects mostly children. A phlycten like lesion is occasionally seen in adults also. The disease is common among communities living in congested localities with higher incidence of tuberculosis and poor nutritional status.

Etiology

It is established that phlyctenular ophthalmia is an endogenous allergic response to tuberculous proteins in the system. Patients with phlyctens usually do not have evidence of active tuberculosis except quiet lymphadenopathy. There may not be a history of tuberculosis and primary complex in early childhood may have passed unnoticed.

Clinical Picture

Phlyctenular conjunctivitis is an acute and recurring condition. Symptoms depend on the stage of the disease and the severity of secondary staphylococcal infection. In early stages, symptoms may be mild like localised redness of the eye, irritation and watering. Once the phlycten surface breaks down, symptoms are severe consisting of photophobia, belpharospasm and lacrimation (Fig. 8.6, Plate 3).

On examination, phlycten presents a small nodular swelling at or near the limbus surrounded by a localised congestion. The nodule is movable over the sclera. There may be more than one phlycten. Once epithelial surface breaks, the conjunctival ulcer causes more redness. The phlycten may remain localised to the conjunctiva or may involve the cornea, the latter is called phlyctenular keratitis. Eczematous conditions may manifest on the lid margin or the skin of the lower lid. The skin may be excoriated below the corresponding nostril. This is due to a proteolytic enzyme liberated as a result of conjunctival inflammation which causes the eczematous condition. An enlarged pre-parotid lymph gland is commonly palpable during the acute phase of the condition.

Diagnosis

Diagnosis of phlyctenular conjunctivitis is easy because of its characteristic clinical features. When away from the limbus, differential diagnosis is from episcleritis which is more common in adults and older people. An episcleritic nodule never breaks down and therefore the symptoms are milder. The conjunctiva is freely movable over the episcleritic nodule. The phlyctenular nodule at the limbus has to be differentiated from other limbal nodules described along with limbal lesions.

Treatment: The age old empirical therapy of insufflation of calomel dust in the conjunctiva is no longer routinely used. Being an allergic manifestation, the most effective treatment is steroid drops used repeatedly. When there is some degree of secondary infection, a combined steroid-antibiotic drops will quickly control the condition. Streptomycin sulphate 25 mg per cc solution as eye drops may be effective where steroids have not controlled the condition. A steroid ointment may be applied on the skin of lids twice a day for eczematous skin around the eyes and the nostril.

Systemic treatment with multi-vitamins and protein is important in all cases of recurrent phlyctenular conjunctivitis.

In persistently recurrent cases, systemic anti-tubercular therapy is indicated even if no clinical evidence of tuberculosis is detected.

SPRING CATARRH

It is also known as vernal conjunctivitis. The term 'spring' catarrh is rather inapplicable in tropical climate where it is better called a summer catarrh because the condition is more aggravated in summer months and is less severe in winter months. There are, however, cases where seasonal variation is insignificant.

Etiology

The cause of spring catarrh is generally accepted as exogenous allergy. Allergens can be anything from pollen to dust, vegetations, food material etc. The allergic etiology is supported by the presence of eosinophils in lacrimal secretion and response of the disease to anti-allergic therapy. The chronicity of disease lasting for years and in some cases without amelioration all the year round has led to the suggestion that there may be an auto-allergen factor, local or systemic. Intestinal parasites may be a possible cause for endogenous allergy.

The tissue changes in spring catarrh are largely a proliferation of epithelium and hyaline and connective tissue degeneration. The characteristic histological finding is the presence of eosinophils.

Clinical Features

There are two distinct clinical forms of the disease. Palpebral spring catarrh and bulbar spring catarrh, both may be present at the same time in the same eye.

The most characteristic symptom is itching of the eyes which may be so severe as to make the person miserable. Every time the eyes are rubbed, the conjunctiva shows marked reaction and becomes congested. The feeling of foreign body sensation is more marked in the palpebral type of spring catarrh. Another characteristic symptom is a sticky and thready discharge in the eyes, which is highly alkaline in nature. In majority of cases, symptoms are more aggravated in summer months and become, milder in colder season. The history of symptoms is usually of months and years with only temporary relief after medication.

Palpebral Spring Catarrh

The diagnosis is made on everting the lids. The lid surface appears rough and irregular. There are greyish yellow vegetations of varying sizes with demarcating lines between each vegetation. This appearance has been described as cobblestone appearance. The vegetations may however, be larger in size and grossly elevated with deeper crevices in between. It is only to be expected that the normal pattern of conjunctival vessels and meibomian ducts is not visible.

Bulbar Spring Catarrh

It presents a characteristic picture. The exposed inter-marginal conjunctiva looks dirty in appearance. The conjunctiva is heaped up near the limbus, more marked in the inter marginal area and may even form a triangular elevation. In severe cases, a cuff of conjunctival thickening may be present all round the limbus. In long standing cases, the heaped up conjunctiva may cover limbus and even encroach into the intra-limbal corneal surface. There is no evidence of active inflammation but the eye reacts to even mild physical handling like everting the lid, by becoming congested (Fig. 8.7).

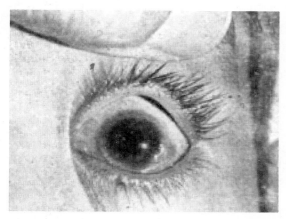

Fig. 8.7: Bulbar spring catarrh showing cuff of conjunctival encroachment over the limbus all round

Diagnosis

Either type of spring catarrh is diagnosed by a clinical examination of the eyes and typical history. It rarely needs to be supported by examination of the conjunctival smear for eosinophils and higher eosinophilia in differential WBC count of blood. In tropical countries, stool examination for any parasitic infestation may indicate the possible source of endogenous allergy and may even help curing the disease by appropriate treatment against the parasite.

Identification of the causative allergen should be done whenever possible. Exposing a patient to a complete series of allergy tests may occasionally be rewarding by desensitising the patient against the detected allergen.

Differential Diagnosis

The main condition to be differentiated is trachoma because both are common in tropical areas and in both the palpebral conjunctiva and the limbus are seats of pathology. The absence of characteristic follicles and cicatrization in palpebral conjunctiva is a very important differentiating feature. Similarly, the absence of Herbert's pits and pannus in the cornea also exclude trachoma. Difficulty however arises when both conditions are present at the same time. Difficulty is further complicated because steroids are the treatment for spring catarrh and not indicated in trachoma.

Prognosis

Spring catarrh is an extremely discomforting disease and may last for years. Occasionally the disease may disappear as suddenly as it came but its disappearance from eye may be followed by another allergic condition like asthma or skin allergy. It does not affect vision. There are however unsupported reports that corneal ulcers and corneal scars may complicate spring catarrh. These cases must be due to incidental secondary infection unrelated to spring catarrh pathology.

The prognosis of spring catarrh is however complicated by indiscriminate and prolonged use of steroids as local instillations. Steroid drops give quick relief and patients continue to use the same without going back to the ophthalmologist. Steroid induced cataract and glaucoma can in such cases cause severe visual loss.

Treatment is symptomatic and the anchor sheet of therapy is topical use of steroids. In severe cases, soluble steroids should be used every three hours 5-7 days. Thereafter and in milder cases insoluble steroids as suspensions should be used three or four times a day till symptoms subside. Patients should be clearly warned of the double-edged sword action of steroids when used over prolonged periods. On one hand they relieve symptoms but can induce cataract and glaucoma. In any case, steroids should not be used for more than 2–3 weeks at a time. Vision and intraocular tension should be recorded every time continuation of steroid therapy is advised. Ocular media under full mydriasis should be examined regularly when repeated steroids are used. Where the use of steroids for longer periods is unavoidable due to the recurrence of symptoms as soon as the steroid drops are stopped, soluble steroid solutions diluted 10 times may be used even for longer periods provided they relieve symptoms. Such highly diluted therapy has less chance of undesirable ocular and systemic complications. Non-steroid anti-histaminic drops containing sodium glycate are available. These can be recommended for prolonged use instead of a steroid solution.

Desensitization of the patient, if allergen is detected by allergy tests, may be really helpful to give the patient freedom from such a chronic disease.

OTHER TYPES OF ALLERGIC CONJUNCTIVITIS

Apart from phlyctenular conjunctivitis as a manifestation of endogenous allergy and spring catarrh an exogenous allergy, the conjunctiva may react to many other sensitising factors, external or internal, physical or chemical.

There are very specific factors which do cause well defined allergic reactions in the conjunctiva. These causative factors are:
1. Allergic reaction to foreign matter like cosmetics in the conjunctival sac or on lids.
2. Allergic conditions like hay fever and asthma.
3. Parasitic infestation in intestines.
4. Allergy to edibles like eggs, milk, fish, meats, certain fruits, and vegetables.
5. Drug allergy to local applications, commonly to atropine but may even be to homatropine, pilocarpine and eserine. Allergy to chemo-therapeutic drugs like sulpha and antibiotics like penicillin, streptomycin, tetracyclin and neomycin has been known.
6. Allergy to medications like an injection of xylocaine is well known.
7. Allergy to chemical substances like plastic contact lenses, prosthetic implants and the plastic of spectacle frames.
8. Allergy due to septic focus elsewhere particularly staphylococcal infection and tubercular focus.

The numerous factors enumerated above cause conjunctival reaction of different grades and different severity. If the reaction is anaphylactic, acute and sudden in onset, the lids are swollen, the bulbar conjunctiva is markedly chemosed and patient is restless due to itching.

The conjunctival chemosis may be concomitant with a systemic allergic attack like acute asthma or acute urticaria. An anaphylactic ocular reaction may also sometimes be associated with similar reaction elsewhere in the body like oedema of the glottis causing severe respiratory distress.

Chronic allergic conjunctival reaction is less dramatic and may sometimes be mild and even symptomless. The special features of chronic conjunctival allergic reaction are redness of the eye, more prominent in the inter-marginal zone.

Treatment: In an acute reaction, soluble steroid eye drops every 1–2 hours and some times oral administration of steroids along with anti-histaminic drugs will help overcome the crisis. While giving the immediate necessary treatment, one should examine the conjunctival sac for any foreign matter which when present, should be removed and the conjunctival sac washed.

Chronic allergic conjunctival reaction is however more taxing to treat partly because it is difficult to detect the causative factor and even if detected, it is not easy to eradicate. Avoidance of the causative factor or its eradication from the system should however be the objective. Symptomatic treatment includes local application of steroids, anti-histaminics and decongestants. Steroids to be used should be insoluble suspensions as eye drops

CONJUNCTIVAL, INVOLVEMENT IN MUCO-CUTANEOUS DISEASES

It is not only because conjunctiva and the skin are both surface ectodermal tissues but also because there is a continuity between the conjunctival epithelium and the squamous epithelium of the skin, that diseases of skin can involve conjunctiva either by continuity or by contamination from the cutaneous material. Similarly, continuity of the conjunctival sac with the lacrimal passages, and through it to the mucous membrane of the nasal cavity and the para nasal sinuses can also cause extension of the pathology from one to the other. Apart from this, the same etiology may independently affect the skin surface and the epithelium of the conjunctival sac.

In every case of non-specific recurrent conjunctival congestion one should look at the skin of the face, look into the nasal cavity, syringe the lacrimal passages, X-ray the para-nasal sinuses and ask the dentist to look for a septic focus before saying that there is no local cause for conjunctival congestion.

The common conditions in this group are:

1. *Pemphigus* with characteristic blisters on face and the body associated with marked conjunctival congestion, ulceration and sub-conjunctival cicatrization leading in most cases to scarred and vascularised cornea, obliteration of fornices, symblepharon and even adhesion of lid margin. It is a disease of unknown etiology.

2. *Steven-Johnson's disease* of obscure etiology of vesiculo-bullous pathology, involves mucous lining of conjunctiva, urethra and synovial sheath of joints.

3. *Reiter's disease* is a disease of obscure etiology involving the mucous lining of the conjunctiva, urethra and synovial sheath of the joints. Non-granulomatous iridocyclitis is an important feature.

4. *Acne rosacea* of the face can be a common cause of recurrent conjunctival congestion either because the infective material enters the conjunctival sac or may be an allergic manifestation. Ariboflavinosis may be an added factor.

5. *Xeroderma pigmentosa* is a serious and malignant disease which not only affects eyes but is fatal. It is supposed to be due to the malignant reaction in the skin to sun rays, and therefore the condition is progressive as the outdoor hours of the child increase. It is distinctly hereditary disease and more than one child in the family may suffer. There may be conjunctival ulcers resulting in a conjunctival symblepharon and false pterygia. Highly vascularised and pigmented nodules form on the bulbar conjunctiva later involving cornea. Histologically changes resemble a basal cell or squamous cell carcinoma.

Granulomatous Diseases of Conjunctiva

The conditions under this category are tuberculosis, Boeck's sarcoid, Parinaud's disease, syphilis, myocosis and leprosy.

Tuberculosis: It affects conjunctiva in two ways. Common tuberculous affections are due to endogenous allergy like phlyctenulosis already described. There may be typical tuberculous nodules or ulcers, chronic and indolent in nature in the palpebral conjunctiva.

Boeck's sarcoid is a nodular lesion of non-specific etiology and involves skin. There may be multiple tumours in the reticulo-endothelial system. The nodules are tuberculoid but with no caseation. The eye involvement includes involvement of conjunctiva, cornea and uveal tissue. There may be granulation tissue formation in lower fornix which may cicatrise to form symblepharon. Uvea is more often involved in the pathology than the cornea.

Parinaud's disease is a conjunctivitis complicated by adenopathy of pre-parotid lymph glands and even the parotid gland.

Syphilitic lesions of conjunctiva. These include chancre and a gumma of the conjunctiva. Soft chancre is a result of direct infection from other infected mucous surfaces like the mouth or genitals. Gumma is a nodular lesion, commonly at the limbus described later.

Leprosy may affect the conjunctiva either in the form of a leprous nodule at limbus, or acute conjunctival reaction along with iritis and keratitis.

Mycotic lesions of the conjunctiva may be caused by various fungi, common in the tropics. Fungal conjunctivitis is however rare. They may cause ulcerations of palpebral conjunctiva or mycotic infections of lacrimal passages, particularly canaliculitis. There may be mycotic granulomatous nodules at or near the limbus.

The treatment of these granulomatous conjunctival lesions is treatment of cause and surgical removal if necessary. The selection of the drug will depend o. id . tification of the cause.

Parasitic lesions of the conjunctiva are not infrequently seen and diagnosed in tropical countries. The commonly reported parasitic infestation of conjunctiva is filarial infestation. Microfilaria may be seen under the conjunctiva intermittently causing symptoms of itching and irritation. Conjunctival condition may be associated with filarial presence in anterior chamber, vitreous, and subretinal space. Eosinophilia in blood and presence of larvae in the circulation are diagnostic features. Hetrazan 2 mg. per kilogram body weight three limes a day (300 mg daily) for fifteen days is effective against microfilaria. If practicable, the filaria under the conjunctiva may be removed.

Onchocerciasis (River blindness) is a blinding disease prevalence in some parts of the tropical world, particularly in central Africa and South America. The causative parasite, like a thread worm, is transmitted by the black fly which breeds in shallow flowing water. In the fly, the larvae develop and microfilaria are transmitted by the fly to human beings causing nodular swellings over the body. The lesions in the conjunctiva may be limbal nodules or conjunctival thickening like in spring catarrh. There may be associated involvement of cornea, sclera, uveal tissue and the lids. Hetrazan (Diethylcarbamazine) is effective against Onchocerciasis also.

Cysticercosis: This is a condition caused by Taenia solium, the parasite causing cysticercus cellulosae. Infection in man is by the ingestion of the eggs of the Taenia solium. The cysticercus from the eggs in the intestines enters the circulation causing cystic growths in many parts of the body. Small cysts may form in the conjunctiva and intra-ocular tissues. Taenia solium may be found in the stool. Treatment of the local cyst is surgical removal. Parasites in the intestines may be eradicated by deworming.

Hydatid cyst is caused by Taenia echinococcus. The natural host is dog but the larvae may become parasitic in the intestines of man from where they migrate into the blood vessels, reaching the liver and other organs. They form cyst which may be large in size with daughter cysts lining the larger cyst. The diagnosis is confirmed by eosinophilia in blood and finding scolices with hooklets in the cyst fluid. A complement fixation test between the serum of the patient and cyst fluid is diagnostic. A Hydatid cyst may be formed in conjunctiva, extra ocular muscles and the orbit. An intraocular hydatid cyst is also reported.

Treatment is surgical removal, taking great care that the cyst does not rupture and the contents do not spill into the tissues because the cyst fluid causes violent reaction and daughter cysts may cause recurrence of disease.

Appropriate systemic therapy for eradicating intestinal infestation should be given simultaneously.

Ocular myiasis (Maggots): With improvement in personal hygiene and available facilities for medical treatment, ocular myiasis is extremely uncommon. In unhygienic environments and neglected cases, the eggs laid by the flies in the conjunctiva may develop into larvae which may be seen crawling in and out of the congested and inflammed conjunctiva. Myiasis may involve deeper tissues and even intra-ocular parts of the eye. The treatment is to kill and remove the maggots with strong drugs like 5% carbolic acid solution or turpentine.

TUMOURS OF THE CONJUNCTIVA

Apart from the inflammatory nodules at or near the limbus, neoplastic growths may involve conjunctiva. The ones which are frequently seen are a congenital naevus, dermoid, haemangioma, malignant melanoma, squamous epithelioma and neurofibroma (Figs 8.8 and 8.9).

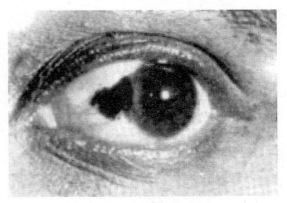

Fig 8.8: Conjunctival naevus

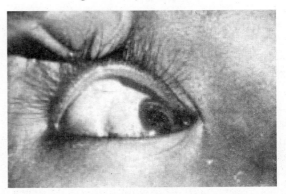

Fig 8.9: Conjunctival Dermoid (Note a few hairs growing out of the upper part)

Congenital naevus is pigmented and mostly seen on the bulbar conjunctiva but can be at the muco-cutaneous junction of the palpebral conjunctiva also. They may be growing in younger age but usually become stationary later on.

Haemangioma of conjunctiva may be an extension from the capillary angioma of the face e.g. in Sturge-Weber syndrome. Markedly convoluted and tortuous blood vessels may appear in bunches in conjunctiva (Fig. 8.10, Plate 3).

Among the malignant neoplasms of the conjunctiva, an epithelioma is more common than a melanoma. An epithelioma of the conjunctiva appears as a flat lesion with a smooth or granular surface. This usually starts at the limbus and may extend on either side. It is locally malignant and does not usually cause metastasis. It should be excised without leaving any part behind. Few healthy lamellae of the corneo-sclera should be included in the dissection. Excision should be followed by beta-radiation. If necessary, a mucous or scleral graft may be needed to support the thin tissue underneath.

When an epithelioma changes into a carcinoma, the disease is more malignant and can cause systemic metastasis.

Conjunctival cysts may be inclusion cysts due to a retained foreign body or a parasitic cyst. Small mucous cysts are common which may sometimes be large in size and extend deep into the orbit. Congenital cysts are frequently seen in children. Parasitic cysts are more common in tropical countries.

Most cysts need surgical removal. The dissection sometimes may have to be more than expected because the cyst may have involved deeper tissues or may be attached to the underlying muscle.

Apart from the neoplastic lesions described above, conjunctival growths may be the usual spectrum of neoplastic lesions from the various other tissues around the conjunctiva. Fibroma, papilloma, lipoma, neuro-fibroma, lymphoma etc. may rarely be present.

Neoplastic growths may extend into the conjunctiva from surrounding tissues e.g. the sclera, the uvea from underneath, dykitioma from the ciliary body. Intraocular retinoblastoma and malignant melanoma may involve the conjunctiva when extra-ocular extension of these has occurred.

Flat nodular lesions of the conjunctiva on either side of the cornea, triangular in shape, muddy yellow in colour, and sometimes pigmented are commonly seen in all age groups. There is no inflammatory reaction. These lesions do not encroach onto the cornea and they are more a cosmetic problem than the cause of any symptom.

The term pinguicula has for long been used and is yet nonspecific in etiology and uncertain as a clinical entity. The common cause, is the irritation by climatic factors like wind and dust.

Nutritional deficiencies are an endemic problem in most of the developing countries. Malnutrition is responsible for many systemic and ocular manifestations and causes these manifestations in two ways. First by being a direct etiological factor and secondly indirectly by lowering tissue resistance to infections and other pathological processes. The factors are deficiency of Vitamin A and other vitamins, protein deficiency, calorie deficiency and iron deficiency.

Ocular manifestations of malnutrition are:
1. Conjunctival changes.
2. Corneal affections.
3. Affections of the rod cells of the retina.

The last two are described in appropriate chapters.

Malnutrition and Conjunctiva: Primary Conjunctival changes due to malnutrition are:
1. Brown pigmentation of the conjunctiva.
2. Bitot's spots.
3. Conjunctival xerophthalmia.

Conjunctival Pigmentation

This is an early stage of conjunctival xerosis. Bulbar conjunctiva in the intermarginal zone shows a brown discolouration and may sometimes be wrinkled.

Bitot's Spots

A white keratinised epithelium of conjunctiva in the intermarginal zone of the bulbar conjunctiva is usually on the temporal side of cornea. 'Kajal' when applied, can stain the Bitot's spot black.

Bitot's spots in children are commonly due to Vitamin A deficiency and are often associated with night blindness (Fig. 8.11).

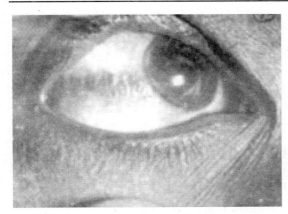

Fig. 8.11: Conjunctival Xerosis—Bitot's spot (Note dry wrinkled conjunctiva on the temporal side)

Conjunctival Xerophthalmia

It is a generalised dryness of the conjunctiva due to malnutrition. The whole bulbar conjunctiva appears dry and wrinkled. Dryness is prominently evident even though there is enough lacrimal fluid in the conjunctival sac. This condition is common in children and is usually associated with corneal involvement from an early to an advanced stage of keratomalacia. Conjunctival xerophthalmia like keratomalacia is a manifestation of multiple deficiency factors like Vitamin A deficiency, protein deficiency, calorie deficiency and iron deficiency. It is a serious condition and should be treated with adequate doses of Vitamin A along with other deficiency factors in therapeutic doses.

Parenchymatous Conjunctival Xerosis

Parenchymatous xerosis of the conjunctiva is usually secondary to cicatrisation in the sub-epithelial tissues which strangulates the goblet cells and mucous glands thereby altering the character of tear film because of the absence of mucous constituent. The conjunctiva appears dry and lusterless. There is shrinking of conjunctival tissue which is associated with shallowing of the fornices and symblepharon.

The common causes of parenchymatous xerosis are:

1. Complicated trachoma.
2. Kerato-conjunctivitis sicca—Sjögren's syndrome.
3. Steven-Johnsons disease.
4. Pemphigus.
5. Chemical burns of the conjunctiva.

CONJUNCTIVAL PIGMENTATION

Conjunctival pigmentation may be congenital or acquired. **Congenital conditions** that can cause pigmentation of conjunctiva are:

1. Localised congenital naevi
2. Congenital melanosis
3. Patches of brown pigmentation around the perforating branches of the anterior ciliary arteries.

Acquired pigmentation of the conjunctiva is due to:

1. Blood pigments following subconjunctival haemorrhage (Fig. 8.12).
2. Bile pigment in jaundice
3. Melanin pigment.
   a. Light pigmentation as in conjunctival xerosis and bulbar spring catarrh
   b. Pigmented melanoma

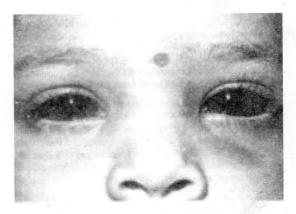

Fig. 8.12: Extensive subconjunctival haemorrhage in both eyes in a child suffering from whooping cough

c. Xeroderma pigmentosa

d. Acanthosis nigricans

4. Copper pigment as in ocular siderosis
5. Silver pigment as in argyrosis.
6. Prolonged use of epinephrine or its derivatives.

Argyrosis: This is a condition where impregnated silver ions get fixed with tissue proteins. Conjunctival argyrosis used to be very common when silver preparations were an everyday treatment for trachoma and conjunctivitis. Silver nitrate 2% or stronger was a routine treatment for follicles in th second stage of trachoma and its daily application continued for weeks and months. The inorganic silver ions become silver albuminate leading to near permanent pigmentation of conjunctiva.

Similarly, organic silver salts like argyrol and protargol were a household treatment for conjunctivitis and continued to be used indiscriminately.

The clinical appearance of argyrosis is dark pigmentation, maximally present in the lower fornix conjunctiva and upper palpebral conjunctiva.

Even now one comes across elderly people who lived in the silver therapy era, and unexpectedly find argyosis. No treatment is needed.

9

Cornea, Limbus and the Sclera

CORNEA

The cornea is the transparent watch glass like disc which is fitted into the anterior opening of the opaque scleral shell. These two structures fused at the limbus together form the outer protective coat of the eye ball. Being transparent, cornea is the most important structure for focussing the light rays on the retina. The cornea and lens together provide a clear image for the retina to be transmitted to the brain.

The cornea is an extremely sensitive structure and is intolerant to insults of exposure, trauma or inflammation. A windy and dusty tropical climate, commonly present bacterial infection, trachoma and malnutrition are all responsible for the heavy incidence of corneal disease. Subjected to continued evaporation from its surface, cornea is the coldest part of the body.

Development

Cornea is developed from anterior mesoderm except the epithelium which is— formed from surface ectoderm.

The ectodermal corneal epithelium and the mesodermal endothelial layers are the first to form by 10 mm stage. The mesoderm thereafter insinuates between these two layers and differentiates to form the stromal part of the corneal thickness which is well developed by 20 mm stage.

The Bowman's membrane formed from the condensation of the superficial stromal layers is evident at the 5th month and the Descemets membrane, a secretory product of the endothelium, by the 6th month.

The limbus is well demarcated by the 65 mm stage (3rd month). The angle of the anterior chamber is evident only by the 6th month and gradually communicates with the canal of Schlemn as atrophy of the mesoderm in the angle takes place.

Anatomy

The dimensions of the cornea are fairly constant. It is 11.5 to 12.5 mm in horizontal diameter and 10.5 to 11.5 mm in the vertical. The cornea therefore is not quite round when looked at from the front. This is due to scleral encroachment into the anterior corneal layers along the upper limbus. Seen from behind, the cornea is however completely circular.

The refractive index of the cornea is 1.345 and the difference in the refractive index of the air and the cornea gives the anterior surface the refractive power of +49 diopters. With -6 dioptres refractive change at the posterior surface, the final refractive power of the cornea is +43 dioptres. The anterior corneal surface has a radius of curvature of 7.84 mm and that of the posterior surface is 7.0 mm, and this explains the anatomical fact that the cornea is thicker at the periphery than at the centre. The corneal thickness at the centre, varies from 0.5–0.8 mm with an average of 0.65 mm and in the periphery 0.9–1.2 mm (Fig. 9.1).

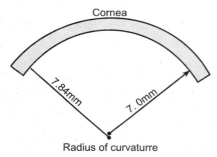

Cornea

7.84mm

7.0mm

Radius of curvaturre

Fig. 9.1: Radii of Curvature of Cornea.
(Anterior Surface 7.84 mm and posterior Surface 7.0 mm)

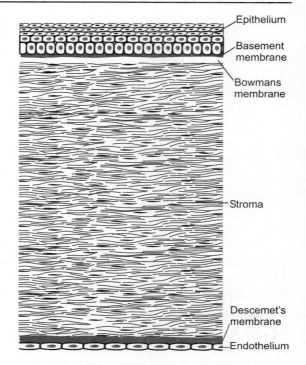

Epithelium

Basement membrane

Bowmans membrane

Stroma

Descemet's membrane

Endothelium

Fig 9.2: Micro-anatomy of Cornea.

The following are the anatomical layers of the cornea (Fig. 9.2).

1. *Epithelial layer.* It is formed of 5 to 6 layers of stratified epithelial cells . Flatter in the superficial layers and poly-hydral and columnar in the deeper layers. The epithelium is continuous with the conjunctival epithelium and its destruction is quickly replaced by the growth of new cells. The epithelium is an important tissue for utilisation of oxygen from the air.

2. *Basement layer of the corneal epithelium.* Identified by electron microscopic studies, it is a homogenous fibrillar structure firmly adherent to the Bowman's membrane underneath. For this reason, whenever the epithelium is peeled off, either surgically or due to bullous formation, the basement membrane remains behind in situ. Pathology in the basement membrane has been attributed to its causative association in keratoconus.

3. *Bowman's membrane: Lying* next to the epithelium and its basement layer, it is a developmental structure formed early in intrauterine life from condensation of superficial embryonic stromal layers. In a fully grown eye ball, Bowman's membrane does not extend upto the limbus but falls short by about a millimetre all round. This is because of the fact that the limbus and the anterior chamber angle develop much later than the formation of the Bowman's membrane. Being an embryonic tissue, it does not regenerate when destroyed.

Stromal layers (Substantia propria). This constitutes the largest part of corneal thickness, 60 to 70 layers of collagen fibres. These fibres are parallel to the adjoining fibres in the same layers but are at right angles to fibres in immediate anterior and posterior layers. The collagen fibres of the stroma are held together by homogenous mucopolysaccharide matrix of an identical refractive index and hence-perfect transparency with uniform refraction of light without defraction. The arrangement of the stroma adds to the tensile strength.

5. *Decemets membrane.* It is the posterior limiting homogenous layer between the stroma and the endothelium. It is a highly elastic layer and can withstand high intraocular pressure even when the anterior stromal layers are destroyed by disease. It is a secretion from the endothelial cells and therefore can be reformed when destroyed.

6. *Endothelium.* Although a single cell layer of flat cells, it is the most important single structure for the maintenance of viability of the cornea. It is a highly sensitive tissue and reacts and suffers when there is inflammation of the neighbouring intraocular structures. Even the autolytic effect of the aqueous humour after death affects the viability of these cells. It has been observed that the endothelial cells start swelling within a few hours after death. When destroyed, the endothelium can regrow by mitosis from the healthy adjoining cells. Functionally, the endothelium is a very important structure which allows selective permeability of nutrients from the anterior chamber into the corneal tissue. It is now established that cornea receives most of the nutrition through endothelium and only limited part from the limbal vascular plexus.

The cornea has a rich nerve supply through a plexus of nerve endings deep in the epithelial layers and this is responsible for the highly sensitive character of the anterior corneal surface. This nerve supply is from the ophthalmic division of the fifth cranial nerve.

The transparency of cornea is maintained by various factors, anatomical, physiological and opticals.

The anatomical factors:
1. Avascularity of the cornea
2. Compactness of the stroma with its regular fibre arrangement
3. A healthy epithelium and a viable endothelial lining.

Physiological factors are:
1. Healthy pre-corneal film
2. Metabolism, partly aerobic and partly anaerobic
3. Adequate nutrition in form of oxygen through epithelium (aerobic), glucose through the endothelium (anaerobic) and other nutrients through limbal circulation
4. Maintenance of water equilibrium by endothelial pump.

The optical factor is the uniform refractive index of the corneal architecture.

Pathological Considerations

The cornea being an avascular structure, responds differently to trauma, inflammations, degenerations and neoplastic invasions than most other structures of the body. Corneal response is also different in the superficial and deeper layers of the cornea, the former being akin to the conjunctiva and the latter to the uveal tissue.

Response to Trauma

Response to trauma will depend on its nature and severity. Any discontinuity of the epithelium is quickly repaired and the gap is covered by new epithelial cells sliding from the healthy adjoining epithelial cells. A simple uncomplicated epithelial break gets completely repaired within 24 hours. A deeper injury involving Bowman's membrane and stroma causes oedema, disturbance to the normal arrangement of the stromal architecture and invites vascularisation from the limbus. Although the Bowman's membrane, once damaged, never reforms, stromal layers have a tendency to rearrange and normal corneal transparency is still possible but only if there is no secondary infection and no scar tissue formation. Infection and vascularisation of the stromal layers usually results in introducing fibroblastic reaction and scar tissue formation which therefore results in some degree of corneal opacity.

Response to Infections and Inflammations

Being an avascular tissue, the cornea should be an easy victim to bacterial invasion but an intact corneal epithelium is a good barrier to bacteria penetrating the corneal tissue. Corneal involvement in any bacterial infection can be facilitated by even a minor epithelial abrasion, for example, rubbing the eyes, or a foreign body or an eye lash abraiding the epithelium. Once bacteria get a foothold, further pathological process can continue if not treated. However, there are some organisms which can penetrate even an intact corneal epithelium, the worst among these are gonococcus and diphtheria bacillus.

Infection of cornea, mostly exogenous, results in oedema, vascularisation, and sloughing of tissue and even an abscess formation. The end result is some degree of tissue loss and scar formation leaving behind a *macular* or *leucomatous* corneal opacity.

If the tissue destruction leads to perforation of the cornea, it results in iris incarceration and consequent *leucoma adherens*. The newly formed tissue is distinctly weaker than healthy corneal tissue and therefore tends to give way under raised intra-ocular tension often caused by moderate to severe degree of iris incarceration in the scar tissue. The resulting ectasia may involve the whole corneal surface if the tissue destruction is extensive and may result in the formation of *a partial or total anterior staphyloma*. The staphylomatous scar is composed of a fibrous layer, without any of the normal anatomical corneal tissue (pseudo cornea) lined on the inner surface by iris tissue. Since there is no anterior chamber and no open channels for aqueous drainage, there is a severe rise of intraocular tension causing gross damage to retinal and optic nerve function.

Neoplasms of Cornea

The cornea is peculiarly free from primary neoplasms of any nature. Neoplastic lesions, benign or malignant, may however extend from limbus into peripheral corneal thickness, for example, a congenital naevus, limbal dermoid, limbal epithelioma etc. Pterygium, specially the recurrent type, also shows histological neoplastic changes like epithelial hyperplasia, hyperkeratosis and racemose type adenoid proliferation of goblet cells. Posteriorly, seedlings of intraocular malignant growths like retino-blastoma may be deposited on the endothelial surface without involvement of other layers.

Corneal Degenerations and Dystrophies

The disadvantage of avascularity of cornea is the higher incidence of degenerations and dystrophies. Corneal degeneration may be primary or secondary to prolonged and chronic intra-ocular pathology. The degeneration may be lipid, hyaline or calcareous in character. Lipid degeneration occurs in lipid metabolic disorders like gorgoylism and Hand-Schuller Christian syndrome. Hyline degeneration as in Salzmann's nodular degeneration, chronic trachoma and salt pan corneal degeneration are fairly common. Among the common calcific degeneration, is band degeneration, primary or secondary.

The cornea is also frequently involved in dystrophic lesions mostly genetic in nature. The dystrophies may involve different layers of the cornea.

Corneal Oedema

The cornea, by virtue of its morphological and biochemical characteristics, has a tendency to develop oedema, localised or diffuse, even on the slightest provocation. The high concentration of mucopolysaccharides in the corneal matrix is the most important single factor responsible for swelling of corneal tissue.

The endothelium behind and the epithelium in front regulate the normal 75% water content of the corneal tissue. Any alteration in this water content, either dehydration or hydration, affect the refractive power and transparency of the cornea causing gross visual disturbances.

Corneal oedema due to endothelial damage is commonly caused by iridocyclitis, which causes endothelialitis. Swelling of endothelial cells allows permeation of fluid through the damaged endothelial layer to cause swelling of stroma. Stretching and tears in the Descemet's membrane are seen in advanced stages of keratoconus and buphthalmos.

A common cause of corneal oedema is following cataract extraction complicated by vitreous prolapse into the anterior chamber and manifests itself as a vitreous touch syndrome. This mechanical damage to endothelium increases fluid inflow resulting in the corneal oedema. Severe rise of intraocular tension in acute congestive and absolute glaucoma also affects permeability of endothelium and hence corneal oedema. Fuchs' dystrophy is primarily an endothelial pathology and stromal oedema is a common feature in this disease. A good example of corneal oedema is graft oedema when the grafted donor cornea has poor endothelial viability. Corneal oedema of the graft is also caused by endothelial based tissue immune reaction. Corneal oedema due to endothelial damage is usually diffuse in nature and when severe, fluid can collect under the epithelium to give rise to bullous formation.

Corneal oedema due to epithelial pathology is usually localised in nature and depends on the extent and severity of the cause. Epithelial corneal ulcers, whether traumatic or bacterial, cause oedema of surrounding corneal tissue. Extensive epithelial damage caused by chemical burns leads to severe oedema of anterior corneal layers. Epithelial based tissue immune reaction in a graft appears as an epithelial graft ulcer commonly associated with oedema of the surrounding tissue.

Causes of corneal oedema may be grouped on morphological basis as follows:

Epithelial causes
- Trauma
- Exposure keratitis
- Chemical burns
- Neurotropic keratitis
- Recurrent erosions of the cornea
- Radiational and thermal exposure
- Tight fitting contact lenses.

Stromal causes
- Interstitial keratitis
- Stromal dystrophies of the cornea
- Stromal based tissue-immune reaction in a corneal graft.

Endothelial causes
- Iridocyclitis
- Fuchs' corneal dystrophy
- Vitreous touch syndrome
- Acute and absolute glaucoma
- Endothelial based tissue-immune reaction in a graft
- Buphthalmos
- Keratoconus hydrops.

Symptoms of corneal oedema: Patients complain of halos and diminution of vision to varying degrees. When there is bullous keratopathy and epithelial breaks, pain, foreign body sensation and photophobia can be very severe. Symptoms are usually worse in the morning soon after waking due to the bullae sticking to the palpebral conjunctiva during sleep and breaking down on opening the lids. Symptoms of the causative pathology are however added to the symptoms due to corneal oedema.

Clinically corneal oedema is evident from the haziness of the cornea and the bedewing of epithelium. In severe cases, there is epithelial bullae formation. Careful slit-lamp examination can identify the grade of oedema, depth of stroma involved and endothelial involvement. The degree of stromal swelling can be quantitatively measured on a slit-lamp with a pachometer which can measure corneal thickness to an accurate 1/50th of a millimeter.

Treatment of corneal oedema: The treatment consists primarily in dealing with the causative factor. Corneal oedema, however needs to be treated in addition to the treatment of the cause.

Simple corneal oedema can be helped by repeated instillations of hypertonic saline (5% sodium chloride). The instillations may be repeated four or five times a day or even oftener. The solution should be freshly autoclaved every week. Hypertonic solution causes relative dehydration and helps reduce oedema. Sterile pure glycerine drops may also be used either as a supplement and supportive therapy or as an independent dehydrating agent. Local steroids, preferably soluble preparations, are quite helpful in reducing oedema.

Oedema with bullous keratopathy needs more energetic treatment. Debridement of the corneal epithelium with tincture iodine in cases with large bullous formation may, in some cases, be helpful but there is always a chance of recurrence of bullous formation. As soon as tincture iodine is swabbed over the surface, the oedematous epithelium gets wrinkled and it is easy to peel it off. Debridement should be effectively done and should be extended to the whole of the oedematous area. Near the limbus or near a graft margin, adherent epithelium may have to be peeled off with a forceps. It may be noted that the epithelium thus removed, does not include the basement layer which is adherent to the Bowman's membrane. Soft contact lens (bandage lens) after debridement of the epithelium helps relieve the symptoms.

Major surgical procedures are indicated in recalcitrant and recurrent cases. Full thickness donor corneal button grafted on a deep dissected lamellar recipient bed (full thickness lamellar graft) is often helpful in preventing recurrence of bullous keratopathy. Considering that the endothelial damage is the basic cause of corneal oedema and bullous keratopathy due to vitreous touch is better treated by a combined procedure of penetrating keratoplasty anterior vitrectomy.

Corneal Vascularisation

Vascularisation of a normal transparent cornea is prevented by the compactness of the tissue and vaso-inhibitory factor, the mucopolysaccharides in the matrix. Normal metabolic activity is also an important inhibitory factor. Vascularisation of cornea is, therefore, always pathological. It is attracted by vaso-formative factors like trauma, inflammation and anoxaemia. Vascularisation is mostly defensive in nature to help phagocytosis and to provide oxygen to an anoxaemic tissue. Neo-vascularisation in cornea is also responsible for an antigen-antibody reaction; the antibodies being carried from the system to the corneal tissue along the vascular channels.

Superficial vascularisation is usually derived from conjunctival vessels. Deeper blood vessels however come from deeply placed anterior ciliary vessels. By and large superficial vascularisation is due to superficial corneal lesions while deep stromal vascularisation is associated with corneal pathology concurrent with anterior uveitis.

It is called pannus. These blood vessels are an extension from the conjunctival vessels round the limbus. Depending on the etiology, superficial vascularisation may be under the epithelium or under the Bowman's membrane.

Corneal vascularisation in trachoma and phlyctenular disease has already been described.

Leprotic pannus: Vascularisation due to leprotic keratitis is more severe and more extensive. There is no particular pattern and the whole corneal surface is involved. Superficial leprotic pannus may also be associated with deep vascularisation of interstitial keratitis caused by leprosy. Poor corneal sensations, leprotic nodules

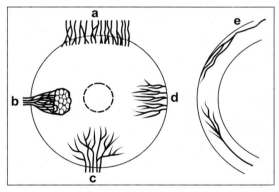

Fig. 9.3: Types of Corneal Vascularisation (a) Trachomatous pannus ending in a horizontal line in the upper cornea. Blood vessels running parallel to each other; (b) Phlyctenular pannus reaching up to the fascicular ulcer from the limbus; (c) Non-specific vascularisation due to any irritation or inflammation in the cornea, [(a), (b) and (c) are superficial types of vascularisation. The continuity of blood vessels can be seen across and beyond the limbus.] (d) Deep vascularisation as in interstitial or parenchymatous keratitis. Blood vessels cannot be traced beyond the limbus; (e) Slit-lamp appearance of corneal vascularisation. (Note the superficial blood vessels under the epithelial layers and deep vessels in the mid-stromal layers

at or near the limbus, associated iridocyclitis and manifestations of leprosy in the body help in clinical diagnosis.

Degenerative pannus: Most corneal scars in trachomatous and tropical countries become vascularised to varying degrees. Even in non-trachomatous areas, tropical climate, poor nutrition and septic foci in the body, common in poorer communities, are factors which help vascular changes of the corneal scars. Degenerative vascularisation is also often present in blind, atrophic and phthisical eyes.

Interstitial Vascularisation

Blood vessels which are situated in stromal layers at different levels, are derived from the intrascleral branches of the anterior ciliary vessels. Their level in the corneal stroma can best be determined by slit lamp examination. The blood vessels usually remain in one plane and do not anastomose anteriorly or posteriorly. When a large capillary net work is concentrated in one area, it gives the appearance of pink coloured patches as seen by oblique illumination and are typically present in syphilitic interstitial keratitis. The empty channels of interstitial vascularisation can also be seen long after the interstitial pathology is controlled. They are best seen in retro-illumination.

Interstitial vascularisation is also a common manifestation of stromal tissue-immune reaction in a graft. These blood vessels invade the graft at different levels. The condition is commonly associated with severe graft oedema.

Deep Vascularisation

Vascularisation at the level of Descemet's membrane or the endothelium is rare. Deep vascularisation in the cornea is present when there is iris adhesion or incarceration following inflammation, trauma or surgery. These blood vessels are responsible for brisk bleeding following a minor surgery like synechiotomy after a corneal graft or any other surgical interference at the angle of anterior chamber.

Apart from the well defined groups of vascularisation described above severe vascularisation of the cornea, intense at all levels of the corneal thickness, is a common association of *chemical burns.*

Treatment of Corneal Vascularisation

Corneal vascularisation is always pathological and secondary to a cause. Appropriate treatment would therefore be treatment of the causative pathology. However, pending eradication and cure of the etiological factor, efforts should be made to minimise the deleterious effects on the corneal transparency.

Steroids are most important local therapy for reducing vascularisation. They probably act by their inhibitory effect on the capillary endothelium. Steroids also reduce oedema and cause some degree of vasoconstriction. They also perhaps act through the muco-polysaccharides. The best mode of administering steroids locally is to instill drops of a soluble preparation every one to two hours during waking hours. Sub-conjunctival injection and systemic administration may be added in severe cases.

Beta radiation has a very definite inhibitory effect on the endothelial cells of newly forming capillaries. Irradiation by beta-rays at intervals of 2-3 weeks, two or three times, will be helpful in controlling neo-vascularisation. Beta radiation however, has no effect on well developed and large blood vessels. The dosage of beta radiation on the cornea should not exceed 1500 in one area because a larger dosage can be harmful to tissue vitality and may retard the healing process.

Surgical procedures for corneal vascularisation include, cauterisation of blood vessels, peritomy, peridectomy and keratectomy. Cauterisation of blood vessels should be limited to only large vascular channels. Too many points of heat cautery may harm tissue nutrition and when too extensively done, may sometimes cause anterior segment necrosis. Peritomy and peridectomy are largely to provide discontinuity between the conjunctival and corneal vasculature and expose the episcleral vessels which can be more precisely cauterised. Following keratectomy, the exposed blood vessels can be more effectively treated with local therapy.

INFLAMMATIONS OF CORNEA

Inflammation of cornea can be epithelial, stromal and endothelial. The process does not however remain localised to one layer for long. Although many of the inflammatory lesions are ulcerative in nature, there are many non-ulcerative conditions where epithelial layer remains intact or may at the worse be passively and indirectly involved due to deeper pathology.

The subject is, therefore, described in two general groups, corneal ulcers and keratitis.

Pathology of Corneal Ulcers

The depth and extent of a corneal ulcer depend on its cause. There are however, certain common pathological considerations which influence the response of the tissue to causative factor.

Marginal epithelium of a corneal ulcer produces an enzyme, collagenase, which plays an important role in digesting and destroying the collagen of stroma and enhances the spread of the ulcer. A continued collagenase activity can lead to recurrent and long standing tissue reaction as for example in chemical burns.

Inflammatory process in the cornea invites blood vessels from the conjunctival plexus to reach the margin of the ulcer. The blood vessels bring in leucocytes to fight the inflammation. The blood vessels are progressive in the beginning and tend to regress as healing starts.

The ulcerative process can be divided into following stages:

a. *Stage of infiltration.* Loss of epithelium and Bowman's membrane occurs in the ulcer area and necrosis involves the corneal stroma. The base and sides of the ulcer are invaded by the polymorphonuclear cells coming from limbal capillaries producing a zone of infiltration.

b. *Stage of progression.* The Ulcer progresses further and this can occur in two directions, i.e., superficially spreading along the surface involving a larger area . Or it may gradually invade the deeper stroma and may ultimately lead to descemetocele and perforation.

c. *Stage of regression.* When, macrophages and leucocytes overcome the invading organisms and also phagocytose the necrotic tissue, the surrounding zone of the ulcer becomes clear with disappearance of the zone of infiltration. Superficial vascularisation has already begun by this time and this helps by pouring in more antibodies and leucocytes.

d. *Stage of cicatrization.* A corneal ulcer heals by scarring. Re-epithelialization of the ulcer area occurs from the surrounding corneal epithelium. In case of a total ulcer, the conjunctival epithelium provides new epithelium. The end result is a corneal opacity, the density and the depth depends on degree of scarring and initial involvement of stromal depth.

Types of Corneal Ulcers

Following types of ulcers are seen clinically (Fig. 9.4).

1. Infected ulcers:
   a. Without hypopyon
   b. With hypopyon.

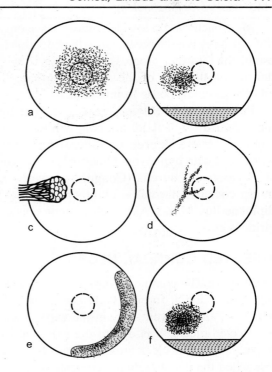

Fig. 9.4: Types of Corneal Ulcer (a) Simple corneal ulcer; (b) Hypopyon corneal ulcer; (c) Fascicular corneal ulcer (phlyctenular); (d) Dendritic (Herpetic) ulcer; (e) Mooren's marginal ulcer; (f) Fungal ulcer with a thick hypopyon

2. Viral ulcers:
   a. Herpes simplex lesion
      i. Herpetic ulcer
      ii. Dendritic ulcer
      iii. Disciform keratitis
   b. Superficial punctate keratitis
   c. Epidemic kerato-conjunctivitis
3. Fungal ulcers
4. Specific ulcers
   a. Phlyctenular ulcer
   b. Mooren's ulcer
5. Neurotropic ulcers
   a. Neuro-paralytic keratitis
   b. Exposure keratitis
   c. Filamentary keratitis
   d. Recurrent erosion
   e. Atheromatous ulcer.

Most bacteria can invade corneal tissue only through an epithelial break. Once the infection is established, further progress of the disease will depend on the type of the causative organism and the tissue response to infection.

Pneumococcus, B.Pyocyaneus and fungi are the organisms which are not only common but cause a severe degree of ulceration often associated with hypopyon. Other organisms are staphylococcus aureus (Coagulase positive), micro-coccus catarrhalis, diphtheria bacillus, diplobacillus Morax-Axen feld, streptococcus viridans etc.

INFECTED CORNEAL ULCER

Symptoms. The common symptoms are watering, photophobia, foreign body sensation and redness. Pain is severe only in the early phase of infected ulcers. It is due to the exposure of nerve endings in ulcer area and may become less when the nerve endings are destroyed.

Irritation or foreign body sensation in the eye and photophobia are also due to irritation of the exposed nerve endings. Excessive watering is due to reflex stimulation and excessive lacrimal secretion.

Defective vision is due to more than one reason. It may be due to the ulcer covering the pupillary area of the cornea. An important cause is iridocyclitis causing a ciliary spasm. It is also due to exudates in the anterior chamber and in the pupillary area.

Signs: The clinical picture of a corneal ulcer will depend on the extent of the ulcer, whether associated with hypopyon or not and whether the ulcer is perforated or not.

A corneal ulcer presents a classical picture of circum-corneal or ciliary congestion. In grossly infected lesions, purulent discharge and infiltrated edge are evident. Circum-corneal congestion is due to associated iritis. More often however, circum-corneal congestion is mixed with conjunctiva, congestion and there may be no area of demarcation.

Grossly infected corneal ulcers are readily visible by ordinary oblique illumination. The base of the corneal ulcer is usually covered with some slough and discharge depending on the severity of infection. The slough and discharge are usually yellowish in colour. A greenish discharge is typical of pyocyaneus infection. Depending on the severity of the infection and the progress of the disease, corneal tissue may be necrosed at the margin and in depth. When most of the stroma is destroyed, the decemet's membrane still withstands intra-ocular pressure and may bulge forwards presenting a condition called *Decemetocele.*

A slit lamp examination can more precisely reveal the depth of the ulcer and the thinning of the cornea, if any. It is important to be forewarned of the latter to prevent perforation when undertaking chemical cauterisation of the ulcer.

Hypopyon ulcer: Any corneal ulcer which is associated with collection of pus in the anterior chamber is called a hypopyon ulcer. The organisms commonly responsible for a hypopyon ulcer are pneumococcus, Ps. Pyocyaneus and Fungal ulcer.

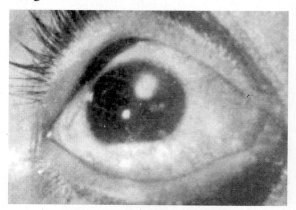

Fig 9.5: Pneumococcal Hypopyon ulcer

The eye is severely congested. The lids are swollen and there is chemosis of the conjunctiva.

A hypopyon is liquid pus and forms a horizontal line of level in the anterior chamber in a sitting position. So long as pus is fluid, it shifts its position with change in posture. When densely fibrinous, these characters may be lost.

The hypopyon is due to associated exudative iridocyclitis and therefore free from bacteria. If however, the ulcer has perforated, the hypopyon no longer remains sterile.

A pneumococcal hypopyon ulcer is commonly caused by type IV and type III pneumococci. Type IV is responsible for 75% and type III for 2% of pneumococcal ulcers. The source of infection many times, is from the lacrimal sac which should, therefore, be investigated in all cases of a pneumococcal hypopyon ulcer. A typical pneumococcal hypopyon ulcer of the cornea has a progressive infiltration at one edge which is undermined and hence it is called *acute serpingenous ulcer or ulcer serpens*. A corneal abscess often forms in deeper layers of the cornea corresponding to the ulcer area with an intervening unaffected tissue. If the ulcer is not effectively treated, the abscess may rupture into the anterior chamber and also extend forwards to join the surface ulcer. This results in perforation and its consequences.

Pyocyaneus ulcer: The causative organism is gram negative Ps. Pyocyaneus (pseudomonas aeruginosa). One of the sources of infection is the use of infected eye drops because the organisms can grow in solutions like fluorescein, eserine, and even in cortisone and penicillin solutions. It is characterised by a greenish coloured discharge and rapid progression. It soon involves the whole cornea and very frequently perforates with resulting complications and consequences.

Fungal ulcers: The incidence of fungal ulcers has in recent years, rapidly increased particularly in tropical countries because of the indiscriminate use of antibiotics and steroids. A mild trauma is usually the starting point and the trauma is commonly from vegetations and thorns etc. Amongst causative fungi, the commonest are aspergillus fumigatus, Fusarium solani and Cadida albicans. Of these, Fusarium solani ulcers are most destructive and those due to aspergillus less so (Fig. 9.6 Plate 3).

The symptoms are relatively mild as compared to the severity of the clinical signs. The ulcer in the beginning may be only a spot of infiltration in the superficial stromal layers. The course of the disease is, however, fulminating. The whole cornea may necrose in a matter of 48 to 72 hours if not quickly treated. A fungal ulcer commonly leads to formation of hypopyon.

It is important to emphasize that fungus as a cause of corneal ulcer should always be kept in mind when evaluating and treating a case of sloughing corneal ulcer. In the absence of appropriate treatment, fungal ulcers perforate with the extension of infection to the inner eye with all its disastrous consequences.

Apart from clinical picture, diagnosis of a fungal ulcer can be confirmed by histological examination of the slough. A quick detection of fungus can be done by mixing a drop of discharge with 10 per cent potassium hydroxide solution on a slide. The hydroxide dissolves all except the fungus which can be seen under the microscope. A smear from the slough stained with PAS stain helps in identifying the fungus. More definitely the diagnosis can be confirmed by culture studies.

Diplobacillary hypopyon ulcer: The causative organism is gram negative diplobacillus of Morax Axenfeld. It runs a mild course, rarely perforates and hypopyon is usually small. Diagnosis can only be made from a smear examination.

Treatment of Infected and Sloughing Corneal ulcers: The principles of the treatment of corneal ulcer are:

 1. Protection and rest to the eye.

2. Relief of symptoms
3. Elimination of causative organism
4. Stimulate healing process
5. Surgical treatment.

Protection and rest to the eye: The eye should be protected from wind and dust. Protection is also needed to relieve the patient of photophobia. It is important that in an eye with profuse discharge, patching will only help multiplication of the bacteria at body temperature in the closed conjunctival sac. Bandaging will also not allow repeated medication in the acute phase of infection. Protection can be provided by sunglasses with protecting shields on the sides. Sunglasses will also relieve photophobia.

More important is rest to the iris and the ciliary body which are concurrently inflammed in most cases of moderate to severe corneal ulcers. Atropine 1% solution should be instilled to begin with once or twice a day. Once the pupil is dilated, further instillation of atropine should only be to maintain dilatation. The effect of atropine is to relieve pain which is caused by contraction of the inflammed iris and ciliary body muscles. Atropine need not be used in non-infective ulcers where the ciliary congestion is mild because these ulcers do not cause any degree of iritis and heal quickly. The effect of atropine once instilled will continue to cause accommodational disturbance for 10 to 15 days while a simple ulcer may heal much earlier. Atropine should also be used hesitatingly in elderly patients for fear of causing glaucoma. A mild degree of inflammation caused by the ulcer may be treated with 2% homatropine drops two or three times a day. If however, severity of reaction demands, atropine should be used as necessary. It is also important to bear in mind that some patients are sensitive to atropine. Children are particularly prone to develop atropine sensitivity like flushing of the face, hyperpyrexia and even convulsions. Local atropine allergy may develop.

This appears in the form of eczematous condition of the skin of the lids. Local application on skin of a steroid ointment before instillation of atropine helps.

Relief of symptoms: Atropine, by paralysing the muscles of the iris and the ciliary body definitely relieves symptoms where iridocyclitis is evidently associated with a corneal ulcer. Analgesics and anti-inflammatory drugs are very helpful in .making the patient comfortable. Anti-inflammatory drugs and analgesics add to the relief of symptoms. Hot fomentation is helpful not only for relief, but also helpful in the healing process. Dry heat can be applied with a heated napkin or electric pads.

Elimination of infection: Newer antibiotics have provided wide choice of specific treatment of individual causative organisms. This, however, needs a smear examination, culture of organisms and determining their sensitivity to various antibiotics. This is not always possible because the patient may have previously had antibiotic therapy disturbing the scope of laboratory studies. In any case, the treatment has to start immediately without waiting for culture reports.

A quicker procedure is to do smear examination of conjunctival discharge or scrapping from ulcer bed to findout if any organism is present and whether it is gram negative or positive, coccus or bacillus. This guides the type of drugs needed.

One should therefore use clinical judgement to at least exclude herpetic and fungus etiology and start treatment with broad spectrum antibiotics. Depending on the severity of the condition, antibiotic instillations should be repeated hourly at least for the first 24 to 48 hours. It is best to use a preparation which covers both gram positive and gram negative organisms. Combinations are available which contain gentamicin, neosporin and polymyxin-B. Supportive antibiotics orally or parenterally may be indicated in very severe cases but their penetration in ocular tissues has been found to be limited.

For fungal ulcers, the drugs that have specific application are nystatin (mycostatin) for candida albicans, fusarium and aspergillus fumigatus. It is insoluble in water and is therefore used as suspension of 100,000 units/ml or as an ointment 100,000 units/gram. It is an irritant drug and therefore not convenient to use as a sub-conjunctival injection. Oral administration or parenteral use is ineffective because of poor penetration into ocular tissues.

Amphotericin-B (Fungizone) is also effective against Candida albicans and aspergillus fumigatus. It is soluble in water. It can be used as 5% eye drops in distilled water (not saline). As an ointment of the same strength can also be used. It can be given by sub-conjunctival route 4 mg/cc, 0.5 cc every day. It can also be given by intravenous infusion drip daily (50 mg dissolved in 10 cc distilled water and diluted in 500 cc of 5% dextrose with 5 mg heparin added to the drip will make the infusion).

The third specific anti-fungal drug is pimaricin which has a broader spectrum of activity and is effective against all the three; fusarium, candida and aspergillus. It is less irritating and can be used in higher concentration. The drug is only slightly soluble and is therefore used as 5% suspension and as 1% ointment. It is non toxic and well tolerated by tissues.

Chlortrimazole is one more anti-fungal drug which is relatively less toxic and well tolerated but effective only against aspergillus infection. It is used as 1% oily drops or ointment.

Nystatin and amphotericin-B are very unstable and have to be kept under refrigeration while pimaricin can be stored at room temperature. It is advisable to keep the patient under observation for checking liver and kidney functions and electrolyte balance if given by systemic route.

In recent years, silver sulpha diazine drops 1% has been tried and found effective against Candida, Fumigatus, Fusarium etc. It also has an anti-bacterial and antiviral spectrum.

In addition to anti-fungal drugs, broad-spectrum antibiotic drops, ointment and sub-conjunctival injections should be used to fight the commonly associated secondary bacterial infection. Iodine administered orally is indicated as a supportive anti-fungal therapy.

Systemic treatment of corneal ulcers: Systemically administered drugs have limited penetration across the blood aqueous barrier and, therefore, their concentration in the aqueous is also not adequate to fight infection in cornea and influence the inflammatory reaction due to iridocyclitis.

Systemic administration of drugs is sometimes considered useful as a supportive therapy. Systemic antibiotic therapy will, to some degree, be helpful against a septic focus elsewhere in the body which may have contributed to inflammation of cornea. Other important drugs given systemically that are useful are Diamox, anti-inflammatory preparation and ascorbic acid.

Stimulate healing process: Diamox is an extremely important and useful therapy where the ulcer is threatening to perforate. Even otherwise, by keeping the intra-ocular tension lower, it facilitates healing of corneal ulcers. It also neutralises the possible harmful effect of mydriatics in elderly patients where there may be a tendency for rise of intra-ocular tension. It should be kept in mind that when diamox is necessary over a longer period, potassium chloride should be administered for the sustained action of diamox by preventing potassium depletion.

Steroids if at all, with the specific therapy should be combined to reduce inflammation and minimise cicatrisation, corneal scarring and formation of posterior synechiae. When necessary, they should be given either sub-conjunctivally or as repeated instillations.

In critical situations like decemetocele, a daily I.V. infusion of hypertonic drugs like 20% mannitol may be given to keep intra-ocular tension at a lower level and prevent perforation.

Vitamin C (ascorbic acid) is an important constituent for cementing character of the matrix of corneal collagen and is actively involved in the metabolic processes of this tissue. It is therefore a useful therapy in all corneal ulcers. The dosage should be on the higher than the lower side and administered orally.

Surgical treatment of corneal ulcers: Many corneal ulcers with destruction of tissue leave behind simple to complicated scars for which the last option of treatment is only surgery. Ulcers threatening to perforate need urgent surgical intervention. The surgical procedures ranging from minor to the most complicated ones that have proved to be useful can be listed as follows:
1. Chemical cauterisation:
   a. Carbolic acid
   b. Trichlor acetic acid
   c. Tincture iodine.
2. Paracentesis.
3. Saemisch's section (discarded but still mentioned).
4. Chouvattage (has been discarded).
5. Conjunctival hooding.
6. Temporary central tarsorrhaphy.
7. Therapeutic lameller keratoplasy.
8. Therapeutic penetrating keratoplasty.
9. Tectonic keratoplasty.

Chemical cauterisation: Apart from specific and supportive therapies, it is always a rewarding practice to treat sloughing corneal ulcers with chemical cauterisation. The most suitable chemical agent is pure carbolic acid. Carbolic acid is a weak acid and does not penetrate deeper. Carbolic acid becomes crystalline in the winter months and needs to be warmed to make it liquid before use.

Carbolisation of a sloughing corneal ulcer, when indicated, should be done adopting a deliberate and effective approach without fear of over carbolisation. The slough should be coagulated with the acid and removed. The base of the ulcer should be painted. It is important that the progressive margin of the ulcer should be thoroughly carbolised particularly the undermined pockets. Sometimes overhanging necrotic edges are better excised so that carbolisation can be done more effectively. Carbolisation of an ulcer acts in more than one way. It coagulates the proteins of the slough. It acts as bacteriocidal agent and it stimulates healing by scarring.

It is important that before carbolisation, the ulcer area should be swabbed to remove any fluids and after carbolisation, it should be swabbed again to soak any excess acid which may otherwise spread over to the conjunctival surface. The proper method of using carbolic acid is to use a pointed matchstick wrapped with a thin layer of dry cotton wool. The size of the tip will depend on the size of the ulcer to be carbolised. After dipping the point of the cotton stick in pure carbolic acid, it should be lightly touched to a wet cotton swab to remove excess acid. The point is then touched to the ulcer surface. One should not use a bare match-stick point. Carbolisation of a corneal ulcer can be repeated. In hypopyon and fungal ulcers it may have to be done daily for two or three days. Carbolisation is an eye saving procedure: Chemical cauterisation can also be done with 10% trichlor acetic acid. It is particularly indicated where the base of the ulcer is very weak and where there is no gross infection. Tincture iodine as a chemical cauterising agent is used for superficial herpetic ulcers, small ulcers after removal of a superficial corneal foreign body.

Paracentesis: It used to be practised in the pre-antibiotic days for draining hypopyon. Paracentesis should be considered only when an ulcer is threatening to perforate and when better indicated surgical procedures, like penetrating keratoplasty, are not feasible.

Chouvattage or cooking of the ulcer surface: It is indicated in cases of decemetocele and large sloughing ulcers. This is done by holding a red hot ball cautery half a millimetre above the ulcer surface (without actually touching the tissue). The radiated heat cooks the slough and the infected tissue. In case of a decemetocele, it coagulates the surface and reduces the chances of perforation.

Conjunctival hooding: It is indicated in ulcers where the infection has been controlled but the ulcer refuses to heal. For the conjunctival flap to stick to the ulcer area, it is important that it should be without pull from the periphery. It sticks best when the cornea surrounding the ulcer is de-epithelialised. Ideally speaking, the Gunderson type, a very thin conjunctival hood flap, is very appropriate.

A thin conjunctiva allows permeation of medication to the ulcer area underneath. It acts by providing a protective layer and helps healing by providing fibroblasts through the blood vessels.

Temporary central tarsorrhaphy has been described elsewhere.

Corneal grafting: Indications of therapeutic corneal grafting are becoming more and more favourably considered.

A. A therapeutic lamellar graft is indicated in:
   1. Indolent ulcers where the deeper stroma and limiting membrane are unaffected.
   2. Recurrent corneal erosions.
   3. Atheromatous ulcer.
B. Therapeutic penetrating graft is indicated for:
   1. Descemetocele.
   2. Large sloughing and hypopyon ulcer of cornea after the acute infection has been controlled.
C. Tectonic penetrating graft is indicated where the eye is threatened with perforation and a total sloughing perforated ulcer is not responding to antibiotic or antifungal therapy.

VIRAL LESIONS OF THE CORNEA

Herpetic lesions of the cornea are a frequent occurrence. More and more ulcers will be diagnosed, if one not only keeps its possibility in mind but is also conversant with its clinical features. The most significant feature of herpetic ulcers is their tendency to recur over months and years.

There are two groups of viruses concerned with corneal diseases. One group is the dermotropic viruses which involve the skin and mucous membrane, e.g., the viruses causing smallpox, chickenpox and herpes simplex. The others are neurotropic viruses, a typical example being the virus causing herpes zoster. This virus also causes superficial punctate keratitis, nummular keratitis and epidemic kerato-conjunctivitis.

Laboratory diagnosis of a virus lesion can be made by demonstration of inclusion bodies in epithelial cells and by innoculation in animals.

The herpes simplex virus is the commonest causative agent for viral ulcers of the cornea. The clinical conditions include, dendritic ulcers, amoeboid or geographical ulcers, disciform keratitis and metaherpetic keratitis. The source of the herpes simplex virus is in the genitals, oral cavity and the lacrimal gland. They can remain dormant in the corneal epithelium also.

Herpetic ulcer: This is a common corneal manifestation of herpes simplex virus. The lesions are superficial involving epithelium, Bowman's membrane and superficial stroma.

The onset is sudden and symptoms are redness, photophobia, lacrimation and pain. The symptoms are far out of proportion to the actual clinical condition.

On examination, there is moderate to severe circum-corneal congestion. The corneal lesion is typical. There is superficial ulcer of the cornea. The lesion may spread to form an irregular, shallow, geographical or amoeboid-shaped ulcer which can be readily demarcated with fluorescein. Being a non-suppurative condition, there is no slough or mucous discharge. On slit lamp examination, there is minimal epithelial oedema at the margins of the ulcer. The ulcer does not extend deeper than superficial stroma. In later stages, there is moderate to intense superficial vascularisation. The corneal sensation in ulcer area is diminished. The most characteristic feature is the recurrence at intervals of weeks or months. The condition does not respond to antibiotics and is aggravated by steroids.

As the pathology does not extend to the deeper stroma, the ulcer never perforates.

Disciform keratitis: It is a viral interstitial keratitis forming a circumscribed lesion in the stroma. The condition may spread to involve the whole stroma and cause folds in decemet's membrane and endothelialitis. When it involves the whole thickness and all layers of cornea, it is called *keratitis profunda*. As no virus has been demonstrated, the condition is considered to be a tissue immune reaction caused by antigen-antibody interchange. A slit lamp examination reveals stromal oedema of considerable degree (Fig. 9.7).

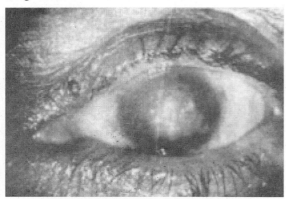

Fig 9.7: Disciform viral keratitis

Dendritic ulcer: Although a dendritic ulcer is a classical example of a superficial herpetic lesion, unmatched by any clinical similarity, it is not as commonly seen as a geographical herpetic lesion. When present, the clinical picture is unmistakable. The irregular branching shape, hence the name dendritic ulcer, with rounded ends of the branchings is suggestive that the lesion is a conglomeration of small individual lesions. The disease is progressive. A small lesion to begin with, it may involve a large extent of the corneal surface (Fig. 9.8, Plate 3).

Superficial punctate keratitis: Superficial punctate lesions of the cornea due to virus are mostly epithelial. They faintly stain with fluorescein. The symptoms are usually mild but long standing. Individual lesions may coalesce forming different shapes. Their special character is recurrences over long periods. They usually do not leave behind corneal nebulae. An identical clinical entity has also been named as Thygeson's superficial punctate keratitis.

Epidemic kerato-conjunctivitis: It is a common condition in congested localities. It comes in an epidemic form with more than one member of the family and many families in the area are affected.

The clinical picture is characteristic: It starts with symptoms of mild nonpurulent conjunctivitis. As conjunctivitis subsides, mistiness of vision starts. On examination, thin superficial, small flat lesions are seen in the central cornea. The lesions are sometimes so small that one may miss them unless the eye is examined under magnification and bright illumination or with a slit lamp. The spots faintly stain with fluorescein and become clinically more evident.

Superficial punctate lesions of the cornea have also been described in South India, an area with a high incidence of malnutrition, particularly deficiency of the riboflavin factor of Vitamin-B complex.

Treatment of viral lesions: IDU (5 iodo-2 deoxy uridine) has been used as eye drops for many years. It is important that in progressive stage, drops should be used 5-6 times daily. It is however to be noted that IDU is not effective in all cases. It is also toxic to tissues. New drugs which have been developed are Vira-A (Vidarbine) used as 3% ointment and Viroptic (Trifluridine) used as 1% solution. These drugs are less toxic to the tissue and are effective in larger number of cases. Other lines of treatment should be the same as for non-suppurative corneal ulcers.

Steroids in the treatment of viral ulcers should be used only if the condition does not respond to pure anti-viral therapy for a week and then too along with an anti-viral drug. Steroids are better indicated for deep viral lesions like disciform keratitis.

The treatment of superficial punctate keratitis and epidemic kerato-conjunctivitis is on palliative lines. The conditions usually resolve without any residual effect on the cornea in most cases. Simple antibiotic drops may be used four to five times a day for 10–15 days. Atropine should be used only if there is significant ciliary congestion.

SPECIFIC TYPES OF ULCERS

Marginal ulcers: There are a variety of marginal ulcerative conditions which are inflammatory or degenerative in nature located near the limbus. Because of their proximity to the limbus, vascularisation to the ulcer margin is common. The tissue nutrition does not suffer to the same extent as in a central ulcer and therefore the ulcers remain superficial and do not perforate (Fig. 9.9A and 9.9B Plate4).

Recurrent phlyctenular keratitis often remains marginal. Multiple phlyctens at the limbus may coalesce to form a marginal ulcer.

Phlyctenular keratitis: It is also called scrofulous or eczematous kerato-conjunctivitis. It is now generally agreed that phlyctenulosis is an ocular manifestation of endogenous allergy to tuberculous protein and corneal manifestation is a tissue immune reaction. Staphylococcal infection is a common association and because of this fact, staphylococcus as an etiological factor was considered for a long time.

Phlyctenular ophthalmia is a common condition in developing countries: It affects small children in ill-nourished states and living in unhygienic environments. The condition is more often bilateral but may manifest in one eye at a time. It is of a recurrent nature and may continue for months and years. Occasionally, a phlyctenular picture may be seen in adults but with very few symptoms.

Corneal manifestations of phlyctenular ophthalmia are of three types:
1. Punctate micro phlyctens along the limbus.
2. Phlyctenular ulcer of the cornea.
3. Fascicular ulcer of the cornea.

Punctate micro phlyctens: This condition is less common than the other types. Punctate yellowish spots are seen just inside the limbus. The micro-phlyctens may be anywhere along the limbus rather than along the upper limbus as in trachomatous pathology. Some of these punctate phlyctens may enlarge and involve the deeper tissue of the cornea near the limbus to leave behind punctate opacities. Multiple such opacities give the limbus a crenated appearance which is characteristically diagnosable even years after the disease has healed.

Symptoms are usually mild in nature: The condition becomes quiet with improvement in nutrition and health of the child.

Phlyctenular ulcer: A phlyctenular ulcer of the cornea is also typically present near the limbus. There may be more than one in one eye and there may be phlyctens in both eyes.

The symptoms in the beginning may be mild but once phlyctenular surface has broken down to form an ulcer, the symptoms are severe and include, lacrimation, photophobia and blepherospasm. Pain of moderate degree is usually present. Associated conjunctivitis due to staphylococcal infection may further add to the symptoms.

The clinical picture is easy to diagnose. One or more ulcers of the cornea near the limbus in an ill-nourished child are characteristic. The excoriated lid margin and eczematous conditions of the upper lip under each corresponding nostril is often seen and is due to the proteolytic enzyme formed at the phlyctenular lesion. Vascularisation is a constant feature of phlyctenulosis.

This type of phlyctenular ulcer usually extends to deeper layers and a perforation is not uncommon, leaving behind a small round dense corneal opacity to which iris is adherent. The presence of one or more such lesions, if traced to childhood, are diagnostic of previous phlyctenulosis.

Fascicular ulcer: It is a characteristic phlyctenular pathology which extends along the surface of the cornea. It starts as a small ulcer near the limbus and extends towards the centre. An infiltrated advancing margin of the ulcer is towards the centre. As it progresses, it leaves behind a relatively clearer cornea over which a leash of blood vessels extends from the limbus to the ulcer. A true fascicular ulcer rarely perforates. When healed, it leaves behind a typical tongue-shaped scar from the limbus. Numerous ghost vessels can be seen extending from the limbus on a slit lamp.

Treatment of phlyctenulosis has been described under phlyctenular conjunctivitis. Treatment for local ulcerative involvement of the cornea due to phlyctenulosis is as for a non-sloughing corneal ulcer. General supportive therapy is also very important. With adequate local and systemic treatment most cases quickly respond. Systemic anti-tubercular therapy may be helpful in recurrent cases.

Mooren's ulcer: This is a chronic ulcerative condition in elderly patients which remains, by and large, localised to the marginal cornea although it may extend all round and may involve all but the central island of corneal tissue. The process causes destruction of Bowman's membrane and superficial stroma. The deeper stroma and Descemet's membrane remain intact.

Mooren's ulcer is a degenerative condition: No specific cause has been attributed although metabolic and nutritional factors, tuberculosis, syphilis and intestinal parasites have been reported to be associated with the condition.

The ulcer begins as a small patch of infiltration, breaking down to form a crater. It extends along the limbus to form a partial or complete ring ulcer. The conjunctiva adjacent to the ulcer is congested and vascularisation extends to the ulcer margin. The ulcer may become broader and a stage may reach that only a small central island of corneal tissue remains unaffected. In the full-fledged stage, the clinical condition is unmistakably characteristic. In spite of severe and extensive nature of the disease, perforation is extremely rare (Fig. 9.9B, Plate 4).

Considering the severity of the disease, the symptoms are not as pronouced but the patients frequently complain of photophobia, watering and redness. Vision is affected when the disease has progressed and caused oedema of the adjacent central cornea.

The condition usually starts in one eye but involvement of both eyes is not uncommon. The end result of the condition in most cases, except those who respond to therapy and surgery, is totally scarred and vascularised cornea with total loss of vision.

The treatment of Mooren's ulcer is very unsatisfactory. No specific local therapy is helpful. Chemical cauterisation of the progressive edges can be tried. Corneal grafting in most cases is the only surgery that may save some of these eyes. Unfortunately the pathology can invade a corneal graft also which therefore limits its scope.

Interstitial Keratitis

Any keratitis where the inflammation primarily starts in the mid-stromal layers is called interstitial keratitis or parenchymal keratitis. The inflammation does not primarily affect the epithelial or endothelial layers. The three granulomatous diseases which primarily cause interstitial keratitis are syphilis, tuberculosis and leprosy. Each of these three cause deep keratitis with differentiating features of their own and hence need to be described separately.

Syphilitic interstitial keratitis: The incidence of syphilitic interstitial keratitis varies widely in different regions of the globe.

Most of the cases are due to congenital syphilis. Acquired syphilis is known to cause a similar condition only in a small percentage of cases and involves cornea in the second clinical stage of syphilis.

It is bilateral in most cases, but in cases due to acquired syphilis, it is more often unilateral and milder. Keratitis due to congenital syphilis becomes clinically manifest between the age of 10-20 years. Along with corneal involvement, the stigmata of congenital syphilis are present, common ones being frontal bossing, depressed bridge of the nose, Hutchinson's teeth and periosteal nodes on the tibia. There may be associated deafness and cicatrices at the angles of the mouth. Some patients are often mentally and physically retarded. The triad of interstitial keratitis, deafness and Hutchinson's teeth is called Hutchinson's triad.

Pathologically, Treponema pallidum, the causative organism of syphilis, have rarely been demonstrated from corneal tissue although some have reported its presence in corneal epithelium. The pathogenesis of the condition has been considered as an antigen-antibody reaction. Cellular infiltration, mainly lymphocytes, along with deep vascularisation affect the posterior layers of cornea. The vascularisation is in form of patches of fine anastomosis of large number of capillaries in the infiltrated area to give the appearance of pink discolouration called Salmon patches.

Clinically, the condition is keratitis and anterior uveitis both together. The cornea looks like uniformly ground glass due to oedema with folds in the descemet's membrane. Keratic precipitates and posterior synechiae are present due to iridocyclitis.

Symptoms vary with the stage of the disease. In the progressive florid stage, the patient complains of redness, lacrimation, severe photophobia and dimness of vision. The eye is painful and tender. The symptoms become milder and may disappear when the disease has regressed.

The disease in some respects is self-limiting and prognosis, therefore, is not bad. In absence of active treatment in the early stage, residual corneal opacity, posterior synechiae and consequent lens changes cause loss of vision.

Treatment: Local treatment along with systemic therapy for syphilis is very important. Effective atropinization is indicated at the earliest. A subconjunctival injection of soluble dexamethasone should be given every day for 8–10 days after which a weekly sub-conjunctival injection of insoluble steroid should be continued till the slightest congestion persists. Hot compresses help relieve pain. For residual opacity, after the disease has remained quiet for at least 9–12 months, a penetrating keratoplasty has a good chance of restoring visual acuity.

Tuberculous interstitial keratitis: Although tuberculosis is considered to be responsible for a very small percentage of cases of interstitial keratitis in the Western world, it is not necessarily so in tropical and developing countries where incidence of tuberculosis in some communities is very high. Tuberculosis is responsible for interstitial keratitis by causing endogenous allergy to tuberculous proteins. The corneal manifestation is an antigen-antibody reaction. In all cases of interstitial keratitis with negative serological reactions for syphilis, investigations should be done to exclude tuberculosis as a cause. A chest X-ray, erythrocytic sedimentation rate, Mantoux tuberculin test, examination for tuberculous glands and evidence of past tuberculosis elsewhere in the body, should be routinely done.

Clinically, the condition differs from syphilitic interstitial keratitis in some respects. Tuberculous interstitial keratitis is more often unilateral. Lesions are more nodular. The keratic precipitates are big. Vascularisation is localised in different sectors. The condition is more progressive and not self-limiting as syphilitic keratitis. The residual corneal opacity is dense.

The treatment is effective atropinization and systemic anti-tubercular treatment. If the eye responds to initial therapy indicating tuberculous etiology, anti-tubercular drugs should be continued for 9-12 months. Desensitisation with fractional doses of old tuberculin is considered useful even in these days. Steroids should be used only locally and should not be used systemically for fear of activating a silent tubercular lesion.

Lepromatous interstitial keratitis: Leprosy is a common disease in India. The two clinical forms are nodular or tuberculoid and lepromatous. Violent iridocyclitis is the commonest ocular manifestation of leprosy. Serious corneal involvement, though infrequent, manifests in the following forms:

1. Limbal nodule.
2. Lepromatous pannus

3. Punctate keratitis
4. Interstitial keratitis.

Limbal nodules and Lepromatous pannus due to leprosy are described elsewhere.

Interstitial keratitis due to leprosy is always associated with iridocyclitis.

The cornea is oedematous and the lesion is more peripheral than central. The flare-up of a lepra reaction can cause aggravation of the corneal oedema which, however, is transitory in nature. The symptoms are mild because of corneal anaesthesia.

Treatment: Although specific treatment of leprosy has provided an opportunity to cure the disease, unfortunately, the persistence of social stigma has kept leprosy patients at a distance from the remedial measures so readily available. Effective and prolonged sulphone therapy will save cornea from ths damage which the disease can otherwise cause. Superficial punctate keratitis due to leprosy is usually associated with some degree of anaesthesia. The symptoms are therefore very mild. There are numerous fine punctate opacities involving epithelial and sub-epithelial layers of the cornea. They have sometimes to be looked for, when the systemic condition is lepromatous leprosy. A slit lamp examination is often necessary to differentiate them from keratic precipitates of iridocyclitis, if present.

Local treatment includes effective atropinisation and topical and sub-conjunctival steroids. Tarsorrhaphy is necessary in cases where there is exposure keratitis which demands protection of the cornea because of lack of corenal sensation.

TROPHIC ULCERS OF THE CORNEA

The conditions that fall under this category are, exposure keratitis, neuroparalytic keratitis and atheromatous ulcer.

Exposure keratitis: The common causes of exposure keratitis are:

1. Facial paralysis.
2. Severe degree of axial proptosis of eye ball.
3. Ectropion of lower lid.
4. Lagophthalmos.
5. Destructive lesions of the lid like severe trauma and acid burns.
6. Non-closure of the eyes as in toxic and comatose conditions.
7. Anaesthesia of cornea leading to less blinking as an after-effect of herpes zoster and the lesions caused by leprosy.

Clinically, the exposed cornea becomes dry with epithelial keratinization. The superficial stroma may become hazy. Abrasion and secondary infection may cause infective ulceration of cornea. The corneal condition is indolent and improves only when the exposure is remedied or sensation returns.

Treatment: This will depend on the causative factor. The patient should be advised protection from dust and wind by use of goggles. Drying of cornea, can to some degree be prevented by using lubricating drops. As a temporary measure, central tarsorrhaphy may be performed. In conditions where exposure due to marked proptosis is irreversible, a permanent lateral tarsorrhaphy is indicated.

Neuroparalytic keratitis. The principal cause of neuroparalytic keratitis is the lesion of the trigeminal nerve either at the level of the Gasserian ganglion or in the peripheral part of the nerve.

The consequences of sensory loss of the cornea are:
1. More chances of trauma or foreign bodies on the cornea because of the lack of protective lid reflex.
2. Poor healing of ulcers of the cornea.

Clinically, cornea in neuroparalytic keratitis looks lusterless and oedematous. There may be fine bedewing of the epithelium which faintly stains with fluorescein.

Circumscribed epithelial ulcers may involve a large part of the cornea. Secondary infection may invade. Perforation and its consequences may result.

Typically, the symptoms are minimal. The patient mainly complains of diminution of vision. Pain is conspicuously absent. Collection of mucoid secretion is common.

Treatment: The eye should be protected at the earliest. A prophylactic central tarsorrhaphy should be done to prevent corneal damage. The band of tarsorrhaphy need only be 2–3 mm in breadth and the patient should be able to see through the inter-marginal space on either side. The patient should be informed that the tarsorrhaphy will need to stay for 9–12 months. After 6–9 months it may be opened to see if eye develops any reaction or not. If the lesion recurs after undoing the tarsorrhaphy, a fresh tarsorrhaphy may be needed. These surgical procedures do not need any anaesthesia; topical or infiltration.

Atheromatous ulcer: It is a chronic ulcerative process in old and gross corneal scars in which iris is usually incarcerated. The term is a misnomer because they are neither atheromatous nor primary ulcers. Old corneal scars like leucoma adherens, partial and total anterior staphyloma have been known to undergo degenerative changes like keratinisation of the epithelium and ulcerative breakdown of the pseudo cornea. Most of these eyes are blind need to be enucleated with orbital prosthetic implant.

Filamentary keratitis: This is a non-specific condition which is chronic and recurring in nature.

The clinical conditions in which filamentary keratitis is seen are recurrent viral keratitis, traumatic debridement of epithelium, kerato-conjunctivitis sicca, neuroparalytic keratitis, complicated trachoma and absolute glaucoma. Filamentary keratitis sometimes appears in the upper part of the cornea near the cataract section during post-operative period. A neurotropic factor in the corneal epithelium probably plays an important role.

The lesion starts as a break in the epithelial surface, and oedema raises the epithelial edge to form a tag. This epithelial tag becomes elongated and coiled remaining attached to the cornea at one end. The movements of the lids contribute to the process of elongation of epithelial thread. The filament and the area of corneal surface where it is attached stains with Rose Bengal and fluorescein.

The symptoms are severe. The patient complains of acute discomfort due to a foreign body feeling. Watering and photophobia make the patient very uncomfortable. The condition may subside only to recur again and again.

If a cause cannot be found, which is often the case, the treatment is to pull away the filaments, desquamate the epithelium around its attachment and cauterise the raw area with tincture iodine. This may have to be repeated. Soft contact-lenses may give long standing relief.

Recurrent corneal erosions: This is a very painful condition which can come on suddenly and recur from time to lime. It may be idiopathic, possibly associated with mild trauma or a neurogenic factor. Recurrent erosions can also supervene on degenerative and dystrophic conditions of the cornea or old corneal scars. This is probably due to a less firm attachment of epithelium to the basement membrane. The patient gets up in the morning with sudden irritation, pain, watering and photophobia. The morning symptoms are possibly due to the oedematous corneal epithelium sticking overnight to the palpebral conjunctiva and peeling off with the first movement of the lids. The symptoms are milder during the day. The defect in the epithelium stains with fluorescein. The condition may sometimes change into filamentary keratitis.

Treatment of the condition is chemical cautery with tincture iodine of the oedematous area followed by pad and tight bandage. Homatropine or atropine may be used once or twice if there is evident ciliary congestion. Oily antibiotic drops at night may be helpful.

A therapeutic lamellar graft may be needed where the condition persists over a long period and does not respond to local therapy.

DRY EYE SYNDROME

For adequate protection of the conjunctival and corneal surface, adequate lacrimal secretion and a healthy precorneal film are an essential requirement. The pre-corneal film is a tri-lamellar layer consisting of a superficial layer of oily Meibomian secretion, a middle watery layer of lacrimal gland secretion and a deeper mucoid layer from the secretions of the goblet cells of conjunctiva. The superficial oily layer prevents excessive evaporation of the middle aqueous layer. The deeper mucous layer adheres firmly to the corneal surface and helps adsorb aqueous layer. The presence of a healthy pre-corneal film is not only essential for a comfortable feeling but also for protecting corneal surface from environmental effects. Any disturbance in the pre-corneal film is harmful and causes discomforting symptoms.

The lacrimal secretion bathing the conjunctival and corneal surfaces can be quantitatively determined by Schirmer's test. The test is performed by using a strip of Whatman filter paper No. 41,55 mm in length and 5 mm width. The strip is folded at 5 mm from one end. The folded part is hooked into the lower fornix over the lower lid margin at the junction of outer one-third and inner two-third. The patient is asked to keep the eyes open. Normally a 15-20 mm length of strip from the fold should get wet in 5 minutes.

Wetting of less than 15 mm in five minutes indicates deficiency of lacrimal secretion. This test is called Schirmer's test-I.

If Schirmer's Test-I shows negligible wetting of the strip, or no wetting at all, the test may be repeated while nasal mucosa is irritated with a stick swab or ammonia vapour to cause reflex lacrimation. If there is adequate wetting of the strip now, it excludes pathology of the lacrimal gland. This test is called Schirmer's test-II.

Dry eye syndromes are caused by various pathological processes, some of which are peculiar to tropical environments. The pathological conditions that can cause dry eye syndromes may be listed as follows:

1. Collagen diseases like rheumatoid arthritis, disseminated lupus erythematosis and polyarthritis nodosa.
2. Absence of lacrimal secretion either congenital or due to a lesion of the seventh nerve between the nucleus and geniculate ganglion where the nerve supply to the lacrimal gland passes through.
3. Complicated trachoma in which sub-conjunctival cicatrisation strangulates the goblet cells and hence disturbs the mucous content of the tear film.
4. Ocular pemphigus, Steven-Johnson's disease and chemical burns.
5. Vitamin-A deficiency by causing keratinization of epithelial layers of conjunctiva and cornea.

The clinical condition of the cornea and the conjunctiva will depend on the cause. There may be history of systemic disease, for example, polyarthritis and stomatitis sicca as in Sjogren's disease and evidence of skin and other mucous membrane lesions as in pemphigus.

The cornea looks dry and lusterless. There may be xerotic patches on the conjunctiva adjoining the limbus as Vitamin-A deficiency. There may be shallowing of fornices, adhesions and symblepharon between the bulbar and palpebral conjunctiva, as in ulcerative conjunctivitis and complicated trachoma. Moderate to intense vascularisation of the cornea is always present. Trophic epithelial corneal ulcers may complicate the condition.

The treatment of dry eyes is to treat the cause which is not always feasible. The first important thing to do is to keep the corneal and conjunctival surface wet with artificial tears. Cauterising the lacrimal puncta has been suggested. However, it is important to remember that fault is not the deficiency in lacrimal secretion but the constituents of tear film that are abnormal. In eyes where lacrimal secretion is less as indicated by Schirmer's test, transplantation of the parotid duct in the fornix was practised in earlier years. This surgery has been given up for obvious reason that parotid secretion is no substitute for lacrimal fluid.

Idiopathic Tear Film Anomaly (ITFA)

The conditions causing dry eye syndromes described above are clinically evident and easy to diagnose. There is however a condition that is fairly common with symptoms which are more aggravated than the clinical picture presents. This condition used to be less frequently thought of and therefore very often not diagnosed. The condition is idiopathic tear film anomaly.

Tear film is made up of three constituents in three layers. It is usually the fault in oily and mucous layers that is responsible for this tear film anomaly. Normally the tear film maintains its unbroken continuity for 15-20 seconds or longer and as soon as it tends to break, the blink reflex restores its continuity so that for all practical purposes, the cornea is constantly covered by a tear film.

The tear film break-up time can be determined by putting a drop of fluorescein, (better to use a fluorescein strip) asking the patient not to blink and examining the tear film on a slit-lamp through a cobalt blue filter. The time between the last blink and the first break in the film is seen as patches of cobalt blue colour in the green fluorescent background. In moderately severe cases, the time may be as low as 1-3 seconds or the tear film may not form at all. The test is readily done as an outpatient procedure and in fact should be done whenever symptoms cannot be explained by any evident clinical findings in the anterior segment.

The symptoms of tear film anomaly are nonspecific and rather vague. The most common complaints are burning in eyes, a pricking sensation in the eyes, mild redness and frequent blinking. The symptoms are more severe when outdoor and have usually been complained of for months and years, in spite of continued local treatment with various eye drops. In chronic and advanced cases, stringy discharge in the fornices is usually seen. On direct enquiry many times the patient himself complains of a thread-like mucous flake in eyes.

On examination, there may or may not be mild congestion. There is no evident cause in the palpebral or bulbar conjunctiva. The cornea does not look as bright and shiny as it should. Some impression of dryness or lustrelessness, can always be discovered if one keeps the possibility of this condition in mind. A tear film break-up test will confirm the diagnosis.

Many patients suffering from this condition have had long therapies, with antibiotic solutions, steroids, decongestive drops without any relief of the symptoms. The condition is becoming more frequent due to environmental changes and is possibly related to more than one factor may be climatic, radiational and atmospheric pollution.

Treatment is mostly symptomatic: The only therapy that relieves symptoms is the use of tear substitutes. Artificial tears with a synthetic base are more useful and their effect lasts longer. They are marketed as Tearisol, Tears Naturelle and Tears plus. Number of tear substitutes are now aviable. The frequency of instillation of the drug depends on the severity of the condition and the lasting effect of the drug. Topical therapy needs to be continued over long periods. Bandage soft contact lens is veryuseful in advanced cases.

CORNEA IN TRACHOMA

Trachoma used to be considered a major cause of corneal blindness in large parts of northern India and in countries with identical dusty and windy climate. Since the advent of chemotherapeutic and antibiotic drugs, the involvement of cornea by trachoma has become less serious. The cornea is however involved to varying extent in all stages of both early and complicated trachoma.

Corneal lesions due to trachoma may be listed as follows:
1. Trachoma follicles at the upper limbus and in the upper cornea.
2. Trachomatous pannus and corneal vascularisation.
3. Superficial punctate keratitis.
4. Marginal ulcer of cornea.
5. Corneal ulcers.
6. Trachomatous cornea.
7. Corneal trachoma.
8. Trachomatous keratectasia.
9. Dry eyes and defective tear film.
10. Exposure keratitis of lower part of cornea.
11. Corneal astigmatism.
12. Corneal scars.

Most of them are described in detail in the section on trachoma. A short description of corneal involvement in trachoma is given here. Trachoma follicles are commonly seen either along the upper limbus or in the upper cornea arranged in a row. After healing, the follicles at the limbus leave behind brownish pits called Herbert's pits. Corneal follicles and pannus heal leaving behind a thin haze with ghost vessels ending in horizontal line just above the pupil.

Corneal scars in trachomatous eyes are due to a trachomatous lesion getting secondarily infected and developing a clinical picture of an infected ulcer of cornea. Trachoma in these cases is the starting pathology providing a nidus for bacteria to invade. In areas where trachoma is endemic, infected corneal ulcers have a close bearing to *trachomatous pathology*. The resulting, scars of these ulcers are more due to secondary infection than due to trachoma.

Apart from a typical trachomatous pannus of the upper cornea, intense vascularisation may involve the whole corneal surface. This is usually due to complications of trachoma like entropion and trichiasis.

A moderate degree of corneal involvement may heal leaving behind a large part of the cornea transparent. The healing process however causes changes in the corneal curvature, resulting in visual defect due to corneal astigmatism.

When a diffuse trachomatous corneal pathology heals, it leaves behind a thin haze in the cornea with large number of ghost vessels. This is called a *trachomatous cornea*. By this time the pathology in the lids has also healed and become quiet (Fig. 9.10, Plate 4).

Trachomatous pathology may heal and leave behind a thin cornea which may become ectatic and is called *trachomatous keratectasia.*

An interesting corneal lesion due to trachoma is localised discrete superficial nodules exactly identical to Salzmann's corneal degeneration. This nodular degeneration is associated with Herbert's pits at the limbus and healed trachoma in palpebral conjunctiva and tarsal plate.

Extensive cicatrisation in the tarsal plates may cause exposure of the lower cornea. The condition is made worse if there is associated entropion of the lid margin and trichiasis. The lower cornea may become hazy, vascularised and keratinised.

MAL-NUTRITION AND THE CORNEA

The cornea suffers from the effects of mal-nutrition more than other tissues of the body with grave consequences. Corneal blindness is therefore the commonest cause of blindness in children in developing countries.

The deficiency of Vitamin A may cause hyperplasia of the epithelial cells and keratinisation of the corneal epithelium, Riboflavin deficiency can cause superficial vascularisation of the cornea. Severe degree of malnutrition due to multiple deficiencies of Vitamin A, proteins, iron and calories cause keratomalacia. Mal-nutrition may indirectly be associated with other corneal lesions, for example, an ill nourished cornea is an easy victim to bacterial invasion aggravating the consequences of infective conjunctivitis and infected corneal ulcers.

Keratomalacia: This is a manifestation of severe degree of systemic malnutrition. Vitamin A deficiency is an important deficiency factor but not the only one. It is severe protein and caloric deficiency along with deficiency of Vitamin A which causes keratomalacia. It is a multiple deficiency syndrome. It is, therefore, incorrect to presume that mass administration of Vitamin A will eradicate or prevent kerato-malacia in the population. What is needed is to deal with other nutritional deficiencies.

Keratomalacia is common in poor communities and usually affects children in very young age. The deficiency is either due to lack of nutrition or due to the child suffering from recurrent gastro-intestinal parasitic disorders and diarrhoea over long periods. Many such children are therefore marasmic. Some of them, instead of being marasmic, are flabby and severely anaemic due to associated iron deficiency. Generally the child appears listless-and dull.

On examination, the eyes have a dull, luster-less appearance. The conjunctiva may show dryness, wrinkling, brown pigmentation and

Bitot's spots on the intermarginal bulbar conjunctiva. The corneal picture depends on the stage and severity of the disease. In the early stage, dryness, poor sensation and haziness of the cornea may indicate impending disaster. Once the disease has advanced, the corneal stroma melts rapidly. A stage may come when the whole cornea has melted away and only decemet's membrane and endothelium cover the iris. It appears as if the whole iris diaphragm is bare and exposed. Most of these eyes end up as total leucoma adherens, partial or total anterior staphyloma or atrophic bulbi. If, however, a timely and energetic treatment improves the nutrition of the child, the result may be less devastating. The cornea may then heal to form a total corneal opacity and this is amenable to restoration of vision with corneal grafting at a later stage.

Along with the corneal condition, other systemic clinical manifestations of malnutrition are also evident. Dry lusterless hair, dry scaling skin and a flabby anaemic or marasmic condition of body are commonly well developed by the time the eye has developed keratomalacia.

Treatment: The treatment of corneal complications due to malnutrition should be undertaken at the earliest and with emergency. Appropriate therapy before the cornea has started melting, may restore the cornea to complete transparency. Once the corneal melting has started, the struggle is to save the eye.

In early stage, the therapy should include an aqueous solution of Vitamin A administration in therapeutic doses by parenteral route because absorption from the gastro-intestinal tract of these patients is always uncertain. Therapy must also include multi-vitamins and protein administration. The treatment should continue till the cornea returns to normal lustre and transparency and *general health improves.*

Once the cornea has started melting, the treatment should include plasma transfusion by intravenous route and Vitamin A along with other vitamins also by parenteral route. Haematinics, if indicated by the blood picture are also an important supportive therapy. The parenteral treatment may be shifted to oral therapy only after the cornea has regained its thickness and integrity.

It is important to bear in mind that the condition may recur if the child returns to its normal poor environments and more so if there is gastro-intestinal disorders which may recur off and on. Not only should the treatment for malnutrition be maintained for long periods but gastro-intestinal disorders like parasitic infections should be simultaneously treated and eradicated.

Local eye therapy is only limited to antibiotic drops to prevent secondary infection and keep the eye protected to prevent damage or perforation of the remaining corneal tissue.

PTERYGIUM

Pterygium is a pathological fleshy conjunctival encroachment on the cornea. Although the tissue originates from the conjunctiva, it is not correct to describe it as a conjunctival disease for more than one reason. Firstly, because it is not called a 'Pterygium' till cornea is involved. Secondly, there must be a reason for the conjunctiva to encroach on the cornea and the reason is obviously in the corneal tissue. Thirdly, the recurrence is more common when dissection of pterygium from the cornea is inadequate. Pterygium is, therefore, primarily a corneal pathology which attracts the conjunctiva to invade it.

Pterygium is much more common in tropical countries. It is distinctly more common amongst outdoor workers exposed to dry and dusty winds. It is, therefore, more common in males than in females. A true pterygium is much more common in adult to old age, and extremely rare in children.

Pterygium has provided enough material for histological studies. In earlier years, it was considered a degenerative pathology. It has also been considered a chronic inflammatory process. More critical histological studies of primary and recurred pterygia have shown marked epithelial papillary down growths, convertion of unicellular goblet cells into tubular glands and heavy vascularization are prominently seen. These and its tendency to recur after surgical excision is highly suggestive of the neoplastic nature of this pathology.

Clinically, a primary pterygium is nearly always seen in the inter-marginal zone mostly on the nasal side of cornea. It may however be on either side of the cornea, when it is called a double pterygium. Pterygium is often in both eyes but different in its extent.

Pterygium is morphologically described to be composed of three parts. The head of the pterygium on the cornea has a progressive margin which infiltrates into and destroys Bowman's membrane and superficial stroma. Behind the head is a slightly narrower part, the neck of the pterygium, about the level of the limbus. Beyond the limbus is the body of the pterygium in the bulbar conjunctiva.

The pterygium may be thin with minimum vascularisation. This type of pterygium is very slow in progress. A fleshy and vascular pterygium is rapidly progressive and extends towards the centre of the cornea but it rarely encroaches onto the central pupillary area. Double pterygia may grow and encroach the pupillary area from either side.

The symptoms of the patients are more often cosmetic than affecting vision. A thin pterygium and an early stage of fleshy plerygium cause no visual defect. When pterygium has however extended 2–3 mm beyond the limbus into the cornea, the pull of the pterygium may alter the curvature of the cornea and cause corneal astigmatism which results in some visual defect. Vision is however, grossly affected when a recurrent pterygium encroaches the pupillary

area or when two pterygia on either side are growing towards the pupil.

Types of pterygium: The different nomenclatures of the pterygium are indicative of the pathological definitions. *A true pterygium* is one which is primary in nature and located in the inter-marginal zone on one or both sides of the cornea and has a characteristic shape with a head, neck and body. A true pterygium on the medial side of the cornea is called *typical true pterygium*. A true pterygium conforming to the above morphology but situated in a position other than the medial side is called an *atypical true pterygium*. The incidence of atypical pterygium is very small and when present, the commonest site is lateral to the cornea in the inter-marginal zone. When there is pterygium on either side of cornea in the same eye, it is called *double pterygium*. When there is one pterygium in each eye, it is *bilateral pterygium* (Fig. 9.11, Plate 4 and 9.12).

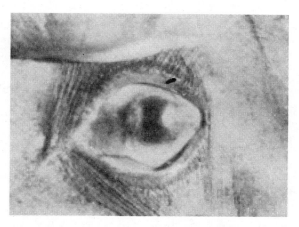

Fig. 9.12: Double Pterygium : One on each side of cornea

A false pterygium is an active pathological process of inflammatory origin resulting in an adhesion between the conjunctival and the corneal surface. It has no characteristic shape and may be present anywhere round the limbus (Fig. 9.13). It occurs frequently after chemical burns and ulcerative conjunctivitis. It is rare that

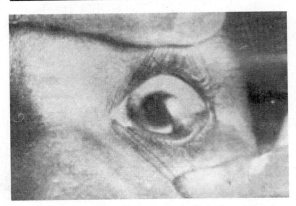

Fig. 9.13: False temporal pterygium. Note the obliquely growing character.

a false pterygium is a bridge between the conjunctiva and the cornea and it is therefore, not correct that one of the differentiating points between a true and false pterygium is that a probe can be passed under a false pterygium as used to be stated.

Pterygium which recurs repeatedly it is called a *malignant pterygium* and this usually does not conform to the shape of a primary pterygium. It is more fleshy and rapidly progressive.

Treatment: Non-surgical treatment like sub-conjunctival injections of hydrocortisone and hylase under the body of the pterygium, followed by doses of beta-radiation to the fleshy part of pterygium have been tried out but the result is uncertain and unsatisfactory. Treatment when indicated is however only surgical.

It is important to bear in mind that a thin and minimally vascularised pterygium in an elderly patient need not be operated at all. A quiet pterygium is like a sleeping tiger better left alone because if provoked, the result may be unpleasant. A more vascular pterygium should however be operated but only when the patient is anxious about the cosmetic part and/or when it is progressive and has introduced corneal astigmatism. It is also extremely important that when surgery of pterygium is indicated, it should be planned and executed with full realisation that

a recurred pterygium is more violent than the primary pterygium and surgery should therefore be adequate to minimise chances of recurrence.

Many surgical procedures have been adopted by various surgeons in various countries. No single surgery has, to date, provided hundred percent prevention of recurrence. Over the decades, the following operative techniques have been used:

1. Simple excision of the pterygium.
2. Dissection and transposition of the head of the pterygium.
3. Dissection and invertion of pterygium.
4. Excision and mucous grafting.
5. Dissection with keratectomy and episclerectomy leaving peri-limbal bare sclera.
6. Partial peripheral lamellar corneal graft.
7. Corneo-scleral lamellar graft.
8. Total lamellar graft for double pterygium.

For a primary pterygium which is fleshy and progressive, the most effective surgical approach is dissection of the pterygium leaving 3 mm of bare sclera beyond the limbus, cauterisation of all bleeding points and Beta-irradiation of the bare area, two to three times at 3-4 weekly intervals. The most important surgical step in this operative procedure is dissection of the head. The incision should start half a millimetre ahead and around the infiltrating margin of the head of pterygium in cornea. It should be deep enough to include few healthy lamellar layers of cornea deeper to the head. The dissection should be carefully extended towards the limbus and carried beyond the limbus up to about three millimeters into the superficial sclera. The head and neck of the pterygium are excised concentric to the limbus. The cut edges of the body are anchored by fine sutures to the sclera in front of the medial rectus insertion.

Dissection of a recurred pterygium is more difficult: Previous surgery leaves scarring and adhesions to the sclera and in some cases to the medial rectus. Dissection has to be much more extensive in a pterygium that has recurred af`er repeated surgery. Such a dissection from the cornea should be wide enough and deep enough as described above. Dissection beyond the limbus has to be more careful because of sub-conjunctival adhesions. One should be careful to avoid scleral perforation at or beyond limbus. Dissection may have to extend even as far as the insertion of medial rectus. Inadvertant inclusion of the insertion of medial rectus in the scleral dissection can cause post-operative diplopia and paralytic squint. It can best be avoided by identifying the extent of muscle insertion and adhesions to the sheath of the muscle by passing a hook under the muscle and then proceeding with further dissection of the pterygium. As in a primary pterygium, the cut edges of the conjunctiva are anchored to the sclera along a concentric line just anterior to the insertion of the medial rectus.

After dissection, the scleral surface should appear clean and smooth. Blood vessels, many of which appear to come from deeper sclera should be cauterised with a hot point. The bare sclera may be irradiated 24-48 hours after the operation. Some surgeons prefer to cover this area with a mucous graft from the cheek or lower lip. The convex edge of the semilunar mucous graft is sutured to the conjunctival edge nasally and the other concave edge to the sclera one millimetre away and concentric to the limbus.

An optical lamellar graft is indicated for a double or single pterygium enchroaching the pupillary area. A therapeutic corneo-scleral lamellar graft may be undertaken where pterygium has repeatedly recurred and a corneoscleral dissection is likely to leave behind a thin tissue due to deep dissection.

Special techniques of partial peripheral lamellar corneal graft, partial corneo-scleral graft and total lamellar graft need modifications depending on individual cases.

CORNEAL DEGENERATIONS AND DYSTROPHIES

Generally speaking, dystrophy is a condition which has a hereditary background usually not present at birth but being *hereditarily predetermined*, becomes clinically manifest later in childhood or adolescence unlike a congenital condition which is present from birth. On the other hand degenerations are acquired conditions either primary or secondary becoming manifest later in life. Inflammation is entirely absent in dystrophies while in degenerations, inflammation may in some cases be a precipitating cause.

Classification of corneal dystrophies and degenerations must necessarily be sufficiently elastic to include some of the known corneal conditions and accommodate the increasing number of atypical cases. The variety of clinical appearances is so enormous and complex that a comprehensive and enduring classification has defied many. Attempts have been made since 1890 to group these corneal conditions. A most detailed classification of primary degenerations of cornea was presented by Franceschetti and Forni which is relatively less important from the clinical point of view.

The corneal dystrophies and degenerations may however be considered in a general sense in four groups:
1. Age changes
2. Degenerations
3. Metabolic disturbances
4. Dystrophies

Age changes: There is a group of corneal conditions which occur with advancing age. It is at times difficult to differentiate correctly between conditions which can be termed as 'physiological' senile changes and those which come under the heading of primary degenerations Difficulty is also encountered to demarcate between physiological senile changes and 'dys-trophic' conditions, e.g. cornea guttata affecting the peripheral endothelium is a physiological change due to advancing age but when it occurs in the central endothelium, it is recognised as pathological endothelial dystrophy.

Degenerations: These are essentially pathological in nature and are similar to degenerative changes occurring in other body tissues. Avascularity and transparency of the normal corneal tissue perhaps make their appearance more dramatic and incidence more frequent. These degenerations are as a result of disease elsewhere in the body and are commonly lipid, hyaline and calcareous.

Metabolic disturbances: The cornea is secondarily involved by infiltration in its layers, of abnormal metabolites due to gross metabolic disorders, for example, gargoylism due to faulty carbohydrate metabolism. Hand-Schuller-Christian disease is due to lipid disorders and cystinosis due to protein disorders.

Dystrophies: Corneal conditions of a hereditary and familial nature come under this group and a number of classifications have been put forth but none of them is quite satisfactory. Characteristic features of dystrophies are that these are bilateral, symmetrical, central and slowly progressive lesions and are devoid of vascularisation. These are sometimes present congenitally but most frequently appear in the first two or three decades of life with one or more members of the family also showing the same clinical picture.

Hereditary tissue changes in cornea as elsewhere, can be *dominant* or *recessive* in character. It is therefore important to carefully take family history (if necessary with leading questions) when a corneal dystrophy patient is examined.

It is best to group dystrophies according to the tissue layers involved in the dystrophic process. The following is a useful classification, for clinical purpose of diagnosis and treatment, of commonly seen corneal dystrophic conditions:

A. Dystrophies affecting the anterior limiting membrane
  a. Primarily affecting the epithelium
    i. Recurrent erosion (dominant)
    ii. Juvenile epithelial dystrophy, Meesmann (autosomal dominant)
    iii. Microscopic cystic dystrophy of epithelium, Cogan
  b. Affecting Bowman's membrane
    i. Cornea verticillata
    ii. Mosaic dystrophy
    iii. Annular dystrophy of Reis & Buckler (dominant)
B. Dystrophies affecting primarily the corneal stroma
    i. Granular dystrophy, Groenouw's Type-I (Dominant)
    ii. Lattice dystrophy, (Dominant)
    iii. Macular dystrophy, Groenouw's Type-II (Recessive)
    iv. Crystalline dystrophy (Dominant)
C. Dystrophies affecting primarily the posterior membranes
    i. Cornea guttate
    ii. Posterior poly-morphous dystrophy
    iii. Annular endothelial dystrophy
D. Combined oedematous dystrophies:
    i. Primary corneal oedema
    ii. Combined dystrophy of Fuchs.
E. Ectatic condition.
    i. Keratoconus (Dominant and recessive, also).

The following pages are devoted to describing some common degenerations and dystrophies which are seen in routine clinical practice.

Age changes

1. **Arcus senilis** is a condition of lipid infiltration of neutral fat and phospholipids in limiting membranes of cornea, particularly in peripheral part of Bowman's membrane. Found in about 80% of people above the age of 60,

it starts as a greyish zone concentric to the limbus commonly in upper periphery but can be in the lower periphery and even along the whole circumference just inside the limbus. A clear zone is always present between the limbus and arcus because Bowman's membrane stops short within a millimetre and half inside the limbus. The inner margin of arcus is ill-defined unlike the clear cut outer margin. It does not impair vision. A similar condition, in children and young people, *Arcus Juvenilis*, is a congenital condition.

2. **Hassal Henle bodies** are hyaline excrescences in peripheral decemet's membrane projecting in the anterior chamber and best seen by specular reflection on slit lamp.

3. **Cornea guttata.** This is a slow senile degenerative change in endothelial layer of the cornea. It can be clinically detected only if routine silt-lamp examination is done in all elderly patients to detect vacuolations and pits in the endothelial surface. A specular microscope shows the condition of the endothelium in greater detail and in better perspective.

Cornea guttata is a symptomless condition. It does not affect vision. The condition however has clinical significance because cornea with guttata changes is likely to react to operative or inflammatory trauma and develop full fledged clinical picture of Fuchs' endothelial dystrophy

The condition by itself does not need any treatment but cornea with guttata changes should be handled with respect during intra-ocular surgical procedures. The endothelial surface of the cornea should be spared undue mechanical trauma, as for example during a cataract operation.

Corneal degenerations: These are mostly non-familial, acquired and progressive. These can be fatty, hyaline or calcareous. A notable example of calcareous degeneration is *Band shaped keratopathy.* This is mostly found in eyes with advanced anterior segment disease like chronic iridocyclitis, absolute glaucoma and phthisis bulbi. It can rarely be primary in healthy eyes. It starts from the periphery of the cornea in the inter-palpebral zone and the two lesions meet in the centre.

Salzmann's nodular degeneration is typically hyaline in nature. These nodules of Salzmann degeneration are superficial involving only the epithelium and Bowman's membrane and rarely the superficial stroma. Histologically, they are thick acellular plaques between the epithelium and Bowman's membrane.

Clinically they are multiple bluish white nodules seen on the cornea which are discrete and raised from the surface with clear cornea in between, lamellar grafting gives very good optical and cosmetic results (Fig. 9.14).

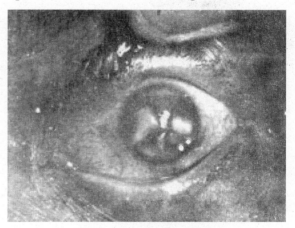

Fig. 9.14: Nodular dystrophy

Terrien's marginal degeneration starts as punctate opacities close to the limbus associated with some vascularisation, spreading circumferentially and ultimately resulting in thinning of the peripheral part. They may cause ectasia of the central cornea (Fig. 9.15).

An epithelial degeneration with characteristic features is seen in dusty and windy coastal towns called *salt-pan keratitis or geographical kera-*

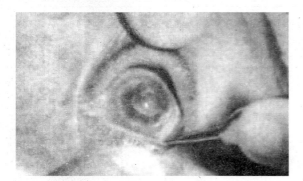

Fig. 9.15: Terrien's marginal degeneration

topathy. The lesions are translucent sago grain-like and raised from the surface. They often start from either side of the limbus in the inter-marginal zone and slowly extend towards the centre forming a band shaped lesion. The lesion assumes dirty brownish colour in due course. The condition is common in elderly patients and affects mostly the males exposed to rigors of the climatic environments. It is primarily an involvement of the epithelial and sub-epithelial zone and most superficial stromal fibres.

Corneal dystrophies: There are classical dystrophies of cornea, granular, macular, Fuchs and lattice which are not uncommon in general population. They have fairly distinctive clinical features to be more or less correctly identifiable by careful clinical examination.

Granular dystrophy Groenouw's type-I. It shows a dominant hereditary trend and appears in one or more offsprings of the same generation. It is never present at birth but makes its appearance in the first decade of life. The lesions appear as small white dots in the central cornea. The cornea in between these lesions is characteristically clear, so also the peripheral cornea. The white spots may appear in different arrangements. They are typically under the Bowman's membrane and in the anterior stroma. The deeper stroma, Descemet's membrane and endothelium remain healthy (Fig. 9.16).

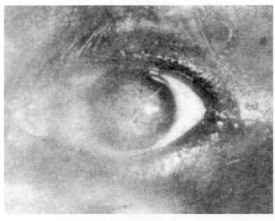

Fig. 9.16: Granular dystrophy

Visual acuity, if at all, is only minimally affected. Corneal sensation remains normal.

Histologically granular dystrophy is a disorder of the corneal mucopoly-saccharides. There is a deposition of hyaline material in the corneal lamellae which get separated. The epithelial layer over the lesion is thinned.

Treatment for granular dystrophy is usually not sought for because visual acuity remains good. However, when needed either for optical or comestic purpose, a partial thickness lamellar corneal graft suffices.

Lattice dystrophy: A dominant hereditary form of corneal dystrophy, first becomes evident towards the end of first decade or early in the second decade of life. The changes become macroscopically obvious at about 20-25 years of age when the cornea loses its lustre and stroma becomes cloudy. In the hazy stroma opacities in the form of stars, dots, filaments and flakes are seen. In the mid-peripheral zone, typical lattice like lines appear which run in all directions but never reach the limbus. They are in different layers of stroma. A disciform opacity is seen in advanced cases which extends from the sub-epithelial zone through practically the whole thickness of the stroma (Fig. 9.17, Plate 4).

Corneal sensation is affected early. Recurrent epithelial erosion is a common occurrence and may be the presenting symptom. The epithelial surface is frequently irregular.

Visual acuity diminishes progressively due to a cloudy cornea and the irregular surface. In the third and fourth decades, these patients become severely handicapped and dependent.

Histologically the essential change is a deposit of amorphous material along with a strongly basophilic substance which is aggregated in and around the stromal lamellae. The lattice network is supposed to represent the hyalanised remains of corneal nerves. Much of the Bowman's membrane is absent or gets covered by a layer of collagen fibrils.

Treatment is sought for recurrent attacks of pain and photophobia due to epithelial erosion. Corneal grafting has to be undertaken in order to improve visual status and get rid of symptoms. A full thickness penetrating graft is needed.

Macular dystrophy (Groenouw's type II): It is a heredo-familial affection inherited as an autosomal recessive trait with frequent consanguinity. It appears in the first decade of life as a fine diffuse opacity in the anterior stroma of the central cornea. Slow progression takes place in the second decade when the corneal haze extends towards the periphery as well as to the deeper stroma. The deeper extension can be right up to the decemet's membrane. Soon dots and irregular forms of opacity appear. The intervening cornea is always hazy. Extension up to the limbus is the rule. Corneal sensation is reduced (Fig. 9.18A, Fig. 9.18B, Plate 4 and Fig. 9.18C and 19.18D, Plate 5)

Visual acuity is affected early in the disease. Most of the patients are severely handicapped by the third decade.

Histologically, the fixed corneal corpuscles become swollen and appear as if they formed a syncytial mass joined by large pseudopodia.

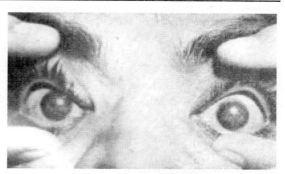

Fig. 9.18A: BE macular dystrophy

Hyaline degeneration is present in the anterior stroma with the overlying epithelium thinned out and cells vacuolated, a change due to recurrent erosion. Mucoid degeneration of stromal lamellae may be a prominent feature with accumulation of acid or neutral mucopoly saccharides.

Differential histochemistry with Masson's trichrome, PAS and colloidal iron stains has shown that Granular dystrophies are mucopolysaccharide defects. Macular dystrophies have hyaline changes and lattice dystrophy is amyloid degeneration.

Patients seek an ophthalmologist's help at an early stage because of visual handicap and recurrent erosion of the corneal epithelium. Nothing short of a corneal graft helps. A careful slit-lamp examination goes a long way in deciding whether the individual needs a full thickness or a partial thickness graft. More often a full thickness graft is needed. Some cases of macular dystrophy may remain limited to the anterior half or two thirds of corneal substance. These can be improved with a partial thickness lamellar graft.

Endothelial dystrophies:

1. *Essential corneal oedema:* The main feature is the oedema of stroma associated with and caused by pathological changes in the endothelium. This may be unilateral or bilateral, occurring in adults and affecting particularly the central cornea. Occasionally a familial occurrence suggests a dystrophic character but

many cases perhaps represent atypical or abortive form of Fuchs' dystrophy.

2. *Fuchs' dystrophy:* Characterised by epithelial and stromal oedema and reduced corneal sensitivity. A slit-lamp examination clearly shows endothelial changes. Cornea gultata as a precursor of Fuchs' dystrophy further confirmed that the endothelium was primarily affected and involvement of the stroma and epithelium was secondary.

The clinical progress of Fuchs' dystrophy can be described in four stages:

1. Uncomplicated degeneration of endothelium, stage of cornea guttata.
2. Oedema of stroma and epithelium causing a bullous Keratopathy.
3. A late state of sub-epithelial connective tissue formation leading to vascularisation and scarring.
4. Stage of complications like cataract and glaucoma.

The early stage is likely to be overlooked unless routine slit lamp examination is done in all elderly patients. The stage of stromal oedema starts with oedema in the posterior stroma which goes on increasing till the whole stroma is involved and bullous formation takes place in the epithelial layer. These are small and central initially but soon coalesce together to form big bullae and also extend towards the periphery. Vision is affected, more so in the mornings when fluid has collected under the epithelium. Irritation and foreign body sensation persists. A bullous may burst and cause an attack of acute pain. Corneal sensation is defective or even absent. As oedema continues, the changes extend towards periphery. Dots and linear opacities occur in the stroma which becomes hazy and thickened. The epithelial bullae become scarred and after a long rather painful course the whole cornea becomes opaque, insensitive and vascularised to varying

degrees. Fuchs' dystrophy causing cataract and open angle glaucoma is too frequent to be overlooked (Fig. 9.19, Plate 5).

Mention must be made of a *secondary Fuchs' dystrophy.* Senile endothelial changes with corneal guttata flare up to manifest similar features as described above. This may happen after a surgical procedure, commonly after an operation for cataract extraction. Operative trauma caused by an intra-ocular lens implant may also end in a similar condition. (Fig. 9.20 Plate 5).

A full thickness corneal graft has been the most effective treatment if undertaken at a relatively early stage of the disease. If successful, graft remains clear for a long time.

Congenital endothelial dystrophy: Although regular Fuchs' dystrophy is a disease of old age, we do see cases in small children with similar clinical appearance. This is Congenital Hereditary endothelial Dystrophy (CHED) (Fig. 9.21 Plate 5).

There is diffuse haze cornea and no vascularisation. The cornea is oedematous and on slit-lamp examination, the endothelial layer is irregular.

The condition may be present at birth or appear soon after. It has to be differentiated from buphthalmos in which the cornea and eye ball are bigger in size and there is marked diminution of vision.

Treatment is only a full thickness penetrating grafting which should be done at least in one eye even before the age of one year to prevent nystagmus.

KERATOCONUS

Keratoconus is also known as conical cornea due to the cone shaped ectasia of the axial part of the cornea. It is a non-inflammatory condition, that usually manifests early in adolescence. It results in considerable visual defect early in its progress due to irregular astigmatism.

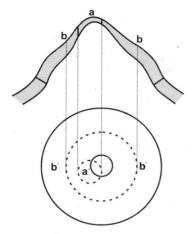

Fig. 9.22: Keratoconus. Sketch shows the corresponding parts of the apex (a) and base (b) of cone. The apex is not exactly in the centre

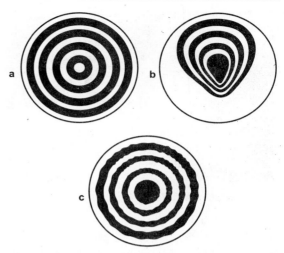

Fig 9.23: Keratoconus. Corneal reflex of Placido Disc: (a) Normal anterior surface of cornea (b) Anterior surface in keratoconus (c) Irregular corneal surface

A number of theories have been put forward from time to time to account for development of keratoconus. No single theory has been found to be satisfactory. Developmental anomaly, degeneration secondary to other disease, lowered nutrition, the endocrinal process and heredity—all have been blamed for keratoconus. In some cases definite hereditary occurrence suggests that it may be a dystrophy. The nature of heredity transmission is not certain. It has appeared as a recessive as well as a dominant heredity. Consanguinity has at times been present.

Electron microsocopy has indicated that early changes are in the anterior layers. Changes in the basement layer of the epithelium and in Bowman's membrane play a significant role in the pathogenesis of keratoconus.

Clinical appearance: Keratoconus is invariably bilateral although unilateral cases are seen, but rarely. Clinical manifestation in adolescence is heralded by defective vision. In very early stages, the cone may be difficult to see with naked eye. Attention may be attracted by irregular retinoscopy observations or by retinoscopy reflex going round and round the central part. Diagnosis is supported by keratoscopy with Placido's disc, where the reflected rings are typically distorted (Fig. 9.23). Later on the cone is conspicuous and easily recognisable. A common clinical test (Munson's sign) is to lift up the upper lid and ask the patient to look down. The cone distorts the lower lid margin. The steeper and bigger, the cone, the more the deformation of the lower lid margin. The anterior chamber depth is increased proportionate to the height of the cone (Figs 9.24, 9.25, and 9.26).

The condition is gradually progressive. It may sometimes get arrested and remain so or may

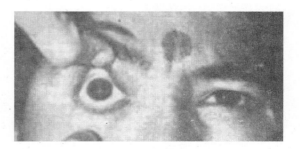

Fig 9.24: Keratoconus. (Front view; note the central haze due to scarring as a result of healed hydrops

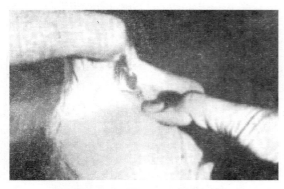

Fig 9.25: Keratoconus (side view; note the forward projection of cone)

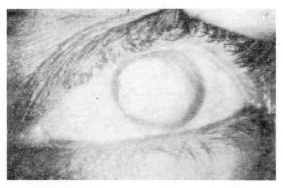

Fig. 9.26: Advanced Keratoconus with recurrent acute hydrops with extensive scarring

reactivate later. An acute episode due to rupture of decemet's membrane can occur during its progress and result in the collection of fluid at the cone causing a localised oedema (hydrops). This localised oedema tends to regress as soon as the endothelium regenerates to bridge the gap. The cornea tends to clear and may regain transparency. However, if stromal oedema is massive and persists or recurs again and again, it leaves behind scarring which is conspicuous in the cone. This further adds to visual impairment.

A slit lamp examination not only confirms the diagnosis but also provides the following information:

1. Thinning of the cornea at the apex of the cone which varies greatly and may be anything from half of normal to a papery thin cornea.
2. Ruptures in descemet's membrane are seen in some cases.
3. In acute hydrops, stromal oedema and tears in decemets membrane are conspicuous. In very acute cases, epithelial bullae formation may occur.
4. Scarring at Bowman's membrane level and in stroma in cases of healed hydrops.
5. Fleischer's Ring has been reported as a coloured ring at the base of the cone and formed by deposition of iron (haemosiderin) in the sub epithelial zone. It is usually a complete ring. Even when specifically looked for, it can be seen only in few cases.

Treatment: Contact lenses in early cases and in cases without opacities, give dramatic results and so also in those who have become stabilised in the early stage. Most other cases will need full-thickness corneal grafting, indications for which can be more clearly defined as follows:

1. When a contact lens does not improve vision satisfactorily.
2. When a contact lens improves vision but the lens cannot be tolerated.
3. When the disease is progressive as indicated by frequent change of contact lenses.
4. When there is recurrent hydrops.

Epikeratoplasty to flatten the cone, increase thickness of cone and improve vision is possible if there has not been an attack of hydrops and no central scarring.

Deep lamellar grafting has been practised in advanced keratoconus. Recipient lamellar dissection is done deep upto decemets membrane.

CORNEAL PIGMENTATION

Although cornea is avascular and transparent, pigmentation in different layers due to one cause or another is not uncommon. The pigment may deposit into cornea either as a manifestation of systemic disease or may be from an ocular pathology. The following are common sources of pigment in the cornea.

1. Haematogenous blood pigment, hemosiderin from haemoglobin.
2. Metallic pigments like iron, copper and sometimes silver and gold.
3. Melanin pigments either congenital or acquired.

Haematogenous pigmentation (blood staining of cornea). Blood staining of cornea is not an uncommon complication after intra-ocular operative procedure with persistent and extensive hypaema as post-operative complication and injuries. Blood in the anterior chamber behaves differently under different circumstances. The anterior chamber may be full of blood one day and 24 hours later, all may have disappeared. On the other hand, blood may continue to remain unabsorbed for days even when there is no fresh bleeding. The absorption of blood, when it takes place, is from the iris surface and an unhealthy atrophic iris is therefore an impediment to the process.

If blood stays in the anterior chamber beyond 3-5 days, the chances are that the fragmented red cells and haemoglobin granules penetrate into the corneal stroma. It is not easy to explain why in one case cornea starts showing blood staining in less than a week and in another case, it may remain in anterior chamber for over 3 weeks and yet not stain the cornea. One factor which is generally agreed to be favourable to corneal staining is raised intra-ocular tension. An unhealthy endothelium, like in eyes with iridocyclitis and raised IOP facilitates blood staining of cornea.

Once the cornea has acquired blood staining, the clinical picture is characteristics. The stain is brown in colour and involves two thirds or larger area of corneal surface. The absorption process, however, soon starts both from the periphery and the deeper corneal layers by phagocytic process. It is extremely unlikely for a blood stained cornea to become completely transparent. Slit lamp and histological studies have shown that residual staining is limited to the anterior stromal layers.

Treatment: The first important preventive step is not to allow the blood in the anterior chamber to remain beyond 3-5 days. The longer the blood stays, more the chances of blood staining. Hypotensive drugs like diamox to keep intra-ocular tension normal or low further helps to reduce chances of blood staining. If there is no sign of even a partial absorption, the hyphaema should be drained forthwith. Surgery should however not be undertaken as long as spontaneous absorption is taking place which may continue over a few days.

Residual blood pigment is mostly in anterior half or two thirds of corneal thickness (histological observation). A deep lamellar graft should therefore restore transparency. Any visual improvement after lamellar keratoplasty will however depend on the functional and anatomical integrity of posterior structures.

Metallic pigments Iron: Rust staining of the cornea is common with an iron foreign body in the cornea. The deeper the foreign body, more dense is the staining. However staining is usually localised to the tissues deeper to and immediately round the foreign body. It does not cause a generalised siderosis of ocular tissue. It is very important to look for rust staining in every case where an iron foreign body has stayed in the cornea for longer period. If an iron foreign body has been removed and the patient still continues to complain of irritation, one should look for a rust stain.

Treatment: The best way to prevent rust staining of the cornea is to remove an iron foreign body at the earliest. If, however, a rust ring has formed, it should be completely scrapped off immediately after removal of the foreign body. The patient sometimes comes with the rust stain only, the foreign body having been removed. Removal of rust after deeply placed iron foreign bodies or secondary rust removal a few days after the foreign body has been taken out, may need deeper scraping. Special rust removing instruments, manual and electric have been devised which should be used, not only to prevent perforation but also to leave behind a smooth, clean surface of the cornea.

Copper: Copper is the constituent of the pigmentation of the peripheral cornea in hepatolenticular degenerations, Wilson's disease. The ring of pigmentation is called Kayser-Fleischer ring and its characteristic appearance is commonly in the stroma and the Decemet's membrane near periphery. It is best seen with a slit lamp.

Silver and Gold: The prolonged use of silver nitrate application or organic silver preparations like argyroll and protargoll causes argyrosis of the conjunctiva and rarely impregnation of silver irons in the cornea also. Gold is an innert metal and does not undergo chemical change in tissues.

Melanin. This pigmentation of the cornea can take place in various forms. It may be:
1. Congenital melanosis usually localised and an extension of a limbal naevus.
2. Degenerative melanosis in the form of pigment particles on the posterior surface of cornea
3. Pigmented keratic precipitates on the posterior surface of the cornea due to cyclitis.
4. Fine pigment granules from a senile degenerative change in the uveal tissue are sometimes deposited on the posterior corneal surface and appear in a spindle form called Krukenberg's spindle.

5. Uveal pigments as in the case of iris incarceration in corneal scars.

CORNEAL INJURIES

Cornea is the most exposed part of the eye ball. It is therefore a victim of all types of injuries. The row of eye lashes provide some protection by filtering dust particles, and preventing them from reaching the cornea. The blink reflex is the most important protective mechanism that protects cornea from various types of injuries, particularly chemical and radiational. The bony orbital margin and the bridge of the nose also provide protection to cornea and the eyes from the impact of falls.

Industrial accidents, both mechanical and chemical are becoming increasingly common causes of corneal injuries due to rapid industrialisation and high speed industrial activities. Fast moving traffic is responsible for another large group of corneal injuries.

Civilian injuries of the cornea are no less common. Sharp objects in the hands of children are not uncommon causes. Labourers like stone breakers often get foreign particles into their eyes which are more often particle from chisel than from the stone. Farmers and labourers working in fields are commonly exposed to trauma from dust and wind and from vegetation and thorns in the fields. Injuries from the horns of animals can cause grievious trauma to the eye ball and cornea.

Fire work industries and digging tube wells with explosives are not uncommon causes for severe injuries to the cornea, eye ball and the face.

The injuries to the cornea may be grouped as under:
I. Physical trauma
   A. Non-perforating
   B. Perforating
      a. Simple perforation
      b. Perforation with iris prolapse

    c. Perforation with lens dislocation or extrusion and vitreous loss.

    d. Perforation with retained intra-ocular foreign body.

II. Chemical burns with alkalies, acids and gases

III. Thermal burns with hot metals and in generalised body burn cases

IV. Raditional trauma

    a. Welding arcs

    b. X-ray radiation

    c. Atomic radiation.

Non-perforating injuries: Non-perforating injuries of the cornea may be concussion injuries, corneal foreign bodies, superficial abrasions and incised wounds through partial thickness.

Concussion injuries. Concussion injuries to the cornea can be caused by a blast or a fall, hit on orbital margin, impact of a fist, ball or a shuttle cock directly on the eye.

The most common damage to cornea by concussion is tears in the Decemet's membrane. The cornea is temporarily oedematous. There may be hyphema usually from iridodialysis.

Treatment is conservative: Local steroids should be used when there is corneal oedema. Hyphema may need to be drained by paracentesis. Attention is often needed for treating more serious intra-ocular injuries, if any.

Corneal foreign bodies: These foreign bodies can be dust, coal, vegetable particles, metallic particles, wood splinters, stone, glass particles and gunpowder particles etc.

The first symptom of the patient is irritation. Lacrimation and photophobia are complained of and the severity depends on the size of the foreign body and whether it is embedded deep or is superficial.

The diagnosis of a corneal foreign body in most cases is quite evident. A foreign particle is sometimes missed. This is particularly so when a black or transparent particle is lying against the dark iris and pupil background. In any case where the history and symptoms are clear cut and no foreign body is seen in the conjunctiva and the cornea, a fluorescein stain may help in localising the foreign body. A slit lamp examination is necessary to find out whether a spot contains a foreign body or not. It is important to remember that a foreign body may have hit the cornea and may have been washed away by blinking and lacrimation but may have left an epithelial trauma. The patient may persist with the symptoms even though no foreign body is present. A fluorescein stain will help detect the epithelial lesion which otherwise may not be obvious.

In most cases the foreign particle is in the epithelium or superficial layers. Numerous gun powder particles commonly following a blast injury may be found at all levels of the corneal thickness. Some high speed particles can also penetrate through the cornea to lie on the iris without causing any aqueous leakage.

Treatment of a corneal foreign body is to remove it as soon as possible. An iron particle should be the earliest to be removed because even a few hours delay may leave behind a rust stain, the consequences of which have already been described.

The removal of a superficial foreign body may be effected by a firm pointed cotton swab. A foreign body spud may be needed when it is embedded in the epithelium. A deeply placed foreign body will need a sharp pointed needle for its removal.

The area left behind after the removal of the particle should be cauterised with tincture iodine to prevent infection. If the foreign body has remained for sometime and there is an infiltration round it the raw area should be carbolized and a subconjunctival antibiotic should be given. The topical use of atropine following the removal of a corneal foreign body should be restricted to cases where the removal of a particle causes tissue trauma or when there is infiltration round the foreign body, or there is distinct ciliary congestion. Atropine need not be used for very superficial foreign bodies which can be removed with a cotton swab or a blunt spud and the patient saved from the avoidable inconvenience of visual disturbance caused by atropinisation. It however should and must be used if indicated. Patching of the eye after removal of foreign body should be done as long as the fluorescein stains the area. For superficial foreign bodies, the eye need not be patched for more than a few hours since, the epithelium grows over the clean raw area very quickly.

If there are a large number of particles on the cornea especially at different levels in its thickness like gun powder particles, their distribution at different levels can best be studied by a slit lamp. These chemical particles may remain quiet and may gradually migrate to the superficial layers and spontaneously extrude out one by one. If there are no symptoms, it is better to allow time for this process. Tissue trauma caused in removing many particles individually will affect corneal transparency. Such a case can best be treated by lamellar corneal dissection followed by a lamellar graft. This includes most particles.

Superficial abrasions: These are a common occurrence particularly in field workers. These may be caused by twigs of vegetation and domestic accidents, with nails, needles and implements in the hands of children. A defective contact lens can also cause a corneal abrasion.

The importance is whether these abrasions get secondarily infected or not. Clean abrasions should be defined with a fluorescein stain. Most clean abrasions heal within 24–72 hours time if the eye is patched after antibiotic instillation.

Infected wounds, however superficial, are a danger to the eye. The worst amongst the infections are the pyocyneous and fungal infection. Patient may sometimes come late when the infection has extended to the deeper layers and there may even be hypopyon. All such patients need energetic treatment as described for suppurative corneal ulcers.

Incised wounds. Clean incised wounds which have not perforated are commonly caused by the sharp edge of a glass piece or a sharp blade or a knife. Again, if un-infected, healing is quick and complete leaving behind a thin scar line. Infected wounds should be treated as bacterial corneal ulcers.

Perforating injuries: The first consequence of a perforating injury is leakage of aqueous, flattening of the anterior chamber and contact of the iris to the wound. If the injury is associated with some degree of force there may be an iris prolapse which acts as a protective barrier against infection entering the eye. If the impact of the force is strong, and the wound is large enough, the lens may be extruded and vitreous escapes. In a severely lacerated wound, intra-ocular haemorrhage and damage to the posterior segment reduces the eye to a state that functioning integrity is not likely to be restored.

The prevention of industrial injuries is a must. The responsibility is both on the employer to provide protective means and on the employee to use them religiously and not expose himself to hazards out of over-confidence.

Injuries to eye are for all practical purposes, the only emergency in ophthalmology which gets the patient to the doctor at the earliest and demands action at the soonest possible. A first aid kit must always be at hand in all industrial units; big and small. In a simple perforating injury, there is temporary and partial escape of aqueous, and spontaneous closure of the wound, leaving behind a quickly reformed anterior chamber and iris-lens in their normal place. Such an injury need be treated only conservatively. No repair is needed because the scar after repair will be thicker and denser as compared to a thin scar of natural healing.

If anterior chamber is not restored soon enough, a contact anterior synechia usually forms. The iris may be sticking only to the posterior edge of the wound and is not caught between the lips of the wound. Such an eye should be handled conservatively and contact synechia can easily be separated later by a synechiotomy spatula through a point puncture at the limbus. The end result of this would be a linear corneal opacity and intact anterior chamber.

In most perforating injuries, where anterior chamber has remained absent for some time, even though spontaneously restored later, the lens moves forward temporarily and contact of the anterior capsule to wound causes a mild trauma to the capsule and this leads to a small anterior capsular dot of a lens opacity. The remaining lens is otherwise transparent. Sometimes during the process of spontaneous restoration of the anterior chamber after injury, the anterior capsule of the lens is stretched and may result in a pyramidal cataract.

The iris may be caught within the lips of the wound edges or may have prolapsed out. This is indicated by the displacement of the pupil towards the point of perforation and the pupil may appear pear-shaped. Such an eye should receive prompt first aid treatment by washing the eye with sterile saline, removing any debris and eye lashes in the wound, drops of antibiotic and atropine instilled and patched with a sterile pad and bandage. It is not absolutely necessary to undertake reparative surgery instantly. These injuries usually need repair under general anaesthesia. The patient should, therefore, be properly prepared. Repair surgery is better undertaken under more favourable circumstances. A few hours time taken for preparation will not pose any problem.

The first consideration in repair is whether the prolapsed iris should be excised or returned into the anterior chamber. If injury is clean and repair is being undertaken within a few hours after the injury, it should be possible to restore the iris to its normal position. The second important point is the oedematous cut edges of the cornea. It is important to make the posterior cut edges clean with scissors so that the apposition after sutures is on the same plane posteriorly. This will prevent anterior synechia and will also leave the scar as thin as possible. The third most important thing is that, after repair of a perforating injury of the cornea, anterior chamber must be restored by injection of air through an extra limbal knife point puncture. It may be necessary to sweep the anterior chamber from across the limbus to fill the air in whole extent of anterior chamber.

It the prolapsed iris cannot be reposed because it has become adherent to wound edges and the prolapsed iris surface has become epithelialised one need not hesitate to excise the same. This becomes necessary when repair is undertaken a few days after the injury. It is possible to free the iris from the wound edges by careful dissection and excise the prolapsed part so that the cut edges retract into the anterior chamber.

Lacerated wounds, with varying amounts of corneal tissue loss, are difficult to repair with good apposition of the wound edges by edge to edge sutures. An ideal restorative surgery would be an emergency tectonic penetrating corneal graft. As a stand by, one may use a glycerine preserved donor cornea to be replaced by a fresh donor cornea soonest after the same becomes available.

This is feasible only when other posterior tissues are unaffected.

Complicated lacerated wound. Injuries where the lens has been dislocated posteriorly or extruded out and a part of vitreous has been prolapsed, repair efforts are not likely to succeed in restoring even a small degree of visual acuity. Most such injuries extend beyond the limbus into the sclera. The vitreous cavity is full of blood. One should carefully weigh the balance between a fruitless repair and enucleation of the eye ball. Repair may be undertaken only with the hope that it may restore anatomical shape of the eye ball. Even after a good repair procedure, the eye may become pthisical and remains persistently inflamed and irritable. The fear of sympathetic ophthalmitis may also be kept in mind although, the incidence of this complication is far less now because most injury cases are covered by steroids during the post-operative period. Needless to emphasise that appropriate explanation to the patient will facilitate a prior consent for enucleation if the same is considered unavoidable after detailed examination under anaesthesia or if repair surgery is found impracticable on the table.

Chemical burns: With increasing industrialisation and the advancement of chemical engineering, there is extensive use of chemicals and as a consequence, chemical injuries of eye in civilian population are becoming more and more common. Chemical injuries among the soldiers during war can also be a problem in times of such emergencies (Fig. 9.27, Plate 5).

Chemical injuries principally fall in three groups:
1. Liquid alkalies.
2. Liquid acids.
3. Gases.

Alkali burns: Among numerous alkaline agents, which cause corneal burns, lime among domestic agents, liquor ammonia fortis among laboratory reagents and caustic soda among industrial agents, are the commonest.

The special features of chemical burns of the cornea and the conjunctiva is their chronicity, recurrence of symptoms and heavy vascularisation. This is due to the fact that alkali fixes with alkaline tissues in the form of an albuminate and this chemical composition countinues to stay in the tissues and the tissue reaction persists.

Lime: It is a common reagent used for domestic purposes such as white washing. To prepare white wash, water is added to masses of quick lime (Calcium oxide) which is converted into calcium hydroxide (slaked lime) and a lot of heat and gas are liberated during this conversion. Children often curiously look into the bubbling process and due to the pressure of gas, lime blocks sometime burst with force and hot lime (calcium hydroxide) particles are sprayed into the eye. Similarly, accidental splashing of slaked lime fluid can take place during the process of white washing.

The patient develops severe irritation, burning and photophobia. Sometimes the burn initially appears mild but follows the usual course of severe symptoms in due course of time. The cornea becomes oedematous and dull. There is marked congestion and albuminous secretions from conjunctiva. Neo-vascularisation of cornea starts about one week after the accident and may be moderate to severe depending on concentration and quantity of the splash. Later the whole corneal surface becomes completely vascularised. The vascularisation is usually superficial and derived from the conjunctiva. Simultaneously changes are taking place in the surrounding conjunctiva. A symblepharon between the bulbar and palpebral conjunctiva with shallowing of the fornices is a common long-term consequence.

Ammonia burn (Liquor ammonia fortis). A common mode of accident is a splash while opening a fresh bottle of liquor ammonia fortis with its mouth pointing towards the person's face. The fluid comes under high pressure so that the blink reflex cannot prevent its entry into the eye. Ammonia burn, like lime burn, is also highly damaging. The symptoms and the tissue changes are identical to lime burn.

Caustic soda (Sodium Hydroxide-NaOH). An agent commonly used in the manufacture of soap is a cause of industrial chemical injury. It causes more destruction of tissue than lime and ammonia. The tissue changes are identical but more severe.

Prognosis of alkali burns: The ultimate prognosis of alkali burn is always uncertain. Even in apparently mild cases, the ultimate tissue changes may be severe. In addition to tissue changes in the superficial layers, there is evidence that alkali may diffuse into the anterior chamber and may cause plastic iridocyclitis. Severe inflammatory conditions of the eye may also cause cataractous changes.

Treatment. The most important consideration is prophylaxis. Effective steps should be taken in the industry. The supervisor in the laboratory must train students to keep the mouth of the bottle directed away from the face specially while opening a fresh bottle. Children should be prevented from 'enjoying' the process of bubbling of lime.

The first step in the treatment of an alkali burn is to wash the eye profusely at the nearest water tap and as soon after injury as possible. It is mostly impracticable to run for a neutralising agent and waste precious time. When the patient comes to the ophthalmologist, the conjunctival sac should be thoroughly irrigated with a mild acidic solution like boric acid lotion and all visible particles of lime should be carefully removed.

An immediate treatment is to instill a drop of atropine and advise hourly instillation of oily antibiotic and soluble steroid drops alternating with each other. Enough ointment should be placed in the conjunctival sac at bed time. **The eyes should not be patched and bandaged.** The patient should be encouraged to keep the eyes open and let the irritant fluid secretion flow out. Instillations of chemotherapeutic agents like thiotepa, an anti-cancerous and anti-mitotic drug, has been used with limited effect. It has been suggested that the fornices should be kept open by passing a glass rod in both fornices every day during the acute period to prevent symblepharon. This procedure is of questionable utility. Apart from being painful, it actually causes more tissue trauma and aggravates the process. A better procedure to prevent symblepharon is the use of fenestrated large haptic contact lens which prevents contact between the inflammed palpebral and bulbar conjunctival surfaces.

If available and possible, one of the best procedures to prevent consequent vascularisation and formation of epithelial ulcers, is to apply a glued-on contact lens (epikerato-prosthesis). An emergency total lamellar graft, if possible, can remove a large part of the alkali albuminate fixed in the tissue and thus may prevent vascularisation. Amniotic membrane transplant or stem cell grafting has proved very useful.

The following procedures have been practised:
1. Peridectomy
2. Superficial keratectomy followed by beta-radiation.
3. Excision and transfixation of false pterygia.
4. Mucous membrane or amniotic membrane grafting round the limbus.
5. Therapeutic corneal grafting.

An alkali burn case in its late stages is the poorest recipient for a lamellar corneal graft. Fresh vascularisation may develop interface between the graft and the deeper recipient bed. Protected by the tissues in front and behind, it is not reached by local therapeutic agents and therefore persists and flourishes. It is for this reason that it may be preferable to do a full thickness graft where the blood vessels are less likely to invade a compact donor button. It is even suggested that a corneal graft should be done before vascularisation develops, that is, soon after the accident.

Beta-radiation had for sometimes, been enthusiastically used for treating vascularisation of cornea, whatever the cause. Its use was indicated in chemical burns because vascularisation is the principal pathology. It should be clearly understood that Stronium-90 beta-radiation has no effect on large blood vessels. Its effect is only on the newly forming capillaries because it inhibits endothelial cell proliferation. It is, therefore, more useful for newly forming vessels and not for treating well developed vascular channels.

Acid burns: Acid burns are either accidental or happen when acid is criminally splashed into the eyes. Accidental acid burns usually occur in industry or in the laboratory. Sulphuric acid is the commonest acid used in industries and is readily available in the market. Criminal splash of acids is not only to blind a person but also to grieviously disfigure the person. The burns are usually bilateral. Hydrochloric and nitric acid burns are usually the result of laboratory accidents.

Sulphuric acid is highly destructive and causes total disintegration of the tissues involved. The action is so quick that the tissues are grieviously damaged before any help is available. The lids may be partly or completely destroyed. The cornea may be liquefied and iris exposed. There are concurrent acid burns on the face and other parts of the body.

Soon after, the cicatrising process starts. In cases, where the involvement is largely of the skin, lag ophthalmos, ectropion and keloids on the face and body are the common consequences of acid burns. There is no secondary infection for obvious reasons.

When there is enough acid entry into the conjunctival sac, resulting changes are obliteration of fornices, secondary pterygium and heavily vascularised corneal opacity. The lids may be adherent to the eye ball or the two lid margins may be ankylosed. Where cornea had completely disintegrated, the end result is a phthisical eye.

Milder acids like acetic acid cause lighter damage and usually result in a vascularised corneal haze.

There are a number of other acidic liquids and vegetable juices which may accidentally fall in the eye or are used as a therapy. They cause conjunctival reaction, chemosis and epithelial oedema.

Treatment: The stronger acids are so destructive that neutralising the acid is hardly ever practicable. However the eye should be immediately and profusely washed with alkaline solution like 2% sodium bicarbonate to remove free acid, if any.

Local treatment includes an oily antibiotic drop frequently instilled into the eye. As soon as the acute stage is over, skin grafting will be needed to reconstruct the lids if necessary. A tectonic emergency total corneal graft may be undertaken even with a preserved donor cornea in eyes where the whole cornea is destroyed and iris is bare, to preserve the anatomical integrity of the eye ball. This is possible only if the lid coverage of the cornea is adequate. An optical penetrating corneal graft may later be considered if the lids have been only partially damaged or the destroyed lids have been satisfactorily reconstructed. Preparatory to corneal grafting, restoration of fornices, surgery for secondary pterygia by conjunctivoplasty or mucous grafting will often be necessary. The optical results of corneal grafting have however been disappointing.

CORNEAL SCARS

Once the active disease has started regressing, the healing lesion gets epithelialised. The newly formed stromal fibres which, to begin with, are irregularly placed, tend to reorganise themselves in a more regular pattern reducing the density of corneal opacity. The resolution of simple opacity is quicker and to a greater degree in children and adolescents but slow and incomplete in older patients. If however, there is a fibroblastic reaction, the corneal scar is dense and shows no tendency towards resolution. The final result of a healing process of a corneal ulcer may leave behind varying degrees of corneal opacity. The classification of corneal opacity is based on its density and not the depth of opacity. The different grades are classified as follows.

Simple scars:

1. *Epithelial facets.* This does not appear as an opacity but only causes an irregularity of the corneal surface. Retinoscopy indicates irregular refraction due to irregular corneal astigmatism.

2. *Nebular corneal opacity.* This is a thin opacity where the arrangement of stromal fibres has been disturbed. The inner structures of the eye can be seen e.g. pupillary reaction, iris pattern and depth of the anterior chamber etc. but visual loss is out of proportion to the degree of nebular corneal opacity.

3. *Macular opacity.* This is denser in appearance. Vision is markedly impaired. Deeper structures can be seen but not clearly.

4. *Leucomatous opacity.* This is dense white opacity and is the result of thick scarring. Deeper structures are not visible through it. If central, it causes gross defect in vision.

Depth of opacity in the cornea is different from these grades of density of opacity. A thin nebular opacity may be mid-stromal or deeper near the decemets membrane and a dense white leucoma may be limited to only superficial 1/3 or 1/2 of the corneal thickness (Fig. 9.28 and Fig. 9.29A, 9.29B Plate 6).

Corneal scars with Iris involvement-Leucoma Adherens: Incarceration of iris tissue in a corneal scar results if there is perforation of the cornea.

At the time of perforation the aqueous escapes and the iris lens diaphragm moves forward. Iris incarceration depends on how quickly the anterior chamber gets restored after perforation and the extent of the area of corneal perforation. When perforation heals with incarcerated iris tissue, a leucoma adherens results which may be partial or total depending on the size of the corneal scar (Fig. 9.30).

Clinically, the diagnosis of iris incarceration in the scar can be made either when iris pigment is seen in the scar or if shallow or absent anterior

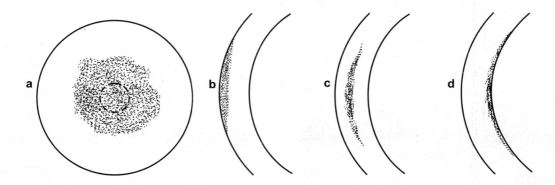

Fig. 9.28: (a) Corneal opacity and its Depth determined by Slit-Lamp Examination; (b) Opacity in superficial stromal layers; (c) Opacity in mid-stromal layers; (d) Opacity in deep stroma near the Descemet's membrane.

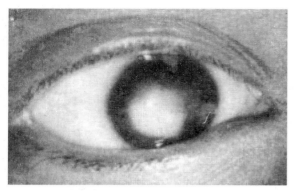

Fig. 9.29A: Simple leucomatous opacity

chamber can be noted through the clear part of cornea as in partial leucoma adherens. Most such eyes have very poor vision.

Corneal scars with ectasia: (a) *Simple keratectasia* is a condition when a corneal lesion heals without perforation but with loss of stromal tissue resulting in reduced corneal thickness. This thinner cornea may yield even under normal intra-ocular pressure and bulge forward, (b) *Deceme-tocele* is when whole thickness of corneal stroma has been destroyed in a localised area and only

the Decemet's membrane persists and bulges forwards (c) *Staphylomatous scars*. When corneal anatomy has been disorganised and the whole corneal thickness is replaced by scar tissue, the result is what is called pseudo-cornea. Pseudo-cornea is weaker than the normal cornea. With extensive iris incarceration, absent anterior chamber and consequent rise of intra-ocular tension, the pseudo-cornea becomes ectatic.

The greater the extent of scarring of cornea and incarceration of the iris, the more is the ectasia. Ectatic corneal scars with incarcerated iris tissue are called *anterior staphyloma* which may be partial or total depending on the extent of the corneal surface involved (Figs 9.31, 9.32 and 9.33).

Long standing corneal scars may undergo degenerative changes. Old scars may break down and cause recurrent irritation. Other

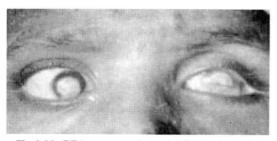

Fig 9.30: RE Leucoma adherens; LE Atrophic bulbi.

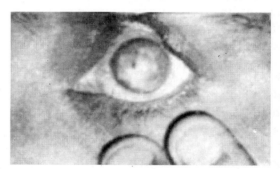

Fig. 9.32: Total Anterior staphyloma; LE front view

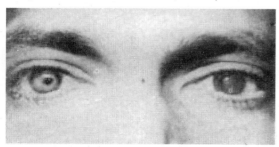

Fig. 9.31: RE Descemetocele

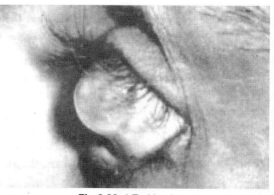

Fig 9.33: LE side view

degenerative changes include keratinisation, calcareous degeneration and atheromatous ulcer formation.

Complicated corneal scars like total leucoma adherence, partial or total anterior staphyloma are often associated with gross tissue changes in the eye. The angle of the anterior chamber is obliterated by extensive peripheral anterior synechiae. The lens is often cataractous and is sometimes adherent to the scarred cornea. Vitreous is fluid and degenerated. There are glaucomatous changes in the disc. All such eyes should be presumed to be glaucomatous even though tonometry is not practicable on the distorted scarred pseudocornea. Most such eyes lose vision and may not have even light perception. Staphylomatous eyes are in many cases, painful blind eyes. Some eyes however retain good light perception and even projection. But that should in most cases not change our outlook of very poor visual prognosis. Even if a total corneal graft (TPK) remains transparent, there is no improvement in vision in most cases. Rarely, however, such eyes have regained vision after TPK but that should not be expected in more than 1 in 5 cases.

Corneal opacity is also often a cosmetic problem particularly in young girls and unmarried boys. An associated squint in uniocular corneal opacities may further aggravate the cosmetic blemish. An advanced protruding anterior staphyloma gives an unsightly appearance. Even a cosmetic shell cannot be fitted on these eyes.

Resolution of corneal-opacity: The resolution of corneal opacity with or without topical treatment takes place to a limited extent but only in simple corneal opacities without iris incarceration. The younger the age and the thinner and more recent the opacity, more are the chances of spontaneous resolution.

Spontaneous resolution of a corneal opacity is possible because the cornea is biologically a very active tissue, even though it is avascular. The collagen fibres have an inherent capacity to rearrange themselves after small to moderate disturbances in its arrangement. This morphological re-arrangement is more significant when the fibrils are in a phase of maturation as in young age. Thin and fresh opacities in young age therefore show a definite tendency to resolve.

The active process of resolution of a recent corneal opacity continues even upto one year. The result may at times be surprisingly pleasant. After a certain time, however, the process of resolution ceases and then surgical treatment may be considered.

Treatment: The treatment of corneal opacities and scars is optical and sometimes only cosmetic.

Optical treatment: Conservative treatment which would help resolution of opacity has been tried with limited results. Dionine (Ethyl morphine hydro-chloride) as 2% drops or ointment, 10% ointment of yellow oxide of mercury, sub-conjunctival injections of normal saline and oxycyanide of mercury were used in olden times when corneal grafting had not become a routine surgery.

Contact lenses may improve vision appreciably when corneal opacity is thin and the visual defect is largely due to irregular corneal astigmatism. A contact lens trial should therefore be done in all cases of thin opacity before considering a corneal graft.

Surgery is indicated in cases of dense and complicated corneal scars. Surgery should however be delayed till the active inflammation persists and enough time, usually 4-6 months, has been allowed for any chance of resolution either with treatment or spontaneous as in young patient.

Optical iridectomy had long been practised to improve vision in eyes with dense central corneal opacities. Optical iridectomy has however, very great limitations. The resulting improvement of vision is limited because the light passes through the peripheral cornea which has irregular refraction and light through periphery of cornea does not focus on the macular area. An optical iridectomy is a distinct disadvantage when a full thickness graft is planned at a later stage.

Optical iridectomy for a corneal opacity should be limited to where a corneal grafting is not indicated or the patient does not want graft surgery. It may also be considered in one eyed patients with complicated corneal scar where there is chance of graft failure and the possibility of the patient losing whatever vision he has.

Optical corneal grafting. In the present era, the ideal treatment for corneal opacity is corneal grafting. Whether a partial thickness lamellar graft or a full thickness penetrating graft is needed can be dependably determined by a careful slit lamp examination which must be done in all cases before deciding on grafting surgery. In complicated scars like total leucoma adherence and partial or total anterior staphyloma, grafting procedure needs to be more complex and one may have to do a sub-total or total penetrating keratoplasty with extraction of the lens and removal of peripheral tags of the iris from its attachment to the ciliary body better called *reconstruction of anterior segment.*

It is possible to repeat corneal grafting and repeat it as often as is needed so long as perfect light projection is retained and the anatomical integrity of the eye ball is intact. In eyes where a corneal graft has repeatedly failed or is definitely not likely to succeed, the surgery indicated is *kerato-prosthesis.*

Cosmetic treatment. This is necessary when optical treatment is either not indicated or is not likely to succeed and where social rehabilitation of the person is important. Social rehabilitation may, in some persons be as important as visual rehabilitation in others.

Tattooing of a corneal opacity has always been an unsatisfactory treatment not only because the colour rarely matches the colour of the iris but also because the pigment impregnated in corneal tissue gets phagocytosed and removed and so the procedure needs to be repeated. When a chemically active reagent as a colouring agent is used, it may excite iridocyclitis which may do more harm. The reagents used for tattooing are Indian ink and platinum chloride for dark black eyes and gold chloride for deep brown eyes.

A cosmetic contact lens shell can be fitted on a opaque cornea provided the corneal surface is regular. It is better than tattooing because the painting of the shell can be matched to the opposite eye.

Corneal grafting as a cosmetic treatment has a definite place although of a low priority as compared to optical and therapeutic keratoplasty. In most cases, a lamellar graft should be preferred for cosmetic purposes even though it may mean leaving behind some deeper opacity. The biological effect of a donor lamellar button will further help resolution of the deeper opacity to some degree. The cosmetic improvement which may be only 50% soon after operation may be come 75% nine months to a year later. Only in very few cases, a cosmetic penetrating graft may be undertaken as in dense leucomatous opacity, in partial and total anterior staphyloma. Total penetrating graft, even if it becomes opaque will provide a uniform corneal surface on which a painted cosmetic contact shell can be fitted.

CONGENITAL ANOMALIES OF CORNEA

Mal-development may affect the size, shape, curvature and thickness of cornea. Some of the common anomalies are described below:

Megalo-cornea: Any cornea which is over 13 mm in diameter is called megalo-cornea. In this condition, cornea remains clear. There are no tears in the Decemet's membrane. Corneal curvature and thickness are within normal limits. The condition is non-progressive and vision is not grossly affected (Fig. 9.34).

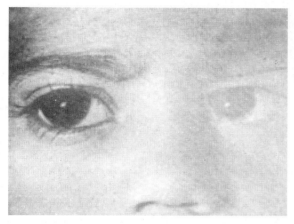

Fig. 9.34: RE Megalo-cornea. LE normal corneal size with macular opacity

Micro-cornea: Any cornea which is smaller than 9 mm diameter is called a micro-cornea.

Micro-cornea is commonly associated with coloboma of iris and choroid. There may sometimes be a coloboma of the lens also. The size of the eye ball is within normal limits. When bilateral, congenital nystagmus is present, vision is impaired but eye is not blind. The eyes are prone to develop lenticular changes with further deterioration of vision by adult age (Fig. 9.35).

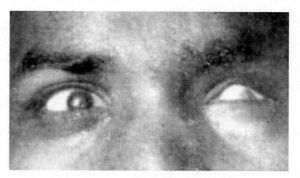

Fig. 9.35: RE Micro-cornea and macular opacity. LE microphthalmos with total opacity

In severe degrees, cornea may be very small 5 mm or less. These eyes are also microphthalmic and are always blind. A very small eye ball with a small cornea may be sitting on a congenital cyst called *microphthalmos with cyst*.

Keratoglobus: Keratoglobus is a large cornea of a large eye ball with increased curvature. The cornea is thinner in periphery but clear. Tension is normal. The condition is usually bilateral and familial. It differs from megalo-cornea in that in keratoglobus the eye ball is larger while in megalo cornea only the cornea is larger.

The table gives the differentiating features of the four conditions which have some common features. These are, megalo-cornea, kerato-globus, buphthalmos and keratoconus (Table below).

	Megalo cornea	Keratoglobus	Buphthalmos	Keratoconus
a. Corneal diameter	Large	Large	Large	Normal
b. Eye ball size	Normal	Large	Large	Normal
c. Corneal curvature	Normal	More convex	More convex	Conical
d. Corneal thickness	Normal	Thinner in periphery	Increased when oedematous	Thinner in the centre
e. Descemet's Membrane	Normal	Normal	Tears all over	Tears in centre
f. Anterior chamber	Normal	Deep	Deep	Deep
g. Angle of Anterior chamber	Normal	Normal	Occluded by embryonic mesodermal tissue	Normal
h. Tension	Normal	Normal	Raised	Normal
i. Vision	Fair to good	Reduced	Markedly impaired	Reduced
j. Other features	Bilateral familial	Bilateral congenital hereditary	Unilateral or bilateral sometimes familial	Unilateral or bilateral hereditary

Arcus juvenilis: It is a peripheral ring of opacity partial or complete which may be present at birth or appear in adolescence. It is usually bilateral, does not involve the central cornea and does not affect vision. It very much resembles arcus senilis excepting the age factor (Fig. 9.36).

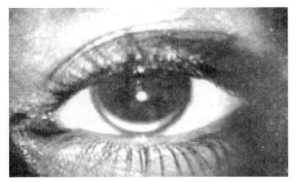

Fig 9.36: Arcus juvenilis with clear corneal rim between the limbus and arcus.

Congenital opacities of the cornea and congenital anterior staphyloma are conditions which are usually the result of intra-uterine inflammations and ulceration of the cornea. These conditions in no way differ from those in adults except that they are present at birth.

LIMBUS

Limbus, in the anatomical sense, is neither the cornea nor the sclera. It is the junctional one millimeter zone of transition between the two. It is however, a very important area both from physiological as well as surgical point of view.

a. The transition from squamous epithelium of the conjunctiva to the stratified epithelium of the cornea takes place here.

b. This is also the zone of anastomosis between the posterior conjunctival and the terminal branches of anterior ciliary vessels.

c. Because of its closeness to the ciliary body, it reacts to the intra-ocular inflammations.

d. The limbus is closely related to trabecular mesh work and the canal of Schlemn, important for aqueous out flow.

It is the engorgement of the anastomotic vessels which is called the circum-corneal or ciliary congestion, a common manifestation of iridocyclitis, congestive glaucoma etc.

Pathologically, conjunctival and scleral lesions may encroach the limbus. To name a few, bulbar spring catarrh, deep scleritis and trachoma. Similarly, corneal lesions may also extend to the limbus e.g. Mooren's ulcer. The reverse is also true. Primary limbal lesions may extend to the cornea or the conjunctiva and sclera like phlyctenular ophthalmia, limbal squamous cell carcinoma, limbal dermoid etc. (Figs 9.37 and 9.38).

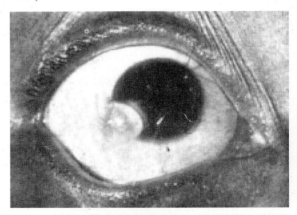

Fig 9.37: Limbal dermoid

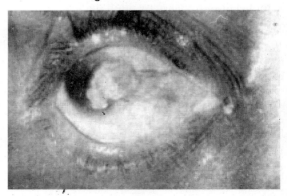

Fig 9.38: Limbal carcinoma encroaching on the cornea. (Note the big blood vessels under conjunctiva reaching the growth).

Clinically, most lesions, primarily limbal in origin, are nodular. A limbal nodule can be present in the following conditions:

1. Congenital dermoid.
2. Foreign body granuloma
3. Retention cyst
4. Phlyctenular nodules
5. Parasitic cysts
6. Syphilitic nodule
7. Tuberculoma
8. Leprotic nodule
9. Limbal epithelioma
10. Post-operative lesion
    a. Cystoid cicatrix
    b. Bleb of glaucoma surgery
11. Extensions from intra-ocular lesions
    a. Syphilitic gumma or tuberculoma
    b. Intra-ocular malignant tumours
    c. Melanoma of iris or ciliary body
    d. Diktyoma of ciliary body

Clinical diagnosis in most cases is not difficult. History, clinical examination under magnification and a slit lamp examination will be helpful. Differential diagnosis is however necessary in conditions appearing identical. Sometimes an excision biopsy is necessary.

The treatment of most lesions has been described at appropriate places. In non-inflammatory conditions, simple excision is possible and safe because, the thickness here is 1.2 to 1.5 mm. However if dissection has to be deep and involves a larger area, the gap may be supported with an identical corneo-scleral graft from a donor eye.

SCLERA

The sclera is the white opaque, protective outer coat of the eyeball forming 5/6th of the outer coat, the remaining l/6th being the cornea.

It is interesting that although both the cornea and sclera are developed from mesoderm, they behave differently in function. The sclera which is transparent in early embryonic life becomes opaque before birth while the cornea continues to retain its transparency. The opaque character of the sclera is due to the irregular arrangement of collagen fibres, scanty matrix between the collagen fibres and gross difference in the refractive index between the collagen fibres and the scanty mucopolysaccharides of the matrix.

The sclera has a diameter of 24 millimeters and a circumference of 72 millimeters. It has an average thickness of 1 mm but is reduced at the attachments of four recti muscles and is very thin where it forms lamina cribrosa through which optic nerve fibres pass.

The sclera on the inner surface is lined by choroid posteriorly and ciliary body anteriorly. On the outer surface, it is covered by Tenon's capsule. The four recti are inserted into the sclera in front of the equator, while the two obliques are attached behind the equator.

The anterior opening of the sclera into which the corneal disc fits, is round and 12 mm in diameter. Just behind the anterior edge of the scleral opening is the circular canal of Schlemn lying within the scleral thickness. The sclera is perforated by various structures, some from inside out and others from outside inwards. These structures from before backwards are:

1. Perforating branches of seven anterior ciliary arteries dipping in at right angles to supply blood to the iris and ciliary body. These arteries perforate the sclera about 3–5 mm from limbus.
2. The four vortex veins, two above, and two below pass from inside out through the sclera obliquely from before backwards, leaving the scleral surface behind the equator.
3. Posterior ciliary arteries, short and long, pass through the sclera from without inwards near the posterior pole around the optic nerve.

4. The structures passing through the lamina cribrosa, the cribriform plate of the sclera, are (a) axons of ganglion cells forming optic nerve fibres, from within outwards (b) central retinal vein from within out wards and (c) central retinal artery from without inwards along with sympathetic plexus.

The sclera is a relatively avascular and acellular structure. The deeper sclera is formed of compact connective tissue fibres, has few blood vessels and few cells. The superficial part, the episclera, is formed of loose connective and elastic tissue with more blood vessels and lymphatics.

Physiologically, sclera is an insert tissue with limited metabolic activity. Its functions are mainly protective and it is likely to give way under high intra-ocular tension.

The episcleral layers being more vascular, suffer from inflammatory conditions more often than the relatively avascular, acellular and inert inner layers. The inflammations of the deeper sclera are usually a part of inflammation of the underlying uveal tissue. Similarly, neoplastic invasion of the sclera is always secondary to intra-ocular neoplasm. The sclera also suffers from pathologies which are systemic particularly the collagen diseases.

Diseases of Sclera

There are three groups of clinical conditions which affect sclera. *Inflammations of the sclera* are either due to a systemic cause or are extensions from adjacent tissues. The second group are *necrotising conditions* which are chronic in nature and in majority of cases are secondary to collagen diseases. The third group consists of *ectatic conditions* where the sclera gives way either due to local pathology or due to raised intra-ocular tension.

Inflammations of Sclera

Inflammations involving sclera are either episcleral or deep scleral and are respectively called episcleritis and deep scleritis. The incidence is common in adults and aged persons. It may involve either one or both eyes. The etiology of primary inflammations is identical in both types of scleritis. Gout, rheumatic fever have, for long, been attributed to be the causes. Most cases of primary scleritis are considered to be due to collagen diseases of the body. Allergy to tuberculous proteins and streptococcal infection in septic foci should also be looked for in cases of inflammations of the sclera.

Episcleritis: This is an inflammation of the superficial layers of sclera.

The patient complains of localised redness and dull pain. Clinically, a localised swelling is seen in the visible part of the anterior sclera. The circumscribed lesion is covered by a congested conjunctiva. The conjunctiva is, however, freely movable over the area of inflammation. The conjunctiva over the area of episcleritis does not break down. Episcleritis usually does not involve cornea and therefore does not affect vision. A characteristic feature of episcleritis is its tendency to recur at intervals.

Although not common, diffuse type of episcleritis may be seen, which may extend posteriorly behind equator. The dull pain, transient and recurring history and diffuse redness of the bulbar conjunctiva in absence of any other cause to explain, may be criteria for diagnosis. Because of these characters, the diffuse episcleritis is called *episcleritis periodica Fugax*. A history or evidence of rheumatic disease or other collagen diseases will help in diagnosis (Fig. 9.39).

Important differential diagnosis of an episcleritic lesion is from phlyctenular conjunctivitis because both are nodular with localised congestion and both have a tendency to recur.

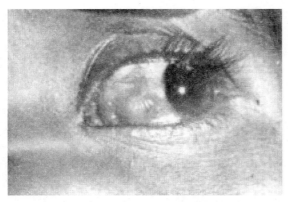

Fig 9.39: Episcleritis. (Note the large nodular lesion with superficial Vascularisation)

Unlike episcleritis, phlycten is in younger children and causes acute symptoms. In a phlycten, the conjunctiva breaks down which never happens in episcleritis. Phlycten may also involve cornea which episcleritis does not.

Treatment: Local treatment consists of repeated instillations of steroid drops which may be started every 2 hours and the frequency reduced as the condition improves. Hot compresses relieve symptoms. Systemic administration of drugs is only necessary in severe cases particularly the diffuse variety. Anti-inflammatory drugs and salicylates help relieve symptoms and help resolution of the condition quickly. Most of the patients respond to this treatment leaving behind very little after effect. In recurrent cases, treatment of systemic pathology, if evident, should be instituted.

Deep scleritis: It is less common but more serious. It lasts longer and causes severe symptoms. It is frequently associated with underlying uveitis and the association is so common that it has been questioned whether uveitis or scleritis is primary.

Clinically, the raised scleral area is larger in size and less defined. The conjunctiva over the area is congested and appears as a pinkish purple discolouration due to deeply placed capillary network.

Deep scleritis when near the limbus may extend into the deeper stromal layers of the cornea. The condition is then called *sclerosing keratitis*. Being associated with uveitis, there is evidence of iridocyclitis like keratic precipitate on endothelial surface of cornea, aqueous flare and posterior synechiae. When deep scleritis involves posterior sclera, there may be patches of choroiditis. Posterior deep scleritis may also sometimes cause orbital cellulitis and proptosis.

Being a lesion in deeper layers of sclera, it leaves behind a dull porcelain colour in the area after healing. The scleral area may sometimes become ectatic and staphylomatous. Systemic investigations to determine the causative factor will help not only diagnosis but also treatment.

Prognosis of deep scleritis so far as vision is concerned is unfavourable unless inflammation is controlled quickly.

Treatment is oral steroids in full therapeutic doses. Steroids should also be administered subconjunctivally or as local instillations. Atropine should be used whenever there is evidence of iridocyclitis. Anti-inflammatory drugs and salicylates will further help reduce inflammation and relieve symptoms.

Necrotising scleritis: Necrotic lesions of sclera, although rare, can cause serious damage to eye ball. The inflammation is usually subacute or chronic in nature and inflammatory reaction disturbs the mucopolysaccharides leading to necrosis, sloughing and exposure of the underlying uveal tissue. When this stage is reached, it is called *scleromalacia perforans*. Depending on the degree of sloughing and the area involved, the eye suffers serious damage. There may be many areas of necrosis leading to disorganisation of the eye ball (Fig. 9.40). Cyclo photo coagulation with Diode laser done for non responding secondary rise of IOP—may cause necrotising scleritis.

Poly-arthritic rheumatoid arthritis should always be looked . In all necrotic lesions of sclera, the possibility of tuberculosis and syphilitic gumma

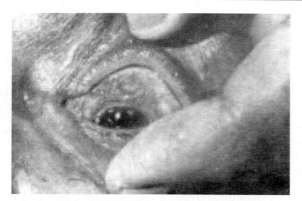

Fig. 9.40: Necrotising Scleritis. (Note the Necrotic Sclera above the limbus)

should be excluded by systemic examination and investigations.

Complications are iritis, vitreous opacities, opacities of the lens, rise of intraocular tension and rarely panophthalmitis if secondary bacterial infection invades the inner eye.

Treatment is very unsatisfactory. Steroids should be given under careful observation. Localised lesions may be covered with a scleral graft. More seriously disorganised eyes need enucleation.

Ectatic Conditions of the Sclera

Being a relatively avascular and acellular structure, it is weaker and can give way following inflammations or following severe rise of intraocular tension.

Being thin and less rigid in infancy, it can undergo generalised expansion with rise of intraocular tension as in buphthalmos. Generalised expansion also exists with total anterior staphyloma.

Localised ectasia of sclera is however a more common clinical observation. These local lesions are called staphylomata. The common types of scleral staphylomata are:

1. **Intercalary staphyloma** is when the ectasia involves the anterior most part of sclera between the limbus in front and the anterior edge of the ciliary body behind. It is commonly present in eyes with absolute glaucoma.

2. **Ciliary staphyloma** is when the sclera covering the outer surface of ciliary body becomes ectatic. It starts at the openings of the perforating branches of anterior ciliary arteries. This is commonly due to inflammatory and degenerative changes of the ciliary body.

3. **Equatorial staphyloma** is when ectasia involves equtorial part of the sclera. The weakest spots there, are the vortex veins passing through the sclera. Most of cases of equatorial staphyloma are due to high intra-

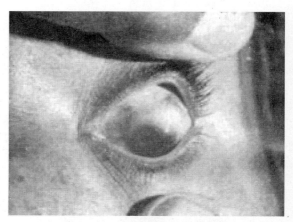

Fig. 9.41: Early ciliary staphyloma

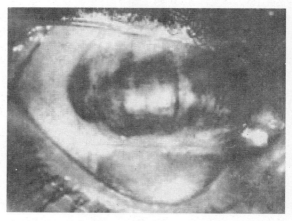

Fig. 9.42: Ciliary staphyloma advanced. (Note the pigmented ciliary body showing through the ectatic thin sclera.

ocular tension either in absolute glaucoma or due to intra-ocular growths.

4. **Posterior staphyloma** is a smooth back-ward bulging of sclera around the posterior pole. It extends to about 4-6 disc diameter area. The main cause is high myopia.

5. **A deep glaucomatous** cupping is ectasia of lamina cribrosa of sclera at the optic nerve head and there being no uveal tissue lining, it is not a staphyloma in the strict sense.

Eyes with inter-calary, ciliary and equatorial staphyloma including the total anterior staphyloma (of cornea) are all lined by uveal tissue under-neath, it being iris in anterior and intercalary staphyloma, ciliary body in ciliary staphyloma and choroid in equatorial staphyloma. Most eyes with these staphylomata are blind due to damage caused by raised tension.

Treatment of staphylomatous eyes is obviously very unsatisfactory. The eyes are blind and PL PR even if present, is rarely accurate. These eyes are better removed at least from the cosmetic point of view so that a better implant or prothesis can be fitted. When it is possible to retain the scleral shell as in anterior staphyloma, intra-scleral spherical implant (after excising the corneal part and thoroughly curetting out all the contents of the eye ball and specially all traces of uveal tissue lining the scleral shell) can be inserted. The anterior opening is closed with sutures. The cosmetic contact shell can be fitted after healing is complete. It is colour matched to other eye. The intrascleral prosthesis with active recti muscles which are not disturbed during evisceration surgery, provides fair motility.

10

Anterior Chamber

It is a space between the cornea in front and the iris and lens behind. The depth of the anterior chamber is on an average 2.5 mm at the pupillary border and 3.0 mm in the pupillary area. The volume of the anterior chamber is not more than .25 to .3 cc. The space is filled with aqueous humour which enters the anterior chamber through the pupil and leaves by the angle of anterior chamber. This flow of aqueous is partly facilitated by the difference of temperature between cornea and lens. This induces a convection current in the anterior chamber. When seen on slit lamp, normal aqueous humour is absolutely clear containing no partculate or cellular material. No light rays are reflected and therefore it is described as *optically empty*.

Angle of Anterior Chamber

Anatomically, actual angle of the anterior chamber is formed by the peripheral part of the anterior surface of the ciliary body and inner surface of sclera behind the limbus. The angle

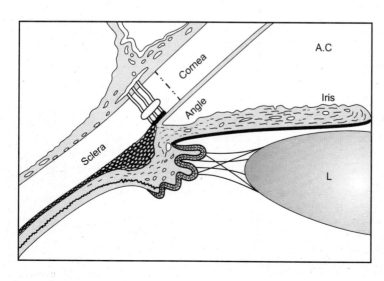

Fig. 10.1: Anterior chamber angle

of anterior chamber is therefore 0.5 mm behind limbus. Functionally it extends from the root of the iris behind to Schwalbe's line in front. On examination with gonioscope, the structures are seen in the following order from behind forwards:
1. Root of the iris.
2. Sinus or dark hiatus of peripheral part of the anterior surface of the ciliary body.
3. Trabecular mesh work underlining canal of Schlemn in deeper layers of sclera posterior to limbus.
4. Dome of cornea demarcated posteriorly by the thick end of Decemet's membrane called Schwalbe's line.

Canal of Schlemn

It is a circular narrow potential space situated within the sclera just behind the limbus. The canal communicates internally with the anterior chamber through the trabecular mesh work and spaces of Fontana. It communicates externally with aqueous veins through a few connecting channels of intrascleral venous plexus, the aqueous draining ultimately into the aqueous veins. Between the canal of Schlemn and trabecular mesh work on the inner surface of sclera, is a thin fibrous band (scleral spur) to which are attached few fibres of the longitudinal muscle of ciliary body, supplied by sympathetic nerve. The scleral spur helps in drainage of fluid from anterior chamber into canal of Schlemn and thus controls maintenance of normal intra-ocular pressure.

The *trabecular mesh work* is a spongy reticular tissue between canal of Schlemn and the angular zone of anterior chamber. The spaces in the mesh work are called spaces of Fontana which are lined by continuation of the corneal endothelium. The aqueous passes through the spaces into canal of Schlemn.

Aqueous veins are venous channels which carry the aqueous into the venous system. They also carry blood from the intrascleral plexus of veins. They can be seen with slit lamp more often beyond the lower limbus and identified by a bilamellar fluid column, half blood and half aqueous. This can be accentuated by pressure on the eye ball.

PATHOLOGY IN ANTERIOR CHAMBER

From clinical point of view, anterior chamber is a poor victim of not only immediate neighbours but also of the distant members of the human body and takes more than its share of suffering. Corneal infections can fill it with pus, the iris can invade the space of anterior chamber, the lens matter can also trespass into it, the vitreous finds it easy to protrude into it after lens is removed, the ciliary body can make the anterior chamber dirty. Even tumour cells from retinoblastoma can find their way into anterior chamber and intestinal parasites can get a joy ride into the anterior chamber.

The Abnormal Contents of Anterior Chamber are Clinically Designated As

1. Blood in anterior chamber—Hyphema
2. Pus and exudates in A.C.—Hypopyon.
3. Foreign body in the anterior chamber.
4. Neoplastic deposits.

Hyphaema

The term indicates collection of blood in anterior chamber. The characteristic clinical feature so long as it is fluid, is the horizontal level of the blood in sitting position which spreads on the iris or goes in the posterior chamber when the patient is lying. If blood is partly or wholly clotted, the clinical appearance changes from bright red to darkish red. If hyphaema has persisted or has not been treated in time, blood staining of the cornea can obscure clear visualisation.

Causes of Hyphaema and Sources of Blood in Anterior Chamber May Be

1. From the conjunctival blood vessels during intra-ocular operative procedure. A sub-conjunctival bleeding following cataract operation, can get into anterior chamber if cataract section has not been securely sutured.

2. Newly formed blood vessels across cataract section may bleed into anterior chamber following post-operative trauma to the eye which may appear mild and insignificant.

3. The radial branches at the root of the iris are a common cause of bleeding into the anterior chamber following traumatic or operative iridodialysis.

4. From iris vasculature: Normally the iris does not bleed even when cut but a highly inflamed iris tends to bleed spontaneously.

5. Neo-vascularisation in iris (rubeosis) for example in diabetes and trunk block of the central retinal vein. These abnormal vessels can readily bleed into anterior chamber.

6. Bleeding in the vitreous chamber, particularly an expulsive heamorrhage from chorio-capillaries may sometimes seep forwards into anterior chamber.

7. Hyphaema may be present without an evident cause. Silent iridocyclitis in elderly patients may cause a symptomless and persistent hyphaema. An intraocular malignancy like a vascularised tumour should be considered in elderly patients if no other known cause can be found.

Fate of hyphaema. In eyes with a healthy iris, hyphaema tends to get absorbed by itself unless there is recurrence or persistent bleeding. The absorption largely takes place through iris tissue. The absorption may sometimes be so quick that the anterior chamber may be full of blood one day and next day it may all disappear. Fluid blood gets absorbed quicker than clotted blood.

Absorption is, however, slowed down if iris is atrophic.

If hyphaema remains or is allowed to remain without surgical interference for more than 4–5 days, blood pigment tends to migrate into the cornea, through the endothelial surface and causes blood staining of the cornea. Cornea staining occurs earlier when there is a co-existing rise of intraocular tension.

Treatment: Whatever the cause, hyphaema should be actively treated. Heavy doses of Vitamin C will help prevent fresh bleeding. Ocular hypotensives will help prevent rise of intra-ocular tension.

Local therapy: The use of atropine has been contested for the reason that by dilating pupil iris surface is reduced which slows absorption. On the other hand, atropine counteracts mild iritis if present and being a vasoconstrictor, it helps reduce fresh bleeding. Atropine should be used if there is ciliary congestion, but in quiet eyes, it may be avoided. An injection of urokinase (an enzyme of human origin) in concentration of 1000 units per cc of saline into the anterior chamber helps break down the blood clots. This is better than streptokinase (fibrinolysin) because the latter can cause antigenic reactions.

Hyphaema should be drained, if it has not shown any tendency to absorb by about fifth day. It should not be delayed, if there is raised intra-ocular tension. In any case, drainage should be promptly undertaken at the earliest sign of corneal staining.

The surgical procedure for drainage of hyphaema is simple. A small Graefe's knife incision is made at the limbus, an iris repositor is introduced depressing the posterior lip of the incision. The liquid blood flows out. Full air is injected into the anterior chamber which by pressure helps prevent fresh bleeding. A suture will need to be applied if the knife opening is large and air tends to leak out.

Clotted blood however does not easily flow out. The section may have to be enlarged at least 3-4 mm and blood clots washed out with saline or aspirated through a large bore canula.

Hypopyon

The term means collection of exudates or pus in anterior chamber. Like hyphaema, as long as the pus is fluid in nature, it shows horizontal level in the anterior chamber when the patient is in sitting position. If, however, the pus is thick and heavily fibrinous, it does not form a level nor change position. Corneal pathology is one important cause for exudates in anterior chamber, when iridocyclitis is associated (Fig. 10.2, Plate 6).

Pus in anterior chamber may also be part of pan-ophthalmitis which is associated with pan-uveitis. A posterior corneal abscess may rupture into the anterior chamber and initiate eyelids and aggravate the hypopyon.

Treatment: Treatment should be concentrated on the cause. Antibiotic therapy by various roots, carbolisation of the ulcer when present are important in treatment of hypopyon. Repeated atropinisation is a must. Hypopyon is rarely drained and it may be indicated only when the anterior chamber is full of pus and causes rise of tension.

Extraneous Material in the Anterior Chamber

A foreign body in the anterior chamber is rarely freely moving. It usually rests on the iris or the lens and remains stuck there. Removal will need picking up a little iris tissue along with the foreign particle and excising the same. A large foreign body like a wooden splinter may be projecting in the anterior chamber. If it cannot be picked up from the corneal surface, it may need to be pushed from within the anterior chamber with an iris spatula introduced through a limbal puncture.

Among neoplastic deposits, retinoblastoma cells are known to float in the anterior chamber and stick on endothelial surface of the cornea. Being an intra-ocular pathology, treatment is directed towards the neoplastic growth.

Among parasites which have been reported to be present in the anterior chamber, filaria and parasitic cysts have been frequently reported. It usually excites iridocyclitis and therefore should be removed promptly.

Angle Pathology

Morphologically, the ultimate pathology of primary glaucoma is in the angle of the anterior chamber. Peripheral anterior synachiae and shallow anterior chamber are manifestations of angle closure glaucoma. Sclerosis of aqueous veins draining from the angle of the anterior chamber is a cause of open angle glaucoma.

Similarly, secondary glaucoma due to loss of communication between the anterior and posterior chamber is caused by ring posterior synechia, swollen lens or vitreous herniation blocking the pupil.

Traumatic glaucoma is also due to injury to the tissues of the angle of the anterior chamber. Blunt injury can cause rise of intra-ocular tension due to lacerations of the trabecular mesh work, tearing off of the longitudinal ciliary muscle fibres from their attachment to the scleral spur, blockage of the supra-choroidal space and recession of the angle of the anterior chamber.

11

The Uveal Tract

The iris, ciliary body and the choroid together are called the uveal tract. They comprise a continuous sheet of pigmented vascular tissue with many common histological features. The iris is like a diaphragm of a camera which controls quantum of light entering the eye. The ciliary body has a dual function, that of accommodation to help focus near objects and it is also the site for formation of aqueous humour which maintains the intraocular tension. The choroid lying underneath the retina serves the function of absorbing light and the chorio-capillaries are the source of nutrition to the functionally most important outer layers of retina.

The amount of pigments in the uveal tissue of normal eyes varies widely in different races and in different environments. A blue and light coloured iris of Caucasian races is characteristic. On the other extreme, the black iris of the Asians absorbs the extra light of a tropical climate. There are intermediate shades of different hues and different density and these variations depend on the mixtures of races all over the world.

The uveal tract extends from the pupillary margin in front to the optic nerve head behind. Anatomically and embryologically, there are common factors in each of the three component parts of the uveal tract but physiologically and pathologically, each of them is a distinct entity. The iris is suspended in the aqueous separating the anterior chamber and posterior chamber. The ciliary body lines the anterior scleral coat and thus exposed to the pathology involving the sclera. The choroid however is more related to retina. There are pathological considerations which are relevant to dividing the choroid in four distinct zones, viz., peripheral, equatorial, macular and peripapillary. Apart from these common and uncommon factors in the three constituents of uveal tract, pathologically also they differ in many respects. The response of the three parts of the uveal tract to trauma, vascular disturbances and inflammations are different.

Pathological Considerations

The iris and the ciliary body are highly vascular and sensitive tissues richly supplied by branches from ophthalmic division of trigeminal nerve. The choroid, on the other hand, is a relatively insensitive tissue. From pathological point of view, the anterior choroid is closer to the ciliary body and is also the seat of anastomosis of the short posterior ciliary arteries and the recurrent branches of anterior ciliary arteries. The anterior choroid, is, frequently affected in irido-cyclitis although clinically not seen. One evidence is the presence of ciliary congestion in anterior choroiditis when there is no iritis or cyclitis. The equatorial part of choroid is the least vascular area. And this is attributed to the cause of *ring scotoma* in retinitis pigmentosa. The posterior choroid, up to the macular area and optic disc is independent of the anterior part and more often involves the retina secondarily or itself gets secondarily involved.

Being a vascular tissue, the whole uveal tract responds to inflammatory stimuli from a mild to the severest degree depending on the cause, whether it is exogenous or endogenous, whether it is traumatic or bacterial and whether it is a systemic granulomatous disease or an antigen-antibody reaction.

An exogenous infection whether due to trauma, perforation of an infected corneal ulcer or post-operative, first causes severe inflammation of the iris and the ciliary body and when it extends into the vitreous chamber, involves the choroid. The iris becomes swollen and inflammatory exudates may collect into pupillary area or pour into the anterior chamber. This severe condition is then called *panophthalmitis*. Exudates from ciliary body collect behind the lens in the hyaloid fossa. Inflammatory cells may diffuse into the aqueous and vitreous. Being the source of nutrition to the important layers of rods and cones, choroidal pathology causes serious disturbance to retinal function and damage to vision.

Vascular Disturbances

Important vascular lesions of uveal tract are neovascularisation of iris, thrombosis of vortex veins and haemorrhage in the uveal tissue or from uveal tissue.

Neovascularisation of the iris is frequently seen in diabetes, Eales' disease and thrombosis of the central retinal vein. Localised neovascularisation may be due to a growth either in the iris itself or in the adjoining uveal tissue behind. Iris neovascularisation may lead to heamorrhage in the iris tissue or in the anterior chamber.

Thrombosis of vortex veins has a serious effect on the eye. It is commonly the result of diathermisation during retinal detachment surgery if the intrascleral portion of the vein is not identified. It can cause solid retinal detachment in the corresponding area with congestion, chemosis and pain in the eye due to back venous pressure.

Haemorrhage in iris is extremely rare. The only site of bleeding following iridodialysis is from the vessels coming from the circulus iridis major at the root of the iris.

Choroidal haemorrhage is due to systemic causes like hypertension, diabetes, arterio-sclerosis and haematopoetic diseases. Highly vascularised tumours like an angioma or a sarcoma can cause a large haemorrhage in the choroid producing a characteristic dark raised area with the appearance of a pseudo-tumour. A massive breakdown of the chorio-capillaries due to a sudden lowering of intraocular tension either due to trauma or during an operation is known as *expulsive haemorrhage* and is the most destructive operative complication during intraocular surgery. As the name suggests, the haemorrhage is so massive that it pushes the retina, the vitreous and lens out of the eye.

Trauma and Healing

The iris being supported by aqueous all round is usually free from the effects of trauma. A rupture of sphincter or detachment from attachment to the ciliary body occurs after a severe non-perforating injury. The interesting feature is that once there is a break in the iris tissue whether at the pupillary margin, iris diaphragm or its attachment to the ciliary body, there is no fibrosis and no healing process. These defects are evident months or years later. The ciliary body and choroid however are not as inactive as the iris. Healing after trauma of the ciliary body and choroid takes place by fibrosis. Indirect trauma can cause rupture of the choroid usually near the posterior pole of the eye ball. It leaves behind a scar with pigmentation at the margin which can be clinically diagnosed as a choroidal tear long after the trauma.

Inflammations of Uveal the Tissue

The iris and ciliary body are the most sensitive tissues of the eye ball and develop an inflammatory reaction following innumerable exogenous causes. The iris and ciliary body are inherently antigenic tissues and therefore hypersensitivity reactions due to dormant and silent systemic conditions are the commonest cause of iridocyclitis.

There are three types of inflammatory reactions, *purulent*, *exudative* and *serous*. Purulent reaction mostly follows exogenous infection and is associated with pus in the anterior chamber, posterior chamber and in the vitreous.

Plastic or exudative iridocyclitis is commonly the result of granulomatous diseases like tuberculosis, leprosy, toxoplasmosis, etc. Exudates collect in the pupillary area, in the retrolental space and permeate into vitreous. Dense posterior synechia and formation of organised membranes is a common feature.

Serous iridocyclitis is commonly the result of tissue hypersensitivity reaction which is caused by a non-granulomatous reaction like a septic focus in the body and allergic reaction. The posterior synechiae are usually thin and tissue disorganisation is less.

The end results of an eye following iridocyclitis will depend on the type of inflammation, its severity and the effectiveness of treatment. The eye may recover leaving behind only a few posterior synechiae which may remain evident for the rest of the patient's life. In severely inflamed eyes or in eyes with extensive peripheral synechiae, glaucomatous process may lead to total loss of vision. Long standing subacute inflammation may result in low tension due to atrophic changes of the ciliary body. Long standing chronic inflammation may leave behind an atrophic bulbi with advanced band degeneration of the cornea.

Inflammation in the choroid is more damaging from the point of view of vision although the discomforting symptoms are few. Choroidal inflammations are arbitrarily described on the basis of four vascular zones. The equatorial choroid, the central choroid, the peripapillary choroid and the anterior choroid. Every inflammatory lesion in the choroid involves the retina in the corresponding area, to some degree. The term most frequently used, therefore, is 'chorioretinitis'. Active lesions in choroid are exudative in nature and patchy in character. It is curious that most lesions in the choroid are due to granulomatous lesions, hypersensitivity reactions being much less common as compared to the iris and ciliary body. Healing takes place by fibrous organisation and results in a healed patch of choroiditis. With choroidal atrophy the sclera is seen through and pigment migrates to the margin of the lesions. The overlying retina is seriously damaged because of its dependence for nutrition on the chorio-capillaris. The healed patch leaves behind a corresponding scotoma in the field of vision.

The choroid at the equator and in front of equator has a relatively poor blood supply. Degenerative and abiotrophic lesions like retinitis pigmentosa with a vascular basis first start in the equatorial part and cause a ring scotoma in early phase of the disease.

Central choroiditis causes oedema in the macular area and in the process of healing results in severe degree of damage to vision.

Choroidal inflammations in the peri-papillary zone of choroid are called *juxta-papillary choroiditis*. The most damaging patch of choroiditis in this area is along the temporal half of disc margin because the pathology involves papillo-macular bundle of nerve fibres and therefore causes large scotoma in the central field.

Atrophic lesions of uveal tissue are also not uncommon. Conditions like essential atrophy of the iris are separate clinical entities. Primary atrophic lesions of the choroid too are clinically seen. *Central areolar choroidal atrophy of macular area, the gyrate atrophy of posterior choroid* and retinitis pigmentosa which is secondarily associated with pigmentary changes are well-known clinical conditions.

The uveal tissue is a common site, for parasitic cysts. Tumours of the uveal tissue include malignant melanoma and dyktioma and are highly malignant. In addition, other tumours arise from the epithelial, muscular and vascular tissues of the uveal tract. The uveal tract is also a favourable site for secondary metastasis from elsewhere in the body.

AETIOLOGY OF UVEITIS

Identifying a causative factor in uveitis has been the most difficult task for saving many eyes from reaching incurable blindness. Although there are a large number of causes which have been identified, it remains unfortunately true that fifty per cent or more cases of iridocyclitis are treated symptomatically and empirically.

Syphilis, tuberculosis and rheumatic arthritis were for long considered major causes of uveitis. The identification of toxoplasmosis was also added among the important causes of uveitis. Streptococcus was also added among the important causes of uveitis. Streptococcus from an unidentified septic focus in the body was still later attributed to be a cause of uveitis where nothing else could be discovered. A more acceptable emphasis has veered round the concept that many cases of uveitis, previously labelled 'etiology not known' are the result of tissue hypersensitivity caused by an allergic reaction. It is now agreed that many causes of uveitis like tuberculosis and septic focus are responsible for uveitis due to the antigens liberated by them which cause hypersensitivity tissue reaction in uvea. Tissue hypersensitivity has been better understood now. The hypersensitivity may be due to extraneous agents or due to auto-immunity. The tissue is sensitised by the first contact of the antigen and a later contact with the same antigen produces hypersensitivity reaction. The importance of hypersensitivity as a cause of uveitis has been emphasized on the basis of an auto-immune reaction wherein an antigen was introduced in the circulation which resulted in the formation of antibodies. The release of a second dose of the antigen excites a more severe antigen-antibody reaction which manifests itself in the form of uveitis. Focal infection, tuberculous proteins in blood, collagen diseases, rheumatic fever are all now considered to be the cause of iridocyclitis due to a hyper-sensitivity reaction. It has also been noted that inflammations due to hypersensitivity are most frequently noted in the iris and ciliary body and much less commonly in the choroid.

In tropical countries, the etiology of uveitis has an added spectrum because tuberculosis, parasitic infestations and septic foci are more common, while conditions like collagen diseases, toxoplasmosis are distinctly less prevalent. The major groups of causes are exogenous, infective and endogenous hypersensitivity. To these may be added the toxic causes and chemical irritants.

Exogenous Infections

1. Perforating injuries with gross infection, the common organisms being pneumococcus, pyocyaneous and fungus.

2. Corneal ulcers, bacterial, viral and fungal in origin.
3. Post-operative infection.
4. Extension of inflammation from the surrounding tissue, e.g., orbital cellulitis, sinusitis.

Endogenous Infections

1. Metastatic diseases
   a. Tuberculosis as a tuberculoma or tubercular iritis.
   b. Syphilis in the secondary and tertiary stages.
   c. Leprosy/Leprotic iritis and Lepra reaction.
   d. Intestinal parasites and infections like filariasis, Onchocerchiasis, Toxoplasmosis, Leishmaniasis, Trepanopsomiasis.
   e. Septic focus.
2. Viral lesions:
   a. Infective fevers like measles, small pox.
   b. Herpetic keratitis, Simplex and zoster.
   c. Behcet's disease.
   d. Vogt-Koyanagi syndrome.
3. Focal infections from teeth, tonsils, sinuses, urinary tract and appendix.
4. Mycotic infections.

Endogenous Hypersensitivity

This includes many causes of endogenous metastatic causes.
1. Immediate anaphylactic reaction.
   a. Serum sickness.
   b. Phako-anaphylactic reaction.
2. Delayed hypersensitivity (allergic irodocyclitis)
   a. Streptococcal septic focus.
   b. Endogenous tubercular allergy.
   c. Rheumatic affections.
   d. Systemic gonococcal infection.
   e Collagen diseases.

Chemical Irritants:
1. Miotics.
2. Gun powder particles.

Systemic and Metabolic Diseases
1. Diabetes mellilus.
2. Collagen diseases.
3. Gout.
4. Sarcoidosis.
5. Diseases of central nervous system.

ANTERIOR UVEA

(Iris and Ciliary Body).

Iris

It is an active tissue with a free central pupillary border and attached in the periphery to the anterior surface of the ciliary body. The latter is called the *root of the iris.* The pupillary border lightly rests on anterior surface of the lens. It is cushioned by the aqueous in front and behind. The spongy tissue of iris has endothelial cell layer anteriorly which is a continuation of the endothelium of cornea. The anterior surface of iris is divided between the outer two-thirds and inner one-third by a demarcating line called the *collarette of the iris.* The unevenness of the anterior surface is caused by crypts more prominently in the central one-third zone. The posterior surface of iris is darker than the anterior surface and is lined by pigment epithelium which is a continuation of the pigment epithelium of ciliary body. Sometimes this pigment epithelium is seen at the pupillary margin as dark round excrescences due to ectropion of the epithelium. In between the two surface layers is the spongy tissue comprised of elastic tissue, the pigment cells, blood vessels and sphincter and dilator pupillae muscles.

The sphincter pupillae is a circular band of muscle tissue along the pupillary border near the posterior surface of the iris. It is intricately mixed with the stroma of iris; each segment acting as if it has a separate entity. This is borne out by the fact that the remaining pupillary margin briskly constricts in cases where a sector iridectomy has been done. It is supplied by parasympathetic fibres of 3rd cranial nerve.

The dilator pupillae muscle is present in iris stroma more anteriorly and relatively peripherally. The muscle fibres are arranged radially and are supplied by sympathetic system via the long ciliary nerves.

The blood supply of iris is from the anastomosis between the perforating branches of anterior ciliary artery and the long posterior ciliary arteries which form the *circulus iridis major.* Branches from this form another vascular circle called the *circulus iridis minor* which corresponds to the collarette on the surface. The veins drain into vena vorticose via the long posterior ciliary veins (Fig. 11.1).

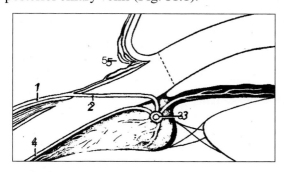

Fig 11.1: Blood Supply of Anterior uvea. (1) Anterior ciliary artery; (2) Perforating branch of anterior ciliary; (3) Arterial circulus iridis major; (4) Long posterior ciliary artery; (5) Anastomosis between the anterior conjunctival vessels round and limbus.

The sensory nerve supply to the iris is from the ophthalmic division of the V nerve through the long posterior ciliary nerves.

Ciliary Body

It is an important structure of the eye ball principally because aqueous is formed through the ciliary processes which is important for maintenance of intraocular tension and nutrition to various structures of the eye. The ciliary body is also responsible for initiating the process of accommodation.

It is a triangular structure with an anterior surface, medial surface and scleral or outer surface. Root of the iris is attached to the anterior surfce. The medial surface extends up to the ora serrata but the ciliary processes are radially arranged only in a 2-mm zone in the anterior part of the medial surface and this is called the corona of the ciliary body. Capillaries in the ciliary processes produce aqueous. The epithelium lining the processes is double layered. The inner layer is non-pigmented and serves as a semi-permeable filter. It allows passage of only soluble substances, (sodium chloride, potassium, ascorbic acid, bicarbonates). No cellular or particulate matter contained in capillary blood is allowed. The process is known as blood-aqueous barrier.

The fibres of the suspensory ligament (the zonule of Zinn) of the lens are attached in a criss-cross fashion in the crypts of the corona of the ciliary body. The ciliary body extends from about 2 mm from the limbus to about 6 mm behind.

The structures that form ciliary body from without inwards are:
1. Longitudinal muscle fibres.
2. Circular muscle fibres or the Muller's muscle of the ciliary body.
3. The stroma consisting of pigment cells and the loose connective tissue.
4. Pigment epithelial layer covering the ciliary processes. The outer layer of the epithelium is pigmented while the inner is unpigmented.

Blood supply: It is derived from the long posterior ciliary and the perforating branches of the anterior ciliary arteries. They form tufts under the ciliary processes. The venous blood drains into the vena vorticose.

Nerve supply: The sensory nerve supply to the ciliary body is from ophthalmic division of V nerve. The motor nerve supply to the circular muscle fibres is from parasympathetic fibres in the third cranial nerve and to the longitudinal muscle fibres from sympathetic fibres.

INFLAMMATION OF THE IRIS AND THE CILIARY BODY

Iridocyclitis

Inflammation of the iris is often associated with inflammation of the ciliary body and vice versa. The term iridocyclitis is commonly used for inflammations of the anterior uvea although iritis and cyclitis are a possibility, however infrequent.

Clinical Features

The clinical features will depend on the type of inflammation, acute or chronic, the causative factors, some of which cause serous iridocyclitis while others cause plastic iridocyclitis, etc. Furthermore, there may be inflammation of iris alone, at least clinically so, or there may be cyclitis alone or both together as is most often the case.

The symptoms of acute iridocyclitis are pain in the eye, redness, photophobia, lacrimation and diminution of vision.

Pain may be severe and neuralgic in acute cases and dull and moderate in chronic cases. The pain in iridocyclitis can be due to more than one cause:

1. Inflammation of the iris and ciliary body causing irritation of the sensory nerve endings.
2. Constant movement of the muscles of the inflamed iris and ciliary body during pupillary contraction and accommodation.
3. There may be secondary rise of intra-ocular tension due to albuminous aqueous or iris bombe resulting in pupillary block.

Diminution of vision: The causes of reduced vision in acute iridocyclitis are many. These are:

1. Oedema of the cornea
2. Keratic precipites on the posterior surface of the cornea.
3. Plasmoid aqueous.
4. Exudates in the pupillary area.

5. Spasm of ciliary muscle causing transient myopia.
6. Cellular haze in the vitreous.
7. Associated macular choroiditis and optic neuritis as an extension of the anterior pathology or independently caused by the same etiological factor.
8. Secondary rise of intra-ocular tension.

In the subacute and chronic stage, reduced vision may be due to:

1. Corneal haze and later band degeneration of the cornea.
2. Organised membrane in the pupillary area with posterior synechia.
3. Secondary complicated cataract.
4. Cyclitic membrane behind lens.
5. Vitreous opacities.
6. Healed central choroiditis.
7. Optic atrophy, post-neuritic type.
8. Hypotension, retinal detachment and atrophic bulbi.

Redness: The typical redness in iridocyclitis is circumcorneal or ciliary congestion.

Signs of Acute Iridocyclitis

Ciliary congestion: It may be anything from a mild ciliary flush to an acutely congested eye. A circumcorneal ciliary congestion is characteristic of anterior uveitis. Even when congestion is more diffuse it can be evidently observed that it is more marked round the limbus and becomes less and less towards the fornices.

Corneal changes: The cornea reacts to inflammations of the iris and the ciliary body in varying degrees. Keratic precipitates (KPs) on posterior surface of cornea are *pathognomonic* of the involvement of ciliary body in the inflammation. The KPs are aggregations of leukocytes which have passed out through the inflamed ciliary epithelium into the aqueous. These stick to the posterior surface of the cornea which is also involved in the inflammatory process in the form of endothelialitis. Partly because of convection currents in the anterior chamber, these KPs are commonly seen on the lower part of the endothelial surface, sometimes arranged in a triangular fashion. Although KPs can be seen with a good illumination and a loupe magnification, these can be best studied on a slit lamp. Fresh KPs as in an acute stage of iridocyclitis are yellowish in colour and round in shape. They are usually the size of a pin head or smaller.

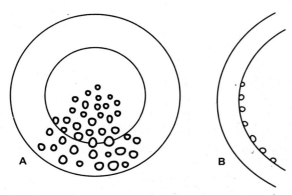

Fig 11.2: Keratic precipitates. (A) Seen with focal illumination; (B) Seen on slit lamp

Large KPs are called 'Mutton fat KPs, and are a feature of cyclitis due to granulomatous cyclitis. Old KPs become lightly pigmented and may shrink in size. They may persist for a long time and in the absence of recurrence, they usually disappear. Corneal oedema is a result of endothelialitis. When associated with raised intra-ocular tension, there may also be bullous formation.

Aqueous flare is a phenomenon of visibility of a light beam passing through the anterior chamber and seen with a slit lamp. The anterior chamber with normal aqueous humour is *optically empty*. Aqueous flare when present, is due to plasmoid albuminous character of aqueous, a change due to acute iridocyclitis when particulate material may be seen in the

illuminated beam of light like the dust particles seen in a narrow beam of light from a ventilator coming into a room (Fig. 11.3).

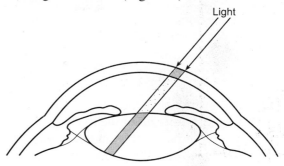

Fig 11.3: Aqueous flare seen with slit lamp. (Note cellular particles seen in the beam passing through anterior chamber.)

Exudates in iridocyclitis. Exudation in iridocyclitis collects in one or more of the following areas:
1. Pupillary area.
2. Anterior chamber.
3. In the angle of the anterior chamber.
4. In the posterior chamber.
5. In the retrolental space.
6. Diffuse in the vitreous.

An exudate may collect in the pupillary area and later organise to form a membrane occluding the pupil *occlusio pupillae*. The exudation may be excessive and collect at the bottom of the anterior chamber to form hypopyon. Aqueous mixed with exudates may block filtration channels in the angle and cause rise of intra-ocular tension even in the early acute phase. When it is severe in degree, it is called *hypertensive iridocyclitis*. Exudation in the angle of the anterior chamber is usually not clinically evident but when organised, it causes obliteration of the angle of the anterior chamber, peripheral anterior synechiae to the cornea, obstruction to the aqueous outflow and secondary glaucoma. Exudation may also be in the posterior chamber and the retrolental space. When this gets organised, it forms a *cyclitic membrane*.

Pupil

In iritis the pupil is smaller due to irritative miosis. The inflammatory reaction in the iris irritates the nerve endings of both, the sympathetic dilator nerves and parasympathetic constrictor nerves. It is a known fact, whenever the nerve endings of both autonomic nervous systems are irritated, the effect of the parasympathetic dominates, and hence the constriction of the pupil in iritis.

The pupillary margin of the iris which rests on the anterior surface of the lens tends to adhere to the lens due to albuminous exudate from the inflamed iris. This is called *posterior synechia*. This may not be clinically evident in a small pupil but mydriatic drops make it visible in the form of an irregular shape of pupillary aperture. The posterior synechia usually becomes evident fairly early in the disease and in early cases, can be an important diagnostic feature (Fig. 11.4A and Fig. 11.4B, Plate 6).

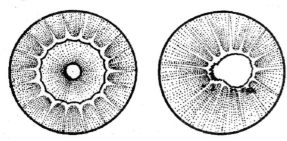

Fig. 11.4A: Posterior Synechia made evident by mydriasis

When the inflammation has become chronic, posterior synechia becomes firm so as to resist effect of a mydriatic allowing dilatation only where there is no synechia. If the synechia binds the whole pupillary margin, it is called *ring posterior synechia*. This prevents communication between the anterior and the posterior chamber, and is, therefore, also called *seclusio-pupillae*. Accumulation of aqueous behind the iris causes a bulging forward of the iris resulting in shallowing of the anterior chamber in mid-peri-

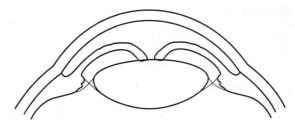

Fig. 11.5: Ring Posterior Synechia with Iris Bombe (seclusio pupilae) Note the adhesion of pupillary margin to the lens and middle part of the iris bulging forward giving the appearance of funnel shape with anterior chamber deep in centre and shallow in periphery)

phery and a relatively deeper anterior chamber in the pupillary area clinically called *iris bombe* (Fig. 11.5). When exudates form and organise behind the whole posterior surface of iris resulting in adherence to the anterior lens surface, it is called *total posterior synechia*. This is clinically evident by absence of iris bombe because iris cannot bulge forward due to its adherence to the lens (Fig. 11.6).

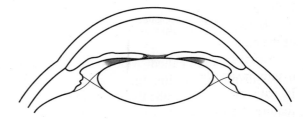

Fig. 11.6: Total posterior synechia (occlusio pupillae). Note the adhesion of large part of posterior surface of iris to anterior surface of lens

Iris

An inflamed iris is thickened. Clinically, the crypts of the iris become shallower and the iris surface becomes smoother, described as loss of normal iris pattern. This is due to interstitial oedema of the iris stroma. In chronic stage, particularly after exudative iridocyclitis, iris becomes thinned and shows patches of stromal atrophy.

Clinical Stages

Iridocyclitis may be acute, subacute and chronic. Ciliary congestion, aqueous flare, fresh keratic precipitates, exudates in the pupillary area, hypopyon, posterior synechia and loss of iris pattern are all clinical features of acute iridocyclitis. Raised intra-ocular tension in the acute stages is a clinical feature of acute hypertensive iridocyclitis. As the inflammation becomes less acute or subacute, the clinical features may becomes milder in nature. Chronic iridocyclitis with healed organised lesions is clinically evident from pigmented keratic precipitates, dense posterior synechia, iris bombe, iris atrophy, organised membrane in the pupillary area and behind the lens and peripheral anterior synechia resulting in a false angle of the anterior chamber and secondary glaucoma.

Iritis vis-a-vis cyclitis: Inflammmation of anterior uvea usually involves iris and ciliary body both. This may not however be so in all cases. It is therefore important at this stage to categorise the clinical features which indicate involvement of the ciliary body as against iritis alone.

Most of the exudative phenomena in anterior uveitis are due to involvement of the ciliary body. In iritis alone exudation is not a conspicuous feature. Ciliary congestion of a milder type, a contracted sluggishly reacting pupil, pigment dispersion associated with pain, photophobia and diminished vision are features of iritis alone. When ciliary body is involved, exudation appears starting with an aqueous flare, exudates in the pupillary area, behind the lens and sometimes hypopyon depending on degree of ciliary inflammation.

Posterior synechia due to iridocyclitis rarely, if ever, breaks with mydriatic drugs while that due to iritis alone often separates when the pupil is dilated with atropine leaving behind pigments on anterior lens surface.

The diagnosis of iridocyclitis may, in most cases, be clinically most evident. However, slit lamp examination helps not only to clarify the clinical features but also helps in determining the stage of inflammatory process. Slit lamp examination may be the only means to establish the diagnosis in very early stages or in cases of iritis alone. The presence of mild aqueous flare, pigment particles on the lens surface in the pupillary area or fine fresh keratic precipitates may be the clinical evidence seen only on slit lamp in early stages of mild iridocyclitis. Early diagnosis with a slit lamp can help institution of correct treatment to give quick relief of symptoms and control of disease.

Tonometry should be done in all cases of acute or chronic iridocyclitis, to help in instituting appropriate hypotensive therapy if necessary.

Once clinical diagnosis of iridocyclitis is made, it is important to look for evidence of systemic disease or history of similar attacks because iridocyclitis is one pathology which is more often of systemic origin than due to local cause. History of syphilis, tuberculosis, leprosy, diabetes, systemic allergy, intestinal disorders, septic tonsil, dental sepsis should all be specially recorded.

Differential diagnosis of anterior uveitis. In spite of the fact that clinical evidence supplied by slit lamp findings is strong enough to make a positive diagnosis of anterior uveitis, it does remain to be differentiated from a few important conditions of the anterior segment. The differential diagnosis of these conditions of the anterior segment is still more important because the therapy indicated in one, may be contraindicated in the other. For example, atropine is the treatment in iridocyclitis while it should NOT be used in glaucoma. Differentiating features of these conditions with congestion of the eye as a common denominator are given in a tabulated form.

Differentiation between congestive glaucoma and hypertensive iridocyclitis needs careful

	Acute iridocyclitis	*Congestive glaucoma*	*Keratitis*	*Conjunctivitis*
Congestion	Ciliary	Ciliary	Ciliary	Conjunctival
Cornea	Keratic precipitates on endothelial surface	Steamy and oedematous	Hazy with infiltration	Clear
Ant. Chamber	Normal or deep	Shallow	Normal	Normal
Aqueous	Plasmoid with flare	Normal with few cells	Normal	Normal
Iris	Loss of pattern	Normal	Normal	Normal
Pupil	Constricted and irregular	Ovally dilated and fixed	Normal	Normal
IOP	Normal or raised in severe exudative cases	Always high	Normal	Normal
Vision	Reduced	Grossly reduced	Reduced	Normal

Note: In Keratitis, association of iridocyclitis will change clinical features.

evaluation of the findings to reach a correct diagnosis. A mydriatic test to make posterior synechiae evident will also help in differential diagnosis. Phenylephrine 10% solution should be used for the test because it is short acting and does not raise intra-ocular tension.

Ulcerative conditions of the cornea with ciliary congestion are not likely to be mistaken for any other condition. However, conditions like parenchymal or interstitial keratitis may need to be differentiated from the corneal involvement in congestive glaucoma and severe iridocyclitis.

Investigations for a Case of Iridocyclitis

The list of investigations needed to determine a definitive etiology is formidable, made worse by the numerous foci from which hypersensitivity reactions can cause iridocyclitis. In the best of laboratories, fifty per cent or more cases still remain etiologically non-specific with the result that often the treatment is empirical and one is still exposed to the chances of recurrence and increasing damage with each recurrence. It is, therefore, not surprising that many eyes become incurably blind in spite of all efforts.

In tropical and developing countries, priorities for investigations have to be so adopted that we exclude first the causes common in tropical environments. The list of investigations necessary for a case of iridocyclitis is, therefore, given below in order of priority:

1. X-ray of the chest for old healed tuberculous lesion.
2. Montoux's test for tuberculous allergy.
3. Blood examinations:
   a. Erythrocytes sedimentation ESR
   b. WBC—total and differential count.
4. Stool examination for parasitic ova and cysts.
5. Serological blood tests for syphilis.
6. Exclude diabetes mellitus
7. Examination for septic focus:
   a. Dental check-up
   b. ENT check-up for infected tonsils, etc.
   c. Genito-urinary check-up.
8. Tests for toxoplasmosis
9. Exclude HIV

Complications and Prognosis of Iridocyclitis

Prognosis of iridocyclitis can best be called uncertain in a majority of cases. A mild attack may come and go without leaving behind any harmful effect.

A moderate degree of iridocyclitis may leave behind permanent posterior synechia and yet the eye may remain quiet and free of symptoms. The most difficult cases are where every recurrent attack adds to the damage already caused. Gross lowering of tension or secondary glaucoma make the prognosis still worse. The common damaging results are organised *exudative membranes* in pupillary area, *peripheral anterior synechia, secondary cataract, cyclitic membrane*, and *atrophy of the ciliary body*. Complications affecting posterior segment include liquefaction of the vitreous, macular oedema, optic neuritis and atrophy. Eyes blinded by iridocyclitis usually present serious manifestations like ciliary staphyloma, atrophic bulbi and band degeneration of the cornea (Fig. 11.7).

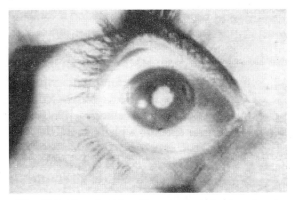

Fig. 11.7: Chronic iridocylitis complicated cataract and early band degeneration of cornea

Treatment

It is truly the most difficult disease to treat and success of treatment depends on whether the case under treatment is of known etiology or is due to indeterminate systemic cause. The treatment includes local therapy, specific treatment for the cause, non-specific treatment, desensitization and surgery.

Local treatment: Effective mydriasis is the anchor sheet of treatment of iridocyclitis. Atropine 1 per cent in the form of drops should be started at the earliest and repeated even up to three times a day till the pupil is dilated to a satisfactory degree. If atropine is not able to dilate the pupil, atropine combined with 10 per cent phenylephrine may be effective. A compound mydriatic is quite often necessary to initiate the process of dilation. A good combination used to be mydricaine which contains atropine, adrenaline and lignocaine.

Atropine destroys the acetyl choline at the myo-neural junction, paralysing the parasympathetic supply to the sphincter and thus allows sympathetic nerves to dilate the pupil.
1. It dilates the pupil.
2. By dilation, it breaks the posterior synechiae.
3. By paralysing the sphincter and ciliary muscle, it gives rest to the eye and relieves pain.

The question is quite often raised whether atropine should be used when there is glaucoma with iridocyclitis. It can, be safely emphasized that glaucoma or no glaucoma, atropine is the drug chosen during the acute phase of iridocyclitis because not using atropine will cause more damage than using it. The rise of intra-ocular tension can be treated by hypotensive drugs like oral acetazolamide or I. V. osmotic agents during the acute stage. Steroids will help control inflammation earlier and therefore will also contribute to controlling secondary rise of tension.

The use of steroids as immuno-superessive and anti-inflammatory agents are the most useful contribution to the treatment of iridocyclitis and next to atropine form the important anchor-sheet. Steroids not only reduce inflammatory process but also reduce chances of damage to vision. Steroid therapy has become particularly important since auto-immune reaction and hypersensitivity have proved to be the basis of many iridocyclitis cases. Steroids however are not a specific therapy and only act as anti-inflammatory and anti-allergic agents.

Steroids are administered as eye drops, ointment, sub-conjunctival injections and by oral therapy. In acute phase, it is advisable to use soluble dexamethasone as repeated eye drops or as a daily sub-conjunctival injection. In subacute stage, hydrocortisone acetate 2.5% can be used as a depot under the conjunctiva.

Other anti-inflammatory and analgesic drugs such as salicylates like aspirin and phenylbutazone are a good supportive therapy to steroids to help relieve pain and reduce inflammation.

Specific Therapy

However limited the scope, investigations may lead to identification of a specific etiology. When so, specific therapy should be added. Broad spectrum antibiotics are specifically indicated in exogenous causes and they can also be given empirically to neutralise any septic focus in the body which may be the starting point of pathology. Anti-tubercular therapy including streptomycin, PAS and isoniazid is often worth a trial particularly in developing countries where systemic tuberculosis is much more common and systemic tubercular allergy is a likely cause. Sulphones in leprosy, penicillin in syphilis, sulphas in toxoplasmosis, arsenic in trypanosomiasis and carbamazine in onchocerchiasis are well-known specific therapies. Similarly, control of diabetes, treatment of septic focus in the urinary tract, teeth, tonsils need a specific therapeutic approach either medical or surgical.

Surgical treatment: One should hesitate to do any active surgical interference in acute inflammatory phase of the disease. One should be conservative rather than enthusiastic when thinking of putting a knife into the eye with active iridocyclitis. It is safer to have atropine and steroids control the inflammation. Small surgical procedures are at times called for either to control rise of intraocular tension, break the posterior synechiae or sometimes improve visual acuity.

Any surgical procedure, in even a healed iridocyclitis case must never be taken lightly. Assessment needs to be meticulously done with all the pros and cons carefully considered. Pre-operative, intra-operative and post-operative modifications have to be pre-planned.

SPECIFIC TYPES OF IRIDOCYCLITIS

Although most cases of iridocyclitis have the same common clinical manifestations, there are some special features peculiar to specific types of inflammations. A few common ones are described below:

Tuberculous iridocyclitis: Tubercle bacillus in the eye is rare. Similarly iridocyclitis due to active lung tuberculosis is also rare. Tuberculous pathology can cause iridocyclitis in two ways:

1. *Tuberculoma* of the iris which is a nodular lesion with characteristic histological changes. The nodules cause varying degrees of inflammatory reaction which ultimately resolve or heal, leaving behind a patch of iris atrophy.
2. Most other cases of iridocyclitis of tubercular origin are due to allergy to tubercular proteins, the characteristic features of which are *chronic granulomatous iridocyclitis* of recurrent nature with mutton fat keratic precipitates. The allergy is due to a protein fraction of tubercule bacillus and the sensitivity is manifested by a strongly positive Mantoux reaction.

The test has its own limitations because most of the population in tropical areas has developed an immunity and therefore Mantoux's is positive in most cases. The Mantoux test, should therefore be repeated in greater dilutions to get more reliable results. A more valuable test however is haemagglutination test between the sheep RBC sensitised with tuberculous antigen and the serum of the patient.

The local treatment of tubercular iridocyclitis is on general lines. Systemically anti-tubercular therapy be given for 2–3 months in identified tubercular cases. Tubercular etiology being much more common in tropical and developing countries, empirical systemic anti-tubercular therapy is worth a trial even though there is no evidence of tuberculosis in the body. This empirical therapy should be given for at least three weeks. If there is no response, it should be stopped.

Desensitisation with tuberculin as an adjunct to other anti-tubercular therapy may help where nothing else has worked. This should be done in consultation and under the supervision of a specialist.

Syphlitic iridocyclitis: Syphilis causes uveal inflammatory reaction in four different ways:

1. Congenital syphilis when plastic iridocyclitis is part of interestitial keratitis.
2. Secondary syphilis, when it causes a severe and acute iridocyclitis with thick posterior synechiae.
3. Syphilitic gumma as a nodular lesion in tertiary syphilis is usually solitary in nature but associated with exudative iridocyclitis. The gumma heals by fibrosis and causes iris atrophy.
4. Anaphylactic iridocyclitis following antisyphilitic therapy with penicillin or arsenic. The reaction which follows 12-18 hours after the injection is due to death of spirochaetes and liberation of their endotoxins. This is called *Herxheimer's reaction.*

Leprotic iridocyclitis: Leprosy causes iridocyclitic inflammation following different pathological modes:

i. Bilateral acute plastic iridocyclitis.
ii. Granulomatous leprotic nodules.
iii. Chronic iridocyclitis with dense posterior synechia.
iv. Anaphylaxis to systemic lepra reaction.

Iridocyclitis is a very common association of leprosy and is a cause of severe visual disturbance due to dense posterior synechiae, exudates in the pupillary area and deposits in the anterior chamber.

In developing countries, particularly in areas where leprosy is endemic, one should specifically look out for leprosy in cases of iridocyclitis.

Iridocyclitis in sarcoidosis. Boeck's sarcoid is a relatively common condition in Western countries but is very uncommon in tropical areas.

Sarcoidosis is not a lesion due to tuberculosis although non-caseating tubercles with epitheloid and giant cells form nodules. It is probably a non-specific antigen-antibody reaction due to some systemic factor. A virus may be a possible cause. Systemic lesions involve the lungs, lymph nodes, mediastinal glands and almost any system in the body.

Uveitis in Western countries is the commonest ocular manifestation of sarcoidosis. It may cause bilateral acute iridocyclitis with systemic symptoms or a chronic granulomatous iridocyclitis with multiple nodules on the iris. An intradermal sensitivity test with a suspension of tissues from affected lymph node may be positive. It responds to steroids.

Iridocyclitis in collagen diseases: The following collagen diseases or related conditions can cause iridocyclitis:

1. Rheumatoid arthritis in adults and older patients.
2. Chronic poly-arthritis in children (Still's disease).
3. Ankylosing spondylitis.
4. Reiter's syndrome consisting of urethritis, poly-arthritis and anterior uveitis.
5. Rheumatic fever.
6. Poly-arthritis nodosa
7. Disseminated Lupus erythematosus.
8. Scleroderma.

Viral iridocyclitis: Viral iridocyclitis can be a complication of herpes simplex and zoster. Viral diseases like mumps, measles, influenza and small pox can also cause iridocyclitis.

Herpes simplex causes herpes keratitis which is associated with a mild allergic type of iridocyclitis. Haemorrhage in the anterior chamber is a special feature of severe viral iridocyclitis. *Herpes Zoster* iridocyclitis is usually of the mild, transient and exudative type.

There are two other clinical entities which are presumed to be of viral origin and are associated with iridocyclitis—*Behcet's disease* and *Vogt-Koyanagi-Harada's disease.*

Behcet's disease is considered to be viral in nature. The features of this clinical complex are ulcers in the mouth, ulcers in genitals and iridocyclitis with hypopyon.

Vogt-Koyanagi-Harada's disease. This is also a clinical combination of various manifestations, probably of virus origin. Vogt (1906) first associated poliosis (whitening of hair) with chronic bilateral uveitis. Koyanagi (1929) added to the syndrome, vitiligo (depigmented patches of skin) round the eyes and on the face, alopecia (patches of baldness) and deafness. Harada (1926) independently described bilateral exudative uveitis with bilateral exudative detachment which was referred to as Harada's disease. These are all now considered one symptom complex, probably of viral origin affecting young adults with gross visual disturbances.

Parasitic iridocyclitis: Various parasites common in tropical countries that are known to cause iridocyclitis, either toxic or allergic in origin are filaria, thread worms, hook worms, cysticercus, hydatid, schistosomiasis, onchocerchiasis, Leishmaniasis, trepanopsomiasis, amoebiasis, etc. *An important parasitic cause is toxoplasmosis.* A granulomatous bilateral macular choroiditis was considered to be commonly caused by congenital toxoplasmosis transmitted to the foetus from maternal circulation. Acquired toxoplasmosis has also been now proved to be of not uncommon occurrence. It causes recurrent type of uveitis, more often choroiditis of granulomatous nature. It is important to investigate for toxoplasmosis as a possible cause of chronic uveitis. Many tests have been developed over the years.

The *Sabin dye test* is based on staining of live parasites with methylene blue when mixed with the serum of a positive patient. *Complement fixation test* is between antibodies in an immune serum and toxoplasma antigen. *Haemagglutination test* is based on agglutination of sensitised red blood cells in presence of specific antibodies. *The fluorescent antibody test* is based on the staining of organisms with specific fluorescein labelled antiserum. The last two tests are considered unreliable.

Mycotic uveitis due to fungi like histoplasmosis, moniliasis, aspergillosis, blastomycosis and sporotrichosis can all cause purulent iridocyclitis as a secondary manifestation of local corneal or systemic mycosis.

SYMPATHETIC OPHTHALMITIS

This is an inflammatory condition of the whole uveal tract and is known as *sympathetic ophthalmitis* because it develops in a healthy eye following severe inflammatory reaction in the opposite eye which can follow a perforating injury or an operative procedure.

Sympathetic ophthalmitis was a dreaded disease and many injured, inflamed eyes were removed for fear of sympathetic ophthalmitis even though there was some chance of visual recovery. The fear was potentially serious because it was believed that once the inflammatory process in the sympathizing eye started, even enucleation of the injured may not save the sympathizing eye and the end result would be blindness in both eyes. Sympathetic inflammation in the healthy eye was feared even in cases where severe iridocyclitis in the other eye did not respond to therapy. The advent of steroids has however reduced the fear of sympathetic ophthalmitis to a large extent. Sympathetic ophthalmitis in the present days is therefore a very uncommon clinical condition. The disease however does pose a threatening problem in some cases.

Factors favouring sympathetic inflammation in the healthy eye are:

1. Perforating injury.
2. Injury in the danger ciliary zone, with incarceration of the uveal tissue in the lips of the wound.
3. Retained intra-ocular foreign body particularly copper and iron.
4. No response to adequate therapy within three weeks. Severe iridocyclitis following cataract operation (surgical perforating injury) which persists or recurs, should also cause concern and fear of iridocyclitis in the other eye which would be favoured by post-operative iris prolapse or incarceration of the iris or the vitreous in the section.

It is curious that an operation like iridencleisis where the iris is deliberately incarcerated in the wound does not cause sympathetic iridocyclitis because except iris incarceration, it does not share any other factors enumerated above. The conjunctival coverage of iridencleisis is also said to be a factor in preventing sympathetic inflammation. The same applies to perforation of the cornea with iris incarceration and long standing leucoma adherence and staphylomata with iris incarcerated in the healed tissues. It is interesting that eyes with intraocular suppuration following perforating injury do not lead to sympathetic ophthalmitis. May be the suppurative process neutralises or abolishes the responsible factors.

Histopathology

The principal pathological change in the sympathizing eye is pan-uveitis with diffuse round cell choroidal infiltration and a preponderance of epitheloid and giant cells aggregating in nodular pattern called *Dalen-Fuchs nodules*. These nodules are seen in choroid.

Etiology

In spite of the disease having been known for such a long time, etiology has still remained obscure.

Hypersensitivity of an antigen liberated from an injured eye (allergic theory) has invited the least objections. The uveal pigment liberated from the injured eye (the antigen) reaches the healthy eye through circulation and sensitises its uveal tissue. A subsequent dose of the antigen precipitates an inflammatory reaction to cause sympathetic ophthalmitis.

Another important factor is the time interval between injury and the onset of sympathetic ophthalmitis. In a majority of cases reported, the interval is 6-8 weeks. Sympathetic ophthalmitis is however possible even up to three months, but rare after that. A recurrence of inflammation in the injured eye however changes the time table.

Clinical Picture

When there is active inflammation in the injured eye, one should look out for evidence of early iridocyclitis in the good eye. The earliest symptoms may be photophobia and disturbance in vision both for near and distance due to accommodative spasm and transient myopia. Mild ciliary flush, aqueous flare and/or fine keratic precipitates should be looked for as long as inflammation in the injured eye persists.

In a full-fledged case, the clinical manifestations in the sympathizing eye may be plastic iridocyclitis, choroiditis, exudation in the retina and the vitreous and even optic neuritis leading to gross visual disturbance.

The diagnosis of sympathetic ophthalmitis is based on details of injury, persistence of inflammation in the injured eye in spite of adequate therapy and early visual disturbances in the good eye. There is no dependable laboratory test. Histology of the uveal tract of enucleated injured eye is only of academic interest.

Prognosis

Corticosteroids have distinctly changed the ultimate prognosis of sympathetic ophthalmia. It is however important to emphasize that enucleation of the injured eye should not be planned in a hurry. It always pays to treat the inflammation in the offending eye conservatively and conduct a regular periodic check-up of the good eye for the earliest signs of inflammation.

Prophylaxis

Even though sympathetic ophthalmia has become less, prophylaxis has not become less important. The important prophylactic steps are as follows:

1. All perforating injuries, specially in the ciliary zone should be surgically repaired meticulously at the earliest. Any prolapse of the iris and the ciliary body should be reposed and if reposition is not possible, it should be excised. The procedure should ensure that no part of the uveal tract remains incarcerated in the lips of the repaired wound.
2. Any retained intraocular foreign body should be removed before severe inflammation develops.
3. Steroid therapy, both systemic and local, should be instituted in full doses and at the earliest.
4. Early removal of the injured eye is to be considered only when the injury is so extensive that due to tissue damage and loss, repair is not likely to result in either restoring some vision to the eye or even help retain anatomical integrity for cosmetic appearance. A more difficult question is the consideration of enucleation when the injured eye has developed severe inflammation but has some vision. Every effort should be made to fight the inflammation so long as there is vision. If there is no response in two to three weeks, an enucleation may have to be considered.

Enucleation may need to be considered if a retained intra-ocular foreign body cannot be removed or its removal involves surgery which is likely to cause serious damage to the eye.

The days of removing an injured eye with a fair amount of vision for fear of sympathetic ophthalmitis are past history because even if sympathetic ophthalmitis has set in and has been diagnosed early, the sympathizing eye can be treated and saved from becoming blind in most cases, thanks to the availability of steroids. The concept that once sympathetic ophthalmitis has set in, in the good eye, enucleation of the injured eye will not serve any purpose is also to be viewed with less seriousness considering the therapeutic possibilities now available.

OTHER TYPES OF UVEAL CONDITIONS

Heterochromic Iritis

Heterochromia is a condition where colour of the iris in one eye is different from the other. The iris in one eye may be blue and in the other brown or dark. In the same eye, the iris may have two different colours in different sectors (Fig. 11.8, Plate 6).

Heterochromia may be etiologically of following types:

1. Simple congenital heterochromia is usually hereditary in type.
2. Neurogenic heterochromia in which case the depigmentation is due to lesions of cervical sympathetic, e.g., Horner's syndrome or operations on the sympathetic trunk.
3. Atrophic heterochromia with patches of discolouration following granulomatous lesions of the iris.
4. Complicated heterochromia.

Heterochromic iridocyclitis is a condition due to non-specific etiology. The clinical picture is of mild iridocyclitis with ciliary flush, minimal degree of aqueous flare, very fine keratic precipitates with no tendency to formation of posterior synechia. The iris surface appears smoother and rarified with areas of atrophy so that the light partially passes through it as is seen by transillumination or by retro-illumination of a slit lamp. The special clinical feature is a frequent association of cataract formation and open angle glaucoma. Local treatment is for the mild inflammatory reaction. Surgery for cataract and glaucoma can be undertaken with good prognosis.

Diabetic Iris

The special features of iris in diabetics are the following:

1. *Tonic pupil*—the pupil in a diabetic patient takes much longer to dilate with mydriatics than in a non-diabetic. This could be due to various possible factors like oedema of the iris stroma, iris atrophy or spasm of the sphincter muscle due to sub-clinical mild inflammatory reaction.
2. *Pigment dispersion*—commonly observed at the time of iridectomy or cataract extraction operation is due to the changes in the pigment epithelium.
3. *Diabetic rubeosis iris*—The condition is characterised by neovascularisation seen on the anterior surface of iris. Diabetic rubeosis is first seen around the pupillary margin and in more advanced cases the blood vessels extending forward from the root of the iris are easily seen. Although haemorrhage from these vessels is very uncommon, there may occasionally be hyphaema and patches of haemorrhages on the iris surface. Extension of neovascularisation into the angle of anterior chamber may cause glaucoma, which like thrombotic glaucoma, is very difficult to treat.

Essential Iris Atrophy

It is an uncommon condition of unknown etiology, probably of hereditary and neurogenic nature. Atrophy involves all the tissues except the sphincter muscle. The condition starts with patchy atrophy and a distorted and displaced pupillary aperture with ectropion of the iris pigment epithelium. The atrophic patches may later appear as holes when atrophic process involves loss of tissue. In due course, all that is left of the iris diaphragm is a few fibrous bands connected to the remains of the sphincter muscle. An incipient glaucoma may supervene which does not respond to conservative therapy.

Iridoschiasis

It is a rare condition is old age. The degenerative changes which are patchy in character cause atrophy of the anterior layers of the iris stroma, which may ultimately become fibrillar strands, the ends of which float in the anterior chamber. The deeper iris stroma and the sphincter muscle remain intact to give a near normal pupillary reaction.

CYSTS AND TUMOURS

Iris and ciliary body, by virtue of being composed of pigment cells, blood vessels, connective tissue and muscle fibres, are particularly prone to develop cysts and tumours.

Cysts

Among the cystic lesions, common ones are congenital cysts, parasitic cysts and cysts due to the prolonged use of miotics. In addition, trauma, foreign body implantation and degenerations may cause cysts.

Congenital cysts of iris although rare, are a distinct clinical entity, seen in young children. The cyst may sometimes be large enough but usually does not reach upto the pupillary margin. The anterior wall is lined by endothelial layer and a few pigmented strands. As long as it is limited to a small sector, it does not result in rise of intra-ocular tension but when extending to larger area, may give rise to secondary glaucoma.

Cysts of the ciliary body usually remain undetected for long. Sometimes a cyst from the pars plana may extend to the ciliary zone and becoming obvious only on dilatation. They rarely need any treatment and are difficult to approach surgically.

Parasitic cysts: The parasites which can cause inflammatory reaction in uveal tissue, can also lead to cyst formation.

Miotic cysts: Prolonged miotic therapy for glaucoma has long been known to cause cysts in iris and ciliary body. Among the miotics that causes cysts is DFP, a drug fortunately much less commonly used. Pilocarpine and eserine can also cause cystic changes rarely.

The cysts are usually small and involve the pigment epithelial layer of the iris. They are never large enough to push the iris forwards or cause secondary rise of tension.

Although the entity of the miotic cyst is well established, their pathogenesis is unclear.

Tumours

These may arise from pigment epithelium, muscle tissue, blood vessels and neurogenic tissue. These are ciliary dysktioma, a leimyoma, haemangioma, neurofibroma and melanoma of iris. Histologically the list can be very large but most of these are extremely rare. In addition, iris and ciliary body may be a seat of secondary metastasis from carcinoma, melanoma, retinoblastoma and sarcoma elsewhere.

CONGENITAL ANOMALIES OF THE IRIS AND THE CILIARY BODY

The common anomalies of clinical importance are described here. The chapter on Congenital Anomalies covers the subject in greater detail.

The congenital anomalies of the uveal tract are due to defective closure of the foetal fissure through which mesoderm enters the secondary optic vesicle. Normally foetal fissure completely closes so that the uvea forms a complete and continuous tract comprising of iris, ciliary body and the choroid.

Faulty closure of the foetal fissure results in colobomatous defect and it depends on the extent of non-closure whether the coloboma involves only the iris, only the choroid or both structures.

Aniridia

It has been reported as a strongly dominant transmission. Complete absence of iris is due to failure of development of the rim of optic cup so that the neuro-ectodermal scaffolding is absent whereby mesodermal iris fails to form. Although clinically it appars like total absence of iris, rudimentary iris tissue can often be seen on fonioscopy (Fig. 11.9, Plate 6).

Congenital Coloboma of the Iris

This is a typical clinical condition which may be present alone or associated with other congenital anomalies, like coloboma of the choroid, coloboma of the lens, microcornea, micro-ophthalmos, etc. The condition can be uni-ocular but may in some cases be present in both eyes.

Corresponding to the position of the foetal fissure, coloboma of iris extends from the pupillary margin downwards. The eyes are hyper-metropic and develop a brown nuclear cataract by adolescence or later. Vision in these eyes, therefore, is always subnormal and the grade of visual defect depends on other associated anomalies and the lens changes.

Differential diagnosis is from surgical coloboma due to a sector or an optical iridectomy. The differentiating features are the location of the coloboma and the anatomy of the collarette of the iris. A congenital coloboma is always downwards while a surgical coloboma may be in any position. The collarette of the iris in congenital coloboma follows the border of the coloboma while it abruptly ends at the cut edges in surgical coloboma (Fig. 11.10).

Coloboma of iris acquires importance when lens extraction is needed later in life. Firstly the

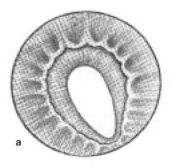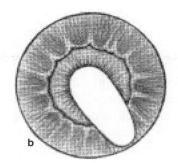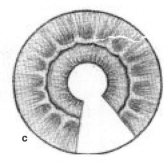

Fig. 11.10: Position of collarette as a Diagnostic Criterion. (a) Congenital coloboma of the iris, the collarette is seen all round the colobma; (b) and (c) Optical iridectomy and complete iridectomy. In both, the collarette ends at the iridectomy margin.

sphincter is non-responsive to mydriatics and secondly the cataract may be removed through the lower limbal section. Sphincterotomy in the 12 O'clock direction may help lens removal.

Persistent Pupillary Membrane

These are remnants of the anterior vascular sheath of the lens. Normally this completely disappears well before birth. Some fibrillar remnants may however persist and be seen in a routine examination.

Clinically they are seen as fine fibrillar net work or strands in pupillary area. The characteristic feature is that they are all attached to the collarette of the iris and not to the pupillary margin. The other end of the fibrils may sometimes be attached to the anterior capsule of the lens. These cases are compatible with normal visual acuity.

Anomalies of the Pupil

The size, shape and symmetry of pupils is an important physiological and clinical fact. However, variations in shape, size and symmetry are sometimes seen. The displacement of the pupil from its central position is called *correctopia*. When more than one pupil is present, it is called *polycoria*. When the size of the pupil in two eyes is unequal, it is called *aniso-coria*. When the pupil is smaller than normal in size, it is called *microcoria*.

An unround pupil which is otherwise normal is however a fairly common anomaly though of no clinical or pathological significance. Similarly a small variation in the size of the pupil of both eyes is also not uncommonly noted if an examination of the pupil is carefully done. Another not uncommon anomaly compatible with an otherwise normal pupil is ectropion of the pigment layer of iris. It is actually the neuro-epithelial part of the iris which at places projects into the pupillary space and is seen as dark black excrescences along the pupillary margin.

Polycoria is however a more significant congenital anomaly because it causes some visual disturbance. There may be two, three or even more apertures in the iris diaphragm. They all differ from the normal pupil in that they have no sphincter muscle. These apertures in the iris may not be complete gaps but embryonic strands of tissue criss-cross, giving it a sieve like appearance. Their significance is that they can cause polyopia and some amount of photophobia. The discomfort can be remedied by using painted contact lens.

POSTERIOR UVEA

Choroid

Embryologically and to some extent histologically the choroid is a member of the uveal family. After the developing phase is over, it gets itself dismembered from the genetic family and joins as a member of the neuroectodermal family of the retina and an important member because the most important rods and cones layer of the retina depends on choriocapillaries for its nutrition. Most of posterior choroid is supplied by the short posterior ciliary vessels while anterior periphery gets nutrition from the long posterior ciliary arteries. The choroid may undergo extensive inflammation and yet iris and ciliary body remain unaffected. Similarly neoplasms of the choroid may remain strictly limited to choroid itself.

The etiology of uveitis already described, by and large covers the inflammatory lesions of the choroid except that lesions due to endogenous hypersensitivity are more common in iris and ciliary body than in choroid. Syphilis and tuberculosis are more often the cause of choroiditis. Pan-ophthalmitis and endophthalmitis which are more choroidal in origin are already described. The clinical features of inflammations, atrophy and degenerations, cysts and tumours of the choroid are described here.

Inflammations of Choroid

Inflammation of choroid is associated with oedema and exudation. During the active stage, inflammatory cells may pass through the retina and cause a vitreous haze. The peculiar feature of the healing process in the choroid is the collection of pigment at the margins of the lesion and atrophy of the remaining elements except the large blood vessels, hence the shine of the sclera through the healed patch.

The retina overlying the healed patch suffers because of disappearance of chorio-capillaries resulting in a relative or absolute scotoma depending on the severity of the pathological change in the choroid.

Clinical manifestation of choroiditis will depend on the site and stage of the disease and whether active or healed. It is important to be able to differentiate between these two stages.

CHOROIDITIS

	Active	*Healed*
Circum-corneal congestion	Mild and only in anterior choroiditis	Absent
Vitreous	Slightly hazy with particulate matter	Clear with few floaters
Lesion	Ill-defined, muddy yellow with oedema	Well defined with marginal pigment, large choroidal vessels and sclera seen
Retinal vessels	Slight elevation over the patch due to oedema	Patch distinctly deeper to retinal vessels.
Vision	Partial diminution due to vitreous haze, severely affected in macular lesions.	Localised scotoma, relative or absolute

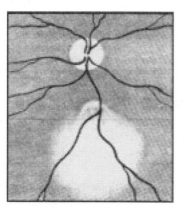

Fig 11.11A: Active choroiditis

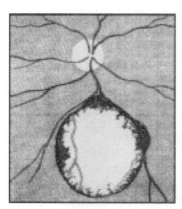

Fig 11.11B: Healed choroiditis

Clinical Types of Choroiditis

Choroiditis may be classified into:
1. Diffuse Choroiditis.
2. Disseminated Choroiditis.
3. Central Choroiditis.
4. Juxta-papillary Choroiditis.

Diffuse Choroiditis: Even though lesions may start separately, they coalesce to involve a large part of the contiguous area. The etiology is more often tubercular than syphilitic. During the active stage vitreous haze is appreciable because of involvement of large area. As healing takes place, clumps of pigment may be present all over the area. Some pigments may be deeper to the retinal vessels while others may migrate to lie along the blood vessels or even in front of them. The field defects correspond to the area of the retina affected and in extensive lesions only central field may remain intact with wide spread pigmentation and intact central field, the condition is sometimes called *secondary retinitis pigmentosa.* The following are the differentiating features between secondary retinitis pigmentosa due to choroiditis and primary pigment degeneration of a hereditary nature.

Disseminated choroiditis: This is a condition where discreet, isolated patches of choroiditis involve chorio-retinal layers with clinically normal intervening tissue. The patches may be few or in large numbers. The lesions, when many, are more often syphilitic than tubercular and when few they are more often tubercular (tubercular allergy or tuberculoma). Being granulomatous lesions, healing by scarring leaves behind atrophic patches with choroidal tissue destroyed and pigmentation at the margins with sclera shining through. A few peripheral lesions may be symptomless but when near the macular area, vision may be grossly affected. Being densely scarred, healed patches leave isolated absolute scotomata in field of vision (Fig. 11.11C, Plate 7).

Central choroiditis: The special feature of central choroiditis is early and severe loss of vision. Bilateral central choroiditis in children should always be investigated for congenital toxoplasmosis. Ophthalmoscopically, macular choroiditis due to toxoplasmosis appears as a round patch of about 2-3 disc diameter size with regular margin. Healing leaves behind an atrophic macular area with pigmentation and a central scotoma.

Juxta-papillary choroiditis: Choroiditis adjoining the optic disc is particularly significant when it is near the outer half of the disc margin because it affects the vital papillo-macular nerve fibre bundle and therefore causes severe visual loss and large field defect out of proportion to the clinical size of the lesion. In active stage, there may be associated papillitis. A healed patch of juxta-papillary choroiditis is associated with pallor of disc adjoining the patch or a full fledged

	Secondary retinitis pigmentosa Diffuse choroiditis (healed)	Primary retinitis pigmentosa
Lens	Clear	Posterior polar opacity in late stage
Vitreous	Floaters	Clear
Optic disc	Normal or atrophic	Waxy yellow
Retinal vessels	Normal	Arteries markedly attenuated
Pigments	At all levels in clumps in the area involved	Always superficial small and spiky, more in equatorial and peripheral area all round along veins
ERG	Normal or subnormal	Extinguished even in early stages
Visual fields	Scotomatous defects in corresponding area	Ring scotoma in early stages and generalised peripheral constriction with tubular field in late stage.

optic atrophy if papillitis occurred during the active stage.

Investigations for a case of choroiditis are on the same line as for anterior uveitis described earlier.

Complications of choroiditis are largely limited to posterior segment and are concerned more with opacities in vitreous and damage to retina. Complicated cataract may be present when associated with anterior uveitis.

Treatment of choroiditis is on the general lines already described for anterior uveitis except that atropinisation is neither required nor necessary. The treatment is more systemic than topical or sub-conjunctival. Retrobulbar or periocular injections may be added. Steroids are vitally needed and in heavy doses so that the lesion gets localised early and the end result is less damaging.

Other Specific Lesions of the Choroid

Metastatic choroiditis: This is due to infective emboli from elsewhere in the body. They cause discrete lesions of severe inflammatory nature with exudation and dense vitreous opacities. When in the macular area, there is severe oedema in the macula indicated by a star appearance all round the central lesion. In very severe cases, the condition may end up as endophthalmitis.

Mycotic choroiditis: Mycotic and fungal lesions of the choroid are usually the result of exogenous infection either due to perforating injury or a perforated corneal ulcer. The infection spreads to all intra-ocular tissues and ends up as pan-ophthalmitis.

Parasitic choroiditis: Toxoplasmosis as cause of choroiditis has already been mentioned. It has been emphasized that the lesion is granulomatous in nature and leaves behind healed pigmented patches. Congenital toxoplasmosis is a cause of bilateral central choroiditis. Acquired toxoplas-

mosis has also been recognised as a cause of patchy choroiditis in adult age. Tests for toxoplasmosis have also been detailed earlier.

Most of the parasites in the intra-ocular tissues like filaria, cysticercus and hydatid cyst first gain entry through choroidal vasculature.

Chorio-retinal Degenerations

The visual cell layer of retina depends on choriocapillaris for its nutrition. This is still more significant in the macular area where there are no retinal vessels. Any degenerative process in the choroid therefore readily extends to macular area of retina.

Damage to vision in these cases is variable. In cases where there is gross macular damage, vision is reduced to 6/36-6/60 with a central scotoma. Patients with more extensive chorioretinal and cerebral degenerations may become totally blind.

Chorio-retinal macular degenerations present a variety of clinical conditions:

1. Heredo-familial degenerations.
2. Central areolar choroidal atrophy.
3. Colloid degeneration of macular area.
4. Senile macular degeneration.
5. Desciform degeneration of macula.
6. Cystic degeneration of macula.

Heredo-familial degenerations: There is a variety of clinical changes in macular area which can be included in this group. The characteristic features are bilaterality and symmetry of the lesion in the two eyes. The conditions may become evident any time from infancy to adulthood.

The following are among the common clinical entities:

1. Doyne's honeycomb choroiditis showing numerous colloid deposits around macular area with pigmentation in the centre.
2. Heredo-familial maculo-cerebral degeneration showing pigmentary degeneration of macula with mental retardation.

3. Infantile amaurotic familial idiocy (Tay-Sach's disease) showing granular degeneration of macular area with cherry red spot in the centre and cerebral palsy. The condition is due to lipid degeneration involving cells of nervous system.

Central areoler choroidal atrophy: There is atrophy of choriocapillaries in macular area involving 2-3 disc diameter area. The pigments in the retina and choroid disappear. Sclerosis of large choroidal vessels is prominently seen in the atrophic area.

Senile macular degeneration: There is a variety of clinical changes in the macular area which fall under this group. They are a common cause of visual failure in old age. There may be associated arterio-sclerotic retinopathy. These macular changes are recognised as age related macular degeneration.

The clinical changes may be:
1. Greyish colouration in the macular area.
2. Stippling in the macular area.
3. Yellowish white patches.
4. Small pigment dots.
5. Small sub-retinal or choroidal haemorrhage in macular area.

Disciform degeneration of macula: It is a circumscribed lesion of 3-4 disc diameters involving macular area and giving the appearance of a pseudo-tumour. There may be haemorrhage and exudates due to arterio-sclerotic changes in the chorio-capillaries. The condition may sometimes be associated with clinical picture of circinate retinopathy. The differential diagnosis from malignant melanoma is important but difficult. A close follow-up of a case will help note any change which may be indicative of malignancy.

Cystic degeneration of macula: Small circumscribed lesions distinctly raised from the surface are not uncommon in old age diagnosed as cystic degeneration. The slit of the ophthalmoscope moved across the lesion distinctly indicates its raised character. The condition is static but if there is a rupture, the picture of a macular cyst changes to a macular hole which may lead to localised macular detachment.

Colloid degeneration of macula: It is not uncommon to find macular area studded with yellowish dots or flat muddy yellow patches. The lesions may sometimes conglomerate to form a drusen. These colloid lesions are compatible with good visual acuity.

Tumours of Choroid

The choroid being principally composed of vascular network and pigment cells, neoplasms of choroid are not uncommon. When small and in periphery, they may remain undetected for a long time. The importance of a choroidal tumour may become highly significant firstly because they can lead to rise in intraocular tension and secondly when melanotic in nature, they may be so malignant that they may be fatal due to metastasis even before the ocular pathology is clinically diagnosed.

Among the common choroidal tumours are:
1. Haemangioma of choroid.
2. Benign melanoma.
3. Malignant melanoma.
4. Secondary neoplasms in the choroid like carcinoma, hypernephroma, chorion-epithelioma and sarcoma.

Haemangioma: They are usually congenital although they manifest clinically later in life. It is seen as a circumscribed greyish yellow lesion distinctly raised from the surrounding retinal surface as seen by the alteration in course of retinal blood vessels over it. The retina round the tumour mass is detached but has a shelving margin and no holes or tears seen which differentiates it from primary retinal detachment. If the tumour mass is large in size, it may cause secondary glaucoma.

The tumour mass is a cavernous type angioma with large blood spaces, covered by a fibrous layer. Can be associated with Sturge Weber syndrome.

A conclusive diagnosis is not always easy particularly the differential diagnosis from malignant melanoma. These cases must be kept under regular clinical review from time to time. If they reach a stage of secondary glaucoma, the eye should be promptly enucleated.

Benign melanoma: Simple benign melanoma, also called naevus is comprised of pigmented spindle cells derived from the neural ectoderm. Clinically, the fundus lesion appears as circumscribed and uniformly bluish in colour commonly seen in the posterior fundus. The lesions are flat and the retinal vessels coursing over them do not get deflected. The condition is usually symptomless and its clinical importance is to differentiate it from malignant melanoma. From this point of view, these lesions should be under constant clinical surveillance to detect the earliest malignant change if any, indicated by increase in size. A photographic record and ultrasonography records will help noting change in size, shape and vascularity from time to time.

No treatment is necessary so long as no change to malignancy is noted.

Malignant melanoma: Malignant melanoma like all pigmented tumours is much more common in white skinned races than in dark skinned population.

Malignant melanoma is usually unilateral, very much more common in the choroid than in the anterior uvea.

It is not clear what initiates the onset of malignant melanoma. A simple pre-existing naevus may change to malignancy.

Histologically, epithelioid cells aggregate round blood vessels forming pseudo rosettes. The neoplastic cells may be pigmented like melanocytes. The reticulin content of the tumour mass indicates the grade of malignancy of the tumour. More cellular with less reticulin is more malignant and vice-a-versa.

Clinically, it starts as a small circumscribed lesion with a clear-cut outline but shelving margins. It is progressive in nature and therefore causes distortion of the retinal blood vessels overlying it with retinal detachment surrounding the mass. Haemorrhage in the vitreous, rubeosis iris and spontaneous hyphaema in an elderly patient in white races often arouses suspicion of malignant melanoma. Malignant melanoma as a possibility in blind and phthisical eyes or in eyes with absolute glaucoma is considered an indication for enucleation in all such eyes even if otherwise not indicated. In its advanced stages the tumour may extend anteriorly to involve ciliary body and may present in the angle of the anterior chamber. It may extend to occupy intra-ocular space and lead to rise of intraocular tension. It may extend through the sclera, particularly along the exits of vortex veins and invade the orbital tissues.

The tumour mass may disintegrate the eye ball and involve structures of orbit giving rise to a large fungating mass.

Secondaries from malignant melanoma are carried via blood circulation. The common sites for secondary deposits are the liver and the brain. This is one condition where metastasis may have taken place even before the ocular disease has been diagnosed because diagnosis is often late as the disease in periphery may not cause any symptoms for a long time. It is often discovered in routine examination.

Clinically, though more theoretically, the progress of malignant melanoma has been divided into four stages with ill defined border lines.

1. Sub-clinical stage with no symptoms and if in periphery, a small tumour is often missed during routine ophthalmoscopic examination.
2. Glaucomatous stage when the lesion has advanced to cause rise of intraocular tension and then the clinical diagnosis indicates unfavourable prognosis.
3. Stage of extra ocular extension.
4. Stage of distant metastasis which is invariably fatal.

Diagnosis of malignant melanoma in susceptible races is sought for in all elderly patients with visual symptoms. Indirect ophthalmoscopy to scan the periphery of the fundus carefully is a routine examination to exclude *early* melanoma. Glaucomatous eyes and solid retinal detachment without a tear arouse suspicion. Fluorescein angiography, transillumination and ultra sonography are done to note progress of the disease. High uptake of radio-active p-32 helps indicate malignancy of the lesion. But it can give false higher readings even in naevi and therefore observations are not dependable. A negative finding is more useful to differentiate between a naevus and melanoma. Examination of aspirated subretinal fluid may show neoplastic cells but it is a dangerous procedure because it may initiate metastatic spread.

Treatment: Enucleation of the eye has been the first choice in all cases where a malignant melanoma of choroid is diagnosed. So long as the disease is strictly intraocular, enucleation with an optic nerve stump alone may suffice. If there is any evidence, however small, of extension into the orbital tissue, an exenteration should be preferred. Although a melanoma is not adequately radio-sensitive, radiation therapy should follow enucleation or exenteration.

In patients where malignant melanoma is diagnosed in the only eye of the patient and the lesion is small, consideration may be given to a less radical therapy, which includes diathermy of the area from the scleral surface or photocoagulation from retinal surface. This approach is possible in small sized tumours. Photocoagulation of a small lesion is also the treatment of choice when diagnosis is in doubt.

In advanced cases where distant metastasis has already taken place local surgery is more palliative than curative in nature.

It is emphasized that melanoma is a slowly growing lesion and enucleation should not be decided in a hurry. There are reports that poorly performed enucleation may throw showers of cells in circulation where there was no metastasis before. This newer thinking suggests:

1. Enucleation for melanoma should not be considered an emergency.
2. Only when the growth is distinctly progressive and increased to a size of 10 mm or more, should enucleation be considered obligatory.
3. Enucleation should be done by a senior person by a very gentle process. Muscles should not be hooked but directly cut with scissors. The lesion should be cryo forzen before enucleation and at no stage of manipulation should the tension be allowed to rise above 50 mmHg. Special cryo probes have been devised which will keep the lesion frozen all through surgery.

Secondary Tumours of Choroid

Among the metastatic tumours, secondaries from carcinoma elsewhere, hypernephroma and a sarcoma can involve the choroid. In most of these cases, the primary tumour is already clinically evident. The tumour mass in the eye follows the same mode of progressing stages, the early stage, the stage of glaucoma and direct extension into the orbital tissues.

The treatment as for all malignant tumours of the choroid, is enucleation or exenteration as the case may be. The prognosis depends on the fate of the primary lesion.

Choroidal Detachment

The choroid and ciliary body both being in contact with the inner scleral surface, are commonly jointly involved in the detachment pathology. Except the firm attachment of ciliary body to the scleral spur and that of choroid at the exits of vortex veins, these two structures are in loose apposition to the scleral surface, the contact being maintained by intraocular tension. When favourable factors develop, the consequence is detachment of anterior choroid and ciliary body

Chorio-ciliary detachment is caused by the collection of fluid in the supra-choroidal and extra-ciliary space. The fluid may be aqueous in nature which may seep into the space through the angle of the anterior chamber. As the fluid is more albuminous in character, another view is that it is exudative in nature derived from choroidal vasculature.

Chorio-ciliary detachment is most commonly seen following an intra-ocular surgery like cataract, glaucoma and full thickness corneal graft operations.

Post-operative Choroidal Detachment

Detachment of anterior choroid is not uncommon following cataract, glaucoma and keratoplasty operations. The precipitating factor is a sudden lowering of tension at operation or a continuing low tension during the post-operative period.

Although detachment process is started immediately or soon after operation, it usually becomes clinically evident 4-6 days or later after the surgery.

Clinical features are characteristics:
1. Flattening of the anterior chamber after it is once formed post-operatively, is an indication of chorio-ciliary detachment.
2. Low tension following cataract operation.

3. Ophthalmoscopically dark round masses are seen projecting all round behind the iris.
4. Detachment of the choroid has a tendency to spontaneously regress as the tension of the eye returns to normal and in most cases it may not leave behind any after effects.

Traumatic and inflammatory detachments are usually flat in nature and more often seen as choroidal detachments rather than chorio-ciliary detachments.

Ophthalmoscopically the retina appears raised with a greyish discolouration. The blood vessels over the raised area are not dark as in a detached retina because it is the detachment of choroid and retina both and not the retina alone. For the same reason, the detachment is a solid detachment with no folds and no tears unlike a primary retinal detachment. When there is vitreous haemorrhage due to trauma or inflammatory exudation in the vitreous, fundus details may not be visible.

Treatment: Post-operative choroidal detachment does not need active treatment in most cases. The patient should however be put to bed and the eye be bandaged. There is however another view that the post-operative routine need not be altered as the choroidal detachment will settle down even otherwise. Any leakage at the section if noted, should however be repaired. Pilocarpine eye drops are used rather empirically. Vitamin C in large doses may help resolution of the supra-choroidal fluid. Steroids may reduce the exudation into the supra-choroidal space.

If the flat anterior chamber persists, restoring the anterior chamber with injection of air may help break the vicious circle. Rarely drainage of the supra-choroidal fluid through diathermy puncture or a scleral incision in the parsplana used to be considered.

Congenital Anomalies of Choroid

Congenital coloboma of the choroid which is a fairly common clinical condition and albinism which usually affects uveal tract as a whole are described here.

Congenital coloboma of the choroid. This is a defect due to faulty closure of the foetal fissure resulting in absence of choroid in the corresponding area. Like coloboma of iris, it is also downwards. It is usually unilateral but may be present bilaterally. When present alone, it is compatible with good visual acuity.

Clinically, coloboma of choroid may present in different grades.

1. An isolated island of colobomatous defect always in the downwards meridian corresponding to the foetal fissure. The inferior crescent when present congenitally is also the mildest form of coloboma of choroid.
2. A coloboma starting a little away from the disc and extending to the periphery. It has a rounded upper end and becomes wider towards the periphery in the line of foetal fissure.
3. Coloboma extending upto the lower disc margin.

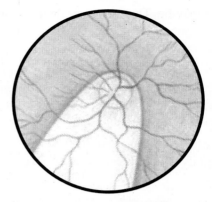

Fig. 11.12B: Choroidal coloboma—enclosing disc

4. Coloboma as in grade III but also engulfing the disc and involving the peripapillary area.

A choroidal coloboma is often diagnosed on routine ophthalmoscopic examination, the ophthalmoscopic picture is characteristic. A white reflex is seen in eyes with grade III and IV colobomata. As fundus details are focussed, the coloboma is seen with clear-cut margins. In coloboma area, the retinal vessels are normal and the sclera shines through there being no choroidal tissue. Some pigment deposits may be seen at the edges of the coloboma.

Vision is usually good because the macular area is away and uninvolved. Visual fields show a scotoma corresponding to the size or a little smaller than the colobomatous defect. The scotoma is due to the fact that even though retinal layers are present in the coloboma, there are no chorio-capillaries to supply nutrition to the rods and cones in the area.

Albinism: The condition indicates absence of the pigment in the uveal tract and is clinically evident in the iris and choroid. It has a definite hereditary and genetic background.

Iris: The iris appears light in colour. It is so thin that fundus glow by retro-illumination can be seen

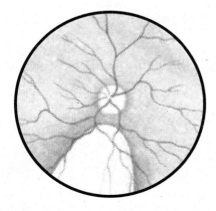

Fig. 11.12A: Choroidal coloboma—close to disc margin

through iris diaphragm. The patients complains of severe photophobia because iris no longer acts as a diaphragm to obstruct and absorb light.

Choroid: Albinotic choroid has also a characteristic clinical picture. The fundus background appears light pinkish in colour. Choroidal vessels are prominently seen through.

Albinotic eyes are usually myopic. Ocular nystagmus is commonly present. Even though vision may not improve beyond 6/24-6/18, near vision is good. Albinism in eyes may be associated with generalised albinism of the skin. These patients not only complain of photophobia but their skin is also sensitive to sunlight.

Refractive errors should be appropriately corrected. Photophobia can be overcome by using tinted glasses. The use of painted contact lens is particularly helpful in preventing light passing through the iris diaphragm.

12

Physiological Lens and the Cataract

PHYSIOLOGICAL LENS

The lens is the second most powerful refracting medium in the eye, next only to cornea. The biconvex human lens and the cornea together help to refract light rays to form a focus on the retina and provide good visual acuity. The second most important function of the lens is the physical part of accommodation, the change in the shape of the lens caused by action of ciliary muscles through the suspensory ligament of the lens. The lens during accommodation, becomes more convex and its focusing power increases.

The crystalline lens is made up of a capsule, the lens matter (the cortex) and the nucleus in different stages of evolution.

Development of Lens

Lens is entirely developed from surface ectoderm. The development starts with the formation of lens plate as early as 4.0 to 5.0 mm stage in the 5th week of embryonic development. Differentiation of cells leads to formation of a lens pit and later the lens vesicle at 10.0 mm stage in 6th week. The lens vesicle of the surface ectoderm invaginates into the primary optic vesicle and thereby leads to formation of secondary optic vesicle.

Further development of the lens takes place by formation of primary lens fibres from the epithelial cells lining the posterior wall of lens vesicles. The primary fibres filling the vesicle cavity ultimately form embryonic nucleus. Thereafter the secondary lens fibres are formed from the equatorial cells.

These fibres surround the embryonic nucleus. These secondary fibres are so arranged that diametrically opposite groups of fibres unite to form the sutures in front and behind the embryonic nucleus. These sutures are visible on the slit lamp within the adult nucleus as an erect anterior Y and an inverted posterior Y.

The capsule of the lens is embryologically present at an early stage of formation of the lens vesicle. This homogenous layer is presumably secreted by the ectodermal cells lining the vesicle and forming the basement layer enveloping the developing lens. The cells lining posterior capsule having already differentiated to form the embryonic nucleus, the cortical fibres are developed from epithelial cells lining the equatorial part of the lens capsule. As new fibres are laid down, older fibres are pushed to the centre and this process continues till adult life to form adult lens consisting of the capsule, soft lens cortex and the firm nucleus in the centre. The capsule in the adult lens is now lined by epithelial cells along the anterior wall only.

The zonule or the suspensory ligament of the lens is developed from the tertiary vitreous which differentiates into anterior and posterior bundles of fibres which are attached just in front and behind the equator of lens on one side and the ciliary epithelium on the other side suspending the lens in position.

It is evident that the development of the lens is actively progressing from the 5th week of intra-uterine life to the age of 20-25 years and even after. The diameter of lens increases from 7.5 mm at 1 year to 9.5 mm in old age and its thickness increases from 2.5 mm at 1 year age to 3.5 mm at 25 years and 4.5 mm in old age.

Any disturbance to this developing process can lead to developmental anomalies depending on at what stage of development the process is disturbed.

Among common developmental anomalies of lens are *spherophakia, microphakia, anterior lenticonus, posterior lenticonus, coloboma of lens* and *congenital subluxation* of lens (Ectopia Lentis). Intra-uterine infection like Rubella (German measles) in first trimester of pregnancy often results in *congenital cataract*, usually in both eyes.

However complete absence of Lens (true congenital aphakia) is extremely rare.

Anatomy of Lens

The lens is situated just behind the iris diaphragm anteriorly and is supported behind by the hyaloid fossa of the vitreous. It is suspended by fine fibres of the suspensory ligament or the zonule. The zonules are stronger in younger age and become weaker in old age. The distance between the equator of the lens and ciliary processes is about 0.5 mm. The circumlental space round the equator within the fibres of the suspensory ligament is called the *Canal of Petit* through which aqueous partly flows into retrolental space.

In the non-accommodative state of the eye, lens has a refractive power of about +19.5 diopters and about +22 diopters when accommodated. It is about 9 mm in diameter and centrally 4 to 4.5 mm in thickness in resting state. The posterior surface of the lens is more convex and the anterior surface is less convex.

The capsule is thinner in the central part and it is through this portion, herniation of the lens substance gives the lens a parabolic shape and brings about accommodation. The posterior capsule has firm adhesions to the hyaloid canal in young age. This adhesion is called the *hyaloid-capsular ligament* which gradually atrophies and becomes insignificant in most cases by the age of 25-30 years.

The lens cortex which is formed from the equatorial capsular epithelium is made up of lens fibres in such a way that the earlier fibres are pushed to the centre and fresh fibres lie in the subcapsular area. It is this process of physical compression of the central fibres by the newly forming peripheral fibres that adult nucleus of the lens is formed by about the age of 20-25 years.

The nucleus of the lens is nearly biconvex. It is embryonic in the early phase of development, foetal soon after birth and adult nucleus by age of 20-25 years. It is soft in early age and becomes harder later on and therefore in older age when there is marked difference in the refractive index of the lens matter and the nucleus, the lens acts as if a biconvex lens nucleus is surrounded by two convaco-convex cortical lenses and this meniscus lens introduces lenticular myopia in older age.

Metabolism of Lens

Like cornea, lens is also totally an avascular structure. The nutrition and transparency of the lens is maintained by anaerobic glycolylic metabolic process.

The transparency of lens depends on the high concentration of soluble proteins, adequate oxidative metabolism and adequate nutrition provided by glucose, amino acids, ascorbic acid, riboflavin and oxygen. The source of nutrition to lens is obviously from the surrounding aqueous humour and the nutrients are utilised by the internal oxidative glycolytic enzyme action.

A cataractous lens is deficient in soluble proteins, potassium, glutathione, ascorbic acid and riboflavin. The poor oxidative system is the cause of poor glycolysis, thereby making the lens an asphyxiated tissue. Another change is higher concentration of calcium and the conversion of cystein into cystine. Even though these biochemical changes have been studied in detail, knowledge of etiological pathogenesis of cataract is still incomplete.

Changes in the Lens with Age

Biologically, the lens is a very active structure. Like all body tissues, it undergoes metabolic and bio-chemical changes and changes in shape, size and transparency. These changes are listed as follows:

1. Globular in infants and biconvex in old age.
2. Increases in size, weight and density with age.
3. Plasticity decreases resulting in weaker accommodation as age increases.
4. The nucleus becomes harder in old age.
5. Difference in refractive index of cortex and nucleus introduces lenticular myopia in old age.
6. Soluble proteins decrease and insoluble proteins increase.
7. The yellow discolouration starting under the posterior capsule and later extending to posterior cortex and nucleus, starts at about 40 years and gradually increases with age.

8. Senile exfoliation of the lens capsule.
9. Degenerative changes in zonular ligament of the lens.

Pathology

Being an avascular structure, the lens does not undergo primary inflammation. Primary neoplasms in the lens are unknown. The lens is however affected secondarily in inflammation of iris and may develop cataractous change. Degenerative changes can cause calcification of the capsule and also cause weakening of the suspensory ligament and spontaneous subluxation of lens.

The lens responds to injury in various ways. Point perforation may seal itself leaving only a small localised lens opacity. Tearing of the capsule results in opacification of whole lens. In young age lens cortex may get largely absorbed leaving a thin membrane. In older age, nucleus, remains of the lens capsule and the cortex may result in membranous cataract. Indirect concussion injury to the lens may cause rupture of the posterior capsule and lead to cataract formation.

Other Senile Changes in Lens

Exfoliation of the lens capsule can be senile in nature or may be caused by inflammations in the eye or may be traumatic in origin by persistent exposure to heat. These exfoliated capsular shreads may hang into anterior chamber attached at one end to lens capsule or may be seen with slit lamp freely floating in the anterior chamber. The condition is not damaging to vision and causes no symptoms.

Pseudo-exfoliation of the lens capsule is however primarily degenerative in nature and results in the formation of thin layer on anterior capsule of lens and on the structures around it. This is not a rare condition if routinely looked for on slit lamp in old age. The powdery deposit first appears on the periphery of anterior capsule so that it can only be diagnosed early by examination under mydriasis with slit lamp. White powdery deposits are also seen on pupillary margin and in angle of anterior chamber. Being slow and symptomless, it is often detected only when it has resulted in open angle glaucoma, in advanced stage. The glaucoma associated with it is called *glaucoma capsulare*.

SENILE CATARACT

Historical

Neither the morphology nor the functioning status of the lens as a structure inside the eye was precisely understood till the beginning of the sixteenth century. In fact, the concept of visual loss in the eye and the spokes of lens opacity against this concept of fluid background gave this disease the term of cataract, a Greek word, meaning a water fall. Greek literature, however, does recognise lens as a solid mass and this ill defined concept was passed on to the Romans and the Arabs and continued to be so understood till about the sixteenth century.

Indian history is however, more precise. The lens has been described as a distinct structure inside the eye in the Vedic book 'Sushrut Sanhita' as early as 3000 years back and cataract called 'Lingnash'.

The history of cataract surgery is fascinating to any ophthalmologist. The couching technique for cataract, first devised by Sushrut; a pupil of Dhanvantari, 3000 years back, has been precisely described in Indian literature. The technique was passed on to Greeks who recorded its practice 300 BC Roman Surgeon, Celsus (25 BC) and Galen (AD 135) followed up the same technique of Sushrut. The Arabs continued with the practice of couching and the same surgery was routinely adopted in Europe till Jacques Daviel immortalised himself by performing the first extraction operation in France on 8-4-1745, published by himself in 1753.

In ancient Indian literature, the difference between a mature and an immature cataract has been mentioned. Reddish cataract, calcified cataract and spokes of cataract have been described. The original description of the operation of Sushrut has a taste of scientific description of that time and it is interesting to enumerate the steps he has described so precisely in the book- Sushrut Sanhita. The criteria for good surgical technique have, in that ancient book, been listed as under.

- Surgeon should keep his beard and hair short.
- Operation should be performed in good weather.
- On an empty stomach.
- In a lighted room.
- In the morning only.
- Patient sitting with steady head helped by the assistants.
- Surgeon sitting with knee high support facing the patient.
- Eye anaesthetised by mouth vapours.
- Rub the eye with thumb (as if to lower tension)
- Wash the eye with mother's milk.
- Patient looking at his nose.
- Probe introduced half finger away from the cornea, (pars Palana)
- Lens manouvered into the space behind.
- Probe withdrawn as soon as the patient sees.
- Bandage the eye with ghee (purified butter) pads.
- Post-operatively, the patient to lie on the opposite side.
- No sneeze or cough for 7 days.
- Dressing after 3 days with ghee pads.
- If operation successful, fomentation.
- **Centraindications to surgery:** Coward persons, indigestion, thirst (probably diabetes)
- Vomiting, headache (probably glaucoma), Ear ache (sepsis near the eye), pain in the eye (infection).

Sushrut even mentioned operating the right eye with the left hand and the left eye with the right hand. Imagine how precise the approach to surgery was even in those ancient days.

The methods of lens extraction devised by Daviel in 1745 was a lower limbal extraction; the lens being pressed out with blunt needle.

Incidence of vitreous loss was fairly frequent in those years and hence further modifications during the last two and half centuries. The historical calender of a few important developments in cataract surgery being as follows:

1. Carlt (1894) introduced extraction by forceps.
2. Barraquer (1917) devised suction method of removal of lens, erisiphake.
3. Use of cocaine as surface anaesthesia was first used by Koller (1884) and retro-bulbar injection was described by Elschnig in (1928).
4. Wright in India (1926) and O'Brien (1929) introduced facial block.
5. The trend between intra-capsular and extra-capsular surgery has been swinging from time to time. The ancient surgery of couching was intra-capsular, though not extraction. The higher incidence of vitreous loss forced the surgeons to adopt extra capsular technique. With development of a retrobulbar injection and facial block, intra-capsular technique re-emerged as a favoured technique about 1930.
6. The development of techniques of suturing cataract section during the last decades has made cataract surgery a really secure surgery with very good prognosis.
7. Intraocular lens implant surgery, though first done in 1949 by Ridley with transparent glass implant, really look off in late nineteen seventies and has become a routine surgical procedure with a number of implant designs and surgical techniques.

Aetiology and Incidence

Cataract formation has been noted from birth to old age; the first being due to congenital or developmental defects, while a senile cataract is age related. Senile cataract is a disease of common occurrence in all geographical areas and in all races. The incidence, however, is distinctly more in tropical countries. The two factors peculiar to tropical circumstances and responsible for this high incidence are higher concentration of actinic rays in tropical sun-light, and nutritional deficiency factors so significant in these areas. It can be generally stated that in developing tropical countries, the age of 50 years and above is considered a cataractogenous age and the degree of incidence increases as the age advances. It is safe to assume that 60% people develop cataract by the age of 60 years, 70% by the age of 70 years, 80% by 80 years and 90% by 90 years of age.

In Western countries where incidence of cataract is relatively less, 22.6% have been reported affected due to cataract in England, 15.94% in Canada and 15.6% in United States. In a statistically dependable National survey in India in 1971-72, it was estimated that 55% of total or partial blindness was due to cataract in some stage of its formation. Of these, incidence in rural areas was 70% and in Urban areas 30%. Similarly, incidence in males was 64.4% as compared to 35.6% in females.

Morphological Types of Senile Cataract

With the routine use of a slit lamp, it has become possible to study lens changes. With clearer identification of the capsule, the lens matter and the nucleus, it is not difficult, to understand that in senile cataract, the changes may involve any one single tissue or may involve more than one of these structures. Common morphological types of senile cataract have been described.

A cataract with the spokes of cortical lens opacities is called the *cuneiform cataract*. Opacity of the nucleus is called a nuclear cata-

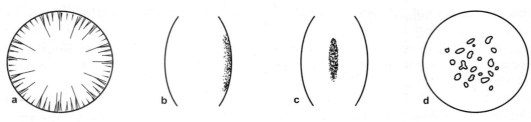

Fig. 12.1: Types of Cataract (a) Peripheral spokes of cortical lens opacity; (b) Central posterior sub-capsular opacity; (c) Nuclear sclerosis; (d) Flecks of anterior cortical lens opacity

ract. Opacity under the posterior capsule is called *cupuliform cataract*. Opacities in the anterior and posterior poles of lens are called *anterior polar and posterior polar* cataracts (Fig. 12.1).

The incidence of morphological types of senile cataract have been reported as under:

Cuneiform Cataract	35% – 50%
Nuclear Cataract	20% – 30%
Cupuliform Cataract	2.5% – 5.0%
Mixed types	15% – 42.5%

The pigmentation of lens nucleus in brown and black cataract has been well recognised. Light crimson yellow colouration of the posterior capsule in older age is also a common senile change in lens. Literature also mentions that the cortical spoke-like opacities mostly start in the equatorial region.

The above data are however from developed countries with low incidence and distinctly different environmental factors as against the conditions in tropical and developing countries. A critical study in India has yielded the following information regarding incidence of morphological types of senile cataract:

Cuneiform Cataract (Cortical spokes)	23%
Cupuliform Cataract (Posterior sub-capsular)	53%
Nuclear Cataract	24%

The majority of cataracts (53%) in tropical countries are cupuliform posterior subcapsular as compared to 5% reported from colder countries. It is also observed from this study that peripheral spokes of the opacities in the lens were mostly anterior cortical and only 17.4% are from equatorial and posterior cortex. The colour changes in the lens were most prominent at the level of posterior subcapsular area, the density of colour becoming less and less towards the anterior zones. Colour changes involved the nucleus only in eyes with nuclear sclerosis and brown pigmentation in brown cataract was noted to extend even into the anterior cortex. All these observations are indicative that a higher concentration of actinic rays in tropical sun light passing through central axial part of the lens and partly getting absorbed there, leads to higher incidence of cataract.

Clinical Features of Senile Cataract

Cataract being the commonest condition causing visual handicap, it is always uppermost in the mind of a clinician when dealing with a patient with defective vision in cataractogenic age. This dominating impression often leads to the presumptive diagnosis of cataract when there may be no cataract. One often overlooks other causes of visual deterioration in this age group. The diagnosis of cataract and actions to follow the diagnosis should therefore be based on sound evaluation of clinical findings. When thinking of cataract as a cause of visual defect, the clinician should face the following questions:

1. Has the eye under examination got cataract, which means precise diagnosis of its clinical and morphological features.

2. Has the patient got cataract and cataract alone or is there any other coexistent pathology which could also affect the vision of the eye e.g. chronic simple glaucoma, vascular retinopathies, senile macular changes and senile optic atrophy.

Having satisfactorily answered, the above two questions to oneself, further questions by the patient will need to be answered:

1. When can the cataract be operated and what can happen if it is not operated?
2. What is the prognosis of operating in a particular case?

   Having made a correct diagnosis and correct evaluation, having answered the questions to the patient and the patient is ready to get operated, a fifth question needs to be answered.
3. What procedure of cataract extraction should be adopted in a particular case to restore satisfactory visual status?

Discussion of answers to the above questions will complete the clinical approach to cataract.

Question One: Has the eye under examination got cataract? *Diagnosis of cataract* is often made very lightly in countries where incidence of cataract is very high. A busy practitioner often presumes cataract as the cause of defective vision in patients of 50 years and above and often omits to exclude other possible causes of visual loss. Many patients are thus deluded into security of a diagnosis of cataract while the patient reaches an advanced stage of chronic simple glaucoma or other progressive fundus pathology. He thus faces disappointment when he prepares himself for operation and is told that the eye is incurably blinded due to some other cause.

It is therefore extremely important that diagnosis of cataract should not only be precise but the eye should be examined in every case in the early stage of cataract formation when a detailed fundus examination is still possible. Apart from excluding other causes, it helps prognostic evaluation and the record is a good guide for comparison when any other condition may subsequently complicate cataract.

The diagnosis of cataract is based on symptoms of the patient and clinical findings.

Symptoms of cataract: Spending a minute or two in eliciting the history of duration of visual disturbance, mode of onset of visual loss, relation to bright light and shade, using glasses if any, visual status before patient developed symptoms related to cataract and surgery if any in either eye will be rewarding. Specific enquiries should be made to exclude diabetes and high blood pressure as a routine. A history of frequent micturition at night, cough and discharge from the ear should be pointedly asked. Personal history regarding smoking and drinking are important to elicit.

Vision: The common visual symptoms of cataract patients are, decrease in presbyopia, hameralopia, polyopia and gross visual loss.

The visual symptoms due to cataract depend on the site of the lens opacity and degree of opacification in the lens. Majority of lens opacities in India being centrally situated, to begin with, the commonest symptom is marked blurring of vision when the patient goes in bright sunlight, a condition, called *hameralopia or day blindness* because the opacity occupies most of the small pupil contracted by brightlight. These patients are relatively more comfortable indoors and at night when the pupil is large and enough light can pass through the clear part of pupil peripheral to the opacity. In eyes with peripheral spokes of lens opacities, visual symptoms are delayed till the spokes have multiplied and extended to the centre of lens. These patients see better in bright light when the small pupil is against a clear part in the centre of the lens while larger pupil in dark causes defraction of light and diminished vision called *nyctalopia or night blindness.* Some patients also complain of polyopia. This is due to the clear segments in a cataractous lens acting like separate pupils (Fig. 12.2).

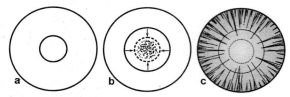

Fig. 12.2: Central and Peripheral Cataract. (Effect on vision in bright light and shade). (a) No lens opacity; (b) Central lens opacity, pupil contracts to bright light, vision diminished (day blindness); (c) Peripheral lens opacity, pupil contracts to bright light, clear lens in pupillary area, no defraction of light, vision improves

Refractive change due to lenticular myopia varying between 3 to 5 dioptres or even more is commonly observed in cases of nuclear sclerosis and nuclear cataract which contribute to visual loss for distance. A common consequence of lenticular myopia is the decrease in presbyopia and the patient who needed convex glasses for near can now read better with less power or even without glasses. This transient improvement in near vision in old age is often interpreted as a sign of improvement in the health of the eye while it is actually the beginning of cataract and a warning of the visual deterioration to follow. Other symptoms due to cataract are halos around lights, black spots in front of the eye and a faulty colour sense.

The vision however is ultimately reduced markedly in all types of cataract when lens opacity has involved large part of the lens by which time the cataract has reached the stage of near maturity. It is important to remember that however advanced the cataract may be, some light does pass through the lens and the iris and reach the retina, and therefore perception and projection of light is always maintained so long as it is cataract and cataract alone and there is no other pathology affecting retinal function. Some patients with intumescent cataract and a shallow anterior chamber may complain of occasional pain which can be due to a transient rise of irttraocular tension caused by the swollen lens.

Examination of eye: *Distant inspection.* An important observation is the presence of squint in some cases, usually a divergent squint appearing later in life in a cataractous eye indicates exophoria turning into exotropia which is transient in nature. It does not influence prognosis of visual recovery after cataract operation. When however the history reveals the presence of squint from earlier age, it could be concomitant squint and the eye may be amblyopic and vision may not improve to a desirable degree after operation.

Oblique illumination: Examination of the eye with a pencil of light is the first step. It is extremely important to emphasise that the grey colouration of the pupil does not necessarily mean that the eye has a cataract. Change of the pupil from black in young age to grey is a physiological change after the age 45-50 years and this is due to increased density of the nucleus with age, which causes some light being reflected back and *causing* grey colouration. An early cataract should therefore never be diagnosed by oblique illumination examination alone. If colour of the pupil is however densely grey or white and no fundus glow is seen with the ophthalmoscope, a diagnosis of cataract may be acceptable.

Oblique illumination also helps in differentiating between an immature and mature cataract by presence or absence respectively of the *iris shadow* on the cataractous lens. A uniformly bluish white discolouration of the pupil and no iris shadow is indicative of hypermature cataract. Oblique illumination can also reveal a brown nucleus of a morgagnian cataract in the lower part of the pupil. Calcific spots on the anterior capsule of the lens also indicate hypermaturity. It is easy to understand as shown in the illustration, the optics of the iris shadow test (Fig. 12.3).

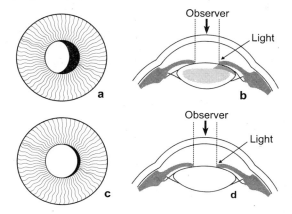

Fig. 12.3:. Iris shadow test, in Cataract, (a) Iris shadow in immature cataract, (b) Optical explanation, (c) Iris shadow practically absent (d) Optical explanaiton

Iris shadow test however has the fallacy that the iris shadow may be absent in the anterior capsular or anterior cortical cataract and may give the impression of mature cataract while the posterior cortex may still be transparent. Fallacious interpretation of oblique illumination examination can nowhere be more deceptive than in eyes with high myopia. The pupil in this condition is typically grey in colour but on examination under mydriasis with the ophthalmoscope, one finds no gross lens opacity and the only change is nuclear sclerosis.

Many myopic eyes are operated under this mistaken diagnosis, without the extra-special precautions necessary for removing a cataract in high myopic eyes. Some of them are lost due to operative or post-operative complications peculiar to cataract operation in high myopic eyes like vitreous loss at operation or post-operative retinal detachment.

Examination under mydriasis: The fear of causing secondary glaucoma due to mydriasis in old patients was to some degree a discouraging factor when drugs like homotropine were used. Mydriatics like phenylephrine are however safe from this point. They dilate the pupil quickly and the action lasts for short time. Being an adrenergic drug, it tends to actually lower the tension of the eye ball.

With an ophthalmoscope, one can define the size, site and number of spokes of lens opacities and the shape and size of the central lens opacity.

Cataract seen with ophthalmoscope presents the following morphological types:

    a. Peripheral spokes of lens opacity.
    b. Central dot or dense lens opacity.
    c. Nuclear sclerosis and nuclear cataract.
    d. Small translucent flecks of lens opacity.

Peripheral spokes of lens opacity are cortical opacities: They are thicker at the periphery and thinner towards the centre. They are commonly located in front or behind the equator. They may be unevenly formed, some short, some long, some thick and some thin. The spokes rarely reach the centre and therefore the vision is affected late.

Central lens opacity forms the largest group of senile types of lens opacity–53%. They are usually dense with a sharp outline. They may be pin head size or occupy half to three-fourth of the pupillary area and therefore can cause gross visual defect in bright light.

Nuclear sclerosis and nuclear cataract: Nuclear sclerosis is a senile change when the nucleus becomes dense and hard which introduces transient lenticular myopia. It is seen as a thin central shadow with a defined outline. With proper adjustment of the lenses in the ophthalmoscope, fundus details can be seen through it although they appear slightly distorted due to refractive change.

Nuclear cataract is a distinct opacification of the nucleus through which the fundus details cannot be seen. It appears as a round dark shadow against the fundus glow. This type of cataract is commonly associated with pigment changes of lens when it is called brown or black, *cataract Nigra*.

Flecks of lens opacity are scattered small flecks of different sizes and shapes seen against the fundus glow. They are translucent and are mostly located in the anterior cortex of the lens. They do not disturb vision and are often noted during routine ophthalmoscopy.

Ophthalmoscopy also helps in examining the fundus details in cases of early lenticular opacity. The condition of disc and blood vessels must be studied as far as possible and the foveal reflex looked for. In cases of central lens opacity, periphery of fundus can be easily examined.

Distant direct ophthalmoscopy, an examination with a retinoscope at 1/3 metre distance, can also reveal the shape and size of opacities of lens against red glow of fundus background. Determination of refractive state of the eye by retinoscopy, if possible done at this stage, will help prescribe correct glasses till further progress of cataract necessitates operation. It will also reveal gross primary refractive condition of the eye like high myopia in the absence of relevant history.

Slit lamp examination: Slit lamp examination of eyes with lens opacity in the early stage of cataract formation is of particular help in determining whether it is in anterior cortex, posterior cortex, in the nucleus or under the posterior capsule. Retro-illumination can also define the shape and the size of the lens opacity (Fig. 12.4).

Clinical stages of cataract. Once cataract has advanced beyond the stage of early lens opacity and a large part of the lens is involved, it is important to differentiate the clinical stages of cataract. These are:

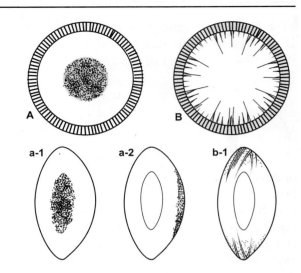

Fig. 12.4: Morphological Sites of Senile Cataract (A) Central lens opacity (dilated pupil), a-1 = nuclear cataract and a-2 = posterior sub-capsular cataract; (B) Cortical spokes—cuneiform cataract, b-1 = spokes of lens opacity starting near the equator.

1. Immature cataract.
2. Mature cataract.
3. Hypermature cataract, (i) Morgagnian cataract, (ii) Membranous cataract, (iii) Calcified cataract, (iv) Spontaneously subluxated cataract.
4. Brown cataract.

Immature cataract: Vision is appreciably reduced. The iris shadow is distinctly seen. The lens may get swollen and become intumescent due to hydration and may make anterior chamber shallow. Fundus glow is either not seen or faintly seen depending on the stage of development of lens opacity.

Mature cataract: Vision is reduced to hand movements or perception projection of light. Iris shadow is absent. The pupil is evenly white in colour. No fundus glow is seen (Fig. 12.5A and Fig. 12.5B, Plate 7).

Hypermature cataract. When the lens matter liquefies, pupil may have uniformly bluish white

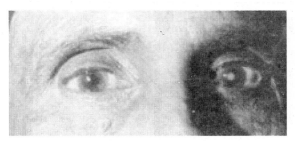

Fig. 12.5A: Senile mature cataract LE

discolouration. Small brown nucleus may be seen in the lower part of the pupil. Dots of calcification may be seen on the capsule. The fluid of the liquefied lens matter may gradually get absorbed and the lens may appear membranous, clinically evident by a deeper anterior chamber some degree of *iridodonesis* due to a space between the iris and the membraneous lens surtace. The capsule of the Morgagnian cataract may rupture and a small brown nucleus may prolapse into anterior chamber leading to severe inflammation and secondary glaucoma. Degenerative changes in the suspensory ligament may lead to spontaneous luxation of the lens (Figs. 12.6, 12.7 and 12.8).

Brown cataract: It is also called hard cataract, *cataract nigra* or black cataract. Brown cataract is due to intense sclerosis of nucleus with pigmentary changes. The nucleus is, therefore, very large and occupies most of the capsular

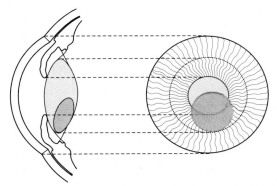

Fig. 12.6: Hypermature morgagnian cataract with displaced nucleus

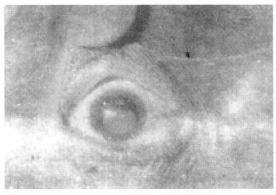

Fig. 12.7: Hypermature morgagnian cataract. (Fluid cortex absorbed and nucleus seen in capsular envelope in lower pupillary area

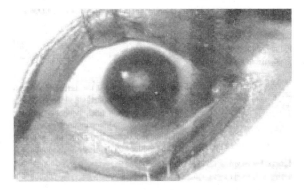

Fig. 12.8: Hypermature calcified cataract showing calcification of anterior capsule

space with very little cortical matter. Brown cataract affects vision out of proportion to the lenticular changes due to lenticular myopia. Brown cataract by itself never reaches the clinical stage of mature cataract. The removal of this cataract depends on the degree of visual loss rather than on the degree of maturity. The colour of the lens may be from light brown to nearly black as the different nomenclatures indicate (Fig. 12.9).

Brown cataract accounts for nearly 10% of all senile cataracts. On oblique illumination the pupil colour is dark brown and the diagnosis may be missed on routine examination.

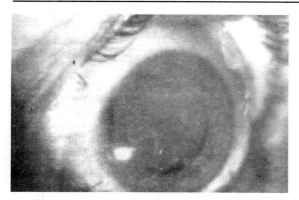

Fig 12.9: Brown cataract

Diagnosis of brown cataract often becomes evident only when the pupil is dilated. Although advanced in stage, a dull fundus glow is seen though details are not visible. Slit lamp examination shows dense brown to black discolouration the nucleus.

Question Two: Has the patient got cataract and cataract alone? Differential diagnosis of cataract: It is not out of place to emphasize that in developing countries with high incidence of cataract, the possibility of cataract dominates the mind of clinician and other conditions causing symptomless defective vision are often overlooked. The condition that is most often neglected is incipient glaucoma in the early stages. The result is that the patient is advised to hopefully wait for the cataract to progress till the vision is reduced to a poor level, and may be, it is only then realised that the patient was all along suffering from glaucoma and that he has reached a stage where the prospects of visual recovery after any surgery have become poor.

The common conditions which are a cause of symptomless deterioration of vision in age are:
1. Senile cataract
2. Chronic simple glaucoma (open angle glaucoma
3. Vascular retinopathies
   a. Diabetic
   b. Hypertensive

4. Vascular optic atrophy due to arteriosclerosis.
5. Senile macular degeneration.

It is important that each one of the above conditions should be excluded before final diagnosis of senile cataract is made. The history of diabetes and hypertension should be routinely asked for. In every case in this age group, intra-ocular tension and blood pressure should be routinely recorded, diabetes excluded and media and fundus examined under mydriasis.

Question Three: When to operate on cataract? If not operated what can happen? How does senile cataract progress? Once diagnosis of cataract has been communicated and the patient is told that it is a progressive condition, he immediately wants to know how soon the eye will lose useful vision and when it should be operated.

The progress of cataract depends on the type of lens opacity. Cortical opacities progress faster. Posterior sub-capsular cupuliform cataract is slow in progress and may take longer before the whole lens is involved. Brown cataract never reaches the stage of maturity. It is also to be remembered that slowly developing senile cortical cataract may, in diabetic patients, sometimes suddenly progress and reach maturity in a matter of few days.

Convention has unnecessarily developed that a cataract should be operated only when it is mature. This concept has not lost ground in developing countries where the quantum to cataract surgery is heavy and number of eye surgeons is relatively small, so that the patient is advised to carry on. The result is that many productive years of life are lost and the eye is exposed to the possibility of hypermaturity and other complications due to cataract. **The correct approach should be that the cataract can and should be operated at any stage of its progress at which it disturbs the routine of** a person's life due to visual handicap. The visual requirement of each individual depends on his profession. A man in active service doing office work cannot wait till cataract matures and must have, at least one eye with good working vision. A businessman with supervisory responsibilities can afford to wait till his daily needs are disturbed. A non technical labourer can probably wait even longer. Skilled professions like driving or sophisticated industrial workers need binocularity as an essential requirement, and the same is possible with newer advances in aphakic corrections. It should however be kept in mind that a cataract should never be allowed to go beyond the state of maturity. It should also be kept in mind that 6/12 vision with accommodation (as in unoperated eye) is better than 6/6 without accommodation (as in an aphakic eye).

Cataract surgery is an elective surgery. Surgeon and patient can both plan with discretion the time of operation within the limits mentioned here. Cataract surgery is, therefore, rarely an emergency except when cataract is the cause of secondary glaucoma in which case the cataract extraction should be undertaken forthwith after controlling the raised tension.

Cataract, if not operated at or before maturity, can cause secondary glaucoma in following manner.

1. **Phakolytic glaucoma** is caused by the intumescence of lens. The lens becomes hydrated, swollen and causes shallowing of the anterior chamber, obstruction of aqueous drainage and rise of intraocular tension.
2. **Phakotoxic glaucoma** is caused by leakage of lens proteins causing iritis, albuminous aqueous in anterior chamber which has difficulty to pass through the angle of anterior chamber and hence rise in tension.
3. **Glaucoma** can also be caused by spontaneous luxation of the lens due to degenerative changes in the suspensory ligament. Luxation is mostly anterior and the severest glaucoma is caused when the lens is caught in the pupillary area.
4. **Glaucoma** is also caused by spontaneous rupture of Morgagnian cataract the nucleus prolapsing into the anterior chamber and causing obstruction of the aqueous outflow and rise of tension.
5. **Glaucoma** can sometimes be caused by dislocation of the lens into the vitreous, although the incidence of this is very small.

Question Four: What is the prognosis of cataract operation? Cataract is one disease where prognosis of surgery has reached a high degree of success. Every patient before cataract surgery wishes to be assured of success and this is now possible with newer developments in technique and instrumentation . The following factors influence the prognosis:

1. **Perception and projection of light (PL and PR).** It must be accurate in all directions. It is good to use a pencil of light to test projection instead of a broad torch light. Hesitant response even in one direction should arouse suspicion of some associated intraocular pathology. A good macular function is an essential requisite for full visual recovery.
2. **Pupillary reaction.** The pupil should be normal in size and shape and brisk in reaction to direct light, indicating good retinal function and normal conducting fibres of the optic nerve.
3. **Anterior chamber depth.** A shallow anterior chamber does not necessarily mean a raised intraocular tension. Moderate degree of shallowing may be caused by the swelling of the lens without rise of intraocular tension.
4. **Intraocular tension.** A raised intraocular tension, even though of a transient nature due to swelling of the lens, must be controlled for good prognosis of cataract surgery.
5. **Systemic conditions.** Diabetes has the well-known disadvantages of low resistance to infection, poor healing and tendency to

bleeding. As in all surgeries, blood sugar can unexpectedly shoot up during and following surgery and may create general health problems.

6. **Enlarged prostate:** A common association in elderly males should always be kept in mind. One does not want, as it can happen, that a patient may develop acute retention of urine due to enlarged prostate post-operatively. Necessary pre-operative treatment should be completed before cataract operation.

7. **Infection** in and around the eye or in the lacrimal passages is a contraindication to surgery till it is cured. An infection around the eye, e.g., sinuses, teeth and ear can be a potent danger and a source of post-operative infection. An endogenous septic focus in the body can excite a post-operative iridocyclitis and affect the prognosis.

8. **Examination of opposite eye** if already operated for cataract and if it shows evident complications, will be a useful guide to improve prognosis of surgery in the eye under review by modifying plans of surgery and taking extra precautions.

Question Five: What procedure of cataract extraction to adopt? *Choice of cataract surgery.* Having made the diagnosis, excluded or controlled any associated pathology, intra-ocular or systemic and having assessed the prognosis, the surgeon must now plan the operative procedure to be adopted.

In older times, extra capsular and intra-capsular extraction of cataract were the only methods available to the surgeon. In last decades, sophisticated techniques such as intracapsular lens implant, phako-emulsification are practiced. These have significantly eliminated post-operative complications and disadvantages of having one eye aphakic and other phakic. Intra-ocular lens implant in uniocular cataract is a distinct advantage. The procedure is akin to having a physiological lens since the implant is placed in the original lens capsule after cataract is removal in an extra capsular procedure. It also takes into account refractive status by pre-operative calculation of power required for that particular eye by biometry. Distant vision having been corrected adequately by the implant, patient has to use only near glasses. Even this can be avoided it implanted lens leaves the eye slightly myopic. This leaves distant vision only marginally under corrected. Small incision surgery has obviated post-operative astigmatism which used to be fairly common with 180° limbal/extra limbal section particularly with interrupted sutures for sealing the large section. Mutlifocal IOLs are coming in vogue which may obviate use of glasses after surgery.

Other Types of Cataract

The lens can develop opacities which might be present at birth or may develop in early childhood. The lens may also become cataractous in adolescence or adult life either due to systemic cause or may be precipitated by direct or indirect trauma.

Types of cataract other than senile cataract may be described as follows:

1. Congenital and juvenile cataract.
2. Traumatic cataract.
3. Complicated or secondary cataract.
4. Pathological or metabolic cataract.
5. Toxic cataract.

Congenital and Juvenile Cataract

A variety of congenital opacities of the lens have been noted. Some are seen only on routine ophthalmoscopy or slit lamp examination while others are evidently large enough to cause visual loss. These opacities may be genetic or due to metabolic or inflammatory disturbances to the eye caused by maternal systemic disease during pregnancy.

Congenital lens opacities may be present at birth or appear during evolution of the lens. The lens opacity may be strictly localised to the embryonic nucleus or whole lens may become opaque by the time child is born. Many of these are stationary and cause no effect on vision while others are progressive and may reach maturity before or soon after birth.

Various types of congenital cataracts can be described as follows:

1. **Total opacity:** The child is born with a completely opaque lens. Some of these are caused by German measles (Rubella), a virus infection affecting the mother in the first three months of pregnancy. These children usually have other congenital anomalies in the eyes and body, e.g., microophthalmos, nystagmus, buphthalmos, deafness, mental retardation and cardio-vascular anomalies.

2. **Lamellar or zonular cataract:** It is usually associated with maternal malnutrition and calcium deficiency and tetany. The lens fibres forming during the deficiency phase become opaque and as soon as the deficiency state is reversed, normal transparent fibres are formed (Fig. 12.10).

3. **Coronary cataract.** These spoke like opacities in the mid periphery of the lens are non-progressive and cause little or no visual disturbance. Unlike spokes of senile cataract, these spokes are in mid periphery and thicker towards the centre and thinner in periphery.

4. **Dot-like opacities** are often seen in cortex during routine slit lamp examination and are static and do not affect the vision.

5. **Nuclear opacity:** The nucleus of the lens develops about the 7th week of foetal development and a nuclear cataract is, therefore, usually present at birth and involves only the embryonic nucleus. It is usually localised and non-progressive. But it can be responsible for appreciable visual disturbance.

6. **Sutural cataract.** Opacity may develop along the suture lines and give a feathery appearance when seen with a slit lamp (Fig. 12.11).

7. **Pyramidal cataract:** It is in the centre of the anterior capsule with reduplication of the capsular epithelium. It can be developmental caused by the contact of the embryonic lens to the overlying embryonic mesoderm or by a corneal ulcer perforation with the lens movement anteriorly when anterior capsule is traumatised by contact with the cornea.

8. **Anterior and posterior capsular opacities** of varying size and shape are

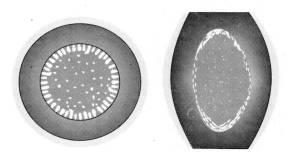

Fig. 12.10: Zonular cataract

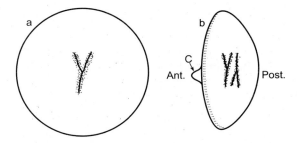

Fig. 12.11: Sutural cataract and pyramidal cataract (a) Y-shaped opacity as seen by oblique illumination; (b) Feathery lens opacity along suture lines as seen on slit lamp; (c) Pyramidal cataract

caused by inflammation or trauma in intra-uterine life. Posterior capsular cataract is rare indeed except when it is associated with the posterior vascular sheath of the lens.

Juvenile cataract is a lens opacity developing later in childhood (not present at birth), is not an uncommon cause of visual disturbance in early age. Hereditary inheritance may be an important causative factor.

Congenital cataract may be associated with other congenital anomalies and therefore prognosis of surgery in congenital cataract should always be guarded. Nystagmus is a common association in children with an advanced stage of cataract and this further limits visual prognosis of surgery.

Traumatic Cataract

The lens may be traumatised and become opaque due to mechanical injury or radiational trauma. Cataract due to these factors can develop at any stage and clinical features will depend on the type and extent of trauma. It may be present in various clinical forms:

a. **Blunt injury** may cause concussion cataract due to sub-clinical tear in the capsule, mostly the posterior capsule. The opacity may either remain localized or may extend into whole of the cortex of lens. The concussion impact of the iris on the lens may leave behind a ring of pigment of the size of the pupil on anterior capsule of lens called the *Vossius ring*.

b. **Perforating injury.** Grade of cataract will depend on type of injury. A needle perforation which may quickly seal by itself may cause a 'localised lens opacity of anterior cortex and the opacity may remain non-progressive. Any sizeable break of anterior capsule will however cause total opacity of lens. The lens may get swollen and lens matter may protrude into anterior chamber. In young age, the lens

may get completely absorbed leaving behind only capsular remains. In older age, inspissated remains of cortex and nucleus may result in membranous cataract (Fig. 12.12, Plate 7). Intra-ocular metalic foreign body can also cause cortical opacity superimposed by changes which are due to dispersion of ions from the foreign body which migrate to different sites in the eye to combine with cellular proteins. Epithelial cells become ready victims thus lens epithelium, ciliary epithelium are commonly involved in the degenerative staining process. It is called *siderosis* when the retained foreign body is iron and *chalcosis* when it is copper or its alloy.

c. **Radiation cataract.** This occurs due to the direct effect of radiation on the developing lens fibres in the equatorial region. This becomes clinically evident after sometime when these fibres have migrated to anterior and posterior cortical area.

d. **Heat cataract:** It occurs due to the absorption of heat by the lens tissue. The opacity is in the form of a disc near the posterior capsule. This is seen commonly in glass blowers and molten iron workers.

Complicated Cataract or Secondary Cataract

Complicated cataract is a lens opacity which is secondary to an intra-ocular pathology.

The common causes are:
1. Inflammations like iridocyclitis.
2. Disease of retina like retinitis pigmentosa, long standing total detachment of retina and disseminated chorio-retinitis.
3. Intra-ocular tumours.
4. Secondary glaucoma.

The inflammation of anterior uvea leads to posterior synechiae and organisation of exudates on the anterior surface of lens. The capsule involved undergoes consequent changes leading to an anterior capsular cataract. Because of damage to the lens epithelium, the anterior cortex may also get involved and develop opacities.

In chronic intra-ocular pathology, the complicated cataract is of the rosette type and on slit lamp examination gives a polychromatic lustre on the posterior capsule.

The myopic change in the lens is nuclear. It is therefore, very important that in all cases of high myopia, examination under mydriasis is a must before making a diagnosis of cataract.

An intra-ocular tumour can cause lens changes in more than one way. The tumour mass touching the posterior capsule may initiate the lens changes. Deposists of tumour tissue on the lens and secondary rise of intra-ocular pressure can also cause cataractous changes.

Pathological Cataract or Metabolic Cataract

Systemic pathologies by causing metabolic disturbance in the body can bring about osmotic changes in the lens, anoxaemia of the lens and disturb transparency of lens resulting in cataract formation. Important systemic diseases which are responsible for cataract formation are:
1. Diabetes mellitus.
2. Parathyroid deficiency (Tetany)
3. Galactosaemia.
4. Myotonic dystrophy.

Diabetic cataract: Diabetes and cataract may co-exist in two ways. One is a cataract caused by diabetes and second is a senile cataract in a diabetic patient. In the latter, the diabetes is only incidental and the cataract in no way differs from the usual senile cataract except that diabetes may hasten maturation of senile cataract.

A true diabetic cataract is a cataract caused by diabetes and is a very uncommon clinical entity. The early change is osmotic hydration of lens and formation of water clefts in anterior cortex. This is caused by higher concentration of sugar in aqueous which disturbs osmotic balance between fluid in the lens and the fluid surrounding the lens. Acidosis caused by diabetes also affects metabolism of lens and hence its transparency. So long as the lens change is limited to this stage, the process is reversible. With the control of diabetes, the lens may get back to normal architecture and transparency.

Typical lens opacity due to diabetes is initially anterior sub-capsular seen with an ophthalmoscope as small droplets and with slit lamp as cleft-like spaces in the cortex. Later, the opacity extends into the whole cortex and then in no way differs from the usual senile cataract. Diabetic cataract is common in juvenile diabetes in which case it may rapidly progress to involve whole lens in a matter of days or weeks.

Galactosaemia cataract: It is error of galactose meabolism causing higher concentration of galactose in blood and is commonly observed in small infants where galactose cannot be converted into glycogen due to deficiency of enzymes. Galactose is passed in urine and infants are marasmic. A high galactose level in serum is toxic to lens epithelium and causes osomotic changes and leads to the appearance of water clefts in lens. The progress of the lens opacity is very fast. If the condition is not controlled early, the whole lens may become cataractous.

Parathyroid deficiency cataract: Cataract due to the parathyroid deficiency is due to hypocalcaemia in blood which also causes convulsive symptoms of tetany. The typical lens changes are zonular in character with a thin central opacity surrounded, by a ring opacity with riders.

Myotonic cataract: It is a bilateral cataract in patients suffering from a congenital form of a myotonic dystrophy with typical facial and mental changes.

Toxic Cataract

Steroid-induced cataract. The prolonged topical therapy of steroids or systemic administration of steroids for long periods can cause progressive lens changes and if therapy is not interrupted, the whole lens may become cataractous. One ocular condition where the severity of symptoms forces the patient to use topical steroids indiscriminately is spring catarrh. Young patients may present themselves with cataract or glaucoma or both, a rather tragic result. From the reports in literature, a continuous therapy for 3 months or more can cause steroid-induced cataract. The incidence will depend on the frequency and the duration of the use of steroid drugs. A prolonged systemic steroid therapy is still more toxic to the eyes. The most common condition for which systemic steroid therapy is understandably prolonged is rheumatic arthritis and post organ transplantation procedures. The ocular complications are the steroid-induced cataract and/or steroid-induced glaucoma.

The earliest steroid-induced lens changes are in posterior cortex and appear in the form of punctate opacities which, in due course of time, may involve the whole lens and the end result is a mature cataract (Fig. 12.13).

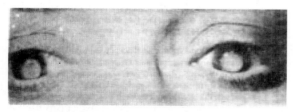

Fig. 12.13: Steroid-induced cataract in both eyes in a young boy

The **anti-glaucoma drugs**, particularly DFP, and phospholine iodide, used for prolonged periods are known to cause lens opacities mostly cortical.

Some chemicals toxic to the lens and therefore likely to cause cataract are naphthalene, dinitrophenol (commonly used for reducing body weight), ergot and thalium. Some of these drugs are used for causing experimental cataract for research.

DISPLACEMENT OF THE LENS: LUXATION AND SUBLUXATION

The lens is held in position by the suspensory ligaments attached just in front and behind the equator of lens. The lens is also supported in its position by the concave hyaloid fossa of vitreous into which the lens rests posteriorly.

The thickest central portion of lens is in line of visual axis of the eye causing maximum refraction of light rays. Any displacement of the lens from its central position will therefore seriously disturb vision.

Subluxation or partial displacement of the lens is more common than complete dislocation. Subluxation is usually in the plane of the lens while complete dislocation may be anteriorly into anterior chamber or posteriorly into the vitreous. The zonular fibres under stress and strain usually give way from their attachment to the lens and not from the cilliary epithelium.

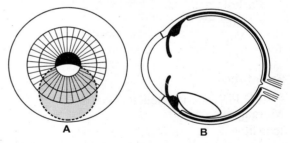

Fig 12.14: Displaced lens (A) Partially subluxated downwards; (B) Complete dislocation of lens into the Virtreous, anterior chamber deepened

Types of Displacement of Lens

1. Total displacement
   a. Into the pupil.
   b. Into the anterior chamber.
   c. Into the Vitreous.
   d. Floating or fixed.
   e. Into the sub-retinal space.
   f. Extruded out.
2. Partial subluxation is in the plane of the lens.

Etiologically, displacement of the lens may be: (i) Congenital, (ii) Traumatic, (iii) Pathological, (iv) Spontaneous, (v) Surgical.

Congenital subluxation is commonly associated with systemic diseases like:

Marfan's syndrome: Haemocystinuria. Oxycephaly. Crouzon's disease (Fig. 12.15, Plate 7).

Systemic clinical features of these conditions are distinctive and not difficult to diagnose.

Traumatic dislocation may be due to:
- Perforating injuring.
- Concussion injury.

The lens may be pushed into the vitreous or may be found lying in the anterior chamber. In cases with extensive injury, the lens may even be extruded out of the eye usually along with the vitreous loss commonly associated with extensive perforating injury of the eye. Extruded lens may be found in subconjunctival space.

Pathological subluxation is present in:
- Staphylomatous eyes.
- High myopia.
- Buphthalmos.

Spontaneous subluxation of lens may be a senile process in cases with hypermature Morgagnian cataract remaining unoperated for long lime.

Surgical posterior dislocation of the cataractous lens can occur by undue pressure with an intra-capsular forceps during an extraction procedure, particularly by a beginner. The lens dislocates and slips into the vitreous.

Clinical Features of the Displaced Lens

Symptoms:

1. Slight tremulousness of lens may not cause any symptoms and may be discovered on routine examination. Also, posterior dis-location of lens is better tolerated by the eye then anterior displacement.
2. Subluxation of the lens, with half the pupil aphakic, may cause:
   - Uni-ocular Diplopia.
   - Lenticular astigmatism.

Complete dislocation of the clear lens into A.C. will cause secondary glaucoma. Posterior dislocation into the vitreous makes the eye aphakic. Wandering lens moving freely in fluid vitreous may be seen as a floating mass in front of the eyes. This may be in high myopic eyes.

On examination:

1. Deep anterior chamber is suggestive of partial or total displacement of the lens. Anterior chamber may be deep in one part and normal in the other part, indicating partial displacement of lens.
2. Jet black pupil in elderly person is clearly suggestive of absence of lens from the pupillary area.
3. Tremulousness of iris (iridodonesis) is a characteristic sign of lens displacement caused by lack of support to iris normally resting on the lens.
4. Examination with dilated pupil may show the lens lying in the vitreous. A clear lens in anterior chamber may appear as a drop of oil.
5. With ophthalmoscope, the border of the lens is seen as a dark semicircular line against the red fundus glow. The fundus details are seen through the aphakic part of pupil only with +10.0 D. lens.
6. Retinoscopy and absence of Purkinje reflexes may confirm diagnosis of total dislocation of the lens.
7. Slit lamp examination not only shows the lens margin clearly but tags of torn zonular fibres may be seen hanging from the equator of the lens.

Complications of Displaced Lens

1. Irritative iridocyclitis may be caused by the lens touching or adherent to the ciliary zone.
2. Phaco-anaphylactic iridocyclitis may be caused by lens protein if the lens ruptures during the process of dislocation.
3. Cataractous changes may start in the displaced lens. One should remember that the lens may be cataractous before displacement as in hypermature Morgagnian cataract.
4. Secondary glaucoma is the most serious and the most damaging complication of a displaced lens. Forward dislocation of the lens caught in the papillary aperture causes acute rise of intra-ocular tension demanding urgent measures. Lens lying in anterior chamber also starts severe glaucomatous process needing quick removal of lens from the anterior chamber.
5. Sympathetic ophthalmitis in the opposite eye has been mentioned but it is very rare. It can possibly be caused when the dislocated lens is lying on the ciliary processes causing repeated attacks of cyclitis.

13

Glaucoma

Glaucoma is a term synonymous with raised intraocular tension, although not universally so. This is the disease which has been mentioned and taken note of even in ancient literature as described by Sushruta, providing the earliest record. Even though not mentioned as a clinical entity, a congested eye which did not respond to treatment and became painful with headache and diminution of vision was termed as ADHI-MANTH, corresponding to what we know as congestive glaucoma.

The ancient Greeks called glaucoma as SUFFUSIO NIGRA from which came the term Black cataract or 'kala motia' because suffusio in Greek meant cataract and nigra black.

The Arabs in the fourteenth century had clearly recognised it as a clinical entity. Richard Bannister differentiated between a cataract and a glaucoma more clearly as early as 1622. It was however William Mackenzi in 1835 who wrote a treatise on glaucoma and explained that, increased water content was the basic pathology of the disease. It was Pristley Smith in 1879 who first explained that it was faulty drainage which was the cause of raised IOP.

It is an enigma that in spite of laboratory and clinical researches, etiopathogenesis of the disease has still remained incompletely understood. This is the disease responsible for a large number of incurably blind the world over. In India and other developing countries, glaucoma continues to be the most important cause of incurable blindness in elderly people.

AQUEOUS HUMOUR AND INTRA-OCULAR PRESSURE (IOP)

The aqueous humour is the optically empty fluid in anterior segment of the eye.

The difference in temperature of cornea and the inner eye is partly responsible for convection current causing movement of the fluid in anterior chamber and its drainage. The balance between its formation and its drainage out of the eye ball, is responsible for the maintenance of normal intraocular pressure (IOP). Decreased formation or leakage of the aqueous can cause low intraocular pressure. The aqueous is also a source of nutrients both for the cornea and the lens.

The aqueous humour is formed from the ciliary body. Plasma passes from the capillary vessels into the sub-epithelial stroma of the ciliary processes and through the ciliary epithelium into the posterior chamber.

It was thought to be a simple filtration and effusion from ciliary epithelium. This however can not be true because chemical composition of capillary plasma and aqueous greatly differs. Can it then be secretion? Probably only part of aqueous formation process. Everything considered, it is reasonable that aqeuous is produced by a combination of ultra filtration, secretion by active transport and diffusion. The important fact is the *semi permeability* of ciliary epithelium which does not allow particulate contents of plasma to pass through thus making aqueous a fluid containing only soluble constituents. The rate of production is controlled by enzymatic action of carbonic anhydrase in the ciliary epithelium.

Aqueous after its formation passes from posterior chamber via the pupil into anterior chamber. Aqueous is drained through the trabecular meshwork in the angle of the anterior chamber, through canal of Schlemn into episcleral aqueous veins and thence via the venous channels into general circulation (Fig. 13.1). A smal part of aqueous is probably drained through cilio-scleral route. Aqueous, across ciliary body passes into supra-choroidal space and via venous capillaries into general venous drainage.

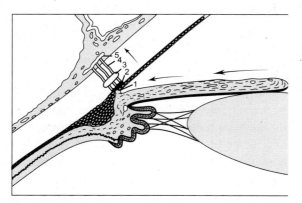

Fig. 13.1: Route of aqueous flow from posterior chamber into the anterior chamber and its outflow. (1) Trabecular meshwork (2) Scleral spur (3) Canal of Schlemn (4) Intrascleral drainage channels (5) Aqueous veins

MAINTENANCE OF INTRA-OCULAR PRESSURE

In addition to the static contents of the eye ball like the lens and the vitreous, the balance between the formation and the drainage of aqueous plays an important role in the maintenance of normal intra-ocular pressure which is extremely important for the nutrition and function of the structures of the eye ball. In addition to the rate of the formation and the drainage of aqueous, the other factors that contribute to the maintenance of the normal intra-ocular pressure are the scleral coat of the eye ball and the blood content in the vasculature of the eye ball.

Scleral rigidity is an important factor that influences the record of intra-ocular pressure. A thin sclera in children may yield under a moderate rise of intra-ocular pressure and therefore a tonometer may not register a high rise of tension. A thin sclera in high myopes is similarly responsible for difficulty in diagnosing early glaucoma in myopes.

The Blood content of the vasculature of the eye can influence intra-ocular pressure. The balance between intra-ocular pressure and the flow of blood into the eye ball is an important factor. The pressure on the eye ball which brings about the pulsation of the central retinal artery, which is normally nonpulsating, is a good clinical proof of the importance of this factor. Similarly pressure in the episcleral veins into which the aqueous drains is also a factor in the maintenance of intraocular pressure.

Depending on these factors, intra-ocular pressure is far from being constant during different functioning states of the body and the different hours of the day.

Normal intraocular tension is so vital for the function of the eye that intraocular tension both higher and lower than normal are harmful for function of the eye.

Normal intraocular tension of eye ball has a wide range and may be anything between 10 to 20-21 mm of Hg with an average of 15-18 mm Hg. Tension 22 and above, and below 10 mm is definitely abnormal. Normal tension has a diurnal variation. It is highest in the early hours of the morning because during sleep, the ciliary muscle has been inactive, aqueous out flow is slowed down and aqueous therefore accumulates in the eye. The tension is lowest in the afternoon for just the opposite reasons. The difference between morning and afternoon tension should normally not be more than 5 to 6 mm Hg. Tension in two eyes is also not always identical. Some variations are within normal limits. A difference of 5 mm or more should be considered pathological for the eye with higher tension. All this suggests that the response of the eye to variations in tension, varies from individual to individual. Effect on the ocular function therefore also varies from individual to individual and from eye to eye. A condition called ocular hypertension may have a fairly high intra-ocular tension and yet all the functions and structures of the eye may be perfectly normal.

RECORD OF INTRA-OCULAR TENSION

There are various methods of recording intra-ocular tension:
1. Palpation tonometry
2. Schiotz corneal tonometry (Indentation tonometry)
3. Scleral tonometry
4. Applanation tonometry
   a. On slit lamp
   b. Hand held Perkins
5. Non-contact tonometry
6. Manometry in experimental animals
7. Electronic Tonography which indicates aqueous outflow facility.

The clinical tonometry can be dependable only when cornea is normal in curvature, thickness and elasticity. A dense corneal opacity will alter the resilience of cornea to the weight of tonometer. The reading will therefore be undependable. Any kind of the corneal tonometry is impracticable on corneas with leucoma adherence or staphylomalous and ectatic corneas.

Palpation tonometry: The intra-ocular pressure of the eye ball can be roughly estimated by palpation of the globe with fingers over the lids. Evaluation by this method can only be dependable in experienced hands. One must have practised this technique on hundreds of patients before one can depend on the interpretation of the feel by one's own fingers. The difference between a normal and moderately high or moderately low tension can be dependably evaluated when the tension in one eye is normal and the other eye is higher or lower.

Schiotz tonometry: This has been an age old method of recording intraocular tension. It is however considered a less satisfactory method mainly because Schiotz readings do not take into account the scleral rigidity factor. In spite of this drawback, Schiotz tonometry is a simple tool in the hands of most ophthalmologists. If it is used with discrimination, the results are fairly dependable.

A Schiotz tonometer is so constructed that the foot plate conforms to the curvature of the normal cornea. The plunger in the foot plate is displaced depending on the corneal resistance and the amount of weight attached to the plunger. The higher the tension, the more is the displacement of the plunger which moves the pointer proportionately on the scale.

Before starting the procedure, the tonometer is assembled and checked on the test block when the pointer should read zero on the scale. The tonometer should be kept clean and the corneal plate should be sterilized before use by dipping in absolute alcohol.

For Schiotz tonometry, a drop of surface anaesthetic solution like 4% xylocaine is enough. The patient is asked to lie down and look at his own thumb held above his face. It is important that the patient keeps both his eyes open. With the lids gently pulled apart, the tonometer with 5.5 gm weight is slowly brought to rest on the centre of the cornea and held there by its own weight and without any pressure. The reading on the scale is noted. The same is repeated on the opposite eye. These readings can be converted into mm of Hg from the conversion tables. If the readings on the scale goes beyond zero, tonometry should be repeated with higher weights of 7.5 gms and 10 gms. Even otherwise, it is a good practice to record tension with additional weights of 7.5 and 10 gms also. Average record will be more dependable. Further more, three readings with three weights will help exclude scleral rigidity factor and give corrected Schiotz tension readings.

The patient should look at the raised left thumb when doing tonometry of the right eye and right thumb when left eye tension is being recorded. This is to avoid the obstruction in seeing the thumb by the examiner's hand holding the tonometer. It is better to support the hand on the forehead of the patient. Tonometry is difficult when one of the two eyes is blind and patient can not fix with the blind eye. It may be helpful to tell the patient that even if he cannot see his thumb, he knows the location of his thumb in space and he should try to look towards it.

For Schiotz tonometry to be dependable, there are certain essential requirements which should be kept in mind:

i. Patient must be relaxed and not squeeze his lids so that no extra effort is needed to keep his lids apart,

ii. The cornea must be in the centre of palpebral fissure.

iii. The tonometer must be held vertical. Inclined position will give wrong readings.

iv. The tonometer should not be kept on the cornea for more than few seconds because continued pressure will reduce the tension.

v. The tonometer should be calibrated from time to time.

vi. In borderline cases and in myopic eyes, Schiotz tonometry should, if possible, be followed by applanation tonometry.

vii. Roughness has no place in Schiotz tonometry because the anaesthetised corneal epithelium may be abraided in which case, the patient will come back with excruciating pain.

Scleral tonometry: This is undertaken when the corneal curvature is grossly altered like in keratoconus or cornea is densely scarred as leucomatous opacities and the leucoma adherence.

Although a special scleral foot plate corresponding to the normal scleral curvature can be fitted on to a Schiotz tonometer, a regular Schiotz tonometer can also be used for scleral tonometry. The patient is directed to look slightly towards the nasal side. The tonometer is rested vertically on the temporal side of the cornea between the limbus and the insertion of the lateral rectus in identical position in both the eyes. It should be kept in mind that scleral tonometry readings of one eye are comparable only with scleral tonometry readings of the other eye. The procedure is therefore more dependable when one eye is normal.

Applanation tonometry is more dependable because it excludes scleral rigidity factor. It has been described in the section on slit lamp examination.

Electronic tonography which records aqueous outflow facility, is important to diagnose low tension glaucoma and hypersecretion glaucoma.

The non-contact tonometer records the rebound of air pressure that is thrust on the cornea from a very close distance but not touching the corneal surface.

Manometry gives a direct record of IOP through a canula introduced into the anterior chamber. The procedure is used only in experimental studies in animals.

GLAUCOMA

The incidence of glaucoma has been generally put at 1 to 2% in persons above the age of 40. In a national survey conducted in India, glaucoma has been attributed to 5.6% of total blindness. The figure could be higher if the methods of detection of early glaucoma are adopted. Most of the other data are largely projected from patients attending hospitals. The fact, however, remains that glaucoma is the most serious cause of blindness.

Aetiology of Glaucoma

Glaucoma continues to be a disease, the aetiology of which is undetermined. In spite of extensive laboratory researches, it is still unclear as to what brings about the local tissue changes in the eye which lead to the rise of intra-ocular tension.

We know what is happening in the eye but unfortunately we do not know what is causing it. There is probably a tension control centre in the brain which is causing the disease, controlling its progress and taking it to blindness in spite of treatment and surgery.

Important considerations in relation to glaucoma are heredity, age incidence, refractive state of the eye, the anatomy of the eye and the physiology of the eye.

Heredity: Although there is no definite evidence, glaucoma has been known to run in families.

Age: Glaucoma is by and large, a disease of old age. Most patients are in the age group of 50 and above. Glaucoma in young age, is however, not uncommon. This does not include congenital and developmental glaucoma.

Refractive State of Eye

Glaucoma has long been associated with hypermetropia. A hypermetropic eye is a small eye with a small anterior segment, more spherical lens and a relatively shallow anterior chamber. Although less common, glaucoma in myopic eyes is not rare and it is often overlooked. This is due to more than one reason. Myopic eyes do not record a high intraocular tension because of thin sclera and therefore low scleral rigidity. Myopic eyes may have myopic cupping of disc which is not always easy to differentiate from glaucomatous cupping. Furthermore, myopic retinal degeneration can cause field changes similar to field changes due to glaucoma. The comment that *hypermetropia reveals glaucoma and myopia conceals glaucoma* is very appropriate. Generally speaking, it holds true that angle closure glaucoma is definitely more common in hypermetropic eyes and open angle glaucoma is as common in myopic eyes and emmetropic eyes.

Intra-ocular Pressure (IOP)

The term glaucoma means raised intra-ocular tension. Normal intra-ocular tension varies between 10 to 20 mm of Hg. The important question is when do we call a tension raised intra-ocular tension. It is generally agreed that an eye with tension 22 to 25 mm of Hg should be considered a glaucoma suspect eye and all the investigations should be done to exclude glaucoma. Tension 26 to 30 mm indicates a glaucomatous eye but diagnosis should be supported by evidence of other glaucomatous changes and should be considered glaucomatous unless proved otherwise.

Glaucoma is a state of the eye where intra-ocular tension has caused changes like disc changes, field changes and damage to vision. A particular tension, even though not high, may cause glaucomatous changes because that tension is not tolerated and therefore becomes pathological. The tension of the eye can be influenced by the condition of sclera and scleral rigidity factor. In infantile glaucoma, the scleral coat is distensible and rise of intraocular tension will cause enlargement of the globe and the tonometer may not record raised intra-ocular pressure even though the eye has undergone gross damage.

Similarly, sclera in myopic eyes is thinner with low scleral rigidity. Schiotz tonometry in these eyes, may therefore be fallacious and this is the reason that glaucoma is not thought of or diagnosed in myopic eyes.

Apart from structural effects of raised intra-ocular tension, it influences the functioning state of the retina and therefore causes diminution of vision. The most ill understood part of the disease is that even after tension is restored to normal by surgery, vision may continue to deteriorate and end in blindness. It is also anomalous that some glaucomatous eyes lose all useful vision and yet retain a small island of temporal field of vision or a perfect projection of light in all four quadrants for years in untreated advanced glaucomatous eyes.

Provocative Tests for Glaucoma

Glaucoma should be diagnosed early and yet it may not always be easy to do so. The anterior chamber may be distinctly shallow and yet the eye may be otherwise perfectly normal. Tension may be slightly to moderately raised but the vision may be normal, the disc may be normal and there may be no field defects. Disc may be cupped yet the vision may be normal and there may be no field defects. These are anomalous situations when glaucoma may have to be proved or disproved. This is all the more important because the eye may be non-glaucomatous today and may become glaucomatous tomorrow.

Provocative tests have been devised to solve confusion is some such cases. The term 'provo-cative' is used to mean to provoke a glaucomatous process in an otherwise normal eye and this may sometimes create a difficult situation. Provocative tests are therefore not to be used as a routine and when done, one should be prepared to meet the crisis, however mild, promptly so that the patient does not suffer any harm due to the test.

Numerous provocative tests have been practised over the years. Many of them are obsolete and need not be discussed. The important ones are:

Water drinking test which is meant for provoking and confirming primary open angle glaucoma. The patient is called on an empty stomach. The tension is recorded. He then quickly drinks one litre of water. Tension is recorded every 15 minutes thereafter. Any rise of tension more than 6-8 mm of Hg by Schiotz tonometer is suggestive that the eye is glaucoma suspect and should be followed up regularly.

The drinking of water disturbs the hydrodynamic equilibrium of blood-aqueous barrier resulting in more aqueous secretion. If aqueous outflow facility cannot adequately compensate for this extra collection of aqueous, it results in rise of intra-ocular tension.

Although this test is simple and safe, not all ophthalmologists are agreed on its necessity and its utility. Some consider it more contributory if the positive results of the water drinking test are supported by a lower C value by tonography.

Dark room test: This test is indicated in eyes with a shallow anterior chamber and narrow angle. The tension is recorded before starting the test. The patient is then asked to remain in a dark room for one hour so that his pupil dilates, the iris crowds the angle and may cause obstruction to the aqueous outflow thereby causing rise of intra-ocular tension. It is important that the patient does not go to sleep, because during sleep, the pupil contracts. He should, therefore, have with him someone to be talking to. At the end of one hour, tension is recorded in very dim illumination or with a red light. Any rise of intra-ocular tension of more than 6 mm of Hg should be considered abnormal. A gonioscopy could also be done with lower illumination to confirm further narrowing of the angle. This will add to the value of the test.

Mydriatic test: This is also indicated for eyes with a shallow anterior chamber and narrow angle. Tension is recorded before the test. A mydriatic is then instilled till the pupil is fully dilated. The tension record is then repeated. Any rise of more than 6 mm of Hg is considered pro-glaucomatous. Two per cent homatropine solution should be used for the test. Atropine is contraindicated because of its irreversible effect. Phenylephrine dilates the pupil but actually causes some lowering of tension because of its vasoconstrictive effect. It is important that the patient must have miotic drops to counter the effect of the mydriatic so that the patient does not remain at home with a dilated pupil and get an angle-closure glaucoma attack.

Classification of Glaucoma

Glaucoma has been classified from different points of view. Etiologically, glaucoma falls in two major groups, *primary* and *secondary*, the former being idiopathic and the latter when it is caused by a known local or systemic cause. Clinically, it has been classified as *non-congestive* and *congestive glaucoma*. The Gonioscopic classification labels glaucoma as open *angle* and *narrow angle glaucoma*. By and large the following classification adopted.

Primary Glaucoma
1. Chronic simple glaucoma (open angle or non-congestive glaucoma)
2. Congestive glaucoma (angle closure glaucoma)
3. Low tension glaucoma
4. Congenital glaucoma.

Secondary Glaucoma
1. Inflammatory—Iridocyclitis (i) Acute (ii) Chronic
2. Lens induced
   a. Phacolytic glaucoma (i) Intumescent cataract (ii) Hypermature cataract (iii) Displaced lens.
   b. Phacoanaphylactic glaucoma
   c. Exfoliative glaucoma
3. Neovascular glaucoma (i) CRV Occlusion (ii) Diabetic retinopathy
4. Traumatic glaucoma—Contusion injury
5. Steroid induced glaucoma.
6. Miscellaneous
   - Aniridia
   - Essential atrophy of Iris
   - Sturge-Weber's syndrome
7. Aphakic glaucoma
8. Malignant glaucoma
9. Pigmentary glaucoma
10. Ciliary block glaucoma
11. Intra-ocular tumours

Chronic Simple Glaucoma

It is a primary glaucoma due to an indeterminate etiology. The incidence is much more common than narrow angle glaucoma. Because of its quietness, the patient does not go to the eye surgeon early enough. This type of glaucoma therefore has to be looked for in every eye patient above the age of 35 to 40. An emphasis is therefore necessary that in every case over the age of 35 to 40 years chronic simple glaucoma should be excluded by careful examination repeated when so advised.

The disease is distinctly more common in males and is essentially bilateral although it may be more advanced in one eye than in the other eye. The disease is known to have a hereditary background.

Pathology

The pathological changes are located in the trabecular mesh work through which aqueous is drained into the aqueous veins. Sclerotic changes have been noted which result in obstruction to aqueous outflow which in tonographic terms is called reduced aqueous outflow facility.

Histological observations have been as under:
1. The collagen of the trabecular meshwork extends into the canal of Schlemn.
2. The proliferation of endothelial cells in trabecular meshwork.
3. The narrowing of trabecular spaces.

In addition, narrowing of intrascleral spaces and aqueous veins add to the obstructive factor. Perhaps the sluggishness of scleral spur due to inertia of ciliary muscle is also a contributing factor.

Clinical features: The onset is slow and insidious. Clinical diagnosis is based on symptoms and objective findings. It has been emphasised that it is far more important to diagnose glaucoma in the early stages to save the eye from ultimate fate of blindness.

Symptoms: In the early stages there may be no symptoms and the disease may be discovered on routine examination.

Transient obscuration of vision is sometimes complained of and is usually related to a rising phase of diurnal variation. Persistent diminution of vision becomes an important complaint only when, the disease has progressed to fairly advanced stage, and vision may be appreciably reduced.

In chronic simple glaucoma, heaviness of the head, particularly in the morning can be an important symptom. This is due to the fact that IOP is highest in early hours of the morning and these patients often get up with heaviness in the head. Another relevant symptom is frequent changes in reading glasses which is due to rapid increase in presbyopia. This is possibly due to the effect of the raised IOP on the action of the ciliary muscle.

The person may have *defective dark adaptation*. Feeling of delayed adjustment when coming from bright light to a shaded room is not an uncommon symptom. It is due to decreased light sensitivity of retina in glaucoma.

Signs: A positive diagnosis of glaucoma is made on the basis of the findings of various examinations like tension, disc changes and field of vision combined with provocative tests if necessary. Special tonography, static perimetry, angio-scotometry are helpful but not always necessary

Intraocular pressure: It has already been emphasized that an eye with IOP 22-25 mm Hg should be considered a glaucoma suspect. Persistent tension of 26 mm of Hg or more is glaucoma. Importance is also attached if diurnal variation is more than 8 mm of Hg. It is also significant if difference in tension between the two eyes is 6 mm of Hg or more. It is, therefore, important that in early glaucoma one reading of IOP will not exclude the possibility. It is advisable that repeat tension records are done by the same tonometer and the same person taking a minimum of three readings each time.

Applanation tonometry has a distinct advantage over Schiotz tonometry in that it excludes scleral rigidity factor and is therefore particularly useful when looking for glaucoma in myopic eyes.

In spite of what has been stated above, the tension may be within normal limits and yet the eye may be glaucomatous as substantiated by disc and field changes. This is labelled as *low tension glaucoma*.

There is a well recognised and identified term called *ocular hypertension*. These are eyes where the tension remains persistently raised but the disc and field changes are absent and visual acuity is normal. There are no diurnal variations and no abnormality in the angle.

This non-glaucomatous ocular hypertension has been evaluated differently by different persons. The question arises whether this eye will later become glaucomatous. There is evidence that this is a possibility and the condition should therefore not be overlooked or neglected. Follow-up over a long period is necessary.

Disc changes: The optic disc area is the weakest part of the scleral coat and cannot withstand raised intraocular tension. Under influence of high tension, disc yields to pressure and develops cupping. It is important to understand that majority of normal discs have some amount of cupping. It is therefore extremely important to differentiate between physiological and pathological cupping.

Physiological cupping of the disc is central. It does not involve the disc to its margin (Fig. 13.2B and 13.2B Plate 8).

Glaucomatous cupping has characteristic features. A glaucomatous cupping extends to the disc margin at least in one sector. A more important criterion is that the part of optic disc which is not involved in cupping is greyish in colour and ischaemic. A still more significant consideration is the direction of the extension of cupping. A cupping which extends in a vertical direction, is significantly glaucomatous. These points should be critically observed when analysing disc changes. Importance is also given to the ratio between the size of the cupping and the size of the disc. This is known as cup: disc ratio. If the diameter of the cup is more than half the diameter of the disc, it is more likely to be glaucomatous than physiological. The significance of it becomes more important if this ratio is more in the vertical direction.

In advanced stages of glaucoma, the disc appearance is very characteristic. The whole optic disc surface is cupped which reaches the disc margin. The cupping has overhanging margins so that retinal vessels are partly obscured during their course from the centre of the disc to

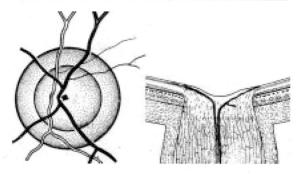

Fig 13.2A: Normal optic nerve head with physiological cupping of disc

the disc margin. The disc is pale and atrophic at this stage. A circum-papillary halo round the disc may be noted in advanced cases of glaucoma (Fig. 13.3A and Figs 13.3B, Plate 8).

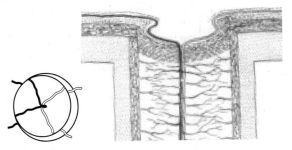

Fig 13.3A: Optic nerve head with deep cupping. Note deviation of blood vessels as they come up on surface

The visual field changes are important criteria of diagnosing early glaucoma. Record of peripheral field of vision with Lister's perimeter is not useful in detecting these early changes which can be recorded by examination on Bjerrum screen or on Goldmann perimeter.

The field changes in glaucoma are nerve fibre bundle defects because of the peculiar anatomical arrangement of retinal nerve fibres as they reach the disc (Fig. 13.4). The nerve fibre bundles above and below the papillo-macular bundle are first to suffer the effect of raised IOP. Inferotemporal bundle is first to be affected and hence the field defect appears first above the horizontal raphe in nasal quadrant.

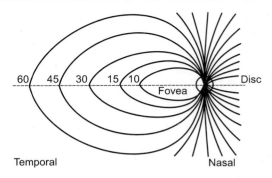

Fig 13.4: Arrangement of nerve fibres in the retina reaching the disc margin explaining the pathogenesis of field changes

The visual field defects in early glaucoma have special features. The earliest field defect is a *paracentral scotoma*. An equally significant change is the *baring of the blind spot* which means that the central field in the area of the blind spot has been so depressed that the blind spot is lying outside the recorded field. As the field changes progress, the paracentral scotoma may extend around the fixation point above or below or on both sides and may form an *arcuate scotoma* (Fig. 13.5). Further extension of field defect may give rise to *Ronne's nasal step* which is a sector defect extending to the periphery of

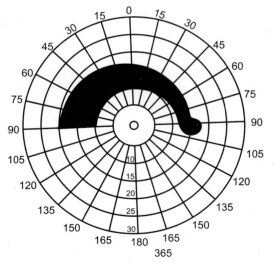

Fig. 13.5: Early field changes in chronic simple glaucoma arcuate scotoma

the central field more often above the horizontal level. Once the field defect has reached this level, the disease has already reached a fairly advanced stage.

In still more advanced stage of glaucoma a large part of the peripheral field has been obliterated and in the end only a tubular field or a small island of temporal field is left (13.6 and 13.7)

The anterior segment of eye: Glaucoma should always be considered during a routine anterior segment examination and findings may lead to further investigations to prove or disprove glaucoma.

Pupil: Pupillary size and shape are usually within normal limits in early glaucoma. However, certain pupillary changes in glaucomatous eyes are known. A large pupil with sluggish reaction is associated with well developed glaucoma. The pupil may be widely dilated and fixed and there may be patches of iris atrophy.

The anterior chamber is usually within normal limits in chronic simple glaucoma.

Similarly, cornea is clear except in advanced absolute stage when cornea can be hazy due to oedema and bullous formation.

The lens changes. Glaucoma by itself is not responsible for cataractous changes. Patients with glaucoma often do not develop cataract though they are in the cataractous stage.

Fact remains that an early glaucoma is as difficult to detect as it is important to do so. A positive approach is needed if we are to save the patients coming for treatment when it has already reached an advanced stage. It should be a regular practice that every patient attending the Eye OPD above the age of 35, should have a tonometry done. Any case that falls in the glaucoma-suspect group should be investigated to exclude glaucoma. Any patient with raised intra-ocular pressure with no other pro-glaucoma

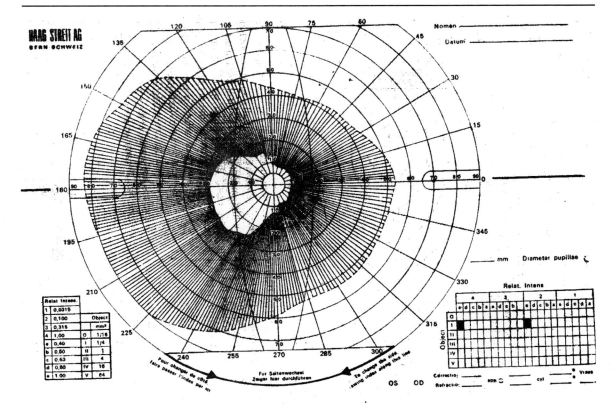

Fig. 13.6: A case of advanced stage of chronic simple glaucoma. Field of vision reduced to tubular stage but vision may be 6/9

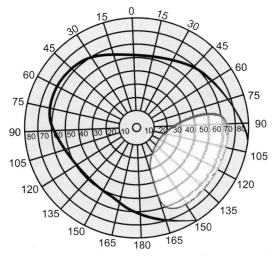

Fig 13.7: Residual field in terminal stage of chronic simple glaucoma. (Only a small island in temporal area remains. Eccentric Vision finger counting 3-4

evidence, should be followed up regularly. Importance should be given when there is difference in tension of the two eyes and cupping in one disc is larger than the other disc because this asymmetry is significant for diagnosis of glaucoma. It is easily said than done, in a country like India were patients are not conscious of the importance of diagnosing early glaucoma and where follow up in the absence of severe visual symptoms is not readily available. For the ophthalmologist, it is always wise to think of glaucoma unless proved otherwise because that is the only way to reduce the number of patients going totally blind due to glaucoma.

Differential diagnosis: The most important differential diagnosis is from incipient cataract because both conditions are insidious in onset and relatively symptomless. Furthermore, an erroneous hasty diagnosis of cataract with grey pupil leads to missing glaucoma. Most important differentiation is the tension record and examination of the media and fundi not only to exclude lens opacity but also to discover glaucomatous cupping if any.

Prognosis: Prognosis depends on the stage at which glaucoma is diagnosed. Full visual acuity for the rest of the life is possible if they are diagnosed at an early stage and before atrophic changes in the optic disc have set in and before field changes have reached an irreversible stage.

The prognosis becomes uncertain once the disease has reached a clinically well developed stage because from this stage onwards glaucomatous pathology is in an irreversible phase: Tension may be restored to normal by surgery with prolongation of sighted life but pathological changes continue and they end up in blindness early or late in majority of the cases.

It is not out of place to emphasize here that glaucoma if not diagnosed and treated at its onset when visual involvement in terms of acuity and/or field defects has not occurred or is minimal, the loss is irreversible and any treatment medical or surgical is an attempt to only save the remaining functional integrity and not regain what is lost.

Treatment: The glaucomatous eye is a sick eye in a sick body. From treatment point of view, glaucoma is, therefore a medical disease treated by medical therapy if diagnosed early. It becomes a surgical proposition if response to medical therapy is unsatisfactory or progress continues in spite of medical therapy.

Medical Therapy

Drugs used locally in glaucoma treatment are:
1. **Miotics:** Pilocarpine, a parasympathomimetic drug is used as 1% to 4% drops depending on response. If stronger than 4% drops

are needed to control IOP and changes in field progress, then surgical intervention should be considered. When used in cases with central lens opacity, diminution of vision becomes problematic due to pupillary contraction.
2. **Epinephrine** a sympathomimetic adrenergic drug used as 0.5% to 1% drops. It does not contract pupil, actually causes moderate dilatation and therefore does not pose a problem in central lens opacity. It also enhances outflow facility.
3. **Betablockers** used as 0.25% to 0.5% drops. Available preparations are Timolol, Betaxolol levobunolol etc. These are contraindicated or used with great caution under guidance of a physician in patients with pulmonary and cardiac disease. An advantage is that these can be combined with miotics when a patient does not respond to a single drugs.
4. **Prostaglandin** derivatives—Latanoprost Travopost are synthetic drugs used as 0.0005%. It can be used with pilocarpine as well as timolol. These also enhance outflow facility.

Drugs used Systemically for Glaucoma Treatment

1. **Carbonic anhydrase inhibitors:** Acetazolamide, Ethoxzolamide and methazolamide. They act by reducing production of aqueous. They are available as tablets 250 mg. Acetazolamide (Diamox) is most commonly used. It is also available as parenteral solution for IV use.

There was a gap of over 40 years between demonstrated effective oral Acetazolamide therapy and introduction of topical carbonic anhydrase inhibitor.

Dorzolamide hydrochloride, first topical carbonic anhydrase inhibitor lowers IOP by reducing aqueous formation. Used as 2%

drops three times a day, it is effective in open angle glaucoma and ocular hypertension, an effect similar to Betaxolol 0.5% twice daily. Effectivity of Timolol is enhanced by use of 2% Dorzolamide twice daily.

It does not produce systemic side effects and is not contraindicated in asthema or cardiac disease. Since it does not cause miosis, there is no visual disturbance.

2. **Hyperosmotic agents:** IV mannitol and urea and oral glycerol are used as additional therapy when rapid lowering of intra-ocular tension is needed as in acute congestive glaucoma, pre-operative to get a more or less normotensive eye for anterior segment surgery. The dose depends on body weight of patients (1-2 gms per kg body weight). IV mannitol is available as 20% solution. Glycerol is prepared in lemon juice as 'Sherbat' for oral ingestion. IV urea is not recommended because of its side effect of nausea. All these hyperosmotic agents act by reducing osmotic pressure and changing osmotic gradient at ciliary epithelial level to reduce aqueous formation.

Surgical management: If conservative treatment cannot control raised IOP and if field changes continue to deteriorate, surgical interference is called for. It is not always a failure of therapy that operation is indicated. People who do not follow the treatment as advised and who cannot come for follow up for reasons of distance and economy, surgical treatment may have to be considered in preference to medical therapy. Surgery would have to be the first choice in cases with advanced stage of glaucoma. Operative procedure is also indicated as a prophylactic measure.

The common operative procedures for chronic simple glaucoma are: *Filtering surgeries to enhance aqueous drainage.*

Older procedure like *Iridencleisis,* Trephining, *Schie's operation* and different *sclerotomies* are abandoned with development of modifications in *External Trabeculectomy, trabeculotomy* and *Trabeculoplaty.* Advances in LASER have further added to surgical therapy of glaucoma.

1. *External trabeculectomy* is now the operation of choice for open angle glaucoma. The advantage of this operation over other procedures is that it avoids avascular, papery thin filtering blebs which have been a source of infection in other procedures. Blebs in trabeculectomy are of a diffuse nature and malignant glaucoma rarely follows this surgery. The routes of drainage in this operation are more than one:
   i. Absorption in the intra-scleral space,
   ii. Diffusion into the subconjunctival space.
   iii. Drainage through supra-ciliary space.
   iv. Possibly through the cut end of canal of Schlcmn and cut edges of iridectomy.

The procedure can be repeated at different site when needed.

It is important to keep in mind that a glaucoma surgery may need to be repeated and therefore the first surgery should always be done on either side of the 12 O'clock position. It is also important to keep in mind that the filtering area should not be disturbed by any other surgery like cataract operation which when needed can be done either through temporal or lower sectors.

There may be a situation when chronic simple glaucoma co-exists with senile cataract. The choice is whether to do glaucoma surgery first and then a cataract operation or do both together. If glaucoma surgery is done first, cataract may be done three or four weeks after by the lower limbal route. It is however feasible to combine external trabeculectomy with cataract extraction at the same sitting along the upper limbus. This combined procedure must always be planned only with normotensive state of the eye preoperatively to avoid intra-operative complications.

Congestive Glaucoma

It is also known as *angle closure glaucoma* or *non-compensated glaucoma*. Congestive glaucoma usually brings the patient to doctor unlike chronic simple glaucoma where the ophthalmologist has to look for it. Because it is diagnosed early and therefore treated early.

Aetio-pathogenesis: In congestive glaucoma obstruction to drainage of the aqueous is primarily at the angle and not beyond the angle and this is facilitated by pupillary block. The later pushes the iris forward and closes the already narrow angle thereby further raising the IOP. Angle closure excites inflammatory reaction which produces peripheral anterior synechiae in part or whole of the extent of the angle of the anterior chamber.

Certain anatomical factors are associated with angle closure glaucoma. These eyes are usually hypermetropic and therefore small. The lens is more spherical and larger in size in proportion to the size of the anterior segment. Aqueous remains collected in posterior chamber causing displacement of iris diaphragm forwards consequently causing shallowing of anterior chamber and narrowing of angle.

Vascular engorgement is also an important precipitating factor in such eyes. Vasomotor instability is a special feature of angle closure glaucoma and is possibly a part of the factors like emotional shocks and accidents which precipitate an attack of angle closure. A satisfactory explanation is also not available for the vertically oval shape of pupil in glaucoma, more prominent in congestive type of glaucoma. It has possibly something to do with the arrangement of dilator muscle fibres or the distribution of nerve fibres.

Clinical features: Angle closure glaucoma presents itself in different clinical forms and stages. These are described as:
1. Prodromal stage.
2. Stage of chronic instability.
3. Acute congestive.
4. Chronic congestive.
5. Absolute glaucoma.

1. **Prodromal stage** is a clinical condition where patients with a shallow anterior chamber occasionally complain of halos around light and some transient mistiness of vision. They return back to normalcy after these temporary disturbances. Not all patients with these symptoms come to the ophthalmologist and this stage is often missed. A few such episodes may lead to chronic instability or the patient may develop an acute attack.

2. **Stage of chronic instability** is a stage where the patient develops symptoms from time to time. These symptoms are halos of rainbow coloured rings around light, mistiness in vision and headaches. The symptoms are usually precipitated by certain environmental factors like going to a movie, working in dark for longer hours or by emotional stress and strain. These eyes when examined during an attack may show semidilated pupil, slight haziness due to corneal oedema, mild ciliary congestion and raised IOP. The symptoms and findings disappear after the attack subsides and tension comes down. The optic disc is normal. Provocative tests are positive but do not need to be done as diagnosis is clear when examined during an attack. Each attack may leave the eye in the normal stage but may initiate a process of peripheral anterior synechia. Iridecto my should be considered to prevent an attack of acute congestive glaucoma.

3. **Acute congestive glaucoma** is the fulminating stage of congestive glaucoma. In pre-diamox and pre-mannitol days, it was a major emergency when patient had to be operated in the middle of the night. In some patients, generalized reaction like vomiting and severe headache overshadow ocular symptoms and hence the recorded example that a patient first went to a surgeon who removed his appendix. Acute congestive glaucoma has a sudden onset. It is more common in females than males.

The basic pathology of the condition is in the angle which is closed in more than half the extent. So that a pre-existing pathology is present before acute attack comes on in most cases.

Clinical features: There is an acute onset of symptoms. The patient complains of severe headache and marked diminution of vision and neuralgic pain in the area of distribution of the trigeminal nerve.

On examination, the lids may be swollen. There is marked ciliary congestion, often with generalized bulbar congestion. The cornea is steamy. The anterior chamber is shallow. The pupil is dilated, not reacting to light and vertically oval. Tension is markedly raised. Vision is reduced to counting fingers at a few feet. Fundus details if at all visible, show hyperaemia, arterial pulsation and blurring of disc margins. There is no glaucomatous cupping. On the other hand, physiological cup may be filled up. Small white flecks (glaucomflecken of Vogt) are often seen on the anterior capsule of the lens in the pupillary area and are definite evidence of an acute attack of glaucoma, past or present.

The acute phase subsides as quickly as it comes, following proper treatment. Cornea clears, vision improves and tension reduces from very high to moderate level. There is no necessity for an emergency surgery.

The severity may not be as acute as described above. Less acute cases are more often seen than the fulminating cases though with the same clinical findings. After relief from the acute phase, the opposite eye should also be examined in all cases. It is not unusual to find evidences of glaucoma in the other eye also, like shallow anterior chamber and narrow angle. It is inadvisable to perform a provocative test for proving this because this may precipitate an acute attack in the other eye also.

Differential diagnosis: Although the clinical features are fairly constant and evident, milder cases of congestive glaucoma have been confused with acute iritis and acute conjunctivitis. Differentiating features have been tabulated in chapter on uvea.

When glaucoma is suspected in eyes with corneal oedema, a few other conditions should be kept in mind which can be a cause of secondary rise of IOP. These are uveitis, Fuchs' dystrophy, glaucomato-cyclitic crisis and severe degree of exfoliative and pigmentary glaucoma.

Prognosis: Prognosis is not as bad as in chronic simple glaucoma. Reasons are that the patient has symptoms of acute nature and seeks advice and treatment early. Furthermore, condition responds to therapy before permanent changes in the optic disc and field are caused.

However, cases of congestive glaucoma with mild recurrent attacks if neglected or improperly treated may develop peripheral anterior synechia and pass on to the more complicated stage of *chronic congestive glaucoma.*

Treatment: The important consideration is to quickly control the IOP by all means at our disposal. Therapeutic doses of diamox by mouth and mannitol as infusion should be started immediately. Miotic like pilocarpine 2 percent is instilled frequently, the frequency depending on severity. Pupillary contraction must be achieved.

Quick control of the acute condition however has one disadvantage because the patient is relieved of symptoms and his vision returns to normal. He, therefore, avoids or declines surgical procedure necessary for permanent control. Many such patients will come back with another acute attack and more damage to the eye. It is, therefore, important that acute congestive glaucoma patient should be hospitalised and the treatment should be completed as necessary.

Peripheral iridectomy is the most consistently used operation for acute congestive glaucoma. It is the operation of choice after a first attack which quickly responds to conservative therapy. In eyes with repeated attacks the choice may have to be made between iridectomy and filtering operation. In such cases, iridectomy may restore tension to normal temporarily, but persisting peripheral anterior synechiae will lead to a stage of chronic congestive glaucoma and filtering operation may then become necessary. The choice will be for filtering operation in cases of long duration, repeated attacks and poor response to medical therapy.

It is nearly imperative that when one eye has suffered from an acute attack of glaucoma, the other should not be left uncared for. A prophylactic peripheral iridectomy should be considered. Iridectomy acts by providing a communication between the posterior chamber and anterior chamber directly. Anterior chamber deepens, the angle opens up and the vicious circle is broken. It is no longer necessary to do a broad basal or sector iridectomy as was previously recommended.

Chronic Congestive Glaucoma

This is a condition which is a result of milder attacks of subacute nature. Each attack leaves behind some amount of peripheral anterior synechia. With successive attacks, a large part of angle is blocked and gives rise to persistently raised intraocular tension.

Clinically, there is a history of intermittant attacks, gradual diminution of vision and persistent mild circum-corneal congestion. The eye may develop cupping of disc. There may be patches of iris atrophy. The pupil remains dilated and non-reacting to light. There may be cataractous changes in the lens. Gonioscopy will help in the differentiation between chronic simple glaucoma and chronic congestive glaucoma, the latter showing the presence of peripheral anterior synechiae. Tonography may be helpful. Very low 'C' value is in favour of chronic simple glaucoma.

Treatment: These cases do not adequately respond to miotic therapy. A filtering operation is the operation of choice (Fig. 13.8, Plate 8).

Absolute glaucoma: It is a stage of glaucoma with absent perception of light. These are blind eyes with no hope of restoring vision. It may follow a chronic simple glaucoma or chronic congestive glaucoma. Patients usually have headache with total loss of vision. The eye is stony hard to feel and tonometry readings are very high. Perforating branches of anterior ciliary arteries are markedly prominent. There is ciliary congestion. Corneal sensation is dull. The cornea is hazy. There may be band of degeneration in cornea. The pupil is widely dilated and fixed. Fundus, if can be seen, shows total atrophic cupping of the disc.

Many of these eyes develop an equatorial staphyloma located at the exits of the vortex veins.

When the condition has lasted for a long time with atrophy of intraocular tissue, intraocular tension may come down to normal or subnormal.

Treatment: Even though incurably blind, the patient may not agree to enucleation. Headache, which sometimes may be very severe, can be relieved with retrobulbar injection of alcohol as a temporary measure. Once equatorial staphyloma has developed or the eye has bullous keratopathy, it is better to enucleate the eye with proper cosmetic implants and artificial prosthesis with good cosmetic results.

Congenital Glaucoma

Glaucomatous condition of the eye from birth can be either primary and developmental in origin or is secondary and often associated with other ocular anomalies.

Primary congenital glaucoma: It is also called *buphthalmos or infantile glaucoma.* It is either present from birth or becomes clinically evident a few weeks after birth. The cause of the condition is the pathological changes in the trabecular meshwork. Either the spaces of Fontana have not opened up as they normally should or there may be pathological abnormalities in the scleral spur or an aberrant position of root of iris. Congenital glaucoma in the morphological respects is identical to chronic simple glaucoma. In both, the obstruction is in the drainage channels. The further evolution of the disease however differs because in the former, eye ball is distensible while it is not so in the latter.

Clinical features: Congenital glaucoma in a majority of cases affects males, though not exclusively. In most cases, the condition is bilateral.

Symptoms: Photophobia in the infant should always arouse suspicion of congenital glaucoma as one of the causes. Usually a large cornea and rapid increase in the size of eye ball arouses attention of the parents, particularly when the disease is predominant in one eye.

Signs: *Corneal diameter.* This is more than 12 mm and disproportionately becoming larger as shown by repeated measurements. In advanced cases cornea may be oedematous and there may be tears in Decemet's membrane. The overall thickness is relatively and evenly reduced.

The anterior chamber is deeper than normal. Eyes become myopic because of the increase in the antero-posterior length. There may be sub-luxation and/or dislocation of lens because of the stretching of zonules. Disc in early stages may be normal. But later, glaucomatous cupping is seen which does not usually reach atrophic stage.

The tension of the eye may not be significantly raised because of the distensible character of the outer scleral wall. Higher tension may however be recorded if disease develops later in infancy. The eye ball as a whole is enlarged and enlargement may be evident even from a distance and attracts attention when one eye is affected more than the other.

Gonioscopy findings are not significantly specific. There may be abnormalities in the trabecular meshwork and position of scleral spur. The ciliary band may be narrow. Sometimes a whitish membrane is seen bridging the angle structures. This is known as **Barkan's membrane** and is due to embryonic mesodermal remnants.

Differential diagnosis is from megalocornea and keraloglobus. Reference may be made to table in the chapter on cornea.

Differentiation from secondary congenital glaucoma is made evident by the special features causing secondary glaucoma. Changes due to ocular anomalies such as aniridia, ectopia lentis as in Marfan's and Marchisani syndrome.

Prognosis: Prognosis is not very good. The eye may retain fair to good vision if treated in the early stages but restoration of vision to normal after gross enlargement of the eye ball, is very unlikely.

Treatment is surgical: Miotics and carbonic anhydrase inhibitors are used as an interim measure prior to surgery.

The operative procedures are:
1. External trabeculectomy.
2. Internal trabeculotomy.
3. Goniotomy.
4. Goniopuncture.
5. Other filtering operations.

External trabeculectomy can be performed easily in the early stage when the sclera has not become very thin. In later stages with very thin sclera, there may be difficulty in scleral flap dissection (Fig. 13.8, Plate 8).

Internal trabeculotomy is a procedure in which the canal of Schlemn is cut open into The anterior chamber on the inner surface. This is a procedure nearer the physiological state.

Goniotomy is a procedure where the trabecular meshwork is opened in part of the angle of anterior chamber with a goniotome. This procedure is done with the help of a goniolens. Goniotomy is preferred to external trabe-culectomy.

Goniopuncture is a less satisfactory procedure because in this procedure, a puncture is made through the trabecular meshwork and adjoining sclera in the hope that the aqueous will continue to seep through this puncture into the subconjunctival space.

Among the filtering procedures, a small trephining of 0.5 to 1 mm size was a common procedure before the above operative procedures developed.

Glaucoma and Aphakia

Because of high incidence of cataract in tropical countries, aphakic eyes are seen in large numbers by every surgeon.

The presence of glaucoma in aphakic eyes can be divided into two distinct groups — *Aphakic glaucoma* and *glaucoma in aphakic eyes*. Aphakic glaucoma is the condition where aphakia is the cause of glaucoma as in complicated aphakia giving rise to raised IOP. These complications can be listed as follows:

1. Pupillary block because of an intact vitreous face obstructing the round central pupil.
2. Vitreous in the anterior chamber.
3. Anterior synechia to the section with capsular remnants of the lens or with the vitreous.
4. Iris prolapse not adequately treated.
5. Persistent hyphaema.
6. Epithelialization of the anterior chamber.
7. Post-operative inflammation with persistent shallow AC causing peripheral anterior synechia.

Most of these conditions cause a congestive type of secondary glaucoma. Oblique illumination examination shows the complicating factor. The pupil may be notched indicating pull due to vitreous or capsular band hooking the pupillary margin. The pupil may be eccentric and drawn up due to synechia to section. There may be hammock pupil where complete iridectomy is done following vitreous escape. The pupil is bow shaped where the upper iris is inverted. Capsular remains adherent to the section and membranous sheet following epithelization can easily be identified. Tension is always on the higher side. Proper identification of the cause and satisfactory evaluation can best be done alter examining these eyes on a slit lamp. Slit lamp examination will identify:

1. Broken or intact anterior vitreous face.
2. Vitreous in anterior chamber.
3. Vitreous adherent to section.
4. Synechia between capsular remains and section.
5. Peripheral anterior synechia.
6. Epithelialization of anterior chamber seen as a membrane which grows along the endothelial surface of cornea and/or anterior surface of iris.

Vitreous touch syndrome is not uncommon in eyes where vitreous is in anterior chamber. Vitreous touch to endothelium causes traumatic endothelialitis, folds in descemet's membrane, oedema of cornea and epithelial bullae formation. Vitreous touch syndrome is responsible for many post-operative problems and causes persistent irritation, congestion of the eye and discomfort to the patient. These cases in the end result in corneal scarring and opacification.

A good cataract surgery with undisturbed vitreous or appropriately handled when disturbed, will go a long way in preventing aphakic glaucoma. Furthermore, any post-operative complications should be identified and suitably corrected. It is possible in most cases to repair these complications and restore the eye to normal condition free from persistent inflammation and freedom from agonising symptoms.

Treatment: In most cases of aphakic glaucoma, some surgical procedure will be needed. Medical therapy can only help in the transient control of tension. A persistent pupillary block can best be treated by removal of vitreous fluid through pars plana with reformation of the anterior chamber by air injection. For anterior synechia to the section surgery includes opening the section separating or excising synechia and resuturing the section. Vitrectomy is a very useful additional procedure.

The above details pertain to the era when intra/extracapsular extraction of cataract without intra ocular implant used to be a routine surgery. With IOLs having become a routine procedure, all these complications are not prevalent after cataract surgery any more.

However, sometimes an AC-IOL may move forward and touch cornea with the haptics iris tissue. The result is likely to be same as described.

Glaucoma in aphakic eyes: This is a condition where glaucoma co-exists in an aphakic eye but is not due to aphakia. Most of these cases have had chronic simple glaucoma prior to cataract surgery. Clinical findings evident of glaucoma like disc changes can be seen after cataract operation. In these eyes vitreous face is intact, the anterior chamber is uniform and the pupil is central. There is no reactionary congestion. It is also possible though very uncommon that a chronic simple glaucoma may set in sometimes after an uneventful cataract surgery and a good aphakic eye.

The question often arises whether the removal of lens compensates for moderate degree of elevated IOP or not. It has been established that in non-glaucomatous eyes, tension after cataract extraction is relatively lower than prior to surgery. Removal of lens may, therefore, compensate pre-operative raised IOP to a limited degree.

Treatment: Treatment of glaucoma in good aphakia can be by medical therapy. Pilocarpine may be substituted by phospholine iodide which maintains better control of IOP and instillation once a day is adequate. Phospholine iodide is a cataractogenous drug but can be safely used in aphakic eyes. Cycodialysis is a satisfactory surgery in good aphakic eye because there is no vitreous in the anterior chamber.

External trabeculectomy can also be performed in such eyes. However there is always a risk of blocking of the scleral window by the vitreous face.

Low Tension Glaucoma

This is a condition where the tension of eye ball persistently remains within normal limits (below 22 mm of Hg) and yet the eye develops glaucomatous disc changes and field changes. These changes are presumably due to the fact that the tension of the eye ball even though within usual normal limits, is high for that particular eye. Tension record is dependable in these eyes only if Schiotz tonometry is done with three weights and scleral rigidity factor corrected (differential tonometry). Applanation tonometry, however, is more useful in such a situation. A diagnosis of low tension glaucoma should only be confirmed when provocative tests are normal, diurnal variation and outflow facility are normal and the angle is open as seen gonioscopically. Low tension glaucoma is more often associated with myopic state of the eye because of the thinning of the scleral coat and low scleral rigidity which can compensate for moderate pressure changes.

The diagnosis of low tension glaucoma is therefore a ticklish proposition and one should hesitate to make this diagnosis unless he has excluded other causes leading to optic disc and field changes seen in low tension glaucoma. A large and deep cupping of disc with atrophic changes seen in such cases, has been called *Schnabel's cavernous optic atrophy.*

The causes which can mimic disc and field changes of low tension glaucoma may be:
1. Myopic cupping with degenerative changes.
2. Primary optic atrophy.
3. Tumours of optic nerve and chiasma.
4. Congenital anomalies of disc cup.
5. Juxta papillary choroiditis.

The treatment of low tension glaucoma should be aimed at reducing the tension to lower limits tolerable to the eye. One may aim at lowering the tension to 8-10 mm of Hg. The treatment is, therefore, largely surgical and external trabeculectomy with small window is the most suitable procedure.

Malignant Glaucoma

Malignant glaucoma means rise of intra-ocular pressure following glaucoma surgery. This mostly follows after a fistulising operation and commonly in eyes where tension before glaucoma operation either was not controlled or could not be controlled. It can however sometimes occur following glaucoma surgery in controlled eyes also.

The basis of pathogenesis of malignant glaucoma is movement of the lens forwards. The sequence of events follow one after another. On opening the hypertensive eye at operation, there is sudden and severe imbalance between the posterior segment and the opened anterior segment with the result that lens moves forwards. This increases contact between the lens and the posterior surface of the iris. Aqueous collects in the space behind lens with the result that the lens cannot move back to its original position.

Consequently, anterior chamber persists to remain shallow or absent during the post-operative period with high tension.

Patient's symptoms become worse with headache, congestion and pain. Use of miotics aggravate the condition.

Although malignant glaucoma is a glaucoma in an eye operated for glaucoma, a few clinical conditions may present a clinical picture akin to this glaucoma. There are:
1. Ciliary block glaucoma.
2. Thrombotic glaucoma.
3. Too tight a scleral buckling for detachment surgery.
4. Choroidal haemorrhage.
5. Subluxated lens.
6. Severe uveitis and scleritis.

All these need to be kept in mind when evaluating a case of malignant glaucoma. It is imperative that filtering glaucoma operation should NEVER be done unless tension of the eye is preoperatively controlled and brought to near normal level by every possible means. Hypotensive drugs both oral as well as infusions will usually help control tension before glaucoma operation in most cases.

Treatment: Once malignant glaucoma sets in, non-surgical treatment is only temporary. Diamox, glycerol and mannitol may cause lowering of the IOP. Cyloplegics like atropine 1% with phenylephrine are helpful.

Surgery is most frequently required when a shallow anterior chamber persists in spite of medical therapy. Aspiration of 1 to 2 cc fluid from the middle of vitreous cavity through a pars plana puncture, combined with injection of air in the anterior chamber and use of cycloplegic may help reverse the vicious cycle. If this does not succeed, lens removal is the next alternative procedure. This is likely to be associated with vitreous disturbance and therefore anterior vitrectomy will have to be done following the lens extraction.

Ciliary Block Glaucoma

This is a pathological process where a glaucomatous eye does not respond to hypotensive medical therapy and miotics make it worse. This condition should be thought of whenever glaucoma cannot be controlled before surgery and when there is no other factor in the eye causing a picture akin to malignant glaucoma.

In this condition shallowness of anterior chamber and rise of IOP is caused by collection of aqueous in the space behind the lens, the swelling of ciliary body with the result that lens and ciliary body move forwards and block the angle of anterior chamber. Use of miotics increases lens-iris contact and aggravates the condition.

Clinically, it presents a picture of mild congestive glaucoma with shallow anterior chamber. The tension is moderately raised and does not respond to hypotensive drugs.

Treatment is cycloplegic with or without epinephrine. Cycloplegics relax ciliary body, pull the lens back, and facilitate passage of aqueous, cyclogel is better than atropine.

If a person comes with a recurrent attack peripheral iridectomy followed by use of cycloplegic will keep the condition under control.

SECONDARY GLAUCOMA

It is a symptom complex rather than a distinct entity. The one common factor to the various conditions which can cause this disease is raised IOP. Clinical picture, etiology and pathology, and therefore the treatment differ for each cause.

The clinical conditions that can cause secondary glaucoma in order of importance are:
1. Lens induced glaucoma.
2. Intraocular inflammations.
3. Thrombotic glaucoma and neovascular glaucoma.
4. Steroid induced glaucoma.
5. Traumatic glaucoma.
6. Epidemic dropsy glaucoma.
7. Intraocular tumours.
8. Essential atrophy of iris.
9. Aniridia.
10. Following keratoplasty.
11. Following scleral buckling.
12. Glaucomato-cyclitic crisis.
13. Miscellaneous.
    a. Heterochromic iridocyclitis.
    b. Enzymatic glaucoma.

Lens Induced Glaucoma

The lens by its presence or following its removal is the leader amongst causes for secondary glaucoma. Many eyes remain unoperated even beyond the stage of maturity and glaucomatous consequences follow in many such eyes.

The mechanism of glaucomatous change in cataractous eyes is variable. The following are the modes by which the cataractous or non-cataractous lens can cause secondary glaucoma. These can be classified into two main groups, glaucoma caused by lens in situ and glaucoma caused by displaced lens.

Lens in Situ

1. *Intumescent cataract.* The lens is swollen due to imbibition of fluid. This pushes the iris forward, narrows the angle of anterior chamber, impedes aqueous drainage and causes rise of intraocular pressure. There are probably some other factors, vascular or neurogenic because not all eyes with intumescent cataract develop rise of IOP. The glaucomatous process is more common where intumescence is rapid in onset and the eye has a narrow angle from the beginning. Clinically, it is a congestive type of secondary glaucoma with ciliary congestion, shallow anterior chamber and dilated pupil. The tension is raised. The treatment is removal

of the lens after normalizing tension with hypotensive therapy.

2. *Hypermature morgagnian cataract.* This is a globular lens which can cause secondary glaucoma either by mechanical shallowing of anterior chamber or sometimes when the lens capsule is ruptured and small hard nucleus lies in the anterior chamber. The nucleus can sometimes be caught in pupillary aperture when the glaucomatous, process is more acute. The lens fluid induces inflammation of anterior uvea further complicating the situation.

3. *Phacolytic glaucoma.* So long as the capsule of lens is intact, a lens can only cause obstructive glaucoma. If, however, lens protein can seep out through the lens capsule through subclinical pores, it excites inflammatory reactions and causes phacolytic glaucoma. These lens proteins can cause rise of intraocular pressure either by collecting in and occluding the angle or by causing tissue reaction of inflammatory nature. Cataract extraction is rewarding in these cases.

4. *Exfoliative glaucoma.* This is a condition much less common in tropical countries. It is clinically identified by slit lamp and gonioscopy. Exfoliated capsular material can collect in the trabecular meshwork and cause obstruction to drainage of aqueous.

    Treatment is removal of the lens combined with glaucoma surgery.

Displaced lens causing secondary glaucoma: Subluxation or dislocation of a normal or cataractous lens can be the cause of severe secondary glaucoma usually congestive in nature. The subluxation or dislocation of the lens may be anterior or posterior. The whole lens may occupy the anterior chamber and cause severe congestive glaucoma. When transparent, it looks like a blob of oil. When cataractous, it is seen evidently as a white mass in the anterior chamber obscuring iris and pupil.

The treatment is to quickly remove it under mannitol infusion.

The lens displaced forward may be caught in the pupillary aperture causing severe glaucomatous reaction. This is relieved by mydriasis and hence it is called *glaucoma inversus.* Removal of lens is the only remedly.

Subluxated lens can cause secondary glaucoma by partly shallowing anterior chamber or by vitreous prolapse in anterior chamber. Subluxated lens causing secondary glaucoma should always be removed. It is likely to be accompanied with vitreous loss which should be managed adequately by vitrectomy.

Posterior dislocation of the lens can happen spontaneously or following attempted regular intracapsular cataract extraction when vitreous presents before the lens is taken out.

Treatment in these cases is very guarded. Various procedures have been practiced, many are obsolete.

1. Removal with vectis: Not a very desirable procedure.

2. Cryo extraction with specially designed insulated probe.

3. With Diathermy needle specially insulated.

4. Two needle techniques one supporting, the other pushing the lens forward.

    Whatever the, procedure adopted, the results are uncertain.

    Pars plana lensectomy with vitrectomy is the one procedure of choice.

Intra-ocular Inflammation Causing Secondary Glaucoma

Intra-ocular inflammation can be acute or chronic. They can cause rise in the pressure by different mechanisms.

Acute iridocyclitis, whatever be the cause, can cause rise of tension in one of the following ways:

1. Albuminous aqueous which cannot easily pass through trabecular mesh

2. Exudative collection in the anterior chamber, with hypopyon blocking the angle.
3. Hypersecretion of aqueous, due to irritation of ciliary body.

Treatment in these types of secondary glaucoma is primarily of iridocyclitis. Mydriatics should be used unhesitatingly and effectively. Control of inflammation will normalise quality of aqueous and relieve glaucoma. Mydriatics will not only control inflammation but also prevent the synechia formation. Hypotensive therapy, will help prevent damaging effect of secondary glaucoma.

Chronic iridocyclitis can cause glaucoma by causing posterior synechia (*ring synechia or total posterior synechia*). It can also cause secondary glaucoma due to organised exudate blocking the pupil. In these conditions aqueous collects in the posterior chamber due to occlusion or seclusion of the pupil leading to the iris bombe, shallowing of the anterior chamber and the narrowing of the angle. It can also cause peripheral anterior synechia in long standing cases of chronic iridocyclitis when angle can be blocked all around. Treatment in cases with posterior synechia is complete iridectomy which is not always easy to perform. Iris may be so fragile that it may be pulled in pieces. Sometimes even when an iridectomy can be done, the posterior pigmentary layer of iris remains stuck to the lens. Filtering operation are indicated where there are extensive peripheral anterior synechiae.

In cases of iris bombe a procedure called transfixation of iris or four Iridotomies used to be done to flatten iris diaphragm and establish communication between posterior and anterior chamber.

Thrombotic Glaucoma and Other Neovascular Glaucoma

It is inappropriately called haemorrhagic glaucoma. Because it is not the haemorrhages which cause glaucoma but it is the blockage of central retinal vein which causes neovascularisation and haemorrhages. It is neovascularization in the angle that is responsible for glaucoma. It is called the 100th day glaucoma because it manifests about 100 days after thrombosis of central retinal vein. Proliferative diabetic retinopathy and sometimes Eales' disease can also cause glaucoma due to neovascularisation in the angle of the anterior chamber.

Thrombotic glaucoma occurs following central retinal vein occlusion usually just behind the optic disc. It is extremely uncommon in blockage of one of its tributaries.

Glaucoma process is caused by the neovascularisation in the angle of the anterior chamber. The most evident clinical manifestation is the vascularisation of iris, *rubeosis,* which may be around the pupillary margin and radial vessels can also be seen on surface of iris. These are clearly seen with slit lamp. There may be haemorrhages on the iris surface.

Starting as *rubeosis iridis,* neovascularistion extends to the angle of anterior chamber causing obstruction to drainage of aqeuous. The abnormal neovascularisation can cause hyphaema with further rise of intraocular tension.

Clinically thrombotic glaucoma causes severe headache. Vision is markedly reduced. Vision loss may be pre-existing due to the original retinal pathology or aggravated by high rise of the IOP.

Treatment: The treatment of thrombotic glaucoma is very unsatisfactory. Filtering operation cannot be done because of fear of haemorrhage from neovascularisation in the angle. Usual procedure is cyclo-cryo therapy and sometimes cyclodiathermy. This has to be repeated more than once. Wherever facilities exist newer procedures like gonio-photocoagulation of the neovascularisation in the angle in early stage may prevent serious consequences.

Pan-retinal photocoagulation of retina is indicated not only to reduce neovascularization thereby reducing chances of thrombotic glaucoma but also to save or restore the vision reduced by retinal anoxaemia and preventing further haemorrhages. This may also be useful if combined with cyclo-cryo therapy to help checking rise of IOP.

In severe painful blind eyes, enucleation may be indicated.

Steroid Induced Glaucoma

With extensive use of steroids, sometimes indiscriminate, incidence of steroid induced glaucoma increases. Steroids induce glaucoma only after prolonged use. Although they may precipitate glaucoma early, if the eye was genetically or inherently pro-glaucomatous.

Steroids cause secondary glaucoma following prolonged oral therapy as is often necessary in arthritis, pemphigus, etc. Prolonged local therapy can also cause secondary glaucoma e.g. use of the steroids for chronic conditions like spring catarrh in which case the patient uses steroids over months and years, without consulting ophthalmologist since the drug gives him relief.

The mode of secondary glaucoma is not clearly understood. It however causes reduced outflow facility and therefore resembles a chronic simple glaucoma.

Steroid induced glaucoma can be associated with steroid induced cataract.

Treatment: If steroids are withdrawn early after the onset of glaucoma, vision returns to normal and the eye becomes normo-tensive in a few weeks time. Reversibility of disc and field changes however, depend on duration of glaucomatous process. In irreversible cases, fistulizing operation is necessary.

Trauma and Glaucoma

Injuries to the eye causing glaucoma are either perforating or contusions. Glaucoma following perforating injuries can be caused by

1. Intraocular haemorrhage.
2. Anterior synechia and iris incarceration.
3. Iridocyclitis.
4. Swelling and rupture of lens.
5. Hyphaema.
6. Peripheral anterior synechia following persistent shallow anterior chamber.
7. Epithelialization of anterior chamber.

Management of these conditions is to deal with the cause. The injury scar, if not properly repaired, may have to be re-done. Incarceration of iris has to be repaired, the anterior synechia separated, and the hyphaema may require drainage.

Glaucoma following contusions: This is a condition which is often over looked, because it is not adequately realised that contusion may cause changes in the angle without any evident external injury.

Contusion causes *tearing of trabecular meshwork, detachment of scleral* spur from its attachment and *recession of the angle* of the anterior chamber. These can be identified by gonioscopy which may also detect iridodialysis.

Glaucoma following contusion can develops early within a few days or a few weeks later. Early glaucoma following contusion is a serious condition and the tension may be very high.

The treatment of early glaucoma is to give usual medical therapy at the earliest. If the eye does not respond, fistulizing surgery should be done. External trabeculectomy is surgery of choice. Late cases are to be treated like any other open angle glaucoma.

Glaucoma caused by contusion resulting in iridodialysis, hyphaema, rupture of pupillary sphincter, swollen cataractous lens, dislocated lens or vitreous haemorrhage is more readily recognised and treatment depends on causative factors.

Epidemic Dropsy Glaucoma

This is a disease peculiar in tropical countries, prevalent in some parts of eastern and central India. It is caused by the toxic alkaloid sanguinarine in the seeds of Argemone Maxicana of poppy family. The seeds are ingested when adulterated with cereals. The glaucoma is caused by vasodilatation in the angle of anterior chamber. It causes non-congestive chronic glaucoma usually bilateral. The tension is very high. Condition should always be kept in mind in endemic areas where other systemic clinical manifestations like odema of feet will explain glaucoma.

If toxic alkaloid is withdrawn, glaucomatous process may be relieved. Glaucomatous changes are reversible if the condition is treated early. In chronic cases, however, regular filtering surgery is necessary.

Intraocular Tumours

Tumours cause rise of intraocular pressure during the second stage of their progress. Any space occupying lesion of eye can cause rise of IOP. either by pushing the iris-lens diaphragm forward or deposits of tumour seedlings in the angle of the anterior chamber. In these cases, tumour pathology is more significant than glaucoma. Therefore clinical features, prognostic outlook and management will depend on type, size and the location of the growth and whether it is benign or malignant in nature.

Essential Atrophy of Iris

Essential atrophy of iris of progressive nature can cause glaucoma. Condition is more frequent in the western countries. Clinical condition of iris is characteristic. There are patches of thinning of iris. Pupil is eccentric. There are areas of peripheral anterior synechia and pigments in the angle. As the condition is progressive the results of the filtering surgery are not very satisfactory.

When the condition is associated with changes in corneal endothelium with oedema and marked reduction in vision it is called *Chandler's syndrome.*

Another bilateral condition is the pigmentary glaucoma with heavy deposition of pigments in the angle of the anterior chamber, first described by Sugar. The cause of pigment dispersion is not known. It is derived from pigment layer of iris which becomes thin and translucent. There may be deposits of pigments on the post surface of cornea. It mimics chronic simple glaucoma in all other respects.

Aniridia

This is a congenital condition when a large part of the iris diaphragm is absent. A small frill of the iris may be present at the periphery. As it is a congenital condition, glaucoma is present from an early age. There is usually associated nystagmus. The treatment is very unsatisfactory.

Glaucoma Following Keratoplasty

Glaucoma in the early post-operative period after the penetrating graft has often been mentioned as the cause of the graft failure. Rise of the IOP in the early post-operative period is more presumed than proved because one would hesitate to do tonometry. There are, however, clinical features which can cause secondary glaucoma. These are:

1. Too tight suturing of graft thereby making the cornea more flat and narrowing of the chamber. For this reason, when doing large sized grafts, donor material should be 0.5 mm larger than the recipient window.
2. Failure to restore anterior chamber on the table at the end of surgery.
3. Severe iridocyclitis
4. Anterior synechia to graft margin.
5. If the iris-lens diaphragm which moved forward during surgery, does not return to its original position.

6. Vitreous in anterior chamber in cases of total penetrating keratoplasty in which the iris and the lens are removed at the time of corneal grafting.

Glaucoma Following Scleral Buckling

Secondary glaucoma following scleral buckling is very rare. Because tension is routinely assessed at the end of the surgery with tonometry or by looking at the disc, the patient is never returned with the raised IOP at the end of the surgery. Scleral buckling causing too much indentation of sclera can also cause glaucoma by pushing iris-lens diaphragm forward and blocking the angle. In these cases, the tension is normal or subnormal at the end of the surgery but may rise after some time.

Glaucomato-cyclitic Crisis (Poshner-Schlossman's Syndrome)

This is a unilateral condition in relatively young patients. There is mild degree of iridocyclitis evident by few keratic precipitates and corneal oedema. A few days after this mild inflammation, tension may rise to high level. Condition is often intermittant and does not leave behind any after-effects. It has to be differentiated from recurrent attacks of acute congestive glaucoma on one side and acute iritis on other side. There is no peripheral anterior synechia thus no angle closure and no posterior synechia to suggest iritis. The treatment is steroids either subconjunctival or as local instillations. Aceta-zolamide may be added if the tension remains high. As the condition disappears after repeated attacks, no surgical treatment is required.

Miscellaneous

Heterochromic iridocyclitis: In this condition mild iridocyclitis is associated with lens changes. There may be abnormal blood vessels in the angle. Heterochromic character of iris is evident.

When these eyes develop glaucoma, it usually persists, even though treated. As cataract is commonly associated, combined cataract and filtering surgery may control the condition.

Enzymatic glaucoma: This used to be more often seen when alpha-chymotrypsin was routinely used in cataract surgery. The tension would rise from 2 to 5 days after cataract operation and last for few days to a week. Glaucoma is caused by the mechanical obstruction in trabecular channels by zonule particles. With advent of extracapsular and IOL surgery this condition is history and use of alpha chymotrypsin is obsolete.

Lasers in Glaucoma

Lasers are being used more frequently as a therapy for all types of glaucoma. The advantages of laser therapy are that it is a non-invasive OPD procedure and can be repeated when necessary. It is a suitable therapy when the patient refuses surgery, when the patient's compliance for prolonged medical therapy is undependable or the eye condition is unsuitable for open surgery. It is also the preferred choice in aphakic glaucoma when there is no vitreous in the anterior chamber and the traumatic glaucoma due to angle recession.

Different lasers are being used as indicated below :

1. a. Prophylactic iridotomy in open angle glaucoma, (ALT) — ARGON LASER
   b. Argon laser trabeculoplasty
2. Iridotomy in congestive glaucoma — YAG laser
3. Iridotomy in congestive glaucoma — ARGON or CRYPTON
4. Laser therapy is also being used for gonioplasty in infantile glaucoma and cyclo-cautery in neovascular glaucoma.

14

Vitreous

ANATOMY

The vitreous body is a clear transparent gel-like substance of semi-solid consistency. The shape is determined by the cavity in which it lies. Anteriorly it presents a concave patellar fossa, a depression caused by the posterior convex surface of the lens. Peripherally, it conforms to the shape of the inner wall of the eye ball. The vitreous body is attached anteriorly to the posterior surface of the lens by the hyloido-capsular ligament of Weigert. This ligament is stronger in younger individuals and as age advances, it atrophies.

Vitreous is comprised of collagen fibrils and glycoaminoglycans supported by hyaluronic acid molecules. The vitreous mass is surrounded by a condensation which is the cortex of the vitreous. The outer covering of the cortex is called the hyaloid membrane (Fig. 14.1).

The hyaloid membrane is the surface condensation of cortex of vitreous gel which surrounds the vitreous body. The posterior hyaloid membrane and inner limiting membrane of the retina cannot be differentiated under normal circumstances. However, in old age and in pathological states as in high myopia and diabetes, the posterior hyaloid face becomes distinctly visible with vitreous detachment.

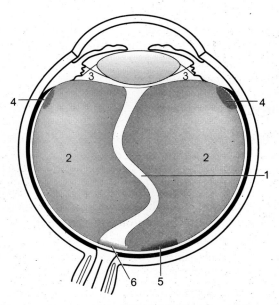

Fig. 14.1: Vitreous Mass (1) Primary vitreous round Cloquets canal, (2) Secondary vitreous forming the main mass; (3) Tertiary vitreous from which develops the suspensory ligament; (4) Normal virtreous adhesion at Ora Serrata; (5) Normal adhesion at macular area; (6) Normal adhesion Optic disc area.

Cloquet's canal represents the remnants of the primary vitreous. It is an 'S' shaped curve extending from back of lens and ending at the optic disc. Remnants of hyaloid (embryonic vascular) system surrounded by glial tissue may sometimes be seen at the disc end of Cloquet's canal. This is called *Bergmister's papilla*.

The vitreous base is an area of adhesion between the vitreous cortex and the pars plana ciliaris region of the ora serrata. It extends 2 mm anterior and 4 mm posterior to ora sterrata and forms a circular band all round. This provides a firm adhesion of vitreous fibrils to the peripheral retina.

The vitreous is also attached firmly to the margin of optic disc without having adhesion to the surface of the nerve head. When the posterior portion of the vitreous body becomes detached, a glial tissue ring from the optic disc can be visualised floating in front of optic disc. There is also a weak attachment of the vitreous body to the macula for 2 to 3 mm in diameter around the fovea. The vitreous is an embryonic tissue neither reformed nor regenerated later in life.

DEVELOPMENT

The development of vitreous body and zonule comprises the development of primary vitreous, secondary vitreous and tertiary vitreous. The primary vitreous is both mesodermal and ectodermal in origin. The lens cells and the retinal cells contribute the ectodermal part in the formation of primary vitreous. The mesodermal component of primary vitreous is contributed by hyaloid vascular system. Eventually the primary vitreous is restricted to the area of Cloquet's canal when mesodermal elements atrophy.

The secondary vitreous is the chief contributor to formation of adult vitreous body and is derived completely from the neural ectoderm. The secondary vitreous is composed of fine dense undulating fibres which arise from the developing retina. The progressive growth of the secondary vitreous causes atrophy of the hyaloid system of vessel, cessation of growth of the primary vitreous and increase in the size of the globe.

The tertiary vitreous develops into zonular fibres (suspensory ligament) during the fourth month of gestation. It is derived from the inner neural ectodermal layer of the developing ciliary body.

After development of the tertiary vitreous, principal changes occur in the hyaloid vessels. The physical and biochemical development of vitreous chiefly concerning its volume, collagen contents, concentration of hyaluronic acid, ascorbic acid and calcium continues after birth and is completed during childhood. The vitreous ultimately becomes a completely transparent gel and allows light rays to reach retina but it has no refractive action. Hyaluronic acid is responsible for viscosity of the vitreous and the gel is formed by the collagen meshwork.

The concentration of hyaluronic acid is highest in the peripheral cortical layers of the vitreous near the retina. The actual function of hyaluronic acid is not known though it has been suggested that it acts as a diffusion barrier protecting the vitreous body from cellular invasion. Hyaluronic acid concentration in the vitreous falls down after an intracapsular lens extraction and therefore the instability of vitreous. This decrease in vitreous stability is a factor of clinical importance.

The total weight of the vitreous in man is 3.9 grams and its volume is about 3.9 ml which is about 60% of the volume of the adult globe. The water content is extremely high between 98 and 99 per cent. The refractive index is between 1.3345 and 1.3348.

CONGENITAL ANOMALIES OF THE VITREOUS

Persistent Hyperplastic Primary Vitreous

The hyaloid vascular system in the vitreous regresses as development proceeds. Failure of this process results in persistent hyperplastic primary vitreous. This condition typically occurs in a microphthalmic eye in a full term baby. The condition is presented with a white reflex in the pupillary area, a shallow anterior chamber and may be associated with glaucoma. A vascularised mass can be seen behind the lens and intra-ocular bleeding can occur from this mass. Long ciliary processes can often be seen dragged into the pupillary space. The condition should be differentiated from retinoblastoma and retrolental fibroplasia. The lens may be cataractous, partially or totally.

Persistent Hyaloid Artery

The hyaloid vascular system may not regress and present three forms of anomalies:
1. The total length of the hyaloid artery may be seen extending from the optic disc to the lens as a fine white thread.
2. The anterior end of the artery may be seen attached 1 or 2 mm nasal to the posterior pole of the lens.
3. The posterior end of the artery may persist and seen attached to the optic disc.

The patients do not have any symptoms. Some may complain of floaters. Ophthalmoscopically, the remnants are seen as white threads attached to the disc, the lens or to both.

VITREOUS OPACITIES

Vitreous opacities are usually secondary in origin due to a degenerative or inflammatory lesion of the structures around vitreous. Subjectively they are seen as black objects in front of eyes freely moving as the eye ball moves. Ophthalmoscopically they are seen as dark spots. They may obscure the view of the fundus if they are numerous.

Symptoms of fine vitreous opacities are common entoptic phenomena even though no opacities are seen with ophthalmoscope. These are called muscae *volitantes* and are common

in later age. These are possibly due to breakdown of the supporting fibrillar network of the vitreous. They are visible to the patients when they look at the sky or against the lighted ceiling of the room. They may however cause disturbing symptoms to nervous patients. No treatment is required. Patients need to be reassured of their harmless nature. They should be advised to overlook them.

Pathological vitreous opacities may be classified according to aetiology:
1. Developmental.
2. Degenerative.
3. Inflammatory.
4. Haemorrhagic.
5. Neoplastic.

Developmental

The developmental vitreous opacities include persistent hyaloid artery. Opacities can also occur in primary vitreous. Usually they do not give rise to any symptoms unless associated with posterior vitreous detachment.

Degenerative

Degenerative vitreous opacities can occur in asteroid hyalitis, senility, high myopia, vitreo-retinal degenerations and amyloidosis.
a. **Asteroid hyalitis** is essentially a degenerative condition which occurs in later age. It is common in males and is mostly unilateral. They are small spherical bodies which occur in bunches or in columns but without any known arrangement. They are seen distributed throughout vitreous but more often in the central cavity. Since the vitreous retains its solid character, the asteroid bodies move only within a small range with the movement of the eye. They are symptomless and vision is not affected. Asteroid bodies are most probably calcium soaps. The condition does not warrant any treatment.

b. **Synchiasis scintillans** may be unilateral or bilateral. They are described as small shining crystalline opacities floating freely in fluid vitreous. These particles are composed primarily of cholesterol crystals. Since these opacities are found in fluid vitreous, they move freely with the movement of the eye ball and settle down rapidly as a shower when the eyes become stationary. They tend to occur secondary to degenerative ocular conditions or can be secondary to trauma, inflammation or haemorrhage. They rarely interfere with vision and need no treatment.

Inflammatory

Inflammatory vitreous opacities result from inflammatory process in the posterior uveal tract or retina. They may be composed of exudates containing inflammatory cells, necrotic tissue and fibrin. The snowball opacities characteristic of pars planitis are typically seen as vitreous opacities. If inflammatory process of the surrounding structures continues, exudates, phagocytic cells and other inflammatory cells may invade the vitreous gel causing liquefaction. Decrease or disappearance of the inflammation may cause diminution of vitreous opacities.

Cysticercosis may cause severe inflammation in vitreous. This is seen as a transparent cystic lesion with invaginated scolex. They may be single or multiple. If these cysts rupture, white deposits occur all over the surface of the retina exciting severe inflammation.

Haemorrhagic

Haemorrhagic vitreous opacities result due to bleeding from normal or abnormal retinal blood vessels. The common conditions associated with vitreous haemorrhage are:

1. Diabetic retinopathy.
2. Eales' disease.
3. Central retinal vein occlusion.
4. Retinal tears.
5. Posterior vitreous detachment.
6. Intraocular trauma.
7. Blood diseases.
8. Hypertension and arterio-sclerosis.
9. Sickle cell retinopathy.

Basically vitreous haemorrhage occurs as a result of traction on the blood vessels. This traction may be due to abnormal vitreo-retinal adhesion. Posterior vitreous detachment may cause tearing of blood vessels. The blood vessels may also get torn due to injury or give way due to increased intravascular pressure as in cases of central vein thrombosis. An intraocular tumour may cause necrosis of the wall of a blood vessel which may rupture and cause massive vitreous haemorrhage.

Vitreous haemorrhages may occur into the sub-hyaloid space or into the substance of the vitreous.

Sub-hyaloid haemorrhage: Sub-hyaloid haemorrhage occurs in the space between the internal limiting membrane of the retina and the posterior vitreous cortex. If the posterior vitreous cortex is intact, blood collects in this space.

Since blood does not clot in this location, it settles down with a definite upper fluid level. The upper layer is less dense than the lower portion. It shifts from one part of the fundus to the other with change in the posture of the head.

Intra-vitreal haemorrhage. If posterior vitreous cortex is disrupted, blood may seep into the vitreous cavity. The cloudiness of vitreous will depend upon the amount of bleeding . If blood is small in amount and occurs in the vitreous gel it remains localised, but if it occurs in a liquid vitreous it causes generalized vitreous cloudiness. A recent vitreous haemorrhage is red in colour appearing dark on ophthalmoscopic examination. It may form dense vitreous membranes in due course of time if it does not absorb.

Vitreous haemorrhage may get absorbed if it is in small amount. Even small repeated haemorrhages are known to get completely absorbed and retain full vision. Repeated or massive haemorrhage is less likely to clear completely and more likely to produce clots, vitreous opacities and membranes. Long standing vitreous haemorrhages not only produce visual defects, but are also likely to produce harmful effects in the surrounding structures such as posterior subcapsular lens opacities and when organised cause retinal detachment.

Neoplastic

Retinoblastoma and other rare retinal tumours may cause opacities either by direct invasion into the vitreous or by causing inflammation or haemorrhage.

CLINICAL FEATURES OF VITREOUS HAEMORRHAGE

Vitreous haemorrhage is one of the common causes of sudden loss of vision. The degree of loss of vision will depend upon the amount of bleeding and the location of the haemorrhage. If it occurs in the posterior pole, the visual loss will be considerable.

Sudden appearance of black spots in front of the eye must give rise to the suspicion of vitreous haemorrhage (Fig. 14.2, Plate 8).

Signs

In a massive vitreous haemorrhage, the fundus glow will not be seen with a direct ophthalmoscope. Indirect ophthalmoscopy may reveal a dark red reflex. A fresh haemorrhage may be red in colour whereas a long standing haemorrhage will look dark.

Blood clots in the vitreous appear as floaters. These floaters disappear with absorption of haemorrhage.

Repeated vitreous haemorrhages and massive vitreous haemorrhages are likely to produce vitreous veils, fibrous bands and membranes.

Treatment depends upon whether the haemorrhage is of recent origin or long standing. Patients with a recent vitreous haemorrhage should have complete bed rest. The head should be elevated so that blood will collect in a dependent position. The blood may clear within a week's time to such an extent that ophthalmoscopic examination is possible to establish the source of the haemorrhage. If this source of bleeding has been identified as a new blood vessel, it can be treated by photocoagulation.

If a retinal detachment is suspected with a retinal tear as the cause of vitreous haemorrhage, it is better to treat it as early as possible surgically. An ultrasonogram and an electroretinogram may be useful to find out the position and functional status of the retina in cases of retinal detachment with vitreous haemorrhage. There is no specific medicinal treatment for vitreous haemorrhage except treat the cause when determined.

Heavy doses of Vitamin C and iodides by mouth or by injection will probably help absorption and preventing recurrence.

If the vitreous haemorrhage has not cleared in 2-3 weeks, it may not clear by itself. Such eyes usually show a dense blood clot or multiple vitreous membranes at different levels. Pars plana vitrectomy is indicated in these cases.

INFECTION OF VITREOUS

Endophthalmitis and Panophthalmitis

The vitreous is a very good culture medium for organisms. Once infection gets into vitreous, it progresses rapidly. This is made easier because vitreous is an avascular tissue and no defensive effort of the body can reach there. The situation is still more serious because any drugs administered systemically or topically, cannot reach vitreous centre and therefore are ineffective. The end result of gross infection in vitreous is therefore unfavourable particularly if timely treatment is not available. Endophthalmitis and panophthalmitis are to some degree synonymous terms with differences in the degree of inflammation. Generally speaking endophthalmitis is an inflammation of the uveal tract in posterior segment of the eye ball, usually endogenous in origin and non-suppurative. Pan ophthalmitis, on the other hand, is a suppurative inflammation of all the inner structures of the eye and is often exogenous.

Exogenous causes are:

1. Perforating injuries with an infected object, e.g., a wooden splinter, iron implements, etc.
2. Perforation of a suppurative corneal ulcer-commonly of pyocyneous or fungal origin.
3. Post-operative infection after intra-ocular surgery when co-existing dacryocystitis has been overlooked or unsterile instruments or solutions are introduced inside the eye. Chances of infection are much greater when vitreous loss occurs during cataract extraction.

Endogenous infection may be initiated by septic emboli carried to the uveal tissue causing exudative choroiditis extending into the vitreous causing endophthalmitis.

Systemic infection may cause metastatic infection of choroid later extending into the vitreous.

Local inflammatory reaction in the choroid and the retina like periphlebitis may also excite vitreous reaction.

Sympathetic ophthalmitis is an aseptic endophthalmitis due to pan-uveitis possibly a result of antigen-antibody reaction.

The clinical picture will depend on the type of inflammatory reaction which may be:

i. Pain in the eye.
ii. Redness of the eye.
iii. Diminution of vision.
iv. Haze in the vitreous.
v. Yellowish or whitish reflex from behind the lens seen with oblique illumination.
vi. Bands and membranes forming in the vitreous and formation of a retrolental membrane giving appearance of pseudo-glioma.
vii. If the condition does not respond to therapy, eye may develop secondary glaucoma or end up as phthisical or atrophic eye.

Suppurative pan ophthalmitis presents a more dramatic picture. The eye becomes a bag of pus within 48 to 72 hours following injury, perforation of an ulcer or operative procedure. There is severe pain, redness of eye, swelling of lids and loss of vision.

The lids are swollen, the conjunctiva is markedly chemosed. The patient has fever. Point of entry of infection is usually infiltrated. In the early stages, there may be hypopyon and in the later stage, the whole vitreous may be full of pus. In severe cases, there is always orbital cellulitis causing some amount of proptosis and optic neuritis. Extension into intracranial cavity along the optic nerve meninges causing meningitis has been mentioned but is extremely rare in this era of antibiotics.

In the terminal stage, the cornea may slough out. These eyes always end up as phthisis bulbi.

Prognosis

In non-suppurative inflammation, it is not always bad. There may be some degree of resolution following effective therapy both systemic and ocular. Some residual effects however persist like vitreous floaters and chorio-retinal scars.

Prognosis of pan-ophthalmitis in most cases is very poor in spite of newer antibiotics and specific therapy being available. The condition is so aggressive that the eye is as good as lost because the results of therapeutic efforts are extremely limited.

Treatment: The best bet lies in identifying the causative organisms by smear examination and culture of the discharge. Appropriate antibiotics should be administered by I.V. infusion or by repeated intramuscular injections. Antibiotics should also be given through the conjunctiva deep into orbit. Antibiotics given directly into the centre of the vitreous have been reported to be helpful in the early stages. Vancomycin 1 mg/0.1 ml and Ceftazidime 2.25 mg/0.1 ml are used intravitreally. If no response is observed in 24-48 hours, vitrectomy has to be undertaken.

If there is no response and if light perception becomes defective, most of these eyes need an evisceration which should not be delayed to save the patient from severe agonising pain.

VITREOUS BANDS AND MEMBRANES

Transparent vitreous gel may be converted into opaque vitreous bands and membranes or sheet of vitreous opacities. The common causes are intraocular diseases associated with inflammation such as pars planitis, iridocyclitis, vitreous haemorrhage, degeneration and penetrating injuries.

The type of bands and membranes may depend on the associated conditions. In long standing vitreous haemorrhage, these will be surrounded by vitreous gel whereas the vitreous will be liquid in degenerative conditions such as myopia and senility. Identification of these membranes will help select the suitable surgical procedure.

Vitreous membranes and bands may arise from different sites, commonest being those which emanate from disc and extend into vitreous in various directions. Vitreous membranes may start from equatorial region and go across the vitreous and may get adherent to the equatorial region of another area. Retrolental membranes usually start from ciliary body or pars plana and give appearance of pseudo glioma. Apart from these three common sites, thin membranes sometimes form in front of the retina appearing as hyaloid condensation of the vitreous and are called pre-retinal membranes. These membranes may be vascularised or non-vascularised.

Vitreous bands like vitreous membranes may involve any part of the vitreous and similarly may arise from optic disc or more commonly pars plana.

The common conditions which give rise to vitreous membranes and bands are:
1. Retrolental fibroplasia.
2. Perforating injuries.
3. Retained intra-ocular foreign bodies.
4. Vitreous loss in cataract extraction.
5. Severe iridocyclitis.
6. Pars planitis.
7. Diabetic retinopathy.
8. Eales' disease.
9. Vitreous haemorrhage.
10. Haemopoitic diseases like sickle cell anaemia.
11. Degenerative diseases like high myopia.
12. Long standing retinal detachment.
13. Coat's disease.
14. Vascularised intra-ocular growths.
15. Phakomatoses.

The treatment of these membranes and bands is called for only when they obstruct vision or when they cause a pull on the retina and cause a tear. Treatment is entirely surgical by vitrectomy which may be open sky vitrectomy in aphakic eyes, anterior or posterior vitrectomy through pars plana depending on location and extent of the bands and membranes. The blood vessels accompanying the membranes and bands can cause severe vitreous haemorrhage during surgery. These blood vessels need to be first coagulated either by laser or by intra-vitreal cryo or diathermy.

POSTERIOR VITREOUS DETACHMENT

The separation of vitreous cortex from the internal limiting membrane of retina is called *vitreous detachment.*

The posterior vitreous detachment is by far the most common condition and is separation of the vitreous cortex from retina anywhere posterior to the vitreous base. It is considered as an ageing process and is common even in normal eyes in older age. The incidence is reported to be higher in eyes with history of posterior uveitis and chorio-retinitis. It also occurs in high myopia and in aphakia. It may be associated with retinal detachment, adult retino-schisis or vitreous haemorrhage.

Posterior vitreous detachment may be complete or incomplete and each of these may be with vitreous collapse or without vitreous collapse.

Complete posterior detachment is separation of the entire posterior cortex from the retina upto the vitreous base. This complete posterior vitreous detachment with collapse of the vitreous body is called *massive vitreous retraction* (MVR) and is of great clinical significance because it adversely influences retinal detachment surgery (Fig. 14.3).

Management

A PVD found asymptomatically on routine examination is benign, but requires monitoring. A patient who presents with a sudden onset PVD without retinal breaks or haemorrhage requires repeat peripheral examination, as the risk of retinal complications is highest following vitreous detachment. If no retinal breaks are seen at that point, routine yearly examination is all that is needed. Prophylactically treat any breaks associated with PVD immediately with photocoagulation or cryoretinopexy.

Symptoms: The symptoms of the posterior vitreous detachment are floaters, *photopsae, metamorphopsia* and blurred vision. Floaters are due to mobile vitreous opacities in front of the retina. The severity and duration depend on location, size and number of floaters and also on the visual acuity of the patient. Photopsae is observed as a spontaneous flash of light by the patient and is of a sudden onset. These flashes of light are most probably due to the traction of the detached vitreous body on the retina at the sites of vitreo-retinal adhesions. It ceases to occur when the vitreous adhesions from the retina are separated or when the retina around the vitreo-retinal adhesion is torn. Metamorphopsia is only an occasional symptom of posterior vitreous detachment and it is due to macular oedema.

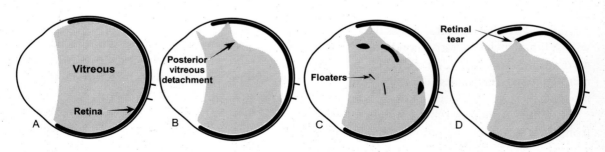

Fig. 14.3: Posterior vitreous detachment. (A) Normal vitreous mass and retina, (B) Posterior vitreous detachment, (C) Posterior vitreous detachment with vitreous floaters and (D) Posterior vitreous detachment with retinal tear

Signs: The signs of posterior vitreous detachment are vitreous opacities, sometimes vitreous haemorrhage and associated retinal changes. The retinal changes include retinal and pre-retinal haemorrhages, macular oedema, and peripheral retinal tears. A complete and accurate diagnosis of the posterior vitreous detachment can be made only after a detailed examination of the vitreous with slit lamp and three mirror contact lens.

Though the posterior vitreous detachment is commonly seen as a part of the ageing process, it is established that more often it is associated with pathological conditions such as retinal detachment, vitreous haemorrhages, macular oedema and retinal tears. It is very important to examine such patients who complain of floaters and flashes of light carefully to rule out this serious condition.

15

Retina

The retina is the principal visuo-sensory layer of the eye and receives light rays refracted by the various refracting *media*. The light reaches the sensory receptors directly (cones and rods) and the stimulus is then transmitted through various neurons to occipital cortex. It is actually the cerebral cortex which sees the object and the retina is only a receptor of visual impulses. It is interesting to note that the images formed on the retina are inverted and the orientation of the objects in the space is interpreted at the occipital cortex.

Developmentally, the retina is essentially a neurogenic layer, except that it has remained outside the skull cavity. The axons of the retinal cells however ultimately reach the brain substance for appreciation and interpretation of the visual stimuli.

The retina is developed from neuro-ecto-dermal layer of secondary optical vesicle. The outer layer of the secondary optic vesicle forms the pigment epithelial layer of the retina while from the inner layer develop the rods and cones and their communicating fibres. It is important to realise this because it is along this embryonic cleavage between the two layers of the secondary optic vesicle that the retinal separation (primary retinal detachment) takes place.

Retina has many functions to perform:

1. It is the seat of image formation. Most of the acuity of vision is in a small one disc diameter area, the macular area, while the remaining large part of the retinal surface is principally responsible for visual field all around.
2. The human retina is especially developed both for day vision and night vision.
3. Colour vision is a function of cones and is therefore best at the macula where population of cones is densest.

Anatomically, retina forms the innermost lining of eye. It is supported by vitreous mass on its inner surface.

The retina extends from the disc margin behind to the ora serrata in front. The ora is 6 mm on nasal side and 7 mm from limbus on temporal side.

The layers of the retina from without inwards are (Fig. 15.1).

1. Pigment epithelium.
2. Layer of rods and cones.
3. External limiting membrane.

4. Outer nuclear layer.
5. Outer plexiform layer.
6. Inner nuclear layer.
7. Inner plexiform layer.
8. Ganglion cell layer.
9. Nerve fibre layer.
10. Internal limiting membrane.

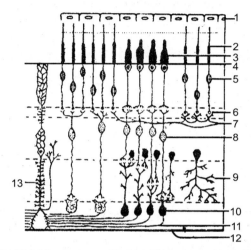

Fig 15.1: Micro-antomy of Retina. (1) Pigment epithelial layer; (2) and (3) Layer of rods and cones; (4) Outer limiting membrane; (5) Outer nuclear layer; (6) Outer plexiform layer; (7) Amacrine cells; (8) Inner nuclear layer—bipolar cells; (9) Inner plexiform layer; (10) Ganglion cell layer; (11) Nerve fibre layer; (12) Inner limiting membrane; (13) Mullers fibres.

Pigment epithelium layer is mainly responsible for absorption of light after it has passed through the transparent anterior layers of the retina. It is through the pigment epithelium layer that the chorio-capillaries supply nutrition to the outer cellular layers of the retina.

Rods and cones form the outermost layer of sensory retina and they are the *first neuron of the visual pathways.* Their nuclei form the outer nuclear layer. Cones are responsible for colour vision and day vision (*photopic vision*) and rods are responsible for night vision (*scotopic vision*). Cones are largely concentrated in the posterior part of the retina. They are heavily concentrated in the macular area. They have a pigment called

rhodopsin (visual purple). The axons of the rods and cones are directed inwards and they relay with the next layer, the bipolar cells, the amacrine cells and the horizontal cells to form the outer plexiform layer. The nuclei of bipolar cells form the inner nuclear layer and their axons form the inner plexiform layer, *the second neuron,* to relay with the next layer, the ganglion cell layer. Ganglion cells form the innermost layer of the cells. These cells have long axons which form the nerve fibre layer of the retina ending into the lateral geniculate body and form the *third neuron of the visual pathways.*

The cells of the retina are held together by Mullers fibres while the nerve fibre layer is held together by glial cells like astrocytes, oligo-dendrocytes and microglia.

The retina is separated from choroid by Bruchs membrane. Internal limiting membrane separates the retina from vitreous.

The arrangement of nerve fibres at the posterior pole has special significance in relation to field defects. The fibres from the macular area with the largest number of cones directly reach the central 1/3 of the, temporal *sector* of disc and form the *papillo-macular bundle.* The nerve fibres of the retina temporal to the macula are demarcated into upper and lower fibres by a horizontal raphe. Those from above the raphe reach upper and outer disc margin and those from below the raphe reach lower temporal disc margin. This peculiar arrangement of fibres is responsible for the arcuate type of scotoma and Ronne's nasal step in field defect.

The macular area is avascular and concave about the size of the disc diameter. The central part is called the *fovea centralis* which is situated two disc diameter temporal to the disc. The retina is thinnest in this part. The fovea contains only the cone layer of retina. The nuclei of foveal cones are heaped at the margin of macula, there-fore the concavity of macular area light rays directly reach the cones and hence the acute sensitivity and visual importance of the foveal area.

The blood supply of the retina upto the outer plexiform layer is from the central retinal artery and the outer layer of rods and cones get its nutrition from the chorio-capillaries.

DISEASES OF THE RETINA

Retinal Haemorrhages

Retinal haemorrhages are a clinical finding which is important from both diagnostic and treatment point of view. Diagnostic, because there are many conditions which cause retinal haemorrhages with peculiar clinical features of different etiologies and from the treatment point of view because they cause visual disturbances.

Retinal blood vessels are situated in the nerve fibre layer of the retina and their arteriolar branches reach upto the outer plexifrom layer. Retinal haemorrhages may therefore be either intra-retinal or pre-retinal. The pre-retinal haemorrhage may remain limited between the internal limiting membrane and the vitreous or it may break through into the vitreous and become a diffuse vitreous haemorrhage.

Pre-retinal haemorrhages also called sub-hyaloid haemorrhages are usually large in size and acquire a shape with a horizontal upper level and a convex lower level. The colour is darker in the lower part and lighter in the upper because the RBCs gravitate to the lower part. The haemorrhage can shift its position by change in the posture.

Intra-retinal haemorrhages are small in size and of varying shapes. The haemorrhages in the nerve fibre layer appear flame shaped, while the deeper intra-retinal haemorrhages may be of any shape from a small dot to a large blotch.

The symptoms of retinal haemorrhage will depend on the area of the retina involved and the size of the haemorrhage. They may cause no visual symptoms till the macula is involved. They may sometimes cause erythropsia in a large-sized haemorrhage. Visual symptoms, however, become predominant once the haemorrhage breaks into the vitreous.

The fate of retinal haemorrhage depends upon its size and location. Pre-retinal haemorrhages, even if they are large, may completely disappear without leaving any after effects. Intra-retinal haemorrhages may, however, organise and leave behind scarred pigmented areas.

Causes of Retinal Haemorrhages

1. *Traumatic:* Due to direct or indirect trauma. Retinal vessels being unsupported by any firm tissue, tend to bleed due to contusions and lacerations.
2. *Obstruction in* conditions like:
   a. Thrombosis of the central retinal vein.
   b. Papilloedema.
   c. Embolism of central retinal artery.
3. *Inflammatory.* The most important conditions are periphlebitis, Eales' disease and Papillitis.
4. *Vascular retinopathies* like diabetic retinopathy, hypertensive retinopathy, arteriosclerotic retinopathy, renal retinopathy, sickle-cell retinopathy.
5. *Blood dyscrasias* like severe anaemia, leukaemia, thrombo-cytopenic purpura and haemophilia.
6. *Vascular malformations* like telangiectasis and Von-Hippel Lindau's Disease.
7. As an extension of sub-arachnoid haemorrhage.

Retinal Vasculitis

Retinal vasculitis is seen in a number of conditions such as sarcoidosis, Behcet's and Eales' disease. The last is the commonest and the most important.

Eales' Disease: Recurrent Intra-ocular Haemorrhage

Eales' disease has been a clinical entity ever since

it was first described in 1882. Initially it was defined as recurrent vitreous haemorrhage. It now denotes cases of retinal phlebitis of indefinite etiology. The disease is distinctly common in developing countries. To start with, it clinically manifests in one eye but in majority of cases, other eye has evidence of pathology without symptoms or develops haemorrhages at a later date. It is a disease, by and large, of young age.

Aetiology: The precise cause of this condition has not been established. The most commonly agreed factor is that it is caused by a tubercular hyper-sensitivity reaction. It is a tissue response to a specific antigen like the tubercular proteins circulating in blood. There is usually no evidence of active tuberculosis but there may be findings which may indicate previous infection like calcified glands, strongly positive mantoux reaction and high ESR. Other causes attributed to this disease may be a septic focus in the body, intestinal parasitic infection, etc.

Pathology: The basic pathological change is periphlebitis in one of the retinal veins. This may lead to damage of the capillary endothelium and blockage of vein resulting in retinal and/or vitreous haemorrhage. This occlusive phenomenon is followed by neovascularisation and later on formation of fibrous bands either along the retina or projecting into the vitreous. Following repeated haemorrhages, there is formation of fibrous bands which on contraction, tend to drag the vessels out of their normal course or into the vitreous producing retinal tears and ultimately retinal detachment.

Clinical features: Clinically, there are two groups of cases:
a. Peripheral
b. Central (Fig. 15.2, Plate 9)

Peripheral retinal peri-vasculitis is usually unilateral to start with. Depending on the degree of vitreous haemorrhage the vision may be mode-rately or severely reduced. There may be history of recurrent such episodes either clearing up spontaneously or leaving behind some after effects.

Examination may reveal evidence of peri-vasculitis with haemorrhages and sheathing along the veins. If haemorrhage has extended into the vitreous, fundus glow may be dull or absent depending on grade haemorrhage. In central vitreous haemorrhage peripheral fundus may be visible through a fully dilated pupil, although details may not be clearly evident.

Small vitreous haemorrhages tend to get partly or completely absorbed. Large haemorr-hages however lead to persisting visual loss and fundus changes due to organisation. Long standing case may show vitreous floaters, fibrous bands with neovascularisation in the vitreous or along retina and sometimes retinal detachment. More important is the examination of opposite eye when evidence of perivasculitis may be discovered in the form of sheathing of veins.

Central Eales' disease is usually unilateral and much less common. The main retinal vein trunk is affected. The optic disc is swollen and the veins engorged and tortuous, with multiple haemorrhages scattered over entire retina.

Every case of Eales' disease must primarily be investigated for tubercular diathesis, a chest X-ray for calcified glands and heavy hilar shadows and the Mantoux test for tuberculin hypersensitivity. Haematological investigations like ESR, total and differential WBC counts may support this possible etiological factor. Repeated stool examination in tropical countries is an important investigation. Serological tests for syphilis should also be done. A fluorescein angio-graphy will help in detecting sites of early periphlebitis and neo-vascularisation.

The prognosis of this disease is unfavourable although few patients may return to normal vision. Most patients get attacks of haemorrhages and each haemorrhage leaves behind additional vitreous floaters and changes in the retina. Some patients who get severe repeated attacks in both eyes, end up being totally blind if not timely and adequately treated. Newer therapies which can prevent recurrence and which can handle vitreous clots and vitreous fibrovascular reactions have brought hope to many patients of Eales' disease.

Complications: The most serious complications are *neovascularization, fibroblastic proliferation* and *retinal detachment*. Fibrous bands may grow into the vitreous and carry blood vessels along with them. Traction by these bands causes a pull on the retina, retinal tears and detachment. Unlike central venous thrombosis, Eales' disease does not usually cause secondary glaucoma except the uncommon central type.

Treatment: The patient should be put to at least one week's bed rest with the head end of the bed raised 45° so that the vitreous haemorrhage settles down in lower part by gravity. This is the most important line of treatment for quick absorption of the haemorrhage. This will also help in early detection of the area of periphlebitis from where the haemorrhage comes so that it can be locally treated. If haemorrhage does not show signs of absorption, pre-equatorial cryo therapy or intra-scleral diathermy may help absorption.

Systemic steroids are indicated when there is active periphlebitis and retinal oedema.

Iodine by injection and iodides administered orally are useful and help absorption of haemorrhages to limited extent. Supportive therapy with vitamin C and vitamin K may also be helpful.

The organised vitreous floaters which do not respond to any therapy and persist, can be treated by vitrectomy. This has brought vision to many young patients who were otherwise nearly blind.

Photocoagulation has also brought hope to many patients with Eales' disease. All patches of neovascularisation should be photocoagulated which is the best therapy to prevent recurrence of haemorrhage. Fluorescein angiography will help in identifying the points of leakage and therefore help in accurate photocoagulation. In patients blinded by fibrous proliferation and retinal detachment, more heroic surgery may restore some amount of vision.

Systemic treatment is important to help prevent newer foci of periphlebitis. Though empirical, anti-tuberculous therapy in established cases of Eales' disease should always be given for at least three months in recurrent cases.

Neovascularization and Vascular Sheathing

Normal retinal arteries are end arteries and do not anastomose with each other. Any anastomotic communications are therefore abnormal. Neovascularisation has characteristic ophthalmoscopic appearance. These are superficial vessels that are markedly tortuous with a cork-screw like appearance. They anastomose with each other and are usually present in bunches.

Neovascularization is caused either due to blockage in circulation e.g. retinal vein thrombosis or due to anoxaemia as in diabetic retinopathy. Important causes of neovascularization in retina are:

1. Diabetic retinopathy.
2. Thrombosis of the central retinal vein.
3. Periphlebitis as in Eales' disease.
4. Angio-matosis retinae.
5. On the surface of a retinal tumour like melanoma or sarcoma.

Being newly formed from endothelial cell proliferation, these are fragile blood vessels and are likely to cause retinal or vitreous haemorrhages. They are amenable to photocoagulation, cryo-coagulation and diathermisation. These treatments are now possible and should be carefully planned and executed. Neovascularization posterior to the equator is best treated by photocoagulation while the same in anterior retina, by surface cryo or diathermy coagulation because the latter cannot be easily reached for photocoagulation. For neovascularization near the macular area, laser coagulation should be preferred.

Sheathing of Vessels

There are three common sites where sheathing of retinal blood vessels is seen:
1. Disc margin.
2. Arterio-venous crossings.
3. Along course of blood vessels.

Sheathing along large blood vessels on or near the disc is usually glial in nature and does not affect the blood flow in the vessels. Sheathing at arterio-venous crossings is an important entity and is most frequently seen in arterio-sclerosis. Sheathing in arterial sclerosis becomes clinically prominent at the crossings because here the artery and the vein have a common sheath. Sheathing of arterio-sclerosis may also extend along the sclerotic arteries. It causes narrowing of the lumen of blood vessel and impedes circulation. Sheathing along the veins, particularly when it is localised in nature, is due to periphlebitis, which may lead to venous obstruction.

Retinal perivascular sheathing in a pathological sense is due to changes in the advantitial layer of the retinal arteries. The result is increased optical density of the arterial wall which causes exaggeration of the arterial reflex. The pathology of anterio-sclerosis causes irregularity in the arterial lumen.

Clinically, neuroglial sheathing of congenital origin extends only a short distance beyond the disc margin and the blood vessels are otherwise normal.

In arterial sclerotic sheathing, one should look for evidence at the arterio-venous crossings and along the arterial walls. In the early stages, the arteries look optically less transparent and the arterial reflex appears exaggerated. Sheathing in this stage is seen as a greyish white line along the sides of blood vessels (*parallel sheathing*). The blood column is completely obscured and the blood vessel appears white cord like a *silver wire* in advanced sheathing (Fig. 15.3, Plate 9).

Retinal Aneurysms

Micro aneurysmal dilatation of the retinal vessels is not an uncommon condition. Originally they were labelled as punctate haemorrhages. Digestive studies of the retina established the existence of capillary microaneurysms. Later, fluorescein angiography established their clinical entity. These microaneurysms affect capillaries and are therefore situated in the retinal layers deeper to the ganglionic cell layer. The conditions where micro-aneurysms of the retina can be seen are:
1. Diabetic retinopathy.
2. Hypertensive retinopathy.
3. Sickle cell disease.
4. Eales' disease.
5. Arterio-sclerosis.

Diabetic retinopathy is the most important cause because it is one of the earliest clinical manifestations of the diabetic effect on the retina. Quite often diabetes is first suspected by the ophthalmologist when he sees a few micro-aneurysms during routine ophthalmoscopy.

Ophthalmoscopically, they appear as red dots with a clear-cut margin and of a size of a pin head. They are frequently seen around the posterior pole of the eye. Depending on the duration of diabetes, only a few may be seen or they may be numerous associated with blotchy retinal haemorrhages. Fluorescein angiography shows these microaneurysms as bunches or clusters in relation to capillaries although only a few are seen ophthalmoscopically.

Retinal Exudates

Exudative reaction of the retina is a common manifestation of many retinal pathologies, traumatic, inflammatory, vascular, degenerative and even neoplastic.

The clinical appearance of exudates depends not only on the chemical composition but also the site of the retina where they collect. The exudates which are dull white in colour and woolly in character, are called soft exudates and are usually in superficial layers of retina. Shining white exudates are hard exudates and located in the deeper layers of the retina.

Soft exudates are characteristically seen in:
1. Hypertensive retinopathy.
2. Renal retinopathy.
3. Pregnancy toxemia.
4. Severe anaemia.
5. Papilloedema.

Hard exudates are typically seen in:
1. Diabetic retinopathy.
2. Arterio-sclerotic retinopathy.
3. Circinate retinopathy.
4. Coats' disease.

Coats Disease: (Exudative Retinopathy)

A non-specific clinical entity was first described by Coats in 1908. The disease was first described as *'external haemorrhagic retinitis of Coats and later' external exudative retinitis of Coats;* also called chorio-retinitis of Leber.

The cause of the condition is unknown. Probably there is a congenital basis in the form of a congenital malformation of blood vessels. Syphilis and tuberculosis have been attributed to the etiology. The condition described by Coats was unilateral for reasons yet unknown and it mostly affected healthy males.

The clinical picture as described by Coats is easily identifiable. There are large patches of yellowish white exudates lying deep to the retinal vessels. It may give the appearance of a pseudo-glioma. There may be shining dots in and around the exudative areas which are crystalline deposits. Haemorrhages are frequently present. The condition is very slowly progressive and may be complicated by exudative retinal detachment. These eyes may sometimes develop iridocyclitis, secondary glaucoma and complicated cataract.

The differential diagnosis is from other causes of retinal exudates but an important differentiation is from retinoblastoma if the patient is young. Ultrasonography may help differentiation between these two conditions. Fluorescein angiography may show dilated capillaries and may also show aneurysmal dilatations. Leakage of dye may indicate the involved capillary bed (Fig. 15.4, Plate 9).

Retinal Vascular Anomalies: Retinal Telangiectasis (Coats' Disease)

Coats disease is now considered a more complex syndrome, comprising not only the entity described above but also including vascular pathologies like retinal telangiectasis and even Von-Hippel Lindau's disease because in both these conditions massive retinal exudates are an important clinical feature. Both these conditions are also non-specific in nature possibly associated with developmental vascular anomalies.

The basic lesion in any of the vascular abnormalities is a loss of integrity of the vascular endothelium leading to abnormal permeability. More advanced cases show total secondary retinal detachment. The vitreous remains clear and dilated aneurysmal vessels can be seen ophthalmoscopically. The end result is usually a blind eye with secondary glaucoma.

The importance of ultrasonography and fluorescein angiography in these conditions has *already* been emphasized. Fluorescein angiography in Coats' disease shows abnormally coarse dilated capillaries, aneurysmal dilatations (micro and macro) and a leakage of dye from the involved capillary bed.

Treatment: Is unsatisfactory and is directed to the particular clinical condition responsible for exudative retinopathy. Photocoagulation of the affected vessels revealed by fluorescein angiography, may prevent progression of the disease and reduce chances of complications like retinal detachment. Nonspecific therapy with steroids and iodine may be helpful.

Angiomatosis Retinae (Von-Hippel-Lindau Disease)

The basic lesion is development of capillary angiomata within the retina. The tumours are derived from the capillary endothelium with proliferating endothelial cells and a feeding artery and draining veins. The condition may be hereditary or sporadic in form.

The earliest recognizable lesion is about the size of a diabetic microaneurysm and as time passes, these lesions enlarge through a process of abnormal hemodynamics, hypertrophy and hyperplasia. A fully developed lesion is formed with a spherical shape and orange-red colour, fed by a dilated tortuous retinal artery and drained by an engorged vein. Single or multiple angiomata may be seen in the same eye and in more than 50% of cases, the condition is bilateral. Whatever the situation of the lesion, abnormal permeability produces changes like exudates, retinal oedema, serous detachment of the retina and intra-retinal deposits of cholesterol. Occasionally, bleeding from angioma results in vitreous haemorrhage.

Retinal angiomatosis may be manifestation of a disease complex and may be associated with angiomatosis elsewhere in the viscera or brain. When associated with central nervous system and visceral angiomatosis, the term Von-Hippel Lindau disease is used.

Treatment: Cryo therapy is ideal. Small angiomata may need only a single sitting, whereas large ones require multiple sittings. Successful treatment is characterised by shrinkage of the mass, disappearance of subretinal fluid and attenuation of the dilated afferent and efferent vessels. Photocoagulation is indicated where cryo-therapy cannot be reached.

Periodic follow up is indicated to watch for recurrence and development of new lesions.

Vascular Occlusive Disorders:

Central Retinal Artery Occlusion

Aetiology: Retinal arterial occlusion is usually found in the elderly, but young individuals can also be affected. The most common cause of central retinal arterial occlusion is embolism of the retinal vascular tree. The emboli may be fatty material from atheromata, calcium deposits from diseased heart valves, fibrin, lipid and platelet thrombi. Bacterial, tumour, parasitic, fungal and exogenous material may also be responsible. The thrombotic causes include athero-sclerosis, syphilitic endarteritis and temporal giant cell arteritis.

The occlusion may be thrombotic in nature or an embolic phenomenon, the former being a slower pathology and latter an emergency. Arterial spasm is an important phenomenon which may be the precursor of occlusion. The common causes of angiospasm are:
1. Systemic hypertension.
2. Migraine.

Females are slightly more prone than males and central retinal artery occlusion is more common than branch occlusions. Bilateral affections are noticed in 2-4% of patients specially when it is secondary to cranial arteritis or carotid artery stenosis. In branch arterial occlusion, the superior temporal branch is most frequently affected.

Clinical features: The typical history of central arterial occlusion is a sudden painless visual loss.

In central retinal arterial occlusion with eyes having a cilio-retinal artery, some degree of corresponding central field of vision is retained. The pupils are sluggish or fixed to direct light reflex but react consensually.

The fundus picture is one of infarction of the inner 2/3 of the retinal thickness. Shortly after the occlusion, the retina appears hazy and takes on a milky colour due to oedema and ischaemic necrosis within a few hours. The arterioles are thinned out and thread like and the most characteristic feature is the cherry red spot in the fovea. This phenomenon is due to the contrast between fovea which is nourished by the underlying choroid and the surrounding markedly oedematous pale area supplied by retinal circulation. In branch retinal arterial occlusion, the infarcted area appears white and can be sharply demarcated from remaining normal retina (Fig. 15.5, Plate 9).

The blood flow through these attenuated vessels is very slow and may show broken column of blood. In sudden occlusion, there may even be reversal of arterial flow in a segment where the red cells move to and fro.

Pathology: The retinal cells undergo necrosis and disintegrate. Gradually the necrotic tissue is resorbed and is replaced by transparent glial tissue.

Arterio-arteriolar shunts develop in branch occlusions and are seen by fluorescein angiography. Though they develop too late to protect retina, they signify presence of an old occlusion and are therefore useful in diagnosis. The disc may go on to total optic atrophy in a central retinal arterial occlusion and sectoral atrophy in a branch occlusion.

Treatment: Treatment is usually unsatisfactory. There is a definite distinction between thrombotic and embolic occlusion in that the former are rarely treatable and their visual outcome is guarded. However, embolic occlusions may be overcome partially using a variety of modalities if promptly treated. Most methods utilise measures to relieve arterial spasm, dilate retinal arteries and decrease intraocular pressure. The first step is a digital massage which lowers intraocular tension. The patient may also be asked to breathe 95% oxygen and 5%, carbon di-oxide which will help to dilate the retinal arteries. Retrobulbar injections of acetylcholine and priscol which dilate retinal arteries, should be given immediately and repeated twice a day. Paracentesis of the anterior chamber or intravenous acetazolamide may be adopted to bring about a rapid reduction in intra-ocular pressure. Improvement can be determined by visual acuity, visual field testing and ophthalmoscopic examination. All this is possible only if the patient is seen immediately otherwise it becomes irreversible and visual loss is permanent particularly in central arterial trunk occlusion.

Central Retinal Vein Thrombosis

Central retinal vein obstruction is a disease of older age group. Men are more frequently affected and it has been noted that the left eye is more commonly affected than the right eye.

Acute obstruction of the central retinal vein is one of the most dramatic pictures in ophthalmology presenting a stormy appearance.

Systemic hypertension is commonly observed in patients with central or branch vein occlusion. It has also been noted to occur in eyes with chronic open angle glaucoma. The other aetiological factors are arterio-sclerotic compression of the vein, inflammation of the vein, periphlebitis or endo-phlebitis of unknown cause. It may occur secondary to orbital cellulitis, sickle cell disease, diabetes, syphilis, tuberculosis and malignant disease. Clinically it may present in one of the three forms.

A. **Impending central retinal vein occlusion.**
It is usually seen as a compression at the

arterio-venous crossing, peripheral venous dilation, occasional intra-retinal haemorrhage and cotton wool spots. Initially the visual acuity is not affected. It can develop into a full fledged central retinal vein occlusion over a period of days or months.

B. **Branch vein occlusion.** The major sites of occlusion are:

1. At the edge of the optic disc.
2. At the arterio-venous crossings.

   The patient frequently experiences a field defect but central vision is maintained. The central vision when affected is due to macular oedema or haemorrhage seeping into the macular area. The fundus picture consists of splashes of intra-retinal haemorrhages along the course of in-volved vessels and extending to periphery of the retina drained by the occluded vein. Sub-hyaloid and vitreous haemorrhage can also occur.

   The natural history of a branch retinal vein occlusion ranges from complete recovery to a progressive situation with permanent visual loss. Poor visual acuity in the branch retinal vein occlusion is due to macular involvement and pre-retinal neovascularisation.

3. *Central retinal vein occlusion.* The pic-ture is more dramatic, with enlarged tortuous veins, extensive superficial and deep haemorrhages all over fundus and numerous cotton wool spots. Often the optic disc margins are not seen clearly due to oedema and overlying haemor-rhages.

Neovascularisation of the iris (rubeosis) is the compensatory phenomenon with development of venous channels because the blood flow in the central retinal vein is obstructed. The newly formed blood vessels may grow into the angle of anterior chamber causing thrombotic glaucoma in due course of times. This has been already described (Fig. 15.6A to 15.6C, Plate 10)

In addition to the characteristic compensatory new blood vessels, on the iris, there may be frank heamorrhage on the iris surface. Hyphaema may appear in the anterior chamber.

Prognosis: The prognosis is bad in central vein thrombosis. It is extremely poor in those cases who develop thrombotic glaucoma.

Treatment: If the patient comes very early, anti-coagulants may help in preventing the extension of the thrombus. Therapy should be started with heparin 5000 units I/V every 4 hours and after 48 hours may be replaced by oral therapy of dicoumerol 0.5 mg tablets, 6 tablets on first day and the dose gradually reduced in 5 to 6 days. During this therapy, coagulation time should be checked up. The prothrombin level should also not increase more than 25-30%. Anticoagulants in central vein thrombosis will help lessen chances of thrombotic glaucoma. In addition, aspirin and persantin, if given by mouth, will retard platelet aggregation and therefore prevent extension of the thrombus.

Steroids in full doses for a short period may help in reducing the periphlebitis factor. They should, however, not be continued for long. Intravitreal steroid and VEGF drug like A vastin have been in use in recent years.

In central retinal vein thrombosis, the most important consideration is periodical check-up of intra-ocular tension. Miotic therapy with pilo-carpine should be maintained for at least three months. If neovascularization has been noted or there is macular oedema, pan retinal photo-coagulation may save some residual vision in the eye.

Once thrombotic glaucoma has developed, the ocular condition is desperate. Fistulising operations are dangerous because of neo-vascularization of iris and angle and may cause intractable hyphaema. The safe procedure is cyclocryopexy. If this does not control tension, partial penetrating intra-scleral cyclodiathermy may be helpful. It should be done in one or two quadrants to begin with depending on the severity of intra-ocular tension rise.

In severely painful and blind eyes caused by thrombotic glaucoma, enucleation may be the only way to relieve agony of the patient.

VASCULAR RETINOPATHIES

The basic mechanism in any vascular retinopathy is abnormal vascular permeability and retinal ischaemia. The latter results in acute intracellular oedema, neovascularization, vitreous haemorrhage, fibrosis and traction retinal detachment.

There are a number of systemic diseases which can cause vascular retinopathy and these are:

1. Diabetic retinopathy.
2. Hypertensive retinopathy.
3. Renal retinopathy.
4. Arterio-sclerotic retinopathy.
5. Toxaemic retinopathy of pregnancy.
6. Sickle cell retinopathy.
7. Retinopathy of prematurity (Retro-lateral fibroplasia).

Diabetic retinopathy: This is a leading cause of blindness in old age. In the European countries and in North America, approximately 1.5% of the population is affected with this systemic disease and diabetic retinopathy.

Diabetic population in the world estimated in 2003 was 194 millions while projected figure by 2025 is 333 millions, an increase of 62 per cent. In south-east Asia, the increase is expected to be from 43 millions to 75.8 millions.

In India, estimated increase is expected from 19 millions in 1995 to 57 millions in 2025. Studies in the last decade indicate that 23 to 36 per cent of all diabetics, irrespective of duration of the disease will develop retinopathy with its associated micro-vascular complications leading to visual impairment.

Three important facts about diabetic retinopathy are that:

1. It is definitely related to the duration of the disease.
2. The relationship of control of diabetes to the incidence and severity of retinopathy is unsettled but it is generally believed that good control at least delays onset of retinopathy.
3. Once retinal complications occur, there is little hope of altering its course through control of diabetes.

Diabetic retinopathy is classified into two major groups:

1. *Simple background retinopathy* which comprises micro-aneurysms, haemorrhages, hard exudates; all three of which are predominantly present in posterior fundus. Another important accompanying factor of background retinopathy is macular oedema which is a major cause of reduced visual acuity. It results due to leakage from micro-aneurysms and shunt vessels and is seen ophthalmoscopically as hard lipid exudates or cystoid maculopathy.
2. *Proliferative retinopathy.* When sufficient time has elapsed, about 5 to 10 years or more, the changes noted in the background type are no longer limited to intraretinal space but lead to proliferative changes. This occurs in 5% of patients with diabetic retinopathy, more commonly in juvenile diabetes. The earliest vascular change is reduction of the intra mural pericytes thereby weakening the vessel wall. This results in localised dilatation of lumen of vessels which develops into micro-aneurysms. Due to an alteration in tissue metabolism, there is hypoxia and new blood vessels develop.

Ischaemia which renders retina anaemic further elaborates vaso-proliferative factor which also stimulates neovascularization. This is followed by fibro-blastic repair and fibrovascular proliferation leading to traction retinal detachment.

Ophthalmoscopic appearance: In simple background diabetic retinopathy, changes are by and large limited to the posterior fundus. The first finding that draws attention to diabetes as the cause of retinopathy is a pale disc. The next commonest finding is microaneurysms which appear as sharp pin head size red dots seen mostly around the disc and macula. These two may often be the only observations and it is not unusual that these ophthalmic findings may be the first which might lead to diagnosis of diabetes that may have remained undiagnosed.

The arteries are sclerotic and rather tortuous. The veins are distinctly engorged. There may be changes at the arterio-venous crossings.

Haemorrhages in diabetic retinopathy may be of different shapes, sizes and location. They are usually located in the deeper layers of retina and are therefore irregular in shape. These haemorrhages may be scattered all over the posterior fundus. Sometimes one may find sub-hyaloid haemorrhages. The exudates are typically shining hard exudates because of their cholesterol constituent. The exudates may again be of varying sizes and shapes but are mainly located in and around the macular area. When hypertensive retinopathy is associated with diabetic retinopathy, one may also find soft exudates (Fig. 15.7, Plate 10).

Macular oedema is the most important cause of visual failure in diabetic retinopathy. It may not always be clinically evident and a fluorescein angiography may reveal its presence.

Proliferative diabetic retinopathy. Neovascularisation is the earliest proliferative change. It is usually seen on and around the disc. The newly formed capillaries have a peculiar cork-

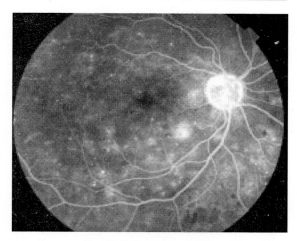

Fig. 15.8: Fl. angiogram DR

screw shape and their anastomosis with each other can be easily seen in contrast to the fact that the normal retinal vessels do not anastomose.

Fibroblastic proliferation is a serious stage of diabetic retinopathy. The fibrous bands may grow along the surface of the retina or project into the vitreous. Newly formed blood vessels usually accompany these fibrous bands, it is important to emphasise that bands of proliferative diabetic retinopathy are mostly attached to or around the disc and always carry new blood vessels with them. In advanced stage this fibrous proliferation with neovascularisation may be so extensive that details of posterior fundus are not visible. They may also be associated with vitreous haemorrhage with fundus glow obscured. Proliferative retinopathy may also be associated with retinal tears and retinal detachment (Fig. 15.9, Plate 11).

Fluorescein angiography is an essential adjunct to diagnosis particularly from therapeutic point of view. It helps to demonstrate anoxic areas, venous changes, intra-retinal vascular abnormalities and areas of neovascularisation which are difficult to detect by ophthalmoscopy.

Treatment: The goal of treatment is to delay onset of diabetic retinopathy or to retard its progress, once it has occurred. The former is obtained by diet, insulin and antidiabetic drugs.

However uncertain the relationship between treatment of diabetes and diabetic retinopathy, it is important even from the visual point of view that diabetes·is wall controlled.

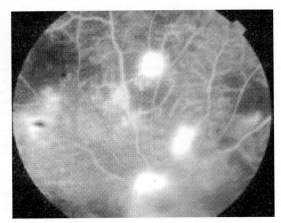

Fig. 15.10: Fluorescein angiogram. Proliferative diabetic retinopathy showing new vessels on the disc

There are no specific drugs which can prevent or treat diabetic retinopathy. There are reports that calcium dobesilate (Doxium or Daxium) given orally, one tablet three times a day for at least 4 months may help in preventing the deterioration of retinopathy, the exact nature of effect is however questionable, anti-oxidants are also given.

Recently, in vitro studies have demonstrated that *Curucumin* isolated from the rhizone of curcuma species (Zingiferaceae Turmeric) has potent antioxidant, anti-inflammatory and anti-proliferative activities in a number of cell types including endothelial cells. The study has also demonstrated in vitro that human retinal endothelial cells proliferation of high glucose pre-treated, is inhibited.

Photocoagulation however is the sheet anchor in the treatment of the diabetic retinopathy which has given many sighted years to people who would have been blind much earlier. Pan retinal photocoagulation and laser coagulation are important modes of treatment.

Vitrectomy is useful in those eyes with long standing vitreous haemorrhage and traction retinal detachments due to diabetes. Ablation of the anterior pituitary by surgery or irradiation is worth the trial in advanced cases of proliferative retinopathy.

In proliferative retinopathy with macular oedema, intravitreal Avastin has been tried. Intra-vitreal Triamcelone also has been used.

Hypertensive retinopathy: The changes due to hypertensive retinopathy are essentially secondary to local ischaemia. Hypertensive retinopathy is classified into four grades using the Keith-Wagner-Barker classification.

Group I. *Consists of only slight narrowing or sclerosis of the arterioles,* producing a focal constriction and a brightened arteriolar reflex. This picture is seen in essential hypertension with adequate cardiac and renal function.

Group II. The arteriolar constriction is more pronounced with *arterio-venous* crossing changes and partial concealment of the venous column. Hard shining lipid deposits and haemorrhages may also appear in this stage. These patients have a continuously higher blood pressure.

Group III. These include patients with *haemorrhages, cotton-wool spots and retinal oedema.* The retinal haemorrhages are flame shaped, and are located in the nerve fibre layer. Cotton-wool spots or soft exudates, represent focal areas of retinal infarction and are seen as grey white patches. These cotton-wool spots mark the accelerated phase of hypertension.

Group IV. *Consists of all the features of the above groups along with papilloedema.* Long standing uncontrolled hypertension often results in the production of macular stars. Large round soft exudates are indicative of adverse prognosis and hence the term *malignant hypertension.* It is often associated with systemic disturbances and progresses rapidly.

Pathology

Main features of hypertensive retinopathy are due to vascular changes. Contributing factors in pathogenesis of retinopathy either due to *Essential* or *Arterio-sclerotic* hypertension are:

1. Vasoconstriction-attenuation of arteries.
2. Arterio-sclerotic-atherosclerotic changes:
   a. A-V crossing changes
   b. Copper wire and silver wire arterial reflex.
3. Flame shaped haemorrhages acquire the shape because they are in nerve fibre layer of retina. Round and/or irregular shaped haemorrhage in arterio-sclerotic retinopathy are in nuclear layer.
4. Soft cotton-wool patches also called soft exudates are due to retinal necrosis caused by areas of infarcts. Hard exudates are lipid and cholesterol deposits in arterio-sclerosis.

Clinical examination of patients with systemic hypertension should first be directed to the blood vessels and arterio-venous crossings. Attenuation of arteries is an important and early observation in essential hypertension. Arteries divide at a more acute angle. The arterial narrowing in early stages is due to spasm and in later stages due to organic changes in the vessel wall.

Arterio-venous crossings should be carefully observed. The changes at these crossings include obscuration of veins under the artery and dilatation of the vein distal to the crossing due to compression of vein.

Patients of hypertension who complain of transient loss of vision and short blackouts have spasms of the cerebral arteries which manifest themselves in retinal arteries also.

Fluorescein angiographic findings of hypertensive retinopathy: In benign hypertension, there is little or no evidence of microvascular abnormalities other than generalized narrowing of the arterioles and capillary bed. In more advanced cases when blood flow is sufficiently reduced, infractions occur which produce patches of capillary non-perfusion.

Prognosis: Serious impairment of vision does not usually occur as a direct result of hypertensive changes in the retina unless there is a local arterial or venous occlusion. Malignant hypertension patients usually die before they become blind unlike patients of proliferative diabetic retinopathy who become blind before they die. The Keith-Wagner-Barker classification is a useful guide in assessing the hypertensive status of the patient and likelihood of damage to the other organs like the heart, kidney and brain. The treatment is mainly directed to control of blood pressure and improvement of renal function if subnormal. No ocular therapy is indicated.

Renal retinopathy. The term 'albuminuric retinitis' was used to describe retinal changes associated with renal diseases. However, it is now known that retinal changes do not correlate with the degree of albuminuria and that they are related to changes or contractions of arterioles rather than to changes within the kidneys.

An important feature of renal retinopathy is neuro-retinal oedema. The disc margin is blurred and the posterior fundus shows a greyish discolouration. There may be a partial macular star. The arteries are spastic in nature and therefore markedly attenuated.

Once acute nephritis has passed on to the stage of chronic glomerulo-nephritis, the renal retinopathic changes become less pronounced and hypertensive retinopathic changes become manifest.

Toxaemia of pregnancy: This is a condition where renal failure and hypertension provide a combined fundus picture. In this condition, retinal vascular changes correspond to severity of the rise in blood pressure. Pre-eclampsia is characterised by generalised narrowing and focal constriction of retinal arterioles.

In uncontrolled toxemia, haemorrhages and cotton-wool spots when seen warrant a termination of pregnancy. An exudative retinal detachment at the level of Bruch's membrane can develop though less common. The detachment subsides after termination of pregnancy. Toxemia recurring in repeated pregnancies causes kidney damage with high blood urea and is a bad prognostic omen both for the mother and for child if pregnancy is allowed to continue.

Arterio-sclerotic retinopathy. Arteriosclerotic changes in the blood vessels of the retina may also be associated with hypertensive or diabetic retinopathy. In such a situation the clinical picture is adulterated by clinical manifestations of hypertensive and diabetic retinopathy respectively (Fig. 15.11, Plate 11).

Arterio-sclerotic retinopathy by itself is not difficult to diagnose. The principal changes are:

1. Thickening of the arterial wall leading to an exaggeration of arterial reflex.
2. Irregularity of arterial lumen, which is due to intimal changes or atheromatous plaques. Irregularity of the lumen can be readily made out with ophthalmoscope.
3. Tortuosity of the arteries which is clinically very evident.
4. Perivascular sheathing is an important observation and is seen with ophthalmoscope as white lines along the arteries. The sheathing extends upto the periphery, unlike physiological/congenital sheathing due to neuro-glial tissue which envelops blood vessels only at and near the disc-margin.

   Arterio-sclerolic sheathing may envelop the whole vessel wall and give the appearance of *copper wire arteries*. Some of the peripheral arterioles may just be reduced to white, threads and give the appearance of *silver wire*.
5. Arterio-venous crossings. A–V crossings develop very significant changes in arterio-sclerosis. The artery obscures the vein underneath it. Because of the pressure on the vein, the vein shows dilatation distal to the crossing.
6. Hard exudates and small haemorrhages are not uncommon in arteriosclerotic retinopathy. The disc remains normal and macular function unaffected.

Sickle cell retinopathy: This is a condition which is common in blacks and almost 100,000 blacks in the United States run the risk of developing sickle cell retinopathy. The disease progresses through various stages starting with peripheral arteriolar occlusion, peripheral arterio-venous anastomoses, neovascularisation, vitreous haemorrhage and finally into retinal detachment.

These phenomena are seen especially during the third and fourth decades of life. Both sexes are equally involved.

The exact mechanism promoting cessation of flow in the peripheral retinal arterioles is unknown, though it is presumed that sickled erythrocytes can act as micro-emboli which can increase viscosity to the point that cessation of flow or thrombosis may occur. Peripheral vessels are more commonly affected probably due to decreased calibre of vessels and the lowered oxygen tension in the periphery in comparison to posterior pole. Ophthalmoscopically, a grey white area in contrast to the normal orange colour of the posterior retina and arterio-venous anatomosis are most frequent at about the equatorial plane mainly supero-temporally. They represent enlargement of pre-existing capillaries rather than true neovascularisation. Neovascular proliferations sprout at the sites of previous arteriolar occlusion and anastomosis. As time goes on, there is an incorporation of additional feeding and draining vessels leading to an arborization pattern and patches of exudation.

Vitreous haemorrhage occurs due to minor ocular trauma at this stage. The haemorrhage may be small and localized or massive. The last stage of the disease is retinal detachment.

Treatment: Consists of photocoagulation of the neovascular tissue. High energy coagulation is best provided by laser coagulation which can also be used for sprouts of neovascularisation into the vitreous.

Retinopathy of Prematurity (Retrolental fibroplasia). Retrolental fibroplasia was the leading cause of blindness in premature children following over use of oxygen in the 1940s. With controlled oxygenation, the disease incidence had a dramatic drop but after its liberalization there is a gradual increase in the number of cases again.

By the 8th month, normal retinal vascularisation is complete nasally, but the temporal periphery does not completely vascularize until shortly after birth. The retina is susceptible to oxygen damage only prior to its complete vascularisation. The changes due to hyper-oxygenation are more pronounced in temporal part. The pathogenesis is vaso-constriction followed by secondary vaso-proliferation. The primary vaso-constrictive response is directly proportional to the concentration of oxygen administered and its duration of exposure. After removal of the infant from high oxygen concentration to room air, a marked endothelial proliferation arises from the residual vasculature. These proliferating endothelial cells develop into new vessels, grow through the internal limiting membrane into the vitreous cavity.

Severity and prognosis of retrolental fibro-plasias (ROP) depends on area of retina involved. Starting with a demarcating line and ridge to extra-retinal fibro-vascular proliferation and ending in retinal detachment, sub total or total, visual prognosis progressively worsens.

Treatment: With the understanding of patho-genesis of the disease, prophylaxis was most successful and the disease was nearly extinct. Efforts to save more and more premature children who are kept under prolonged oxyge-nation still causes stray cases of retrolental fibroplasia.

Treatment is very unsatisfactory. Photo-coagulation may be helpful in some cases. Prophylaxis and follow up is far more important.

Inflammations of the Retina

Inflammations of retina are, in most cases, secondary to inflammations of choroid, the important among them being toxoplasmosis, sarcoidosis and pars planitis.

Septic emboli, fungal retinitis, rubella retinitis even though primarily start in retina, usually become chorio-retinal inflammations.

Ocular toxoplasmosis. May be acquired or congenital. Toxoplasma gondi is an intracellular parasite for which cats are a natural host. Cats shed the organism in their faeces, which in turn can contaminate foods or infect herbivorous animals like rabbits which are eaten by man. Raw and under-cooked meat is therefore a major source of infection.

The diagnosis of ocular toxoplasmosis is based on the ophthalmoscopic picture and serum antibody tests.

Patients with ocular toxoplasmosis complain of blurred vision with floaters and this is due to inflammatory cells and debris floating in vitreous. The seat of inflammation is the inner retina, where the organism multiplies. It classically becomes translucent or grey and then into a white raised retinal lesion with indistinct borders. Vascular sheathing and retinal haemorrhages may occur. These lesions last about 8 to 10 weeks after which a dense white scar with varying amount of pigmentation is left behind. The vitreous usually clears.

Loss of vision when present in ocular toxoplasmosis, is due to:

1. The failure of the vitreous to clear.
2. Direct damage to the macula by the atrophic scar.
3. Traction retinal distortion and detachment due to contraction of preretinal membrane or vitreo-retinal bands.

Recurrences are not uncommon and they can be from the old focus of infection or from new lesions called satellites. Most often they develop from the edge of old scars where there is a breakdown of toxoplasma cysts with release of viable organisms.

Congenital toxoplasmosis: In an infected pregnant woman, organisms cross the placental barrier into foetus and affect multiple organs of which eye is the most characteristic. Large atrophic macular scars are often seen in these infants. These are bilateral and heavily pigmented. Any healed bilateral chorio-retinal lesion in macular area in a child, should therefore always be considered to be due to toxoplasma as an etiological factor which should be confirmed by laboratory tests (Fig. 15.12, Plate 11).

The diagnosis of ocular toxoplasmosis is confirmed by Sabin-Feldman Dye test where even small amounts of anti-toxoplasma antibodies can be detected. Any positive dye test titre regardless of level is significant. The other tests that can be employed are the indirect fluorescein anti-body test and hemagglutination test.

Treatment:

1. A combination of pyrimethamine (daraprim) and sulphanamide is still the treatment of choice.
   a. Pyrimethamine—150 mg, loading dose followed by 25 to 50 mg daily for 6 week, orally.
   b. Sulphadiazine—4 grams loading dose followed by 1 gram 4 times a day for 6 weeks.

2. A newer agent is Clindomycin which is used in resistant cases in doses of 150 mg 6 hourly.
3. Cortico-steroids as an anti-inflammatory supportive therapy is given preferably as a depot in retrobulbar space, and is a valuable adjunct.

Pars Planitis: This is otherwise called peripheral uveitis and is usually bilateral. The condition is more common in young and is characterised by bilateral vitreitis and retinal periphlebitis. The inflammatory cells in vitreous accumulate anteriorly in the retrolental space and ora serrata, producing the typical 'snow banking' appearance. The latter phenomenon is most typically seen along the inferior ora and posterior pars plana overlying the vitreous base.

Retinal periphlebitis is a prominent feature of the disease and can be demonstrated by fluorescein angiography.

The visual acuity is usually not reduced. Vision when affected is due to macular oedema and micro-cystoid degeneration. A characteristic feature is tenderness of eye ball in ciliary zone. Other complications that can occur are posterior polar cataract, fibrovascular proliferations at vitreous base, inflammatory vitreous membranes, neovascularization, vitreous haemorrhage, preretinal membranes, traction retinal detachment and cyclitic membranes. When fibrovascular proliferations occurs in the far periphery, rubeosis iridis and neovascular glaucoma may also ensue.

Treatment, needs to the continued for a long period of time. Large doses of systemic steroids or subtenon injections is still the preferred mode of therapy. Cryo-therapy is another line of treatment.

Sarcoidosis: This is a chronic idiopathic systemic non-caseating granulomatous disease with protean clinical manifestations. The disease usually manifests itself within the 2nd and 5th decades. Ocular involvement is reported in approximately 50% of the cases with systemic disease. Virtually all the ocular structures can be involved in the disease process with posterior segment affected in 25% of patients.

The vitreous characteristically shows 'fluffy snow ball' infiltrates which are found as whitish nodules along retinal and choroidal vessels. Chorio-retinitis and periphlebitis are other important manifestations of posterior segment. The periphlebitis has a typical appearance of 'candle wax drippings' because of thin yellow waxy infiltrates. Macular oedema and papill-oedema may be seen. Cells and infiltrates are seen in the vitreous.

Histologically, these candle wax drippings consist of granulomata composed of nodular collections of epithelioid cells.

Diagnosis is aided by chest X-ray which is abnormal in 80% of cases with ocular involve-ment.

Patients diagnosed and treated early, have a favourable outcome. Topical steroids are not quite adequate. Systemic cortico-steroids and cycloplegics are required in addition.

Retinal Dystrophies/Abiotrophies

These are genetically transmitted diseases and constitute a group of disorders where mechanism of retinal degeneration is not known. However the basic change in all of them is a premature cell death. These retinal dystrophies are progres-sive and have to be differentiated from the stationary forms like congenital night blindness and colour blindness.

The basic abnormality is in the retinal pigment epithelial-photoreceptor complex with secondary changes in the rest of the retina and chorio-capillaries.

I. Primary retinal dystrophies

Retinitis pigmentosa. (Primary pigmentary degeneration of the retina also called tapetoretinal degeneration). The term retinitis pigmentosa is a misnomer because there is no inflammatory element in the disease. The disease should therefore be more appropriately *called primary pigmentary degeneration of the retina.* This is a hereditary disease starting in young age and responsible for incurable blindness. It is bilateral and may affect more than one member of the family. The disease is a serious problem all over the world and distinctly more common in families with consanguineous marriages.

The pigmentary disturbance is characterised by clumps of pigment occurring in the retinal mid-periphery and often in a perivascular pattern. The lesions are typically called 'Bone Corpuscles' but can occur as irregular clumps as well. Clinically, marked attenuation of arteries is a very important finding.

Optic nerve takes on a waxy appearance. As pigmentary changes increase, retina becomes thinner, the choroid becomes more visible resul-ting in a tassellated appearance. The macular area may be spared or associated with a macular degeneration. Development of posterior polar cataract in long-standing cases is quite common.

The visual fields show marked constriction starting with ring scotoma which gradually extends towards periphery and towards centre, ultimately leading to a tubular central field. The *scotopic electroretinogram* is markedly sub-normal or extinguished. The electro-oculogram also shows an absence of response. An extin-guished ERG is often recorded even before the disease has become clinically significant. This is an important method of evaluating the future outlook for children in families with history of retinitis pigmentosa.

The visual complaint begins as difficulty in adaptation to dark and gradually develops into complete night blindness. As the disease pro-gresses, visual acuity is affected even though central vision is maintained for quite a long time. Ultimately most patients become totally blind. The younger the age at the onset of the disease, earlier is blindness. When disease starts; around adole-

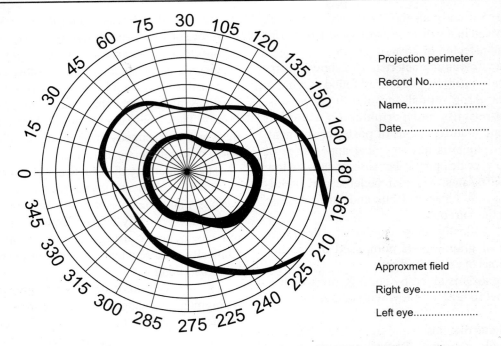

Projection perimeter

Record No....................

Name.........................

Date............................

Approxmet field

Right eye...................

Left eye......................

Fig 15.13: Ring Scotoma in visual field typical of early primary pigment degeneration

scence the patient may retain useful vision till later age. Mental retardation is not uncommon in early onset cases. Deafness may be associated in some patients.

Among the various theories of pathogenesis the most important is vascular theory. The chorio-capillaries are diminished in number and reduced in calibre. This results in poor oxygen supply to the layer of rods and cones with the result that not only is there degeneration in the retinal cells but there is migration from the pigment epithelial layer to the superficial layer of the retina where these pigment masses tend to lie along the retinal vessels, probably because better nutrition is available there.

Another vascular factor in pathogenesis is the relatively poor blood supply in the pre-equatorial region of choroid where there is anastomosis between the recurrent branches of the long posterior ciliary arteries and short ciliary arteries. Hence this part of retina has the least

blood supply from the chorio-capillaries and therefore is the starting point of the degenerative process of retinitis pigmentosa. The same explains the ring scotoma in early phase of the disease (Fig. 15.14, Plate 12).

Heredity: Retinitis pigmentosa can be autosomal recessive, autosomal dominant or sex linked recessive. The large majority is probably autosomal recessive and is the severest form of the disease. The autosomal dominant form has a slower course. The sex linked type is rare, when the females are the carriers and though asymptomatic, may show ocular signs. The hereditary factor should be upper most in the mind of clinician not only for diagnosis but also for genetic counselling.

Pathology: The basic change in tapetoretinal degeneration is disappearance of rods and cones and outer nuclear layers. Pigmentary changes of the retina are secondary and probably related to loss of photo-receptors. The pigment itself is derived from the retinal pigment epithelium and migrates to the inner layers where it proliferates.

Atypical types of retinitis pigmentosa

A. *Sector retinitis pigmentosa.* Pigmentary changes occur in any one quadrant of the eye, the rest of the eye being normal. They are usually autosomal dominant. There are two varieties of the sector form; one being-stationary and the other slowly progressive and representing an asymmetric form of generalised retinitis pigmentosa.

B. *Unilateral retinitis pigmentosa.* Unilaterality of disease although clinically described is pathologically extremely unlikely. In some cases, the evidence of pathology in the clinically normal eye is indicated by a subnormal ERG. In a truly unilateral case one should always think of the condition as a secondary pigment degeneration due to a local vascular or inflammatory cause.

C. *Retinitis pigmentosa sine pigmentosa.* None of the pigmentary changes characteristic of retinitis pigmentosa are seen but symptoms of night blindness from an early age, marked attenuation of arteries, waxy appearance of disc and extinguished ERG are important diagnostic features in cases with family history of the disease.

D. *Inverse retinitis pigmentosa.* This is so named because the pigments which are generally seen in the periphery appear in the macular and paramacular regions. The heredity is autosomal recessive. Although ophthalmoscopically they appear dissimilar from typical retinitis pigmentosa, electro-physiological studies indicate that these are true generalised retinal degenerations.

E. *Retinitis punctata albicans.* The condition appears and behaves electro-physiologically similar to the typical retinitis pigmentosa except that the retina shows white, punctate spots all over. Unlike retinitis pigmentosa, the disease is non-progressive and does not lead to blindness.

Differential diagnosis: Differential diagnosis of retinitis pigmentosa is from conditions which show pigmentation but are acquired and non-familial in character. The condition which may resemble is syphilitic chorioretinitis where pigmentary changes are dominant. This condition is called *secondary retinitis* pigmentosa and is characterised by pigment areas in patches with some amount of scarring. An ERG may be sub-normal but not extinguished. Other conditions which cause pigmentary changes in the retina are gyrate atrophy of choroid and patches following photocoagulalion. History of photo-coagulation will exclude this possibility. Marked attenuation of arteries and early total extinction of ERG in retinitis pigmentosa are important differentiating features.

Syndrome associated with retinitis pigmentosa: The commonest clinical syndrome is Lawrence-Moon-Biedl syndrome characterised by polydactyly, obesity, hypogonadism, mental retardation and retinitis pigmentosa. Look out for an additional finger or toe in obese patients with a history of night blindness.

Treatment: Treatment of primary pigmentary degeneration is very unsatisfactory. The disease is prevalent all over the world and thousands of people are blind at a young age in every country. Numerous therapies have been tried from time to time but with unsuccessful results.

Biological therapy with implantation of 2 × 3 mm size of placental pieces under the conjunctiva were tried for many decades. The procedure is simple. The implant used to be repeated every 6–8 weeks.

Placental extract freshly prepared and used within one month has been given by intra-muscular injection every alternate days for 15 days at a time. The course may be repeated once in 6 months. A German placental preparation was available in 1960s for intracutaneous injection on forehead.

Nicotinic acid as a peripheral vasodilator is the only treatment that makes some sense. It should be given by mouth in maximum tolerable doses and the therapy continued for a few months to a few years. A healthy body can tolerate upto 300 mg per day but the dose may have to be reduced to a level less than the dose which causes tingling of skin and flushing of face. Derivatives of Ribo nucleic acid have been tried in the USSR claiming favourable results but not supported by other clinicians.

Ultrasonic therapy in USSR had been suggested but with questionable authenticity of results. Surgical procedures like fistulising operations for glaucoma have been tried with the hope that lower intra-ocular tension will increase the blood flow through the retinal vessels.

Vitamin A therapy is often given because night blindness is the principal manifestation of this disease. It does not harm even if it does no good.

Genetic counselling is far more important than any form of therapy. The following guidelines should be adopted in the interest of the patient and the family.

1. A genetic family tree should be prepared with the help of parents to the maximum extent of information available. This will indicate the chances of transmission in future generations, depending on whether it is dominant or recessive.
2. If a child has this disease, other children in the family should be examined to detect the disease at the earliest. This will help in planning education and training in a correct direction with future in mind.
3. In the case of suffering children, the ultimate prognosis should be explained which will help in the planning of education and economic-rehabilitation.
4. In case of adults suffering from the disease, they should be advised that they should either not get married and if the marriage is unavoidable or they are already married, they should have no children so that the progeny of the diseased can be limited to the minimum. In any case, the marriages should be strictly with families farthest from any blood relationship, so that genetic influence gets diluted. Cousin marriages in certain communities are responsible for perpetuation of this disease adding many more incurably blind people to the population.

II. Primary macular dystrophies

Primary macular dystrophies, among them Best's disease, Stargardts' disease have definite hereditary traits and are mostly autosomal in transmission. The age of onset is around the first decade but may be detected even earlier. They are usually bilateral and symmetrical. The chief symptoms are early decreased central vision which becomes more severe as the disease process progresses. Ophthalmoscopically, the 'egg-yolk' lesion at the fovea is typical. It may develop sub-retinal neovascularization and ultimately a disciform scar. Bilaterality, symmetrical appearance of lesion starting in adolescence, slowly progressive nature are diagnostic features.

Fluorescein angiography shows typical leak fluorescence and subretinal neovascularisation. Though electro-oculogram is abnormal, the electro-retinogram and dark adaption curves are normal. Visual fields show a relative central scotoma which later becomes absolute.

Fundus Flavimaculatus: It is a non-progressive, benign type of primary dystrophy characterised by yellowish patches all over the posterior fundus. The patches are deep to the retinal vessels. Electrical response is normal. The patches are probably colloidal in nature. The condition requires no treatment.

III. Primary chorio-retinal dystrophy

The best known disorders in this group are sex linked choroideremia, gyrate atrophy (autosomal recessive) and autosomal dominant central areolar choroidal sclerosis.

Choroideremia: It is a bilateral disease and is characterised by night blindness. It is sex linked and predominantly affects males. Females have a mild non-progressive course. Night blindness begins in early youth in males leading to total night blindness after about 10 years age. The earliest signs are seen as a salt and pepper appearance of the fundus due to retinal pigment epithelial degeneration. Later a progressive atrophy of the choroid with exposure of the choroidal vessels is seen. This process involves the entire fundus leaving only a small patch of the retina and choroid in the macula. The electro-retinogram is abnormal showing a loss of scotopic electro-retinogram followed by a progressive loss of photopic response also.

Gyrate atrophy: It is a progressive atrophy of the choroid. The atrophic areas are irregular producing a geographic pattern and spread posteriorly. The retinal vessels appear normal over these patches. The macula is preserved until late in the disease. The onset is around the third decade. Night blindness is the most constant symptom. Visual fields are constricted.

Central areolar choroidal sclerosis: It manifests itself around the 3rd or 4th decade and is characterised by a slowly progressive decrease in central vision. There is gross degeneration of the pigment epithelium and atrophy of the macular region. Ophthalmoscopically it looks like a large well defined atrophic patch involving macular and perimacular area. Choroidal vessels are seen through atrophic retina. The electro-oculogram is normal, whereas the electro-retinogram shows abnormal photopic response and normal scotopic activity. Colour vision is defective and visual fields show non-progressive central scotoma.

IV. Primary vitreo-retinal dystrophies

These dystrophies affect superficial retina and vitreous body and include juvenile retinoschisis, Wagner's disease, Goldman-Favre dystrophy etc.

Juvenile retinoschisis: Was formerly called congenital vascular veils of the vitreous. It is a *sex linked recessive* condition and manifests around the first decade. The condition is slowly progressive and is characterised by decrease in central vision. Ophthalmoscopically, foveal retinoschisis appears as a 'cart wheel' like lesion. Peripheral retinoschisis is associated in about 50% of cases with vitreous haemorrhage and retinal detachment. An electro-retinogram shows a selective decrease in b-wave amplitude electro-oculogram being normal. Colour vision is defective and visual fields may show absolute scotomata corresponding to the area of the schisis.

Wagner's disease: This is transmitted as an autosomal dominant trait and is characterised by mild to moderate myopia, cataract, strabismus, vitreous degeneration, and chorio-retinal changes. The electro-retinogram is subnormal. The cataract starts at puberty as posterior cortical opacity.

The vitreous is liquefied and the cavity appears empty except for a few whitish, translucent, fenestrated membranes at the equator.

The fundus shows choroidal atrophy, peripheral retinal pigmentation along the retinal vessels, retinal vascular sheathing, narrowing and sclerosis. Retinal detachments are common and periodic examinations are therefore mandatory.

Goldmann-Favre Syndrome: It is a rare disorder and is of autosomal recessive inheritance. It can sometimes be sex-linked. This condition is characterised by peripheral retinoschisis in the young, pigmentary degeneration, complicated cataract and retinal detachment.

Degenerative Diseases of Macula

Common and important conditions are senile macular degeneration, central serous retinopathy and epiretinal membranes.

1. Senile Macular Degeneration

Better recognized as Age Related Macular Degeneration (AMD) is a leading cause of bilateral irreversible visual loss in older population. Increasing longevity has caused AMD a significant health problem compromising quality of life.

The predisposing causes are drusen and subretinal neovascular membranes.

a. *Drusen* are otherwise called colloid bodies which are localised depositions of hyaline material between retinal pigment epithelium and Bruch's membrane. They stain densely with Periodic acid Schiff reagent. They occur as an aging process and are seen after the age of 60.

Ophthalmoscopically they appear as small, bright, and sharply defined spots beneath the retinal vessels and are largely confined to posterior pole. They are usually innocuous and besides slight metamorphopsia, do not cause reduction in central vision, unless concomitant degenerative changes of the retinal pigment epithelium and chorio-capillaries occur.

b. *Sub-retinal neovascular membranes or choroidal neovascular membrane.* These membranes can occur either subretinally or may be under the pigment epithelium. This is one of the most important morphological forms of senile macular degeneration.

In early stages, the sub retinal neovascular membrane extends under the intact retinal pigment epithelium when it may not be detected even with fluorescein angiography. When retinal pigment epithelium is damaged, either due to depigmentation or atrophy, the neovascular membrane becomes obvious ophthalmoscopically and is readily appreciated by fluorescein angiography as a typical 'cart wheel' or lacy fluorescence.

The neovascularisation rapidly progresses and eventually blood and exudates accumulate due to leakage at first between the layers of Bruch's membrane and then causes a detachment of the retinal pigment epithelium. Finally, it breaks through pigment epithelium into subretinal space forming a haemorrhagic detachment of the retina. Though the haemorrhage blocks the underlying subretinal neovascular membrane, presence of blood and exudate at macula are reliable signs to suspect its presence. Organization of these haemorrhages gives rise to a typical *disciform macular chorio-retinopathy*.

AMD may be neovascular, wet ADM or non-neovascular dry AMD. Wet AMD is characterized by choroidal neovascular membrane while dry AMD shows drusen, local pigmentation and retinal pigment epithelial degeneration (Fig. 15.15A and 15.15B, Plate12).

Clinical features: Gradual and slowly progressive visual impairment in elderly people with no other cause to explain, is usually attributed to senile macular degeneration. There is no consistent macular picture which could be pointedly labelled as senile macular degeneration. On the contrary it produces a very varied ophthalmoscopic picture. Exudation and pigmentation, combine to present varieties of clinical manifestations. A deep haemorrhage in macular area may cause macular detachment. In long standing cases where scarring has taken place, a disciform lesion is seen. Fluorescein angiography can explain the pathogenesis of many of these macular changes.

Advanced investigative procedures like *scanning laser ophthalmoscopy, optical coherence tomography, Indocyanine green angiography* have shown diagnostic structural changes in AMD.

Clinical course and treatment: These conditions have a poor prognosis, although it never causes total blindness. In selected cases, during the progressive stage, photocoagulation plays a very vital role in arresting the rapid progress of a subretinal neovascular net. The goals of treatment are:

1. To collapse serous retinal pigment epithelial detachment.
2. To eliminate and obliterate subretinal neovascular membranes by photocoagulation.

Newer methods of treatment include intravitreal steroids alongwith photo-dynamic therapy. Intravitreal steroids act as anti-angiogenic, anti-inflammatory and anti-fibrotic agent while newer drugs like Avastin, Lucentis (anti VEGF agents) have a marked effect on choroidal neovasularisation. Trans pupillary thermo and photo-dynamic therapy have been tried.

2. **Central serous chorio-retinopathy (CSR).** Central serous retinopathy is characterized by a serous detachment of the sensory retina due to focal area of leakage from chorio-capillaries through a defect in retinal pigment epithelium. Although the exact etiology of this condition is not established, a tubercular diathesis is a distinct possibility in developing countries.

This disease usually occurs in young adults, preferentially males who present symptoms of blurred vision of sudden onset, metamorphopsia, micropsia, a central dark spot in the visual field and increasing hypermetropia.

Ophthalmoscopically a shallow detachment of the macular area is seen. The oedematous area is circumscribed. In early stage, the raised macular area may show yellowish spots. In long standing cases there may be pigmentary changes. The condition has a tendency to spontaneously resolve but the resolution is slow and takes from few weeks to few months. If oedema does not recur, vision may be fully restored with some minor disturbances in central vision still persisting like metamorphopsia or relative scotoma. Recurrence of the condition may, however, lead to permanent damage of vision if not treated in time. Fundus examination with a slit lamp typically shows a double slit appearance, the convex being from the anterior surface and the deeper straight one from the posterior layers (Fig. 15.16, Plate 12).

Fluorescein angiography shows a typical spot of hyperfluorescence that appears early in the angiogram demonstrating the origin of leak through the retinal pigment epithelium. Later in the course of the angiography, the leak enlarges in size and becomes fuzzy or produces the typical 'smoke-stack' appearance as the dye begins to fill the subretinal space.

As the term indicates, oedema is due to serous retinopathy and there is no inflammatory reaction, the condition has to be

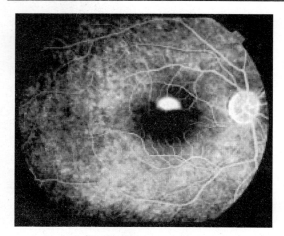

Fig. 15.17: Angio of CSR

differentiated from inflammatory lesion like central choroiditis which does not show a tendency to spontaneous resolution and which can cause more tissue damage and persistent visual loss. Similarly senile macular degeneration needs to the differentiated from CSR. The senile change is not raised and is ill defined as compared to CSR.

Treatment: Most eyes undergo spontaneous resorption with full recovery of vision within 1–6 months though metamorphosia, colour defects or scotomata may persist. The value of steroid therapy is questionable but use of anti-tubercular drugs may help early resolution.

Photocoagulation is a very useful aid in helping early resolution and resorption of the subretinal fluid and is done at the site of fluorescein leakage.

Indications for early photo-coagulation are:

1. Persistence of central serous retinopathy.
2. Recurrence with visual defect.
3. Previous episodes in other eye causing permanent visual defect.
4. Occupational need requiring prompt restoration of vision.

The risks of photocoagulation are accidental foveal burn. The procedure has therefore to be done with great care producing light burns and taking great care to avoid the fovea.

3. **Epi-retinal membranes:** (Macular pucker, premacular fibrosis). These names denote a single disease entity where epiretinal membranes are one end of the spectrum and pre-retinal fibrosis and massive vitreous retraction is at the other end. The basic disturbance is at the vitreo-retinal interface.

The patients present with blurred vision, diplopia, metamorphopsia or positive scotomata. Ophthalmoscopically, the characteristic changes are a wrinkled reflex at the macula with radiating traction lines like spokes of a wheel. There is no medical treatment for the condition. Peeling of the membrane is possible through a pars plana approach.

Cystic Degeneration of Retina

The supporting net work of the retina is the weakest in the outer and inner nuclear layers and to some degree in the ganglionic cell layer. A cystic space can therefore more rapidly develop in these layers. These cysts may ultimately rupture and give rise to retinal holes.

The causes of cystic degeneration are:

1. Traumatic or inflammatory causes like Berlin's oedema and posterior uveitis.
2. Vascular lesions like circinate retinopathy and Coats' disease.
3. Myopic degeneration.
4. Senile degeneration.

The commonest sites for cystic degeneration are the peripheral retina and the macular area.

Cystic macular degeneration gives the appearance of a honeycomb showing quite a few cysts of varying size. The cystic degeneration of the peripheral retina is common in myopes and is not an uncommon finding even though there are no symptoms.

Clinically, cystic degeneration of retina is discovered during a routine ophthalmoscopic examination because they do not necessarily cause any visual disturbances. However when the cyst ruptures giving rise to a hole formation, it may lead to retinal detachment, which, in the macular area is disastrous to vision.

Senile central holes are mostly idiopathic and asymptomatic. The holes may be lamellar or of full thickness. Ophthalmoscopically they appear as round clear cut red areas in or around the macular area. Clinically, a macular hole or a cyst may look alike but they can be differentiated using a slit beam of the ophthalmoscope. In case of a cyst, the slit beam will be seen as curved forwards. In case of a hole, it will appear deeper in the central area with a break at the edges.

Circinate Retinopathy

This is a characteristic fundus condition in which numerous white spots form a girdle round the macular area. This girdle is broadest in the outer side and thinnest between macula and the disc. The macular area in the centre of the girdle also shows pigmentary changes. Vision is moderately reduced. The condition is usually bilateral and commonly affects older people.

The cause of this pathology is considered to be a haemorrhage in the deeper layers of the retina. Senile arterio-sclerosis contributes to haemorrhage as well as macular changes. Field changes show a central scolorna.

Treatment is unsatisfactory. Iodides and ascorbic acid may be helpful to some degree.

Colloid Bodies

Clinically, this is a common condition although rarely affects vision. The colloid hyaline material usually aggregates at the level of the Bruch's membrane. It may be a part of senile degeneration or may be due to inflammatory or vascular pathologies of retina. Ophthalmoscopically they are seen as yellowish dots of the size of a pin head scattered all over the posterior fundus. They do not affect vision and as such are of no pathological significance. The colloid bodies may, however, aggregate to form masses which are called drusens. These drusens are seen like bunches of grapes and are commonly present at or near the disc margin. When they are large in size, they may cause relative scotoma in the field of vision.

Colloid Degeneration of Retina

In this group the condition often seen is *Doynes honey-comb choroiditis*. It is a primary familial disease. The condition is bilateral and mostly affects females. Clinically there are flat small white patches around macula and in the maculo-papillar area. There may be haemorrhages which grossly affect central vision. The condition is probably due to degeneration in the pigment epithelium.

Heredo-macular Degeneration

Macular dystrophies or macular dysplasias. This is a hereditary condition, familial in nature and bilateral. The macular changes present a varied appearance which may include light pigmentation and greyish white spots in the macular area. The characteristic feature is the symmetrical nature in both eyes. The symptoms start in young age and slowly progress. Central vision is affected but peripheral field is always retained intact (Fig. 15.18, Plate 12).

Amarautic Familial Idiocy

This is a familial disease of primary lipid degeneration of ganglion cells of the nervous system including the retina. When infantile in origin, it is called *Tay Sachs disease*. Clinically the mile stones of a child's growth are retarded. The child becomes blind by the time the disease has developed clinical features, Macular area is white in appearance with a central red fovea giving the appearance of a 'cherry red spot'. The condition is usually incompatible beyond a few years of life due to involvement of the central nervous system.

Lipid degeneration in late infantile stage is *'Niemann-Pick disease'* which is associated with lipid deposits in liver and spleen.

Maculo-cerebral degeneration is also an identical condition with a strong heredity. These conditions are also described in further details in the chapter on systemic ophthalmology.

Retinal Detachment

Anatomically, rhegmatogenous retinal detachment is a separation of anterior sensory layers of the retina upto rods and cones from pigment epithelium layer of retina. Embryologically, it is a separation between the structures developed from the two layers of secondary optic vesicle. The term retinal separation will therefore be more appropriate but we will continue to use the term retinal detachment as is being conventionally done.

Retinal detachment is already a major ophthalmic problem in Caucasian races while it is very uncommon in blacks in whom myopia is also less common. With increasing incidence of myopia and enormous number of aphakic patients, the problem is becoming more important and will continue to do so in future years. No statistical data are available from developing countries but it is a disease at present more prevelant in urban communities; correspondingly more frequent in the educated. The disease is distinctly more common in males and the common age incidence is from 30 upwards. Retinal detachment in myopes can however be seen at an early age.

Aetiology: No definite cause can be attributed to the causation of rhegmatogenous retinal detachment. It is said that an eye which is likely to develop a retinal detachment is potentially an eye with certain changes.

Myopia is an important factor and retinal detachment is more common in myopics of -5.0 Diopters and above. Myopia with extensive degenerative changes is however less likely to develop retinal detachment obviously because of the changes that bind the tissues together. Reports indicate that 65% of retinal detachment in phakic eyes are in myopes.

Retinal changes are important precursors of retinal detachment. The common degenerative changes related to detachment are *cystic degeneration, lattice degeneration, retinoschisis* and tears and holes.

Lattice degeneration appears as areas of greyish streaks in the periphery of retina which are indicative of retinal capillaropathy, occlusion of finer retinal vessels. The retina becomes atrophic and pull of the vitreous causes tears and holes.

Cystic degeneration which can be present even in normal eyes may, in older age break down and cause retinal detachment.

Retino-schisis which is a separation within the anterior layers of retina is a senile degenerative process causing cystic spaces. These cysts may break through anteriorly and cause partial holes which may not cause a retinal detachment. If however, degeneration extends to the deeper layers of retina it may cause a primary retinal detachment.

Holes and Tears a hole is round in shape and is commonly a result of cystic degeneration, while a tear is a V or horse-shoe shaped, caused by pull of vitreous on degenerated area like lattice degeneration. Holes or tears may be one or more either near each other or at different distances from the ora serrata. The commonest site is the upper temporal retina. Large sized tears are called giant tears.

Disinsertion or dialysis is also a break but it is detachment of retina from ora serrata. When there is a giant tear extending to 90° or more or there is a large dialysis in the upper part, retina may be inverted and fold upon itself thereby exposing the pigment epithelium layer with rods and cones layer on the inverted flap; a condition which demands a highly complicated retinal surgery.

The vitreous plays an important role in causation of retinal tears and dialysis. The instability of vitreous is an important causative factor and is also an important factor in causation of detachment in aphakic eyes. Some vitreous detachment is present in all cases of retinal detachment but a massive vitreous detachment makes the prognosis worse.

The organised bands and membranes in the vitreous cause a pull on the retina, a retinal tear and retinal detachment which is termed as *traction detachment* of the retina as against rhegmatogenous detachment.

The Refractive State of the eye is also an important factor.

Myopic eyes develop retinal detachment more frequently as compared to emmetropia or hypermetropia because of frequent cystic degenerative changes in the periphery of myopic retina.

Aphakia or phakia: It is generally agreed that aphakia is an added factor to the incidence of detachment. It was a common consensus that retinal detachment is relatively more common after an intra-capsular operation than an extra capsular operation. It would be correct to emphasise that aphakic eyes with vitreous loss at operation are more prone to develop retinal detachment, and still more prone are aphakic eyes where vitreous is adherent to the section and the strands exert a pull on the vitreous mass.

Trauma: A rhegmatogenous detachment is not a traumatic condition. But trauma probably plays an indirect role in initiating the process. Most detachments have a sudden onset and a mild insignificant trauma may have only precipitated the onset of the process.

Sub-retinal fluid: The sequence of events are a tear in the retina followed by seepage of fluid into the sub-retinal space. The sub-retinal fluid is from the vitreous and is more fluid in nature in myopic eyes with vitreous degeneration. The vitreous traction keeps the operculum of the tear pulled up allowing more and more fluid to pass underneath the retina leading to extension of retinal detachment.

Clinical course: Retinal detachment affects one eye. Bilaterality is uncommon although retinal changes are seen in the opposite eye in a majority of cases. The other eye may be affected 5-10 years later.

Symptoms: Although the onset is sudden, most patients have experienced premonitory symptoms like flashes of light (photopsae) seen in the field opposite to the location of the tear. The sudden appearance of black spots or sudden increase in pre-existing black spots is distinctly suggestive of impending retinal detachment. Visual loss due to retinal detachment will depend on the area of retina detached. Vision may not be much affected when detachment is in the periphery and in lower part. Most patients volunteer a statement of sectoral loss of vision explaining that they can see well in one part of the field but not in the other. Patients may complain of a curtain like thing hanging from above in superior detachment. When upper detachment is balloonous and is overhanging macular area, visual loss is marked. Visual loss may otherwise be due to macular oedema which in some cases explains visual deterioration out of proportion to the size and location of the retinal detachment.

Signs: Anterior segment is normal in recent cases. Pupillary reaction may be affected when light falls on the detached area. The tension of the eye may be normal or low. The larger the tear and the detachment, the lower the intraocular tension.

Ophthalmoscopy: An ophthalmoscopy should be done with full mydriasis.

There should be no fear of secondary glaucoma due to mydriasis in elderly patients because these eyes are mostly hypotensive eyes. Vitreous when hazy may be due to vitreous opacities or more commonly due to a retinal haemorrhage extending into the vitreous. These findings are so consistent that a soft eye with hazy vitreous and sudden loss of vision where fundus details cannot be seen, should be presumed to be a retinal detachment eye unless proved otherwise. If such is the condition, both eyes should be patched and the patient put to absolute rest in bed. In a majority of cases the vitreous will clear in 48-72 hours allowing better ophthalmoscopic examination.

Direct ophthalmoscopic appearance of retinal detachment is characteristic. The detached retina appears grey in colour because the red glow from the chorio-capillaries is obscured by the sub-retinal fluid. Retinal vessels appear dark because of the opaque background under the retina. The vessels are also tortuous. The elevation of the blood vessels from the normal retina to the detached retina can easily be made out at the border of the detached retina (Fig. 15.19, Plate 13). In fresh and balloonous detachment, retina appears tremulous and may even change its position with change in posture. A deep groove may be seen dividing the balloonous detachment into two parts, in lower part. Retinal bands are commonly seen in long standing retinal detachments. Chronic detachments with folds and bands are like fixed detachments which neither change in shape nor in position.

Direct ophthalmoscopy, even with full mydriasis dos not allow fundus viewing much

beyond equator. However, efforts can be made to reach beyond equator. This can be achieved to a certain extent if temporal periphery is viewed from nasal side with the patient turning his eye to extreme temporal side. Similarly, nasal periphery can be seen from temporal side.

Indirect ophthalmoscopy is extremely important and equally essential to get a good record of the fundus condition. As majority of degenerative changes, tears and holes and of course dialysis are in the peripheral part of retina, these can only be seen with indirect ophthalmoscopy. Every case of retinal detachment should therefore be examined both with direct and indirect ophthalmoscopy. Indentation of the sclera with a specially designed finger gloved indenter under full mydriasis can help in examining the retina even upto the ora serrata.

Examination is not complete till a hole has been seen or its presence has been definitely excluded. It is a good dictum that every eye should be presumed to have a hole or a tear unless definitely proved otherwise. Sometimes a tear is not seen at the first examination. A repeated examination is therefore necessary. A tear may sometimes become evident only after detachment has become flatter by rest. It is also important that one should not stop examination after a hole is detected. There may be more than one hole and they may be situated in different quadrants and at different anterio-posterior levels. It is not unusual that the detachment may be in the lower part while the tear may be in the upper part. Sometimes a few white linear lines are seen in the detached retina and if they are traced forward they may lead to the location of a tear.

It is equally important to find out if the macular area itself is detached which should not be confused with a balloonous upper detachment overhanging the macula.

Details of the method of direct and indirect ophthalmoscopy have been described in the chapter on dark room examination.

Slit lamp examination will give information which is not possible by either type of ophthalmoscopy. A slit lamp examination can differentiate between a hole and a haemorrhage and in a cyst and a hole. Slit lamp examination with three mirror Goldman lens permits study of the retina upto the extreme periphery and detection of small holes not seen by ophthalmoscopy. Examination with 90° lens is important when looking for posterior breaks as the hand held lens with biomicroscope provides a magnified image of posterior retina.

Examination of vitreous is very important from the prognostic point of view. With the slit lamp one can note the vitreous detachment, vitreous pull on the retina, vitreous membranes and massive vitreous retraction (MVR).

An ultrasonography will be particularly useful where the vitreous haemorrhage or opacities in the media do not permit examination of the retina with the ophthalmoscope.

Electro-retinography will be helpful particularly for prognostic evaluation. Being a composite response of the retina as a whole, ERG indirectly indicates the amount of detachment in relation to the total retinal area and it also indicates the functioning capacity of retina (Fig. 15.20).

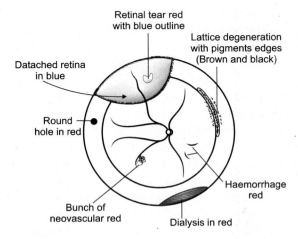

Fig 15.20: Indirect Ophthalmoscopy Charting—How to Chart Different Types of Lesions

Intraocular tension: Most of the detachments have a relatively low intra-ocular tension. A large balloonous detachment with giant tears will make the eye very soft. A tonometry may therefore need to be done only if the eye feels firm and the difference of tension between two eyes is significant.

Visual fields: The field loss is proportionate to the area of retinal detachment. In any case, this is not an important routine examination.

Differential diagnosis: Differential diagnosis is mainly from secondary retinal detachment. A slow onset, absence of tears, sloping edges of the detached area, neovascularization of the retina and raised intraocular tension are indicative of detachment secondary to neoplasms. Transillumination and ultra sonography will be helpful in a difficult situation.

Complications: A long standing detachment can cause silent chronic uveitis. It may cause secondary lens changes mostly posterior subcapsular lens opacities to begin with. An eye with total retinal detachment with a funnel shaped retina usually ends in a phthisical and atrophic eye.

Prognosis: With advances in the technique, prognosis of rhegmatogenous primary retinal detachment, if operated early, has vastly improved. In a favourable situation like the above, in 70–80 per cent of operated eyes, retina is settled, although visual result may not always be equally proportional. One should therefore appreciate the difference between anatomical result and visual result. It is, however, important to note that final improvement of vision may not always be in the immediate post operative period and may take 2 to 3 months to stabilise.

Prognosis is less favourable in aphakic eyes than in phakic eyes due to instability of the vitreous.

Unfavourable Factors Are:

1. When a hole is not detected.
2. When there are multiple tears and at different distances from the ora serrata.
3. Long standing detachment with retinal bands.
4. Giant tears with inversion of retina.
5. Pre-retinal fibrosis and formation of epi-retinal membranes.
6. Massive vitreous retraction.
7. When earlier surgery has failed and diathermy was used.
8. All cases of secondary retinal detachment.

Prophylaxis: Prophylaxis is important and possible when there are fundus findings which indicate a possibility of retinal detachment at a later date. In patients with family history, these predisposing factors should be looked for and treated if necessary. Prophylaxis becomes all the more important when one eye has already developed a detachment because upto 30% of cases are likely to develop detachment in the other eye. Prophylactic measures are:

1. Sealing of a hole without detachment if detected. A hole can be sealed by photo-coagulation if in the posterior fundus and by cryo and light diathermy if situated anteriorly.
2. Lattice degeneration is also better treated by cryo therapy.
3. Cystic degeneration is a senile change and needs to be considered for therapy only if it has caused multiple holes.
4. Vitreous bands or preretinal membranes will need a more complicated procedure like vitrectomy to prevent retinal detachment.
5. A prophylatic consideration in eyes with retinal detachment in one eye and operable cataract in the other eye is pre-equatorial cryopexy in the cataractous eye before cataract surgery.
6. In patients with a family history of retinal detachment and eyes with predisposing factors, physical strain should be avoided particularly lifting heavy weights, jumping or yogic exercises like "sheersasan".

Treatment

The principle of treatment of retinal detachment has long been clearly understood. The first important principle is to seal the hole or tear by cryo or photocoagulation.

The second is to create an aseptic reaction by cryo or diathermy in the choroid and the pigment epithelium layer of the retina so that the retina once approximated, remains attached.

The third is to approximate the retina to its bed by drainage of sub-retinal fluid and indentation of the sclera with silicon bands or rods from the outside.

Sealing of a hole or a tear continues to be the basis of successful retinal reattachment. Most surgeons seal it with a cryo therapy from the outside or a photocoagulation from inside. The aseptic reaction in the choroid and the pigment epithelium of retina is done with cryo or surface diathermy. It is now considered adequate if this reaction is created only in the area of a tear or a hole so that it is not necessary to do an extensive cryo or diathermy which may cause secondary changes in the retina causing secondary tears and redetachment.

The approximation of the retina to its bed is done by drainage of subretinal fluid and identation of the sclera. There is a group of eye surgeons who do not drain the sub-retinal fluid and perform what is called a *dry retinal surgery*. Their contention is that if the hole is adequately sealed, no more fluid will come into the sub retinal space and the preexisting fluid will get absorbed. There are a few reports in literature that even a cryo or diathermy reaction is not necessary because the pressure of scleral indentation itself will create a reaction which will seal the hole provided of course that the indentation is precisely against the retinal tear or a hole. The most important consideration in successful retinal surgery is, therefore, approximation of the sclera by indentation, which should be accurately located corresponding to the position of retinal tears.

With newer surgical approach, the patient does not have to be in absolute bed rest for more than 24-48 hours and is out of the hospital in 2-3 days.

Retinal surgery in previously operated and failed cases or in cases with giant tears and inverted retina need much more extensive surgery like posterior vitrectomy, membranectomy, Intra-vitreal diathermy and cryo-pexy and pealing of epi-retinal membranes. In such eyes one may need to support the operated retina by injecting air, gas (SF6 or C4F8), ringer's solution or sodium hyaluronate (Healon) as an internal tamponade. Silicone oil injection in vitreous in complicated detachment has been in vogue for last few decades.

Traction Detachment

There are a group of conditions which cause a retinal detachment not primarily due to changes in the retina but due to pull by the fibrous bands in the vitreous. Such a detachment is called Traction Detachment.

The common causes of traction detachment are:
1. Injuries causing fibrous organisation in the vitreous, from the periphery.
2. Eales' disease where the fibrous bands are also from the periphery of retina.
3. Proliferative diabetic retinopathy where the bands are attached mostly in the posterior retina.
4. Retrolental fibroplasia, vascular organi-zation of fibroblastic tissue in infants prematurely born and sustained under hyper oxygenation.
5. Coats disease in late stages.
6. Other causes of fibro-blastic organisation in vitreous.

The clinical features are evident from the changes due to the causative pathology in the vitreous. Retinal details are not adequately visible although traction tears may be seen.

The surgery needed in these cases is complicated and the results are unsatisfactory. Peripheral retinotomy helps relieve traction.

Secondary Retinal Detachment

Retinal detachment secondary to a local cause is both clinically and therapeutically a different proposition. Anatomically this is a true detach-ment because here the separation is between the Bruch's membrane and the pigment epithe-lium layer of the retina. The fluid under the retina in this type of detachment is also not from the vitreous but from the chorio-capillary layer of the choroid.

A secondary detachment is commonly due to a tumour in the choroid. Another very common cause is an exudative detachment due to toxamia of pregnancy or hypertensive nephropathy.

Clinical features of secondary detachment are that the detachment is solid, more localised with sloping edges and neovascularization. No retinal tears are seen. The intraocular tension is either normal or raised depending on the size of the growth. A transillumination test gives a dark outline. The vitreous and anterior chamber may show tumour cells.

The exudative detachment is, however, a serous detachment and is reversible with improvement of the systemic condition and of course no retinal tears or holes are seen.

Toxic Retinopathies

There are a wide variety of retino-toxic agents and therefore in the evaluation of a patient with suspected retinal toxicity, a good medical history with careful questioning about the drugs used, is mandatory. A good ophthalmic examination is also important including perimetry with red and white test objects. These enable us to pick up subtle or early scotomata. Electro-physiological studies are useful to determine early toxicity, the earliest sign being a steadily decreasing Electro-oculogram (EOG) and electroretino-gram (ERG).

Common Toxic Agents and Their Effects on Retina

Chloroquine: The toxic effect of chloroquine, used in the treatment of malaria and rheumatoid arthritis was first discovered in 1957. The overall incidence of retinal toxicity was found when total dose exceeded 250 mg a day over long periods as in rheumatoid arthritis. The tissue concentration of chloroquine accumulates over a long period of time and unfortunately toxic effect on the retina does not regress even after withdrawal of the drug.

The mechanism of action of chloroquine is still uncertain, but it has been shown that chloroquine is concentrated in the eye and has a particular affinity for pigmented structures and interferes with metabolism of the retinal pigment epithelium leading to a secondary degeneration of the visual cell layers. The retinal pigment epithelium shows loss of pigment and its migration to the inner nuclear layer. There is complete destruction of the photoreceptors. The ganglion cell layer and bipolar cell layer are within normal limits.

The ophthalmoscopic findings in chloroquine toxicity are characterised by loss of foveal reflex and increased pigmentation in the macular area. Later a de-pigmented ring is surrounded by a hyperpigmented one which is typically called the 'bull's eye lesion' or 'target lesion'. The vessels are narrowed and optic disc atrophies.

The patients usually complain of decreased visual acuity. Central, paracentral and peripheral scotoma may be present. Colour vision is abnormal. An electro-retinogram shows an enlarged a-wave and a reduced b-wave and electro-oculogram shows a definite depression. Adaptation to dark is normal in the early stages thus differentiating it from typical retinitis pigmentosa. A fluorescein angiography may reveal early retinal pigment epithelial atrophy even before they are visible ophthalmoscopically and demonstrates a much larger area of degeneration than is evident from clinical examination.

Treatment: It is usually not successful. The medication has to be discontinued at once. Ammonium chloride or dimercaprol (BAL) can be used as an antidote to enhance urinary excretion of chloroquine. Damage that has been done, however, cannot be reversed. It is, therefore, of utmost importance to be aware of this toxicity when administering the drug on a long term basis and a periodic careful ophthalmological examination is necessary.

Phenothiazines: Toxicity due to phenothiazines used as anti-histaminics and tranquillizer in psychosis has been known to produce ocular toxicity and systemic side effects like agranulocytosis. Doses above 800 mg a day are found to be toxic to retina.

The patients initially complain of blurring of vision and a brownish vision. Ophthalmoscopically, pigmentary deposits appear, scattered between the equator and posterior pole with retinal oedema and hyperaemia of the disc. An eventual loss of night vision is not uncommon. The electro-oculogram is decreased and electro-retinograph is extinguished or depressed. Colour vision is abnormal and visual fields show constriction and central scotoma.

The exact mode of action is unknown. There are similarities between phenothiazines and chloroquine that they produce pigmentary degeneration, but in the former, toxicity occurs after a short while and is reversible, while in the latter, it occurs after a long period and is irreversible.

Treatment: Consists in discontinuation of the drug.

Methanol: Methanol toxicity resulting in blindness has been recognised due to its effect on ganglion cells. It may occur in an acute or chronic form. In the acute form, nausea, headache, and giddiness finally result in coma and if the patient survives, goes onto blindness and optic atrophy.

In the chronic form, the initial symptoms consists of decreased visual acuity, scotoma in the visual field (central, centro-caecal or paracentral), a contraction of the field and finally optic atrophy.

Treatment: Alkalanization of plasma with intravenous sodium bicarbonate is the first step. Milder cases show improvement in 4-6 days. As the severity is directly correlated to the degree of metabolic acidosis and plasma carbon-dioxide, the end result is fatal in severe cases.

Lead: Chronic exposure to lead produces ocular toxicity in only 1 or 2% of cases with systemic lead toxicity.

Ophthalmoscopically, the most characteristic feature is retinal oedema, papilloedema, haemorrhages around the posterior pole, vascular sheathing and exudates which appear as shiny dots in the macula. Optic neuritis may also ensue and may eventually lead to optic atrophy. The condition is associated with systemic involvement including encephalopathy.

Digitalis: The patient usually complains of 'confused vision' with objects appearing in many hues. Visual symptoms are scintillating scotomata, flashes and photophobia. Central scotoma has also been reported. Studies have shown loss of receptors, bipolar cells and ganglion cells in experimental animals.

Indomethacin and phenyl butazone. These are drugs used as anti-pyretic, analgesic and anti-inflammatory agents. These drugs are so commonly and empirically used that it is not uncommon to note their toxic effects. Patients complain of headache, nausea and epigastric pain. The characteristic features of indomethacin toxicity in the eye are macular pucker, central serous retinopathy, macular pigment changes and mottling of the paramacular region. Electroretinograph is reduced, dark adaptation curves altered and central scotomata are not uncommon.

Treatment: Consists of discontinuation of the drug and most patients show an improvement.

Retinopathy in Ocular Trauma

a. **Commotio Retinae (Berlin's oedema):** This is characterised by retinal oedema involving all the layers in the posterior pole following ocular contusion. Ophthalmoscopically, posterior pole appears milky white, with a characteristic 'cherry red spot' in the fovea. Visual acuity is decreased. Secondary changes like macular cyst, macular hole or pigmentary disturbance of the macula prevent complete visual return.

b. **Purtscher's Retinopathy (Traumatic retinal angiopathy).** This usually follows two to three days after crush injuries of chest and long bones. Ophthalmoscopically it presents as bilateral, superficial woolly exudates and haemorrhages around optic disc and macular area. The visual loss is due to macular involvement.

c. **Retinal tears:** Blunt trauma to the globe can cause retinal dialysis leading to retinal detachment. It is commonly seen in the inferotemporal quadrant, since here the globe is most exposed, and retina is thinnest. The next common site is the upper nasal quadrant due to countrecoup effect.

d. **Retinal haemorrhages:** Small retinal haemorrhages which occur following injury disappear without any effect. Severe haemorrhage in vitreous may provoke fibro-vascular reaction ultimately leading to retinal detachment.

e. **Penetrating injuries:** Penetrating injuries often result in vitreous haemorrhage and its complications due to fibro-vascular proliferation. They may also result in endophthalmitis.

f. **Intra-ocular foreign bodies:** Intraocular foreign bodies can produce retinal damage during perforation, resulting in a retinal tear.

Intra-ocular foreign bodies can be inert or irritant depending on the type of the foreign body and the ocular reaction they induce.

Gold, silver, plastic etc., do not produce any specific tissue reaction. Metallic particles like iron and copper incite inflammatory response.

Copper foreign bodies induce suppurative reaction. Copper gets oxidised in the eye and can cause *chalcosis*. Chalcosis manifest as a greenish Kayser-Fleischer ring in corneal periphery. In the lens it produces a greenish discolouration and 'sun flower' cataract. The metallic flecks on the retina cause retinal atrophy. Removal, if successful, arrests worsening of chalcosis.

Iron: Iron is another toxic intra-ocular foreign body as it produces the dreaded condition of siderosis. *Siderosis* is due to electrolytic decomposition of retained iron which interferes with cellular metabolism. The ganglion cells and retinal pigment epithelium are most prone to siderosis.

Siderosis also manifests as corneal and lens epithelium and capsular staining, rust coloured iris, and retinal pigmentation. It may cause optic atrophy and secondary glaucoma.

Electroretinogram in siderosis is diagnostic showing a large a wave with a sub-normal b-wave.

Treatment consists of removal of foreign body after accurate localisation. When direct visualisation is difficult, X-rays combined with ultrasonography and computerised tomography can be utilised. Removal is done trans-sclerally using a magnet or by pars-plana approach with a foreign body forceps and vitrectomy endo-laser.

Tumours of the Retina

Neoplasm of the retina may arise from glial tissue (glioma) or from the retinal blood vessels (Von Hippel Lindau disease). Choroidal tumours often extend into and involve retinal layers. However, the most important primary tumour of retina is *retinoblastoma.*

Retinoblastoma

Retinoblastoma, one of the most important intra-ocular tumours, originally called glioma retina, is fortunately not very common. However, it assumes great importance because of threat to the eye and the high mortality rate.

These are congenital malignant tumours which arise from the embryonic retinoblasts and develop from multiple foci of these cells.

The onset is around two years of age though cases have been reported in older patients too. There is no sex predilection. Approximately 30% of the retinoblastomata are bilateral. This is due to independent multicentric origin in both retinae and not extension from one eye to the other.

Etiology: Retinoblastoma is inherited as an autosomal dominant characteristic of extremely high penetrance. A family history of retinoblastoma may be present. A patient with bilateral retinoblastoma or a family history of retinoblastoma will have a 50% chance of passing the disease to the off spring while patients with sporadic unilateral retinoblastoma have only a 10-15% chance of passing this disease on to next progeny.

Pathology: It appears that retinoblastoma arises from elements in the inner layers of the retina. The retinoblastoma cells have a marked electron microscopic resemblance to primitive retinal cell elements.

Microscopic appearance of retinoblastoma is composed of uniform, small, round or polygonal cells with scanty cytoplasm and hyperchromatic nucleus. These cells grow abundantly around blood vessels forming pseudo-rosettes.

Retinoblastoma never occurs in sites outside the retina. Areas of necrosis and calcium deposition are seen. There is no relationship of cell type to responsiveness to irradiation or prognosis.

Macroscopically retinoblastomata are divided in two groups. Those that appear from the inner nuclear layer grow inwards into the vitreous *endophytic* type and these are distinguished ophthalmoscopically as white or cream coloured fluffy masses with abnormal vessels over it. Like most neoplastic cells, these cells lack cohesiveness and spill into surrounding structures. Seedlings thus appear in vitreous appearing as snow balls' and small white flecks referred to as 'satellite' lesions may be found on retina adjacent to the mass.

When the tumour originates in outer nuclear layer, its growth proceeds outwards and is referred to as the *exophytic type*. These grow into the subretinal space, detaching the retina ahead of it. The choroid is invaded sooner or later when the growth is rapid owing to its high vascularity.

Lack of cohesiveness, is responsible for seedlings on iris, angle of anterior chamber and posterior surface of the cornea. A large number of these cells may aggregate and settle down in the anterior chamber producing a 'pseudo-hypopyon'. Accumulation of tumour cells in filtration angle may cause secondary glaucoma even in early stage of tumour. Distant metastasis occurs via the blood stream. Lymph nodes in pre-auricular region are affected.

Necrosis occurs when cells outgrow their blood supply and die devoid of nutrition. Calcification is a unique feature which can be made out histologically and demonstrated radiologically.

Clinical manifestations. There is usually some delay between onset of the disease and time of diagnosis, specially in children until white reflex becomes apparent.

a. A white reflex from behind the pupil (leucocoria) is the most prominent feature. This has to be distinguished from other causes of leucocoria (Fig. 15.21, Plate 13).

b. A red painful eye with glaucoma is common when the tumour has in filtrated angle of the anterior chamber. The secondary glaucoma may be due to necrosis or haemorrhage within the tumour.

c. In advanced stage, the tumour may extend outside the eye and may appear as a large fungating mass from the orbit (Fig. 15.22).

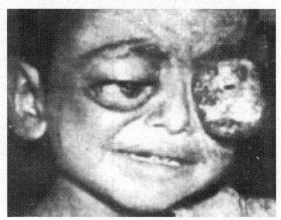

Fig 15.22: Retinoblastoma—Fungating
mass left side

Depending on clinical manifestation, retinoblastoma can be classified into following stages:

1. Localised to retinal layers. The child may be brought for defective vision, an esotropia or leuco-coria in endophytic cases.

2. Stage of secondary glaucoma when tumour mass fills up intraocular space.

3. Extra-ocular extension with the tumour having ruptured through sclera and spread into orbit and anteriorly out of palpebral fissure as a fungating mass.

4. Distant metastasis, via optic nerve to intra-cranial tissues, rarely to remote body organs because of early mortality.

Examination of fundi under general anaesthesia and full mydriasis is the most important step in the early stage. If the tumour is clinically evident in one eye, examination of the other eye and scanning the entire fundus is extremely important.

Diagnosis

1. *Ophthalmoscopy.* Indirect ophthalmoscopy with scleral depression affords a wider field of observation and visualisation of the extreme retinal periphery.
2. *X-ray orbit.* Shows calcification, when present, is a very important sign.
3. *X-ray optic foramina.* Both foramina should be taken and compared. An enlargement of the optic foramen means that the tumour has invaded the optic nerve and spread posteriorly.
4. *Ultrasonography* in cases with opaque media may confirm the diagnosis and lead to prompt treatment. B scan is particularly useful.
5. Higher level in the serum of lactic dehydrogenase (LDH) is supportive of retinoblastoma diagnosis in case of doubt.

Prognosis: Prognosis depends upon the histo-pathological examination report. If the optic nerve is found to be involved at enucleation, and confirmed by histo-pathology, the prognosis is poor and most patients die. If histology of enucleated eyeball shows choroidal extension, then also the prognosis becomes bad as there is a chance for the tumour to have spread through the blood stream. Tumours which are composed of well differentiated cells carry a better prognosis than when they are anaplastic and poorly differentiated. The children die of cachexia, toxaemia and intracranial extension.

Treatment

1. Enucleation is still the treatment of choice in unilateral cases irrespective of the size of the tumour but only after the fellow eye is examined and systemic metastasis has been ruled out. At enucleation, optic nerve is cut as long as possible from the globe. In bilateral cases, with asymmetric presentation, the more advanced eye is enucleated and the fellow eye treated conservatively. The same is the approach when early growth is discovered in the only remaining eye. When retina of both eyes is extensively involved and there is no useful vision the condition is already so advanced that these children do not live. Bilateral enucleation has no scope.

   If histology indicates extension of the tumour up to the cut end of the optic nerve and there is no evidence of dissemination into the orbit, removal of the remaining part of the optic nerve in the bony canal and the intracranial portion may be done by the transfrontal surgical approach.

2. **Photocoagulation.** Small tumours upto 8 mm size near or posterior to the equator are suitable for this treatment. The principle is to cut off its blood supply. Burns are first produced on the normal retina around the base of the mass and summit of the mass coagulated after an interval. The case is carefully followed up. If there is recurrence, it may be close to the previous tumour site and can also be coagulated.

3. **Cryo therapy:** It is equivalent to photocoagulation and is easier in anteriorly located lesions. There is a suggestion that unlike photocoagulation, cryo therapy may leave the lamina vitrea intact and carry less danger of dissemination of the tumour into the choroid. The technique utilised is the triple freeze-thaw method. Cryo therapy destroys tumour cells by destruction of the micro circulation to the tumour.

4. **Radio therapy:** This gives good results when only one quadrant is involved. Cobalt 60 plaques are effective in the treatment of retinoblastoma. The site is first selected using an indirect ophthalmoscope and ultra sonography.

6. **Irradiation of the socket.** This is done when the optic nerve is infiltrated as seen in histology of enucleated eye ball. A cone is placed in the socket with radon seeds in it. The socket may contract and later necessitate a plastic repair.

7. **Chemotherapy:** Triethylene melamine can be given orally or intramuscularly in doses sufficient to cause a fall in blood count. This may be combined with irradiation therapy. It is particularly useful where the tumour recurs in the orbit after enucleation.

All cases, irrespective of the type of treatment, have to be followed up once in three months for three years, once in 6 months for the next two years and every year for five years and thereafter.

Phakomatosis

Phakomatosis is a group of conditions which are congenital in origin and probably hereditary in transmission. The conditions included under this group are:

1. Angio-rnatosis Retinae (Von-Hippel Lindau's Disease).
2. Sturge-Weber's syndrome.
3. Tuberous sclerosis (Bournville disease).
4. Neurofibromatosis (Von Recklinghausan's disease).

Angio-matosis retinae *(Von-Hippel Lindau's disease).* This is a congenital vascular anomaly which results in angio-matosis of the vessels. In retina there is extreme dilatation and tortuosity of the retinal veins. Sacculations may form at some places particularly in the periphery of the retina and large blood vessels may be seen feeding these aneurysmal lesions. Retinal haemorrhages, exudates and retinal detachment may be seen. Neovascularization and gliosis may cover a large part of retina in later stages. Secondary glaucoma may complicate the retinal condition. Similar lesions may be found in cerebellum, medula oblongata and spinal cord. Such lesions are also seen in other tissues of the body like skin, kidneys, bones and pancreas. Photocoagulation of the feeding vessels may help in reducing the aggravations and complications.

Sturge Weber's syndrome is a capillary angiomatosis affecting face, lids and conjunctiva. They are usually present from birth and extend as the age advances.

A fibro-vascular mass may form in the angle of the anterior chamber and cause buphthalmos. Similar lesions are also noted in retina and choroid.

Angio-matosis of the choroidal plexus in brain may cause internal hydrocephalous.

Treatment includes cryo application for smaller lesions on the face, cyclo-cryo-pexy for buphthalmos and photocoagulation for choroidal lesions.

Tuberous sclerosis *(Bournville's disease).* This is a congenital condition where solid tumours appear in the cerebrum and other organs of the body. A peculiar clinical feature is an associated skin condition called adenoma sebaceum with pigmentation. In the eye, small tumours may be seen on and around the disc and appear like drusens. These infants are usually mentally deficient and not many of them live more than a few years.

Neurofibromatosis *(Von Recklinghausan's disease).* This condition has a congenital basis and is a neurofibromatosis of the peripheral nerves of the body. These are Schwann sheath tumours. Small pedunculated tumours may cover a large part of skin in large numbers with pigment spots all over. Neurofibromatosis may involve lids, iris, retina and optic nerve and may cause optic atrophy.

Congenital Abnormalities of Retina

1. **Congenital pigmentation of the retina** *(Bear tracks).* This is characterized by small oval grey spots or greyish black spots scattered all over fundus. They are flat and lie in a plane beneath retinal blood vessels. This is thought to be congenital hyperplasia and heaping of retinal pigment epithelium and usually does not have any significant effect on visual acuity.

2. **Opaque nerve fibres:** The medullary sheaths of the optic nerve fibres normally stop short of the lamina cribrosa, so that in the papilla and retina, the fibres are non-medulated and transparent. However, at times, the medullation does not stop at the lamina, but persists over the optic nerve disc and out into the retina (Fig. 15.23A to C).

   Ophthalmoscopically, they appear as tongue-shaped white patches emanating from or near the disc with a feathery frayed margin. When not continuous with the disc, they may appear isolated but not very far.

   The retinal vessels are at places hidden by these opaque nerve fibres.

   Visual fields show an enlargement of the blind spot or a scotoma corresponding to the position of the patch.

   They do not show any increase in size with time but sometimes may disappear due to degeneration of the medullary sheaths in glaucoma or optic atrophy.

   Small patches of medullated nerve fibres may be mistaken for cotton wool exudates and have to be differentiated.

3. **Albinism:** There are three clinical types of albinism.

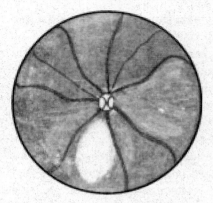

A. Grade-I Isolated opaque fibres bundles away from disc margin.

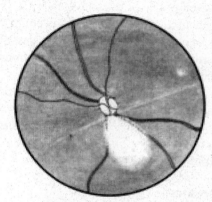

B. Grade-II opaque nerve fibre bundle adjacent to disc.

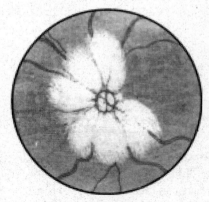

C. Grade-III opaque nerve fibres all round the disc.

Fig. 15.23A to C: Opaque nerve fibres

Oculo-cutaneous albinism:

a. *Type I*. This is the tyrosinase negative type and is an *autosomal recessive* trait. This condition is characterised by a total lack of pigment all over the body including eyelids and eye lashes. A typical red reflex is seen when light is shone into the eye. These patients also have macular hypoplasia or aplasia, very poor visual acuity, high refractive errors, strabismus and nystagmus.

Poor visual acuity and nystagmus are related to macular aplasia and hypoplasia rather than to lack of pigment.

b. *Type II*. This is tyrosinase positive and is transmitted as an *autosomal recessive* trait and is more common in blacks.

These patients are not so badly affected and tend to show some increasing pigmentation as they grow older by which time they may even show improvement in visual acuity.

Ocular albinism:

c. *Type III:* This is a sex linked recessive disorder. The skin colour of the patient, retinal pigmentation and macular involvement are variable. The decrease in visual acuity is usually not so severe as with the other two types.

The great majority of patients are male who have normal pigmentation of the skin and hair but deficient pigmentation of eyes with macular hypoplasia. The females are carriers and have normal visual acuity though they have abnormal iris transillumination and blotchy pigment abnormalities in retinal periphery.

Treatment: Though treatment is unsatisfactory, every attempt should be made to help an albinotic child. Photophobia should be overcome with tinted glasses or coloured contact lenses. High refractive errors and strabismus should be corrected. Since near vision is better than distant vision, they should be encouraged to read with the aid of large prints.

16

Neuro-ophthalmology

INTRODUCTION

Neuro-ophthalmology concerns ocular symptoms and the signs in relation to the diseases of the central nervous system. This chapter will make ophthalmologists familiar with common neuro-ophthalmic problems so that they will be in a better position to help the neurologist or the neuro surgeon.

Neuro Anatomy

The end receptors of visual impulses are the rods and cones of the retina. The first order of neurons are bipolar cells and second order of neurons are ganglion cells. The axons of the ganglion cells from the retina converge towards optic disc to emerge out as the optic nerve. The third order of neuron in the visual path is the cells of lateral geniculate body which project impulses to visual cortex.

Optic Nerve

The optic nerves are true prolongations of brain comprising of nerve fibre tract covered with meningeal sheath which are derived from the coverings of brain. Each optic nerve starts from the eye ball from a point just above and 3 mm

nasal to the posterior pole. It may be described as having four parts:

1. Intra-ocular portion-1 mm long
2. Intra-orbital portion-30 mm long
3. Intra-canalicular or intra-osseous portion-6.0 mm long
4. Intra-cranial portion-10 mm long.

The intra-ocular portion of the optic nerve is the smallest portion, and occupies the posterior scleral foramen. It measures about 1 mm. The intra-orbital portion of optic nerve extends from the globe to the optic foramen and lies as an elongated 'S'. Its diameter in the orbit is 3 to 4 millimeters which is broader than the intra-ocular portion. This long intra-orbital portion allows free movement of the eye ball within the orbit. At the apex of orbit, the nerve passes through the inner part of the common tendinous ring, the *annulus of Zinn*. The origin of medial and superior recti is almost adherent to the dural sheath of the optic nerve and this explains the pain associated with contraction of these muscles in retrobulbar neuritis. Laterally, between the optic nerve and the origin of the lateral rectus are sixth nerve, the two divisions of the oculomotor nerve, naso-ciliary nerve, and ophthalmic veins. Further forwards, the optic nerve lies in the centre of muscle cone formed by the four recti, the orbital fat separates them from the nerve. The ciliary ganglion lies in the orbital fat lateral to the optic nerve 1 cm in front of the optic foramen. The naso-ciliary nerve, the ophthalmic artery and the superior ophthalmic vein cross from the lateral to the medial side just above the optic nerve. The long and short ciliary nerves and arteries surround the anterior part of the optic nerve near the eye ball. The central artery, a branch arising from the ophthalmic artery near the optic foramen runs forwards, enters the dural sheath of the nerve, and crosses the subarachnoid space to enter optic nerve on its infero-medial portion about 1 to 2 centimetres behind the eye. As the optic nerve pierces the eye ball it loses its myelin sheath and this is responsible for the transparency of the nerve fibre layer of the retina so that light can pass through to reach the layer of rods and cones.

The optic nerve enters the bony optic canal through the anterior opening of the canal at the apex of orbit. The optic foramen is formed by the two roots of the lesser wing of the sphenoid. Each canal is directed posteriorly and medially and measures 4 to 9 mm. The distance between the two optic formamina is 28 mm but it is only 14.7 mm between the two cranial openings. This canal transmits optic nerve, ophthalmic artery and some filaments of sympathetic carotid plexus. In the optic canal the nerve is related medially to the sphenoidal air sinus and posterior ethmoidal air sinuses with only a thin plate of bone intervening between them. Because of this close relationship with air sinuses, the optic nerve can be involved in inflammations of these sinuses.

The intracranial portion of optic nerve extends posteriorly and medially to form optic chiasma. The length of this portion of the optic nerve measures 10 mm. The frontal lobe of the brain lies above each optic nerve. On the lateral side of the optic nerve the internal carotid artery and its branches form an immediate relationship of

optic nerve. This accounts for loss of vision and visual field defects in cases of carotid aneurysm.

The sheaths of optic nerve are continuous with meninges of the brain and are termed dura, arachnoid and pia. The dura splits into two layers at optic foramen—the outer layer becomes continuous with peri orbita, and the inner forms the outer sheath of optic nerve.

The sub-arachnoid-space of optic nerve contains cerebro-spinal fluid which is continuous with intracranial space. The pia invests optic nerve and sends fibres into it to form the septa. The special feature of optic nerve fibre is the absence of Schwann sheath and hence the optic nerve fibres once cut or damaged, do not regenerate.

Optic chiasma is formed by the junction of the two optic nerves. The chiasma lies above the diaphragmatic sella measuring 12 mm in transverse and 8 mm in antero-posterior dimensions. Anteriorly related is the anterior communicating artery. Laterally, on either side is internal carotid artery as it comes out of cavernous sinus which is below the lateral edge of chiasma. Infundibulum of pituitary gland lies posteriorly with the gland itself related inferiorly to chiasma.

The optic nerve fibres decussate and cross over in the chiasma before they form the optic tracts. Nerve fibres from temporal half of retina traverse uninterrupted laterally in the chiasma and continue posteriorly in the optic tract of same side. These are uncrossed fibres. Nerve fibres from nasal qudrants of the two retinae decussate and cross over into optic tract of opposite side in a rather intricate manner. Lower nasal quadrant fibres bend back and form a loop in the proximal part of optic tract of the same side then cross over to opposite side tract. Nerve fibres from upper nasal quadrant leaving the optic nerve at its chiasmal end form a loop in the end part of optic nerve of opposite side before it joins the chiasma and then pass into the optic tract of

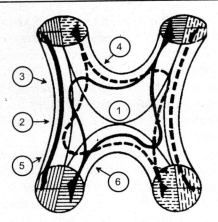

Fig 16.1. Arrangement of fibres in the Chiasma—Pressure Effects. (1) Median pressure—bilateral hemianopia; (2) Lateral pressure—(a) Ipsilateral nasal hemianopia with diagonally quadrantic temporal defects; (b) Ipsilateral blindness and contralateral superior temporal quadrantanopia; (3) Antero-lateral pressure—Ipsilateral nasal hemianopia with contralateral superior temporal quadrantanopia; (4) Anteromedial pressure—(a) Ipsilateral blindness with contralateral superior temporal quadrantanopia; (5) Postero-lateral pressure—(a) Ipsilateral nasal hemanopia. If the posterior looping fibres are also involved, there will be, in addition, an ipsilateral lower temporal quadrantanopia; (6) Postero-medial pressure—hemianopia. If the posterior looping fibres are **also** involved, there will be, in addition, an ipsilateral lower temporal quadrantanopia.

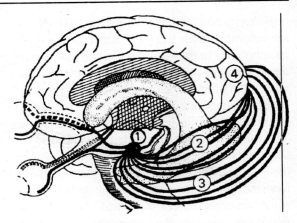

Fig 16.2. Visual Pathway from Retina to Occipital Cortex (1) Lateral geniculate body; (2) Visual fibres directly to occipital lobe; (3) Visual fibres passing through temporal lobe; (4) Visual cortex on the inner surface of occipital lobe

opposite side. Decussation of nasal fibres takes place in the chiasma as they cross from right to left and vice versa.

Thus each optic tract contains temporal fibres from same side and nasal fibres of opposite side after they have decussated in the chiasma.

The ratio of the crossed and the uncrossed fibres is about 53:41. The macular fibres constitute almost two third of the whole nerve whereas the macular area represents only about one tenth of the retina. The macular fibres also have two sets of fibres both crossed and uncrossed. The crossed macular fibres decussate to the opposite side in the most posterior portion of the optic chiasma.

Optic tract: The optic tract connects the postero-lateral angle of the chiasma to the lateral

geniculate body and it runs postero-laterally from the chiasma forming the antero-lateral boundary of the inter-peduncular fossa. Each tract conveys both visual and pupillo-motor fibres both crossed and uncrossed. The posterior cerebral artery runs below and parallel to the optic tract.

Lateral geniculate body: The lateral geniculate body, one on each side, is part of the thalamus and forms an end relay station for visual fibres in the course of the optic tract. The lateral geniculate body consists of alternate layers of white and grey matter. The six layers of grey matter are of cells which receive the visual fibres. The crossed fibres end in layers 1,4,6 while the uncrossed fibres end in 2,3,5. The upper retinal fibres go to the medial half of the lateral geniculate body and the lower retinal fibres go to the lateral half. The macular fibres end in a wedged shaped area confined to the posterior two thirds of the lateral geniculate body.

Optic radiation: The optic radiations are geniculo-calcarine tract, and they extend from lateral geniculate body to the visual area in the occipital cortex, and occupy the posterior part of the internal capsule in front of auditory fibres. The proximity of visual fibres to the sensory and motor fibres in the internal capsule produce *homonymous defects* along with hemi-plegia or hemianaesthesia. The dorsal fibres of optic radiation run laterally straight back into the occipital lobe. The ventral fibres run forwards in the temporal lobe passing around and over the temporal horn of the lateral ventricle and terminate in posterior portion of the occipital lobe. The loop that is formed in the temporal lobe is called the *loop of Meyer*. Thus any space occupying lesion affecting these bundles separately will cause quadrantic field defects.

Visual cortex: Commensurate with the large number of cones and rods and their highly specialised function, the visual cortex occupies a large area on the medial surface of occipital lobe. The most important functional area of the retina, the macular area, occupies a large area of visual cortex surface. The upper retina is represented above the calcarine fissure and the lower retina below the calcarine fissure. The macular area is represented in the posterior part of the calcarine fissure and the posterior pole of the occipital lobe.

Medulated character of optic radiational fibres form white lines in occipital cortex and these are called lines of *Gennari*. Because of this peculiar feature in the grey matter, occipital cortex is called the *striate area of visual cortex.*

The visuo-sensory area is essentially a perceptive centre for (a) appreciation of sensation of light, (b) perception of size, shape and colour of object, (c) the fusion of two separate images in binocular vision, and (d) the orientation of objects in space.

Blood supply to the visual pathway: The retino-calcarine pathway receives its blood supply from two systems of arteries, the carotid system and the vertebral system. These two systems of arteries are connected at the base of brain by arterial *circle of Willis* (Fig. 16.3).

The blood supply to the optic nerve is from ophthalmic artery. The intracranial part is

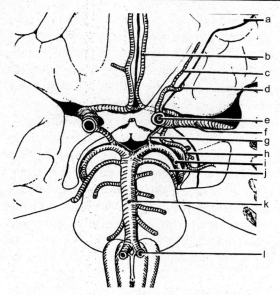

Fig 16.3: Arterial Circle of Willis (a) Eye ball; (b) Anterior cerebral artery, (c) Central retinal artery, (d) Ophthalmic artery, (e) Internal carotid artery; (f) Middle cerebral artery; (g) Posterior communicating artery; (h) Anterior Choroidal artery, (i) Posterior cerebral artery, (j) Superior cerebellar artery, (k) Basilar artery, (l) Vertebral arteries

exclusively nourished by branches from the internal carotid, the anterior communicating artery, the ophthalmic artery and the anterior cerebral artery.

The optic chiasma is supplied by branches of the anterior communicating artery, anterior cerebral artery, internal carotid artery and the posterior communicating artery.

The optic tract is supplied mainly by the pial plexus of blood vessels. The anterior one third of the optic tract is supplied by branches from internal carotid, the middle cerebral and the posterior communicating arteries. The posterior two thirds receives branches from the anterior choroidal and posterior cerebral arteries.

The medial and posterior aspects of the lateral geniculate body are supplied by branches from the posterior choroidal artery while the anterior choroidal branches supply the anterior and lateral parts.

Optic radiation is supplied anteriorly by branches of anterior choroidal, posterior choroidal and middle cerebral arteries. In the middle it is supplied by the penetrating branch from the middle cerebral artery called the *deep optic artery* and posteriorly by the calcarine artery, continuation of the posterior cerebral artery.

The main supply to the visual cortex, is by calcarine artery. The middle cerebral supplies the lateral surface near the posterior pole. There is a well marked anastomosis between the posterior and the middle cerebrals and this accounts for sparing of the macula in cortical lesions (Fig. 16.4).

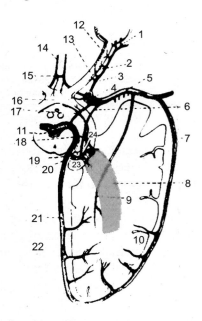

Fig 16.4: Vascular Supply of Visual Pathway from Retina to Occipital Cortex (1) ciliary arteries; (2) Central optic nerve artery, (3) Ophthalmic artery; (4) Internal carotid artery, (5) Middle carebral artery, (6) Anterior choroidal artery; (7) Middle cerebral artery; (8) Optic radiations; (9) Middle cerebral—deep optic branch; (10) Cerebral cortex; (11) Basilar trunk; (12) Central retinal artery; (13) Optic nerve; (14) Anterior cerebral artery; (15) Anterior communicating artery; (16) Chiasma; (17) Posterior communicating artery; (18) Choroidal plexus; (19) Posterior choroidal artery, (20) External geniculate body, (21) Posterior, cerebral artery; (22) Calcarine artery; (23) Thalamus; (24) Optic tract.

METHODS OF CLINICAL EXAMINATION OF NEURO-OPHTHALMIC PATIENTS

Approach to a neuro-ophthalmic patient should be done by an ophthalmologist in a systematic way so that he can, to a certain extent come to a diagnosis of a neuro-ophthalmic problem with the available ophthalmic and neuro-ophthalmic signs and symptoms of the patient. A complete examination of a neuro-ophthalmic patient can be done with the following guidelines.

History

About 85 per cent of the diagnosis in neurological patients is based upon history. Normally, there is a tendency to underestimate the value of medical history, but it often indicates the nature of the problem and frequently leads to a provisional diagnosis saving a lot of elaborate and expensive investigations. The history is best obtained at first hand from the patient but it can also be supplemented by relatives. In an unconscious patient and also in patients who are very sick, the relatives should be depended upon. In history, the chief complaint must be given the primary importance, for example, whether patient has come for headache, defective vision, diplopia, etc. This history could include the onset of the problem, duration, whether the defect gets better, gets worse or stays the same, gets any relief with medication etc. The following information should also be obtained-mental alertness of the patient, his cooperation, his facial expression, his memory power, his speech, his hearing ability etc. Personal medical history about any chronic medication for any other illness should be obtained. The family history is equally important especially in cases of seizures, genetic diseases, familial optic atrophy, retinitis pigmentosa, myopathies, diabetes, glaucoma etc.

Examination

The general appearance of the head and face will obviously indicate hydrocephalus, microcephaly, craniostenosis, myopathies, immobility of Parkinson's disease, the dry indurated skin of hypothyroidism, the contour of the face and limbs of acromegaly, etc.

General examination of the eye consists in looking for proptosis, ptosis, strabismus, or any fullness over the peri-orbital region, etc. Any abnormal movements of the lids should be noted.

Visual acuity includes best corrected visual acuity for distant vision, near vision and colour vision. If the neurologist and the neuro-surgeon are not aware of the refractive error of the patient they may unnecessarily subject these patients for elaborate investigations to find out the cause of the decreased visual acuity.

Colour vision is tested with the help of Ishihara plates: Conduction defects of the optic nerve like optic neuritis typically reduces colour perception.

Pupils: This is a very simple, reliable test, but is often neglected. The pupils are assessed in terms of size, regularity of the outline, reaction to light and reaction to convergence. The light should be introduced from sides with the patient looking straight ahead to avoid the added effects of convergence. While, doing this test, one has to look for character and duration of constriction of the pupils. The size of the pupil could be measured with the use of a ruler calibrated in millimetres. The details of pupillary examination and pupil anomalies have already been described.

Ocular motility: Each eye is manoeuvered by six extraocular muscles, each of which has a partner in the contralateral eye for simultaneous movement of the fellow eye. Muscles which work in pairs for conjugate gaze are called yoke muscles, for example, on looking to the right lateral rectus of right eye and medial rectus of left eye are yoke muscles. Each extra-ocular muscle has an ipsilateral antagonist which must relax if the globe is to move. Therefore, as the lateral rectus contracts to abduct the globe, its antagonist medial rectus is inhibited.

General inspection of the patient must include observation for spontaneous head tilt or face turn in cases of ocular palsy. These patients try to close one eye while narrating the complaints or have difficulty in walking because of diplopia.

The ability of the eye to move symmetrically and synchronously in the same direction, horizontally or vertically is termed conjugate gaze. Conjugate gaze is tested by asking the patient to move the eyes to the right or left. When the patient is asked to look to the right, the right lateral rectus and the left medial rectus should act. If this conjugate movement is not possible then it is termed as horizontal gaze palsy. The testing of convergence should be done by asking the patient to fix a near object directly in front of the eyes. While doing this the pupillary reaction should also be noted. A sure sign of convergence is pupillary constriction. So it will be helpful in using the patient's own finger as a target for convergence. Thus convergence may be examined even in a blind patient due to proprioceptive clues to the nearness of his own finger.

The ocular movements in infants and children should be tested by attracting the infant's attention. Normally, a child will turn the head and eyes towards a sound, but if the child fixes accurately and follows a silent object (toy), the movement can be tested in all directions.

Optokinetic nystagmus is seen when a normal person looks at an object which is moving rapidly or when a subject is in a moving vehicle and looks at a stationary object (railway nystagmus). This can be tested either by using a optokenetic drum or by a tape with stripes. This test is useful in frontal and parietal lobe lesions.

Fundus: Examination of ocular fundus is done in critical detail under full dilatation. Atropine should be avoided as far as possible because the effect takes ten days to wear off and it is confusing for the neurologist or neurosurgeon to follow the case.

Visual fields: A great deal of information may be obtained in diagnosing and localizing lesions by fields alone. The confrontation fields can be very helpful in neurological cases and it provides a rapid, readily available technique which may be utilised at the bed side or in the office. With confrontation, the examiner compares the patient's field with his own in a face to face position. This depends upon the patient's cooperation. The common indication for checking the fields are:

1. Unexplained defective vision.
2. When a patient complains of defective field of vision.
3. Any sign of increased intracranial pressure.
4. Any case referred as a sellar lesion.
5. Whenever the neurosurgeon asks for it.

If the patient's condition permits, field examination is better done by perimetry and tangent screen and it should be done both for white and colour objects. The colour field is important especially in a macular lesion and in suspected chiasmal syndrome. In suspected optic nerve disease, special exploration of the fixation area (central scotoma) should be done. Similarly, in a case of early chiasma compression, peripheral fields may be absolutely normal but central fields may reveal a hemianopic defect.

Test sensations: The best way to do this test is to take a wisp of cotton and to touch the sclera near the limbus and gradually take it to the cornea. With normal corneal sensation the patient will blink. Any decrease in corneal sensation will be detected by comparing both sides. A cotton wisp may also be used to test light touch sensation of the brow and face looking for differences from one side of the midline to the other. Subcutaneous sensory testing is best accomplished with patient's eyes closed. Along with this test, the sense of smell, the fifth nerve and the seventh nerve functions are also tested.

Ophthalmodynamometry: This test is more useful in conditions where one suspects carotid insufficiency. This requires full dilatation of pupil and topical anaesthesia. Pressure is applied to the eye ball using a spring loaded plunger (Bailliart's ophthalmodynamometer). Fundus examination should be done with one hand and the plunger should be adjusted with the other hand. A difference of 20 per cent between diastolic reading is considered diagnostic of unilateral carotid stenosis or occlusion.

Pulsation of the carotid, temporal and facial arteries: The pulsation of the carotid on both sides should be felt and, bruit if any heard. Similarly, palpation of the temporal and facial arteries should be done. Blood pressure should be checked in both arms in the lying down and standing postures.

X-ray studies: The common X-rays that are requested are skull lateral view (evidence of intracranial tension, pituitary pathology, meningioma, etc.). X-ray orbit for evidence of enlargement, any fracture, X-ray of the optic foramen (for glioma and meningioma of optic nerve), paranasal sinuses in cases of mucocele of the frontal sinus, ethmoidocele, maxillary antrum growth etc. As an ophthalmologist one should be in a position to read and interpret the aforesaid X-ray and know what the other conditions are that require special X-rays like angiogram, pneumoencephalogram, brain scanning etc.

Fundus photographs and fluorescein angiography should be done as they will be very useful in follow-up of cases.

OCULAR MOTILITY AND ITS DISORDERS

The muscles of eye movements, their nerve supply, the location and the relationships of their nuclei are described in detail in the section on paralytic squint. It suffices to state here that impairment of lower motor neuronal function results in peripheral nerve palsy of the corresponding muscle with clinical manifestations of restriction of movement and diplopia in the field of action of the particular muscle or muscles. There are however higher centres and associational nerve fibres to and from these centres. One such important nerve pathway is the medial longitudinal bundle which is closely related to the oculomotor nuclei as well as the main motor, sensory and cerebellar fibres. At these supra-nuclear levels, directional movements of the eyes are represented and not individual muscles. Involvement of these higher pathways at supra-nuclear level therefore results in '*gaze palsy*' or loss of conjugate movements e.g. vertical gaze palsy is often associated with a lesion at or near the superior corpora quadrigemina. Cortical or subcortical lesions in the frontal area cause irritative manifestations and result in deviation of the eyes to the opposite side while a destructive lesion causes paralysis of movement to the same side as the lesion.

Nuclear Involvement of Oculomotor Nerves

Involvement of sixth nerve nucleus produces a conjugate gaze palsy of ipsilateral side. A co-existing peripheral seventh nerve palsy suggests a lesion in the area of sixth nerve nucleus because of their closeness in the pons. Lesion of the trochlear nerve nucleus alone is rare.

Lesion of third nerve nucleus, when it occurs, is usually bilateral. Vertical conjugate gaze palsies, internal ophthalmoplegia, bilateral ptosis can result from lesions in the area of oculomotor nucleus. A symmetrical ptosis which progresses rapidly is usually indicative of a nuclear lesion.

Infra-nuclear lesions of Oculomotor Nerves

Abducent palsy: The cause of sixth nerve palsy can be non-localizing or localizing. The peripheral course of the sixth nerve is a lengthy one and it predisposes the nerve to get involved by lesions at all levels from brain stem and base of the skull through the petrous tip and cavernous sinus to the superior orbital fissure and orbit. Paralysis of the sixth nerve is a common accompaniment of raised intracranial pressure, whatever the cause. The sixth nerve is fixed to the pons at its exit from brain substance and it is held firmly over the superior border of petrous portion of the temporal bone by the petro-sphenoidal ligament. Any displacement of the brain stem kinks the nerve over the petrous bone and causes palsy. The sixth nerve palsy has therefore none or very limited localising value.

The non-localising causes where the sixth nerve is involved are:
1. Increased intracranial pressure.
2. Following head trauma.
3. Cavernous sinus thrombosis.
4. Diabetes.
5. Basal meningitis.
6. Middle ear infection.
7. Peripheral neuritis of virus etiology.

The localizing involvement of the sixth nerve occurs in:
1. Pontine lesions (Pontine gliomas, pontine infarction and demyelinization).
2. Cerebellopontine angle lesions (acoustic neurinoma, meningioma, etc.)
3. Tumours arising from the middle cranial fossa.
4. Lesions at the cavernous sinus or superior orbital fissure.
5. Carotid-cavernous fistula.

With the diagnosis of isolated sixth nerve palsy in the absence of other localizing signs, one should suspect hypertension or diabetes.

Trochlear palsy: Isolated involvement of the trochlear nerve is rare. In old age, isolated fourth nerve palsy may be associated with diabetes. The other common cause of the isolated fourth nerve palsy is injury.

In clinical examination, the trochlear nerve palsy is less obvious. In a large number of patients, tilting of the head towards the side opposite to the defective eye is seen. To obtain relief from double vision the head is rotated to the sound side and tilted towards the shoulder on that side. In the presence of complete third nerve palsy, it is difficult to test the trochlear nerve, but the presence of intorsion indicates that the superior oblique muscle is functioning. All these patients show vertical deviation in the primary position with increase in deviation on adduction of the involved eye.

Palsy of third nerve: The lesion could be at the inter-peduncular level, in the cavernous sinus, the orbit or at the myo-neural junction.

Inter peduncular lesion: The common conditions that involve oculomotor nerve are aneurysms (posterior communicating artery aneurysm), meningitis and trauma. Tuberculous basal meningitis is still common in which oculomotor palsy can be bilateral with other signs of basal meningitis.

Cavernous sinus lesions: The oculomotor nerve can be involved at the level of the cavernous sinus due to thrombosis, aneurysm, arterio-venous fistula etc.

Orbital lesions: In lesions at the level of apex of the orbit, the third nerve can be involved with other ocular nerves. A recurrent third nerve palsy can occur in diabetes and is usually associated with severe pain in and around the eye.

Lesions at the Level of Myoneural Junction

Ocular myasthenia: Although myasthenia gravis affects many muscles, the ocular signs, particularly ptosis, are frequently the earliest indications or presentation of this disease. The ocular signs are characterized by bilaterality and asymmetry. There is usually reversal or improvement with cholinergic drugs. The onset of this disease can be at any age although common in older people. Muscular weakness in myasthenia is attributed to pre-synaptic disorder of neuro-muscular transmission. This condition has to be differentiated from chronic external ophthalmoplegia where it is bilateral and symmetrical and will not respond to cholinergic drugs. Intravenous injection of 2.5 mgm prostigmin will produce dramatic recovery for myasthenia. The effect of this drug is quite short lived.

Diplopia: Binocular diplopia is characteristic of extraocular peripheral muscle palsies. The type of diplopia and methods of charting have already been described.

OCULAR MANIFESTATIONS IN INTRACRANIAL LESIONS

Papilloedema, Optic Neuritis, Optic Atrophy

60 to 70 per cent of intracranial tumours produce ocular signs and symptoms and the majority of these are of great diagnostic and localizing value. The ocular effects in intracranial tumours may be general due to increased intracranial pressure or focal that are due to localised pressure effects.

Papilloedema

The term papilloedema was described by Parson in 1906 for a swelling of the optic disc. It is defined as passive oedema of the optic disc. This is an important sign in intracranial disease but can also occur in vascular hypertension, severe anaemia, benign rise in intracranial tension and acute leukaemia.

Pathogenesis of papilloedema: The pathogenesis of oedema of optic disc associated with elevated intracranial pressure has been a subject of interest and controversy for more than 100 years. With new additions of anatomical, physiological and pathological observations, numerous theories have been put forward regarding the pathogenesis. It has been postulated that the swelling occurs because the intracranial pressure is transmitted into the vaginal sheaths, compresses the optic nerve and mechanically impedes the circulation. The concept is supported by evidence that the swelling in papilloedema is primarily intracellular.

Experimental models of optic disc swelling have been produced by ocular hypotony. Sohan Singh Hayreh by introducing progressively distended intracranial baloons produced in Rhesus monkeys a condition simulating the growing intracranial space occupying lesion in man. The occurrence and course of oedema of optic disc depended upon the raised cerebrospinal fluid pressure in the cranial sub-arachnoid space and its transmission into the optic nerve sheath. Another hypothesis is that retinal vascular changes are secondary to the oedema and not the cause of it. Compression of these vessels at optic disc produces stasis in the territory drained by them and thus leads to their dilatation. From the multiplicity of theories for pathogenesis of papilloedema, one can conclude that the mechanism is still controversial and variable. Combinations of one or more of the anatomic, vascular, mechanical and metabolic factors are responsible for development of papilloedema.

Ophthalmoscopic appearance of papilloedema: Hyperaemia of optic disc. This is due to capillary dilatation in the optic nerve head. Conditions like hypermetropia and vascular anomalies of the optic disc can mimic hyperaemic disc.

Blurring of the disc margin: The blurring of disc margin is due to swelling of glial cells surrounding nerve fibres. This swelling usually starts on the nasal side at the upper and the lower poles of the optic disc because of the arrangements of the nerve fibres. The temporal margin is the last to become indistinct.

Filling up of the physiological cup: Some observers have described a veil-like tissue filling up the optic cup as the earliest evidence of papilloedema. These changes are presumably due to the distension of the perivascular spaces with fluid. However, this is not a reliable sign for obvious reasons.

Venous dilatations and tortuosity of veins: Frank B. Walsh and William Fletcher Hoyt considered this sign as the most important single evidence in diagnosis of papillodema and this sign becomes more strong if there is a lack of venous pulsation at the optic nerve head.

Elevation of the optic nerve head: Normally the optic disc lies at the same level as the rest of retina. When there is swelling and oedema in the region, the optic disc protrudes forwards and this protrusion may reach upto 7 to 9 dioptres. Because of this, the edges of the optic disc overlie the surrounding retina so that the vessels are not only bent acutely but may be buried by the swollen tissue and their course may be seen interrupted in some places. This sign may not be taken as a single confirmative finding because it may be seen in conditions like drusen of optic nerve head, pseudo-neuritis etc.

Paton's lines: These lines appear only on the temporal side of the disc and are in a vertical direction concentric with the disc margin. As the disc swells, a slight displacement of retina away from the temporal edge of the disc occurs causing a variation of the reflection from the internal limiting membrane which is seen as Paton's lines and which may disappear when oedema increases.

Haemorrhages and exudates: Haemorrhages are in the nerve fibre layer at the disc margin. When there is a single splinter haemorrhage close to the disc, it means that early papilloedema from increased intracranial pressure is the cause. These haemorrhages usually appear as radial and linear in shape.

If papilloedema persists, optic disc suffers further damage and as a result of a progressive lesion of the nerve fibres, the optic nerve becomes atrophic which leads to *post-papilloedematous optic atrophy*. Ophthalmoscopically the peripheral portion of the optic disc becomes greyish white and the veins are less congested. The arteries are also narrowed and there may be sheathing of the vessels due to glial proliferation.

If intracranial pressure is relieved by any means, resolution of papilloedema occurs following reduction of intracranial pressure. The regression of oedema usually follows immediately after the reduction of the increased pressure. The first sign is resolution of hyperaemia of the optic disc and easy recognition of the physiological cup of the optic disc.

Clinical Symptoms of Increased Intracranial Pressure

The symptoms and signs are variable and they are determined by the aetiological factors responsible for the development of papilloedema. However, symptoms like headache, nausea, vomiting, and diplopia are common.

Headache: This is one of the earliest symptom of increased intracranial. The cause of headache in raised intracranial tension is not very clear, but it is considered to be due to the stretching of the meninges. Sharply localized pains may be explained on the basis of involvement of the sensory nerves at the base of the skull or due to localized involvement of the meningeal nerves.

Nausea and vomiting: This could be explained due to herniation of medulla into foramen magnum due to increased intracranial tension irritating the vomiting centre.

Diplopia: It is a common complaint associated with paralysis of oculomotor nerves, more commonly the abducent nerve.

Transient blurring of vision: This is due to compression of the optic nerves in the optic canals or due to spasm of the retinal arteries. Some attribute the transient blindness in raised intracranial tension due to temporary interference with circulation through the posterior cerebral arteries. If obscuration is unilateral, it is suggestive of cerebro-vascular insufficiency. When intracranial tension is relieved, the patient is relieved of these blackouts.

Visual acuity: Visual acuity remains normal or near normal in the early stages of papilloedema and this enables differentiation between papilloedema and optic neuritis. In persistent papilloedema progressing to post-papilloedematous optic atrophy there is definite deterioration of acuity of vision.

Field changes in papilloedema: Papilloedema produces enlargement of blind spot, the size of the enlargement depends upon the extent of the optic disc swelling. This enlargement of the blind spot is due to (a) slight displacement of the retina away from the optic disc which also causes Paton's lines, and (b) a slight serous detachment of the retina away from choriocapillaries causing relative scotoma of overlying sensory retina. The enlargement of blind spot may be the only sign or it may be associated with field defects due to involvement of visual pathway as a result of compression by the tumour. The peripheral fields remain normal in case of papilloedema but in later stages due to continued compression, the peripheral fields may show concentric contraction especially on the nasal side and this may progress if intracranial tension persists.

Fluorescein angiographic studies in papilloedema. This test is useful in distinguishing the true swelling of optic disc from conditions simulating papilloedema. A profuse and persistent pooling of the dye in optic disc and staining of tissue surrounding the optic disc is characteristic of papilloedema. The staining at optic disc may persist even for ten minutes.

Differential diagnosis of papilloedema: Since the diagnosis of papilloedema is important in raised intracranial tension, the ophthalmologist should be able to give a definite opinion whether papilloedema is due to raised intracranial tension or other factors.

1. **Optic neuritis:** The common differential diagnosis is from optic neuritis which is an active inflammatory involvement of the optic nerve and in this condition there will be swelling of the optic disc, blurring of the disc margin etc. Following findings will help to differentiate papilloedema from papillitis. Papilloedema is usually bilateral even though in certain conditions like localised orbital and ocular conditions, it may be unilateral. Optic neuritis is commonly unilateral but it can be bilateral in cases of demyelinating diseases and also in meningitis. The important distinguishing factor is disturbance of visual functions. In optic neuritis visual acuity is grossly disturbed while vision remains almost normal in early cases of papilloedema. The other factor is pain in the eye ball especially on movement of the globe which is an important sign in optic neuritis because the inflammation of the optic nerve can spread to muscles which are close to the nerve. In optic neuritis the characteristic pupillary reaction is Marcus Gun pupillary phenomenon (an initial constriction followed by persistent dilatation) and this is due to disturbance of conductivity of optic nerve whereas pupil reaction in papilloedema is normal.

The swelling of the optic disc is more in papilloedema and comparatively much less in optic neuritis. The visual field defects will help to differentiate papilloedema from papillitis. In papillitis, due to impairment of papillo-macular bundle, there will always be a *central* or *centro-caecal* scotoma, specially for red colour whereas in papilloedema no such scotoma is seen but there will be an *enlargement of the blind spot*. Flurorescein angiography is another important differentiating feature.

2. **Drusen of the optic nerve head:** It is a congenital condition of the optic nerve head where there is deposition of hyaline like substance on optic disc which produces elevation of the optic disc with blurring of the disc margin. This can easily be differentiated from papilloedema by the following factors: In drusen of the optic disc, the elevation is confined only to the optic disc whereas in papilloedema the elevation spreads to adjacent retina. In drusen one can definitely see irregular yellowish white excrescences which is characteristically described as

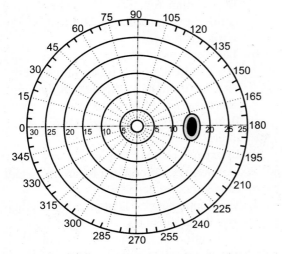

Fig 16.5: Enlarged Blind spot in a case of Papilloedema

mulberry like appearance and is completely absent in papilloedema. In drusen of the optic disc, the veins remain completely normal at the optic disc level and haemorrhages are absent. Both these conditions will show enlargement of the blind spot.

3. **Medulated optic nerve fibres.** It is recognised as white flame shaped streaks of fibres near the disc margin and extending to the adjoining retina. This may give an appearance of blurring of disc margins, but if a person is familiar with the opaque nerve fibres, it is very easy to distinguish one from the other.

4. **Congenital anomalies** of the optic disc like arteriolar malformations, *Bergmeister papilla and coloboma* may mimic papilloedema but other symptoms and signs will help to differentiate one from the other.

Unilateral papilloedema due to intracranial lesion can occur in tumours arising from frontal lobe and olfactory groove. The clinical condition is called *Foster-Kennedy syndrome* which is characterised by papilloedema on the opposite side and optic atrophy on the side of the lesion.

Pressure of the lesion causes atrophy of optic nerve of the side well before intracranial tension is raised. The contralateral nerve responds to raised intracranial tension as the lesion progresses in due course while atrophic ipsilateral nerve does not develop papilloedema.

In case of meningioma of sphenoid ridge and cerebral abscess, papilloedema may be more on one side than on the other.

In an individual who already has optic atrophy due to other aetiological factors, subsequent development of increased intracranial tension cannot produce papilloedema in this atrophic eye but the sound eye can reveal papilloedema.

Inflammations of the Optic Nerve

Inflammation may affect meningeal covering of the optic nerve when it is called *'perineuritis'*.

It may affect the nerve itself, it is then called the *'optic neuritis'*. Inflammation of optic nerve may involve different parts of the nerve from optic disc to optic chiasma. From clinical point of view, inflammation at optic disc level is called *'papillitis'* while inflammation anywhere behind the eye ball is called *'retrobulbar neuritis'*. Wherever the pathology, it causes marked diminution of vision, because it is the principal conducting medium for visual impulses from retina to higher centres.

Aetiology: The causes of optic neuritis are at great variance between those in western countries and those in tropical areas. For example, disseminated sclerosis accounts for more than 60 to 70 per cent cases of optic neuritis in Europe and the United States, while this disease is extremely uncommon in India. The causes of optic neuritis may be grouped as follows:

1. *Systemic causes* like syphilis, tuberculosis, diabetes, virus infections, toxic causes, vitamin deficiency and allergic conditions.

    a. Syphilis causes optic neuritis in the second stage and should be excluded by appropriate laboratory tests in all cases of optic neuritis. Where there is no evident cause, Wasserman reaction of cerebro-spinal fluid may be done in support of the serological reports.

    b. Tuberculosis causes optic neuritis either as a manifestation of tuberculous allergy or a tuberculous pathology in the optic nerve itself. Optic neuritis as an extension from tuberculous meningitis is discussed later.

    c. Intestinal parasites, particularly those circulating in blood can be an important cause of optic neuritis.

    d. Viral optic neuritis is more common than usually appreciated.

    e. A vitaminosis: deficiencies are important causes of optic neuritis. Deficiency of vitamin B_1, B_2, (pellagra), and B_{12} can cause optic neuritis commonly seen in times of famines. Deficiencies during pregnancy and lactation can cause retrobulbar neuritis.

   f. Infectious diseases like smallpox, measles, chickenpox, mumps, Herpes zoster and typhoid can cause optic neuritis.

2. *Extension of inflammation* from neighbouring tissues.

   a. Intraocular conditions: (i) Endophthalmitis and pan-ophthalmitis simultaneously cause papillius, (ii) Posterior Uveitis can extend to involve the optic nerve head to cause neuritis, (iii) Sympathetic ophthalmitis may involve the optic nerve.

   b. Meningeal inflammations extend along the meninges of optic nerve and can cause perineuritis and neuritis. Tuberculous meningitis as a cause of optic neuritis is responsible for blindness in children in many cases. Suppurative meningitis of bacterial origin or meningitis due to viruses can similarly involve the optic nerve.

   c. Paranasal sinusitis of the ethmoids and antrum and periostitis of bones in orbital apex can cause optic neuritis.

   d. Extraction of a septic tooth, if not covered with antibiotics is known to cause optic neuritis.

3. *Demyelinating diseases* are a common cause in western countries. The diseases in this group are multiple sclerosis and neuromyelitis optica (Devic's disease).

4. *Toxic neuritis* or toxic amblyopia due to tobacco, methyl alcohol, lead, arsenic are important causes. Newer drugs are being added to the list which can cause optic neuritis.

5. *Collagen diseases* like temporal arteritis are also associated with optic neuritis.

Clinical picture: The clinical picture of optic neuritis not only depends on the cause but also on the site of inflammation in the course of optic nerve. The main symptom is loss of vision and the signs include ophthalmoscopic appearance and changes in the field of vision.

Vision: Central vision is lost suddenly and to a severe degree. The central field shows central scotoma.

Pain on movement of the eye is due to closeness of origin of extra-ocular muscles and the inflamed meninges of the orbital part of optic nerve.

Pupillary reactions have important diagnostic features: Direct and consensual reactions are present but they are ill sustained and the pupil slowly dilates even when the light is kept on (Marcus Gunn Sign).

Ophthalmoscopic appearance: In retrobulbar neuritis, the optic disc may appear normal and hence the saying that neither the ophthalmologist nor the patient sees anything. In cases of papillitis and when the retrobulbar involvement is close to the eye ball, ophthalmoscopic appearances are characteristic.

– Optic disc is hyperaemic.

– Arteries are narrowed

– Disc margin is blurred, varying from slightly blurred or fluffy disc margins to choked disc but oedema is never more than 2 dioptres.

– Retinal veins are moderately engorged.

    There may be a few haemorrhages and exudates on and around the inflamed disc in acute cases.

– When inflammation of the nerve head has extended to surrounding retina (neuro-retinitis) there may be some amount of retinal oedema and a partial macular star.

– In severe cases, there may be a thin haze in the posterior vitreous.

    If inflammatory process persists, the clinical picture of optic neuritis may change to *post-neuritic optic atrophy.*

Differential diagnosis: Papilloedema is the most important condition to be differentiated. The differentiating features from papilloedema are:

1. No pain on movement of the eye.
2. Central vision is not affected and field changes show only an enlarged blind spot and sector defects due to pressure on visual pathway.
3. Pupillary reaction is normal.
4. Disc swelling is more than 2 dioptres.
5. Veins are markedly engorged.
6. Haemorrhages and exudates are in abundance at and around the disc.

Field studies and radiological examinations will support diagnosis of the papilloedema.

Pseudo-neuritis, commonly associated with gross hypermetropia and irregular astigmatism is easy to differentiate because except the blurring of disc margin, there is no other evidence.

Prognosis: Transient visual improvement is not uncommon but if untreated, the condition goes on to optic atrophy. With effective treatment, the recovery of vision is to be expected unless there is a cause which cannot or has not been treated. Recurrence is common in demyelinating etiology.

Treatment: First consideration is to control the inflammatory reaction to save the nerve from effects of gliosis and permanent damage to vision. Adrenocorticotropic hormone (ACTH) and cortico-steroids are the most important treatment in early and acute stage of the disease. The treatment is best started with ACTH injections twice a day for 5-7 day, followed by full therapeutic doses of cortico-steroids. Antibiotics with heavy doses of Vitamin B-complex by injections are an important supportive therapy in active phases.

Treatment of the cause is *most* important and all positive reports of the investigations should be taken into consideration for long-term treatment. Any surgical interference is rarely if ever, indicated except when the treatment for severe inflammation in sinuses or meninges calls for such interference.

Demyelinating diseases:

1. *Multiple sclerosis or disseminated sclerosis* is a common cause of unilateral retrobulbar neuritis. The fleeting character of neurological manifestations in early stage of the disease show similar transient ocular manifestations. Visual symptoms include transient blurring of vision in one eye which may appear and disappear intermittently. Optic nerve involvement is retrobulbar and therefore optic disc is normal. The characteristic ocular finding is unilateral central scotoma due to involvement of papillo-macular bundle of nerve fibres in retrobulbar course of optic nerve. In chronic stages, vision may be progressively diminished. The temporal pallor of disc gradually changes to optic atrophy.
2. **Neuro-myelitis optica** (Devic's disease). This is also a demyelinating disease with clinical manifestations of bilateral optic neuritis and acute myelitis. Vision is markedly diminished and there is evidence of lower motor neuron type paraplegia.

Optic Atrophy

Optic atrophy is a condition where morphological structure of the optic nerve has been altered and conducting function of the nerve fibres has been disturbed. Clinically the term optic atrophy cannot be precisely defined because there may be good visual function although disc appears atrophic and on the other hand, the vision may be reduced out of proportion to the clinical picture of the disc. The final diagnosis of optic atrophy can therefore only be made with supporting evidence of diminished visual acuity, pupillary reaction and visual field changes. In doubtful cases, ERG, VER and EOG may be helpful.

Clinical confusion can arise when there is a large physiological cupping giving a white central appearance with only a small peripheral rim of normal colour. Generally speaking, optic atrophy is a term used for a white coloured disc. Anything less than white colour is called a pale or very pale disc. It is important to explain that the change in the colour of the disc is largely due to disappearance of vascular capillaries as a result of causative factor. Atrophy of nerve fibres, their sheath and neuroglial degeneration add to the change in the colour of the disc.

Optic atrophy is classified as primary or secondary although this is not a very satisfactory description. The term *primary optic atrophy* is specifically used for optic atrophy due to neuro-syphilis as in Tabes dorsalis and general paralysis of insane. *Secondary optic atrophy* is better classified from the aetiological point of view:
1. Post-neuritic optic atrophy.
2. Post papilloedematous optic atrophy.
3. Consecutive optic atrophy.
4. Vascular optic atrophy.
5. Glaucomatous optic atrophy and Schnabel's cavernous atrophy.
6. Hereditary optic atrophy.
7. Optic atrophy due to miscellaneous causes.

Primary Optic Atrophy

This is a primary degeneration of the optic nerve fibres in fourth stage of neurosyphilis. The ocular changes may be associated with neurological manifestations of lesions in the posterior columns of spinal cord like tabetic gait etc. Optic atrophy may be the first clinical manifestation of tabes dorsalis.

Clinical appearance is of a white chalky coloured disc with central cupping. The margins are clear cut. Blood vessels are usually within normal limits. The fundus is otherwise normal. Vision is reduced and there is peripheral contraction of visual fields. Typical Argyll-Robertson pupil is present in many cases. The diagnosis of tabetic atrophy should however be made only in consultation with a neurophysician because tabes and the GPI as such are uncommon in India.

Post-Neuritic Optic Atrophy

It usually follows papillitis. There is history of sudden diminution of vision followed by transient improvement and then gradually progressive visual deterioration.

Ophthalmoscopically, disc is greyish white in colour, the physiological cup is filled with neuroglial tissue. The disc margin is distinctly blurred but not elevated. Arteries are attenuated and there is perivascular sheathing along blood vessels on disc and upto a disc diameter from the disc margin. Macular degeneration may be seen when inflammatory process has spilled over to the macular area.

Vision is reduced to varying degrees and there is peripheral constriction of field of vision. Pupillary reaction may range from sluggish to absent depending on visual acuity. In unilateral cases, direct reaction is absent but consensual is present in the affected eye.

Post-neuritic atrophy is in some respects akin to post-papilloedematous optic atrophy. The special feature of post-papilloedematous optic atrophy is the *humping of blood vessels* at the disc margin because of the markedly raised level during papilloedema in acute stage, which is not evident in post-neuritic optic atrophy.

Post-Papilloedematous Optic Athrophy

Differs from post-neuritic atrophy by the displacement of blood vessels caused by severe oedema of the disc during acute stage. Perivascular sheathing is usually absent. Evidence of cause of papilloedema is an important differentiating feature. Peripheral constriction of field is identical.

Consecutive Optic Atrophy

Optic atrophy which is a consequence of disease in the neighbouring tissues is called consecutive atrophy. Chorio-retinitis, retinitis pigmentosa, toxic retinopathy, diabetic retinopathy and degenerative myopia cause atrophy because of degenerative process in the nerve fibre layer of retina extends on to optic nerve fibres. The colour of the disc may be anything from waxy pale to greyish white. A clinical picture of chorio-retinitis, myopic degeneration or retinitis pigmentosa will dominate when that is the cause. A pale disc is a very important feature of a diabetic retinopathy even in the early stages.

Vascular Optic Atrophy

A pale disc is a common manifestation in old persons due to arterio-sclerosis and arterial attenuation. This may lead to moderate or severe degree of visual loss. The disc is white when atrophy is due to occlusion of the central retinal artery or following severe anaemia or severe haemorrhage. In addition the arteries may be markedly attenuated or become thready white lines particularly in periphery.

Glaucomatous Optic Atrophy

It is a clinical entity which has characteristic features. There is a large cupping with steep edges and obscuration of vessels behind the cup edge. Raised intra-ocular tension will confirm the diagnosis. It is important to emphasize that the cup and atrophy will persist even if tension is restored to normal by surgery.

Schnabel's cavernous atrophy is a large excavation originally attributed to low tension glaucoma and by some, to degenerative myopia. The condition is however not as specific as originally described.

Leber's Hereditary Optic Atrophy

It is an uncommon disease of hereditary bilateral nature affecting largely males and becoming clinically manifest as about the age of 20 years. Vision is gradually reduced although they do not become totally blind. Central scotoma is an important field change.

Congenital optic atrophy may affect children of a very young age. It is of recessive hereditary origin. Vision is grossly affected. The optic disc is markedly atrophic. Ocular nystagmus is common.

Toxic Atrophy

It is usually the result of toxic amblyopia. The changes in the disc are consequential to degeneration of ganglion cells of retina with atrophy of nerve fibre layer.

Optic Atrophy Due to Deficiency

Temporal pallor of the disc is a common manifestation of deficiency syndrome due to deficiency of Vitamin B_1 and riboflavin.

Temporal pallor of the disc as an abnormal finding is often diagnosed rather indifferently. It is important to emphasize that a shallow physiological cupping often extends to the temporal margin and often gives white appearance.

Treatment of optic atrophy is essentially treatment of the cause of optic atrophy. Once the atrophy has established, vasodilators and Vitamin B complex factors are only a placebo treatment.

TUMOURS OF THE OPTIC NERVE

Common tumours of the optic nerve are gliomata and meningiomata.

Glioma

The glioma is usually evident in the first decade of life and commonly arise in the intraorbital portion of optic nerve. The next common site is chiasma and intra cranial portion of optic nerve.

When the tumour extends towards the optic disc it will be seen ophthalmoscopically. These gliomata are either *astrocytoma or spongioblastoma.* The common symptomatology of these tumours is loss of visual acuity. The loss of visual acuity is likely to be earlier in glioma than in meningioma. *Proptosis is another cardinal sign* in glioma. Radiologically glioma produces enlargement of optic foramen. Field defects start as a central scotoma and may enlarge with growth of the tumour. The course of the tumour is quite slow and treatment is surgical removal through transfrontal route.

Meningioma

Meningioma arises from optic nerve sheath occurring after 30 years of age. These tumours are now known to arise from arachnoid although they are attached to the dura. They are composed of cells similar to fibroblasts and some authors have described them as fibroblastoma. The meningioma arises either near the optic foramen within or outside the muscle cone or near the periorbita. The common symptomatology of these cases is *eccentric proptosis* with restriction of ocular movements. Visual acuity is affected at a later stage. Radiologically these tumours are likely to produce enlargement of optic foramen and optic canal. These tumours do not respond to irradiation and the only treatment is surgical removal either through transfrontal cranial approach or orbital approach depending upon the site.

Apart from these tumours, pigmentary tumours of optic disc are observed infrequently and are called *melanocytoma.* They are seen ophthalmoscopically as darkly pigmented lesion close to the optic disc. *Haemangioma* of the optic disc usually presents as elevated dark red mass over the disc. *Neurofibroma* of the optic disc has also been reported.

The optic nerve can be involved by *secondary tumours* as elsewhere in the body and also from adjacent structures like melanoma of the choroid extending towards the optic disc and retinoblastoma during its intracranial extension.

Visual Fields in Neuro-ophthalmic Conditions

Examination of visual fields helps in localising intracranial lesions along the visual pathway. In some cases, visual field defect may be the only sign indicating presence of an intra-cranial lesion. The examination of the visual field is completely a subjective test and therefore the patient's understanding and co-operation are important for interpretation of the field record.

Common Field Defects in Neuro-ophthalmic Conditions

Blind spot. The blind spot is a physiological scotoma representing the optic nerve head where there are no sensory elements. The scotoma is enlarged in conditions where there is increase in the size of the optic disc, for example, papillo-edema, congenital lesions of the optic nerve head like opaque nerve fibres and drusen of the nerve head.

Central scotoma: It means presence of a non-seeing area at the central fixation spot. This occurs in lesions of macula and also in some lesions of optic nerve.

Centro-caecal scotoma: When the scotoma extends from the fixation point to blind spot, it is called *centro-caecal scotoma.* Such defect is seen in toxic amblopia and tobacco amblyopia.

Homonymous hemianopia: *Homonymous hemianopia* is encountered in lesions of posterior portion of the optic chiasma, optic tracts or optic radiations upto the calcarine cortex. Here the nasal field of one eye and the temporal field of the other eye are affected. This is designated as right or left depending upon the side of the temporal defect. This field defect may be quadrantic instead of hemianopic when corresponding quadrants of field are affected and is called *homonymous quadrantanopia.*

Sparing of the macula: In homonymous hemianopia, when the central line of hemianopic field skirts the central part instead of bisecting it, it is called the sparing of the macula. Macular sparing occurs in lesions of the optic radiation and occipital cortex.

Splitting of macula: The macular splitting is more likely to occur in association with homonymous hemianopia produced by lesions in anterior portion of the optic tract. In macular splitting, there is absolute bisection of fixation point for all the test objects.

Bitemporal hemianopia: This, defect is characteristic of chiasma lesions. Here the temporal fields of both are affected.

Binasal hemianopia: In this defect the nasal fields are lost due to involvement of the uncrossed temporal fibres in each eye. The defect occurs only at the level of optic chiasma with pressure effect at lateral angles of chiasma. This defect is comparatively rare and is seen in aneurysm of one internal carotid artery with displacement of the chiasma against the normal artery on the opposite side, intra ventricular tumours and rarely in meningioma arising from lesser wing of the sphenoid.

Altitudinal Hemianopia

In this condition, either the upper or the lower halves of the fields in both eyes are affected. This defect is commonly due to vascular lesions at the level of the calcarine cortex. It can also occur rarely following a lesion at the level of the optic chiasma.

Importance of Visual Field Defects in Localising Intracranial Tumours

The visual field examination in all neuro-ophthalmic patient is indicated irrespective of whether they complain of defective vision or not Figs 16.6 to 16.9).

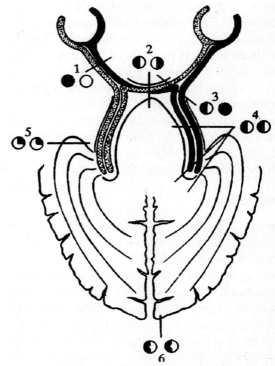

Fig 16.6: Visual Pathway Showing Sites of Total Interruption of Nerve Fibres and Various Abnomal visual Field defects produced by such Interruptions, (1) Optic nerve—blindness on side of lesion with normal contralateral field; (2) Chiasma—bitemporal hemianopia; (3) Optic nerve chiasmal junction, blindness on side of lesion with contralateral temporal hemianopia; (4) Limb of internal capsule—contralateral homonymous hamianopia; (5) Optic radiation—anterior loop in temporal lobe-superior quadrantanopia; (6) Occipital cortex calcarine fissure lesion—contralateral congruous homonymous hemianopia with macular sparing.

Field Defects in Optic Nerve Lesions

The defect can be as a result of congenital lesions, injuries, inflammations, vascular diseases, toxic factors, due to degenerations or by pressure. The field defect due to optic nerve lesions can be best studied by dividing the nerve in three parts:
1. Optic nerve head.

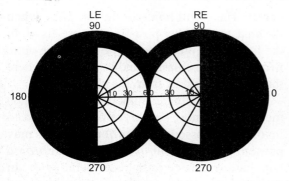

Fig. 16.7: Typical bitemporal hemianopia caused by pressure on chiasma from below and behind.

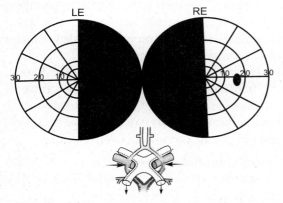

Fig. 16.8: Typical binasal hemianopia due to lesion at the lateral angle of chiasma

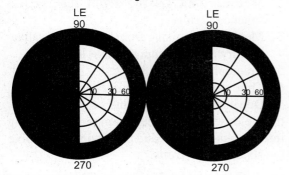

Fig. 16.9: Left homonymous hemianopia due to optic tract lesion

2. Retrobulbar portion of the optic nerve.
3. Intracranial portion of the optic nerve.

Lesion of the optic nerve head: Coloboma of the optic nerve is a result of defective closure of

the foetal cleft. In this condition there will be a nerve fibre bundle defect and this defect depends upon the extent of the coloboma which remains permanent.

Blind spot will be enlarged in cases of congenital drusen of the optic disc.

In myelination of the optic nerve fibres, there may be enlargement of blind spot and if myelination extends well into the retina, there will be corresponding scotoma.

Feld defects in papilloedema: Whatever may be the cause of papilloedema, there will be enlargement of blind spot. This enlargement of blind spot is generalised in all directions and its size varies according to the severity of the condition. Repeated measurement of the size of the blind spot will help in the follow-up. In cases of papilloedema going on to optic atrophy, there will be contraction of peripheral fields due to atrophy. Reduction in the size of the blind spot may be noted due to subsiding oedema.

Field defects in papillitis: There is central, paracentral and centro-caecal defects because of the nerve fibre involvement. Invariably, there will be central scotoma because of macular oedema. Even in cases of retrobulbar neuritis, the characteristic field defects will be central scotoma or centro-caecal scotoma depending upon the axial or peripheral involvement of the nerve.

Field defects in optic nerve lesions: The tumours of optic nerve can cause a central scotoma in early stages but when the scotoma enlarges it breaks into the periphery in the form of sector defect. When tumour involves the chiasma the field defect may occur in the other eye also.

Field defects in intracranial portion of the optic nerve. The lesions which compress the antero-superior aspect of the chiasma (olfactory groove meningioma, aneurysm of the internal carotid artery, dilated third ventricle etc.) the field defect may be a small scotoma or a picture of Foster Kennedy syndrome can be manifested.

Field Defects in Lesions of Optic Chiasma

The optic chiasma is the only portion of the visual pathway where an accurate diagnosis of the intracranial lesion could be made by careful examination of visual fields. This defect differs according to the anatomy of the optic chiasma, fibre arrangements and also in relation to the surrounding structures.

In 80 per cent of cases the optic chiasma lies over the posterior two third of the sella. In 12 per cent of the cases it lies directly over the centre of the sella. In 5 per cent of the cases the optic chiasma is prefixed with short optic nerves and in 3 per cent of the cases the chiasma is post-fixed with long optic nerves. The field defects are produced in lesions of optic chiasma as a result of direct compression, traction, vascular disturbances and lacerations. The field defects may be classified according to whether pressure on chiasma is from below (Infrachiasmatic), from above (Suprachiasmatic), from sides (Perichiasmatic) or Retrochiasmatic.

Infra-chiasmatic: The most common infrachiasmatic lesion comprises of pituitary adenoma which exerts pressure on the postero-inferior part of chiasma. The typical field defects in most cases is a symmetrical bitemporal hemianopia. Chromophobe adenoma is the most frequent infrachiasmatic lesion (75%). It is characterised by the classical *bitemporal defect*, *primary optic atrophy* and the *enlargement of sella turcica* with hormonal disturbances. As the pressure is from below, the defect starts from the upper temporal quadrant gradually extending on to the lower. The colour fields, especially for red, are important for early diagnosis of sellar lesion. In early cases of chromophobe adenoma peripheral fields may be normal for white test objects but colour fields may reveal bitemporal

defect. There will however be variations when the chiasma is either post-fixed or pre-fixed. In the former the pressure will be where the optic nerves join the chiasma and in the latter where the optic tracts start from the chiasma.

Sometimes pituitary tumours may press upon the posterior most portion of optic chiasma to involve the crossed macular fibres and this may present with *bitemporal central scotoma* without any change in the peripheral fields. In such cases the diagnosis will be obviously missed if central fields are not recorded. The prognosis for vision in pituitary tumour will depend upon duration and the grade of compression. Even large field defects may recover provided duration of the compression is short.

If the visual acuity is grossly reduced and if the field defect extends beyond the centre of fixation, the visual prognosis is guarded because hemianopic defect may extend into the nasal field and ultimately lead to total loss of vision.

Supra-chiasmatic lesions. The lesions which commonly involve antero-superior aspect of optic chiasma are:
1. Olfactory groove meningioma.
2. Meningioma arising from the medial sphenoidal ridge.
3. Meningioma arising from tuberculum sallae.
4. Aneurysm at the supraclenoid level.
5. Craniopharyngioma.
6. Third ventricle dilatation.

Depending on the type and site of the lesion, the field defect may be bitemporal involving inferior quadrant first and proceeding to involve the superior quadrants.

Peri-chiasmatic lesions: The common conditions that produce peri-chiasmatic lesions are basal meningitis, basal arachnoiditis and aneurysms arising from the circle of Willis.

Aneurysms of internal carotid artery may give rise to lateral pressure on chiasma whereas the supraclenoid aneurysm causes pressure from above and causes corresponding field defects. Aneurysm of anterior cerebral artery may give rise to a bilateral field defect or blindness in one eye and temporal hemianopia in the other eye.

The chiasma is closely related to sphenoid sinus inferiorly. Floor of sphenoid sinus forms roof of the nasopharynx. Tumours of the nasopharynx can compress the optic chiasma by eroding the floor of the sphenoid sinus.

Field Defects in Lesions of Optic Tract and Behind

This group includes optic tract, lateral geniculate body, optic radiation and the visual cortex. Vascular lesions play an important role in the post-chiasma visual pathway. Lesions of optic tract are uncommon because it is relatively protected by the overlying brain. The characteristic visual field defect produced by lesions of optic tract is homonymous hemianopia which is incomplete and incongruous with no macular sparing and sometimes with actual macular splitting.

Aneurysms arising from the posterior communicating artery or from the internal carotid artery may press upon optic tract and cause field changes. Basal inflammations like meningitis may involve optic tract by infiltration or by endarteritis and produce field defects.

When there is a homonymous hemianopic defect either congruous or incongruous with no macular sparing, with no fundus pathology and no pupillary abnormality, one should think of optic tract involvement.

Lateral geniculate body: The visual field changes due to lesions in the lateral geniculate body are difficult to diagnose because they are identical with those caused by lesions in posterior part of optic tract or anterior part of optic radiations. Because of the close association of geniculate body with thalamus, features like

hemi-anaesthesia may be seen on the side of the field defect and *hemiplegia* on the opposite side due to pyramidal involvement.

Field defects in lesions of the optic radiations: A vascular lesion at optic radiations is fairly common at internal capsule level. Occlusion of branches of middle cerebral artery can account for hemianopia of congruous type, hemiplegia and hemi-anaesthesia.

If the lesion is in the upper portion of the optic radiation which is situated in posterior inferior parietal lobe, the resulting field defect will be contralateral inferior homonymous quadrantic defect. The lesion in the lower part of the optic radiations passing through temporal lobe produces an upper quadrantic field defect and a lesion in the upper part of temporal lobe results in complete hemianopia which is quite indistinguishable from an occipital lobe lesion.

Field defects in lesions of the occipital cortex: The visual cortex is mainly supplied by posterior cerebral artery and also small portion from the meningeal plexus formed by the middle, anterior and posterior cerebral arteries.

The characteristic visual field defect in occipital lobe lesion is congruous homonymous hemianopia with macular sparing. When the lesion compresses the upper or lower lip of the calcarine fissure, the resulting field defect will be of quadrantic or altitudinal type.

Vascular lesions are much more likely to produce field defects than tumours. An isolated and complete hemianopia is commonly due to occlusion of posterior cerebral artery. The macular area escapes because of dual blood supply from the middle cerebral artery. The pupillary reactions are normal.

Radiology of the Sellar Region

In 90 per cent of tumours in and around chiasma, there are some changes in the bone. The pituitary fossa may be enlarged with decalcification and in some cases it is deformed with definite shortening or truncation of the dorsum. Suprasellar calcifications are seen approximately in 56 per cent of cases. In chromophobe adenoma, the sella is definitely enlarged in all measurements—linear, area wise and volumetric. Adenoma tends to round pituitary fossa giving rise to the feature known as ballooning. Erosion of clinoid processes is a common early pressure effect (Figs 16.10 and 16.11).

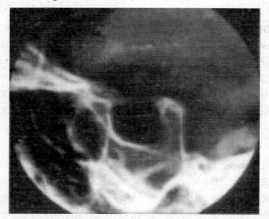

Fig. 16.10: X-ray showing Ballooned Sella due to Intra-sellar pituitary Adenoma

Nystagmus and Nystagmography

Nystagmus is involuntary oscillating movement of eye balls. It may be horizontal, vertical or rotatory nystagmus depending on the direction of the excursion of the eye. The common causes of nystagmus are:

1. *Congenital nystagmus* is due to congenital anomalies like albinism and spasmus nutans.
2. *Ocular nystagmus* is due to gross retinal dysfunction caused by binocular pathology before the age of 1 year. It is usually pendulous in nature with to and fro excursion of movements being equal in extent and speed.

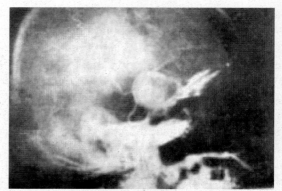

Fig. 16.11: X-ray showing a suprasellar Aneurysm causing Bilemporal Hemianopia. (Note the feeding blood vessels

3. *Vestibular nystagmus* is jerky in nature with a fast and slow component. The nystagmus is enhanced when looking in the direction of the fast element and inhibited when looking in the direction of the slow component. As the term explains, the vestibular nystagmus is due to disturbance in the cochlea and semicircular canals of the ear.
4. *Cerebellar nystagmus.* It is irregular saccadic movement of the eyes and as the term explains, it is due to cerebellar lesions.
5. *Cerebral nystagmus.* Due to lesions in basal ganglion and supra-nuclear palsies and is typically present in Huntington's chorea.
6. *Opiokinetic nystagmus* is a nystagmus artificially induced by making the patient look at a drum with alternating white and black lines. It is used in detecting malingering and evaluating whether the child is blind or has some vision.

Apart from clinical examination, nystagmus can be objectively recorded by an amplifier indicating the electrical potential produced in muscles during the different components of nystagmus. The procedure is called *nystagmography*.

17

Systemic Diseases and Important Ocular Manifestations

The eye ball is an integral part of the body and, therefore, shares advantages of good health and suffers from ill effects of many systemic diseases. It is true to say that having become an ophthalmologist one cannot cease to be a physician. This background is important because many a times a physician is dependent on the ophthalmologist whose findings and their interpretations are important for clinching a diagnosis. Similarly, an ophthalmologist sometimes cannot co-relate his findings without the help of examination by the physician.

Tuberculosis, syphilis and leprosy are diseases which can be responsible for many ocular lesions. Many of these lesions are directly or indirectly responsible for blindness.

The next group of systemic diseases, lesions of the nervous system are closely related to ophthalmic findings and hence the importance of the subject of neuro-ophthalmology. Vascular pathology, metabolic diseases and endo-crinal disorders are particularly significant for the ophthalmologist who should understand fundamentals of these diseases if he were to dependably guide the physician in co-relating the findings of both. Lastly, congenital anomalies of the eye ball and its adnexa are not uncommonly co-existing with congenital and developmental systemic anomalies.

It is not possible to discuss the whole of medical ophthalmology in a book like this. Those systemic conditions which cause significant ocular changes and which call for a frequent reference from the physician to the ophthalmologist or from the ophthalmologist to a physician are discussed here.

TUBERCULOSIS

Tuberculosis in developing and poorer countries continues to be a major health problem. Poor nutrition, congested localities with poor ventilation are some factors which help spread of tuberculosis and its persistence.

Tuberculous infection may affect any tissue of the eye ball except the lens and indirectly even the lens. Tuberculous pathology may present various clinical manifestations.

A. **The primary complex** in children is a tubercular infection before the system has time to develop immunity. Many children pass through this process under a mistaken diagnosis of typhoid or other non-specific illnesses. Most of these children develop some degree of immunity and become tuberculin positive for the rest of their lives. The Mantoux reaction is therefore more often positive even in otherwise normal individuals in countries like India.

B. **Acute milliary tuberculosis** is an acute dissemination of the disease in different tissues of the body. Milliary tubercles of very small size may involve lungs and be seen on the iris, choroid and the retina.

C. **Tubercular nodules** with caseation in the centre affecting primarily the lungs cause generalised tubercular manifestations. These tubercles may also be in conjunctiva, uveal tissue, retina, optic nerve, orbit and extraocular muscles.

D. **Tubercular lymphadenopathy** which is commonly present in the mediastinum and the triangles of the neck, even though there is no infection in the lungs, is another common tubercular affection.

E. **Tubercular allergy** is responsible for many lesions which for long had been considered idiopathic and non-specific. Tissues develop sensitisation to tuberculous proteins circulating in blood but the lesions do not show any characteristic histology of tuberculosis.

F. **Tuberculous ulcers** of the skin (lupus vulgaris) may involve the lids and conjunctiva in ulcerative pathology.

G. **Bovine tuberculosis** of the intestines does not cause any ocular manifestations and is, therefore, not important for an ophthalmologist.

Tuberculosis as a possible cause for ocular inflammations should, therefore, be uppermost in the mind of an ophthalmologist practising in a tropical country. It should be emphasised that ocular tissues are highly sensitive to tuberculous allergy. The list of allergic ocular manifestations is important.

a. Phlyctenular ophthalmia.
b. Episcleritis and Scleritis.
c. Interstitial keratitis.
d. Iridocyclitis
e. Disseminated choroiditis.
f. Exudative retinitis.
g. Retinal periphlebitis.
h. Central serous retinopathy.
i. Coat's disease.
j. Optic neuritis.
k. Tuberculoma; orbital, conjunctival, iris etc.

Tuberculosis as a cause of these specific lesions of ocular tissues has been referred to and discussed in appropriate places.

For the reasons that tuberculosis is a common possible cause of ocular lesions, anti-tubercular therapy should be considered where no etiology is defined and where other non-specific therapies have failed. Whatever therapy is given, whether by parenteral or oral routes, a minimum of three week's course is necessary to evaluate the response. If the response is favourable, the treatment should be continued for at least three months. Guidance of a physician in this matter will always be helpful.

LEPROSY (Hansen's Disease)

The word Hansen's is commonly used for exchange between medical personnel when the patient need not hear the word 'leprosy'. Leprosy has unfortunately been considered synonymous with a 'bad' disease in 'bad' people. This is neither true not correct. Although believed to be so, leprosy is not transmitted from one individual to other unless there is a prolonged physical contact.

Leprosy is a disease much more common in tropical countries and in poorer communities living in congested areas. Lepra bacillus, the causative organism, is a neurotropic organism and its infection is a significant and indolent cause of blindness in leprosy patients.

There are two clinical types of leprotic manifestations:

1. Nerve (tuberculoid) type.
2. Nodular (lepromatous) type.

The nerve or tuberculoid type of leprosy is relatively quieter and a chronic disease. Anaesthesia of the skin, peripheral neuritis with facial paralysis and *consequent paralytic ectropion* and *lagophthalmos* cause corneal complications. Thickening of the ulnar nerve is commonly looked for, for diagnosis.

Lepromatous nodules are a mass of granulation tissue with giant cells and lepra bacilli in abundance. These nodules are commonly seen on the face, giving the characteristic repulsive appearance. The nodules may appear in the conjunctiva and may cause deep parenchymatous keratitis. Leprotic pannus and corneal anaesthesia are commonly associated with keratitis. Subacute or chronic iridocyclitis is the most disabling cause of visual loss in leprosy patients. Leprotic nodules may involve choroid and retina. The presence of lepra bacilli can be microscopically identified in most of these lesions.

Lepra reaction as a manifestation of an acute tissue reaction, like the Herxheimer reaction in syphilis, can become an acute problem requiring urgent anti-anaphylactic treatment.

SYPHILIS

Syphilis is common in all countries; developing or developed, though at different phases in different environments like tabes dorsalis in neurosyphilis is common in Europe and extremely uncommon in countries like India. On the other hand, manifestations of primary and secondary syphilis are uncommon in Europe where treatment is taken early in the disease, while neglect, poverty and ignorance make people suffer from early stages of the disease, in tropical countries.

Syphilis can readily be transmitted from parents to children and, therefore, may present as a manifestation of congenital syphilis. When acquired later in life, syphilis passes through the stages of *primary chancre, secondary syphilis,*

tertiary syphilis and *neuro-syphilis*. It is understandable that congenital syphilis first presents as a stage of secondary syphilis because the primary stage is in parents.

Although an untreated syphilitic infection can be readily confirmed by serological tests, it is not uncommon to come across negative reactions because of penicillin therapy so frequently taken by parents for one or the other body infections. A negative serological reaction, therefore, should not always be accepted as absence of syphilis. Wasserman reaction performed on cerebrospinal fluid may sometimes give a positive result where a Kahn's test or VDRL have been reported negative.

There is no system in the body which escapes syphilitic affection and so also no tissue of the eye ball. The clinical manifestations due to syphilitic infection of different tissues of eye ball are described in appropriate places. A concise list of these is however given for various stages of syphilis:

A. *Primary chancre* in the lids is mentioned though hardly ever seen
B. *Secondary syphilis,* when serological reaction becomes positive, may cause:
   i. Ulcerative blepharitis.
   ii. Granular conjunctivitis.
   iii. Dacryoadenitis.
   iv. Alopecia and vitiligo.
   v. Iridocyclitis.
   vi. Exudative Chorio-retinitis.
   vii. Optic neuro-retinitis and post-neuritic atrophy.
   viii. Disseminated choroiditis
   ix. Macular choroiditis.
   x. Syphilitic basal meningitis with ocular palsies.
C. *Tertiary or gummatous stage.* Clinically appears two to ten years after infection, the serological reaction continues to be positive though less frequently. The ocular manifestations may be:

i. Gummatous ulcers of the lids.
ii. Syphilitic tarsitis.
iii. Alopecia of lashes and brows.
iv. Orbital periosteitis causing superior orbital fissure syndrome with ocular palsies.
v. Interstitial keratitis.
vi. Episcleritis and scleritis.
vii. Scleral gumma.
viii. Sclerosing keratitis.
ix. Chronic iridoyclitis—granulomatous.
x. Disseminated choroiditis, secondary retinitis pigmentosa and salt pepper fundus.
xi. Gummatous nodules in iris, ciliary body and choroid.
xii. Heterochromia iris.
xiii. Retinal haemorrhages.
xiv. Central vein thrombosis.
xv. Ocular manifestations due to syphilitic arteritis like pulseless disease and carotid arteritis.

D. *Neuro-syphilis:*
a. Tabes dorsalis with characteristic tabetic primary bilateral optic atrophy, Argyll-Robertson pupil and neurogenic heterochromia.
b. General Paralysis of Insane (GPI) with Argyll-Robertson pupil and rarely primary optic atrophy.

Congenital Syphilis

Congenital syphilis starts with manifestations of secondary stage although the primary infection has already caused certain changes.

An ophthalmologist should be able to identify stigmata of congenital syphilis which should attract his attention to the possibility of syphilis as a cause of ocular manifestation.

Stigmata of Congenital Syphilis

i. Frontal bosses.
ii. Depressed bridge of nose.
iii. Perforated nasal septum.

iv. Cicatrices at the angles of mouth.
v. Hutchinson's teeth which are widely spaced apart, narrower at apices with notches in the crown.
vi. Hard-shotty lymph glands in neck.
vii. Pigeon chest with protruding sternum.
viii. Sabre tibia with periosteal nodules.

Ocular Manifestations Are

i. Typical bilateral interstitial keratitis with salmon patches of vascularisation in the cornea,
ii. Salt-pepper fundus.
iii. Though less commonly, other manifestations of secondary and tertiary syphilis may be manifest.

GONORRHOEA

Gonococcal infection has, in the pre-penicillin era been the cause of ophthalmia neonatorum in most cases and an important cause of corneal blindness in children. The original Crede's method of prophylaxis by routine instillation of 1% silver nitrate in eyes of new born infants (replaced by penicillin drops 10,000 units per cc) reduced the incidence of ophthalmia neonatorum. Better maternity facilities, more hygienic methods and the effectiveness of penicillin as a therapeutic agent against gonococcus have now reduced the incidence of ophthalmia neonatorum to a rarity in most countries.

Apart from ophthalmia neonatorum, gonococcal infection can cause purulent conjunctivitis (blenorrhoea) in adults where the infection is transmitted from the genitals to the eye through hands or clothes.

The most important ocular manifestations are due to metastatic endogenous gonorrhoeal infection with arthritis, dacryoadenitis, tenonitis and iridocyclitis. Gonococcal iridocyclitis has characteristic features of gelatinous exudates in the anterior chamber and hyphaema.

DISEASES OF THE NERVOUS SYSTEM

1. *Intracranial Space Occupying Lesions*
   These are conditions which often cause ocular manifestations in which the neuro-physician/surgeon and the ophthalmologist very often need the help of each other. The subject is dealt with in the chapter on neuro-ophthalmology giving details of ocular findings and visual field changes.
2. *Inflammations of Meninges and Brain*

Meningitis. This is due to inflammation of the meningeal coverings of the brain and is commonly associated with febrile reaction and its manifestation in other parts of the body. The meningeal coverings of the brain continue as meningeal coverings of the optic nerve. Infections, inflammations and tissue reaction from meninges can therefore easily extend into the orbit and the eye ball. Furthermore, meningitis may involve cranial nerves during their course across the intracranial cavity and cause ocular palsies.

Meningitis is commonly viral, meningo-coccal or tubercular. Viral and meningo-coccal meningitis can cause:

a. Conjunctivitis.
b. Keratitis.
c. Uveitis.
d. Retinal periphlebitis.
e. Papillitis.
f. Optic neuritis.
g. Muscle palsies, usually the sixth nerve.

Tubercular meningitis is more common in tropical countries and is an important cause of blindness in children. The ocular manifestations in tubercular meningitis are:

a. Optic neuritis.
b. Consecutive optic atrophy.

It is as important to minimise loss of vision as to save the life of the patient, if a situation is to be avoided that the patient has survived but has to live a blind life.

Encephalitis is an inflammation of the brain and the systemic manifestations usually overshadow the ocular findings. Encephalitis is commonly of viral origin. It can also be caused by bacteria and parasites.

The ocular manifestations of encephalitis are:

a. Papillitis.
b. Optic atrophy.
c. Visual pathway lesions causing field changes.
d. Ocular palsies.
e. Cerebral blindness.

Hydrocephalus means blockage to the circulation of cerebro-spinal fluid and consequent accumulation within the cranial cavity. The blockage commonly takes place either in the aqueduct of Sylvius between the third and fourth ventricles or in the foramina of Magendie and Luschka which provide a communication between the cerebro-spinal fluid in the meningeal space and intra-cerebral ventricles. It may rarely be caused by blockage at the level of the foramen magnum.

Hydrocephalus is usually congenital but may be acquired later in life. The clinical manifestations, therefore, depend on the age at which it develops.

Congenital hydrocephalus is associated with an enlarged skull and separation of the sutures. Ocular manifestations are:

i. Optic atrophy.
ii. Proptosis.
iii. Limitations of eye movements.

Papilloedema is not a common manifestation because the enlargement of the skull compensates for the rise of intra-cranial tension.

Acquired internal hydrocephalus may be inflammatory in origin or can also be due to brain tumours. As the skull sutures are firmly closed, it causes symptoms of raised intra-cranial tension like headache and vomiting. The important ocular manifestations are:

i. Papilloedema.
ii. Visual field changes characteristic of the site of lesion.
iii. Ocular palsies, commonly sixth nerve.

Devic's disease (Neuro-myelitis Optica). This is a demyelinating disease of visual pathways and the spinal cord, commonly affecting children and adolescents. The important systemic manifestation is paraplegia. The ocular manifestations may be:

i. Acute optic neuritis, usually bilateral,
ii. Consecutive optic atrophy,
iii. Nystagmus.

Disseminated sclerosis (multiple sclerosis). The disease is extremely uncommon in India while it is common in Europe and largely affects adults. This is a demyelinating disease, probably viral in origin affecting the myelin sheath covering of nerves. The lesions are usually patchy with intermittent exacerbations. Systemic manifestations are both sensory and motor.

The ocular manifestations are:

i. Optic neuritis, usually retro-bulbar and fleeting in character.
ii. Central scotoma.
iii. Consecutive optic atrophy.
iv. Argyll-Robertson pupil.
v. Muscle palsies, sometimes conjugate in nature.
vi. Nystagmus.

Syringomyelia: This is a degenerative disease causing cavities in the cervical spinal cord and the brain stem. The typical neurological manifestations are due to cervical cord lesions causing sensory loss and muscle palsies in the face and upper extremities. The ocular manifestations are:

i. Horner's syndrome.
ii. Neuroparalytic keratitis.
iii. Heterochromia iris.
iv. Ocular palsies.
v. Nystagmus, usually rotatory.

Poliomyelitis: This is a virus disease affecting children and involves spinal cord. The disease may ascend upwards and may involve brain-stem when it is called bulbo-myelitis. The ocular manifestations more often seen in bulbo-myelitis are:

i. Ocular palsies III, IV and VI nerves.
ii. Pupillary and accommodation paralysis.
iii. Rarely optic neuritis and papilloedema.
iv. Ptosis due to sympathetic lesion in cervical poliomyelitis.

Horner's syndrome: This is a syndrome caused by a lesion in the course of the cervical sympathetic chain. The lesion may be in the superior cervical sympathetic ganglion and cervical sympathetic plexus along the internal carotid artery in the neck. The manifestations are commonly unilateral causing decrease in sweating of the face and flushing of the skin on one side. The unilateral ocular manifestations are:

i. Ptosis on the side of the lesion.
ii. Miosis of the pupil on the same side.
iii. Inequality of accommodation in two eyes.
iv. Slight lowering of intra-ocular tension on the same side.

Myasthenia gravis: This is a disease of unknown etiology caused by defective formation or storage of acetyl choline at myoneural junctions resulting in weakness of muscles. The manifestations are usually transient and symptoms are relieved with rest.

The ocular manifestations are:

i. Intermittent ptosis.
ii. Deficient convergence.
iii. Accommodation palsy.
iv. External ophthalmoplegia involving one or more muscles.

The characteristic transient nature of the manifestations should always invite consideration of this possibility when no organic cause can be detected. The symptoms are more common after exertion and ocular complaints present themselves in later part of the day. A diagnostic test is the injection of neostigmine, an anti-cholinestrase drug, following which myasthenic ptosis promptly disappears.

Parkinsonism (Paralysis agitans): This is an old age degenerative disease involving corpus striatum. The characteristic systemic manifestations are a typical blank facial expression, Parkinsonian gait due to rigidity of the muscles and tremors in the hands. The ocular manifestations may be:

i. Facial spasms or twitchings.
ii. Ocular palsies.
iii. Ptosis.

Cerebellar Ataxia, Friedreich's is a hereditary disease, commonly affecting young children. Degenerative pathology is in spino-cerebellar tracts and therefore causes progressive ataxia. The ocular manifestations are:

i. Nystagmus,
ii. Pupillary paralysis,
iii. Gaze palsy,
iv. Optic atrophy.

Chorea is a degenerative condition involving basal ganglia and cerebral cortex. The Huntington's chorea is hereditary in nature and is associated with mental deterioration. Ocular associations are:

i. Facial spasm,
ii. Lid retraction,
iii. Irregular eye movements.

Cerebral diplegia (Little's disease). The condition is a bilateral spastic paralysis of the limbs since birth caused by abiotrophy of cells of the cerebral cortex and the cerebellum. The ocular associations are:

i. Micro-ophthalmos.
ii. Congenital cataract.
iii. Retinal degeneration.
iv. Optic atrophy.
v. Nystagmus.

Epilepsy: This is a fairly common condition with recurrent fits of transient unconsciousness and spastic rigidity of the limbs. The disease may be idiopathic or secondary to intra-cranial lesions. Ocular manifestations are usually noted during an attack and are:

i. Conjugate deviation of the eyes.
ii. Squint.
iii. Nystagmus.
iv. Pupils are first small and later become dilated.
v. Visual hallucinations may precede an attack.
vi. Pigmentary retinal dystrophy may be coincidental.

Hepato-lenticular degeneration (Wilson's disease): This is a hereditary disease due to disturbance of copper metabolism with accumulation of the metal in liver, brain and the kidneys. The systemic manifestations are cirrhosis of liver and neurological features due to lesions of cerebral cortex and basal ganglia. The ocular manifestations are:

The pigment ring in the cornea called the *Kayser-Fleischer ring* best seen with a slit lamp intralimbal deep near the descemet's layer. It may be an incomplete or a complete ring. The colour of the ring is a mixture of red-green-blue and yellow shades.

ENDOCRINAL DISEASES

The pituitary, thyroid and parathyroid glands cause ocular changes either directly or indirectly.

Pituitary Disorders

The pituitary as the leader of endocrinal orchestra is the most important endocrine gland for ophthalmologist because it not only affects the eye through endocrinal systemic disorders but can also affect visual functions due to its close anatomical relationship to optic chiasma and optic tracts.

The pituitary gland is located in the pituitary fossa on the upper surface of body of sphenoid bone and is covered by a fibrous sheath called *diaphragmatic sella*. The pituitary gland is nearest to the posterior and inferior surface of optic chiasma in front and lies medial to optic tracts as they emerge from optic chiasma.

Pituitary gland consists of two parts: The posterior and anterior lobes. The posterior lobe secretes pituitarin which is a vasopresser, anti-diuretic and a contractor of the smooth muscles. All these actions of the posterior pituitary do not directly concern the ophthalmologist.

The anterior lobe which develops from the Rathke's pouch as an ectodermal invagination from the roof of mouth concerns ophthalmologist in more than one way. The anterior lobe of pituitary has two types of cells, the acidophilic cells and the basophilic cells. The acido-philic cells are mainly concerned with skeletal growth, the hypersecretion of which causes *gigantism* and *acromegally* while hyposecretion from them results in *dwarfism* and *cretinism*. The basophilic cells secrete various hormones like thyrotropic hormone, excess of which causes exophthalmos and the adrenocortico-tropic hormone, which stimulates the production of corticosteroids by the adrenal cortex. The anterior pituitary also controls pancreas through glycotropic hormone. Other hormones of the anterior pituitary like lactogenic, gonadotropic hormones are not important in ophthalmology.

The clinical manifestations of anterior pituitary endocrinal disorders cause the following conditions:

1. Hyper-pituitarism
   a. Gigantism in childhood.
   b. Acrogemally in adults.
   c. Thyrotoxicosis.
   d. Thyrotropic exophthalmos.
   e. Hyperglycaemia and Glycosuria.
2. Hypopituitarism.
   a. Dwarfism.
   b. Cretinism.
   c. Hypothyroidism.
   d. Hypogonadism.
   e. Adreno-cortical insufficiency.
   f. Simmond's disease.
   g. Frolic's dystrophia-adiposo-genitalis as in Laurence Moon-Biedl syndrome.
3. **Pituitary tumours cause visual field and optic nerve changes**: Most of the tumours are chromophobe adenomata of the anterior lobe and cause enlargement of pituitary fossa, pressure on optic chiasma and anterior part of optic tract and systemic endocrine changes.

Ocular Changes due to Pituitary Tumours Are

a. Typical field changes commonly starting as upper temporal quadrantic hemianopic defect developing into full bitemporal hemianopia. An atypical field change may be due to altered anatomical relationship of optic chiasma or when the tumour presses more on the optic tract.
b. Optic atrophy.
c. Ocular palsies when the tumour has markedly grown laterally.
d. Papilloedema is not a common manifestation of pituitary tumour but may rarely develop if the tumour is so large as to cause raised intracranial tension.

Pituitary tumours are often first diagnosed by an ophthalmologist on the basis of field changes, X-ray of pituitary fossa and sometimes systemic endocrinal manifestations. The importance of early diagnosis is to indicate radical treatment of tumour before visual loss has become irreparable. Once optic atrophy sets in, vision does not return even if the tumour is successfully removed surgically.

Thyroid Disorders

The thyroid gland is of particular importance to the ophthalmologist. The secretions of the thyroid gland are thyroxine and tri-iodo-thyronine, both act by increasing basal metabolism.

Hyperthyroidism with excess secretion of thyroxine causes thyrotoxicosis as in Grave's disease. Hyperfunction of thyroid is the result of disorders of pituitary-thyroid axis, the thyrotropic hormone of pituitary controlling the formation of thyroxine. The whole symptom-complex is probably an auto-immune reaction originating in hypothalamus which produces thyrotropic release hormone which in turn releases thyrotropic hormone from pituitary which controls thyroxine formation. The pathological change in tissues is deposition of mucopolysaccharides. Neuro-muscular manifestations are due to increased sympathetic tone.

Hypothyroidism causes cretinism in children and myxoedema in adults. Cretinism is characterised by retarded skeletal growth and mental retardation. The infant is lethargic with a broad puffy face, flat nose and epicanthus, the tongue is enlarged and skin dry and thickened.

Myxoedema presents a similar clinical picture in normally grown adults with a hoarse voice, loss of eyebrows and goitre due to iodine deficiency.

Parathyroid Disorders

Parathyroid gland secretes parathormone, an excess of which causes hyper-calcaemia, increased absorption of calcium from bones and renal failure.

Hypoparathyroidism causes hypocalcaemia, increased phosphorus in the serum causing increased excitability of nervous tissue. The clinical condition caused is *tetany with muscular spasm* in the hands and feet and cataract. A diagnostic feature is twitching and spasm of the face and lids when the facial nerve is lightly hit with the finger as it crosses the neck of the mandible.

Adrenal Gland Disorders

Although a small structure situated at the upper pole of kidneys, the adrenal glands play an important role in the well-being of the body and are responsible for the capacity to withstand stresses and strains of life. The adrenal glands act under the influence of pituitary and pituitary gland in turn is controlled by hypothalamus. The important secretion from adrenocortex is corticosteroids. The adreno-corticotropic hormone of anterior pituitary controls adrenocortex activity. The medulla of the adrenal glands secrets adrenaline which is a vasoconstrictor and a stimulant to sympathetic nervous system.

Hyperfunction of adrenal gland causes Cushing's syndrome, the ocular manifestation of which may be hypertensive retinopathy. Hypofunction causes Addison's disease, the latter is clinically manifested by low blood pressure, hyperpigmentation in lids, conjunctiva and mucous lining of the mouth.

METABOLIC DISORDERS

The important metabolic disorders which cause ocular changes, fall in three categories, carbohydrate metabolic defect, the lipid metabolic defect and protein metabolic disorder. Some metabolic disorders are inborn. Typical examples are alkaptonuria, cystinuria, albinism, etc.

Carbohydrate Metabolic Disorders

Diabetes Mellitus is the commonest carbohydrate disorder. The incidence of diabetes is rapidly increasing with increasing urbanisation and industrialisation. So much so that in Western countries it is one of the major causes which can lead to incurable blindness in elderly people. There is already enough evidence that it is happening in India too and blindness due to diabetes is acquiring national significance.

Diabetes mellitus is due to deficiency or non-utilisation of insulin which is produced from beta cells of the islets of Langerhans in the pancreas. Insulin is necessary for utilisation of glucose which is a vital source of energy. Failure of proper glucose metabolism leads to increased production of fatty acids resulting in excessive fatty acid and acetone accumulation in blood which can produce acidosis, ketosis and coma.

There are two type of diabetes.

    I. Insulin dependent

    II. Insulin resistant

Type I: This diabetes is due to failure of pancreas to produce enough insulin and is therefore called *insulin dependent diabetes.*

It is common in young patients suffering from juvenile diabetes. It is acute in onset with symptoms of polyuria, polydypsia and loss of weight. Diabetic retinopathy becomes manifest 15-20 years after onset of diabetes. This type of diabetes is best treated with insulin.

Type-II: This type of diabetes is due to non-utilisation of insulin. Enough insulin may be produced by pancreas but it is not utilised to metabolise sugar and carbohydrates. It is therefore called *insulin resistant nondependant diabetes.* Diabeto-genic hormone of anterior pituitary is an important factor controlling utilisation of insulin and metabolisation of glucose. The onset of disease is insidious with mild symptoms. It may be discovered only on routine check up of blood or during fundus examination. It can be partly controlled by control of weight, exercise and diet. Oral anti-diabetic drugs are often sufficient.

The pioneering work of Banting and Best leading to isolation of insulin in 1921 made control of diabetes a possibility for the first time. Insulin has controlled diabetes, saved patients from carbuncle and diabetic coma but blindness due to diabetic retinopathy is on the increase. The increasing span of life in 20th century has led to a higher incidence of blindness due to diabetic retinopathy.

There is some hereditary tendency for diabetes mellitus to be carried on in successive generations. Obesity, sedentary habits and emotional tensions have a close bearing on the incidence of diabetes. Dietary habits with excessive intake of fats and carbohydrates is a distinct contributory factor in families with a diabetic history.

Clinically, senile diabetes which appears at the age of 50 years and after, is less harmful than diabetes starting earlier. It is responsible for majority of blindness cases due to diabetic retinopathy.

Diabetes is one disease which can affect any tissue of the body. Of all the tissues, the eye suffers the most. Possibility of diabetes in a patient is first thought of on finding peculiar lens opacities and/or observing micro-aneurysms in fundus. It is not unusual that diabetes may be first discovered on routine blood examination before eye surgery.

The ocular changes caused by diabetes form a long list as noted below: (The clinical details of these changes are discussed in the respective places.)

    a. Xanthoma of lid skin and recurrent styes.

    b. Subconjunctival micro-aneurysm and haemorrhages.

    c. Corneal dystrophy of lipid type.

    d. Rubeosis iris, spontaneous hyphaema and haemorrhagic glaucoma.

    e. Diabetic iritis.

    f. Iris pigment dispersion.

    g. Diabetic cataract.

    h. Vitreous haemorrhage.

    i. Fibro-vascular proliferation in vitreous.

    j. Diabetic retinopathy—simple or proliferative.

    k. Diabetic optic neuritis.

    l. Pallor of the disc and optic atrophy.

    m. Orbital haematoma causing proptosis.

    n. Peripheral neuritis causing ocular palsies.

    o. Lipaemic retinitis.

    p. Choroidal haemorrhage.

    q. Sub-arachnoid haemorrhage leading to peripapillary haemorrhages.

    r. Transient myopia.

s. Gaze palsies due to supranuclear lesions.

t. Congenital ocular defects in infants of diabetic mothers.

Galactosaemia: This is a hereditary disease of young children due to defective metabolism of galactose which is not converted into glucose as it should be. It results in high galactose levels in serum. The systemic manifestations are hepatomegally, jaundice and mental retardation. The important ocular change is bilateral cataract. Galactosaemia cataract is a reversible cataract if systemic condition can be restored to normal galactose metabolisms.

Mucopolysaccharidosis: This is a metabolic disorder due to defective mucopolysaccharide metabolism. Gargoylism or Hurler's disease is a typical example of mucopolysaccharide defect. The clinical manifestations include skeletal dysplasia, cardiac anomalies and mental retardation.

The ocular manifestations are:

a. Corneal dystrophy.
b. Congenital cataract.
c. Congenital glaucoma.
d. Optic atrophy.
e. Exudative retinopathy.

LIPID METABOLIC DISORDERS

A lipid metabolic defect results in heavier deposition of lipids in body tissues, many times associated with dementia and paraplegia. Typical clinical manifestations of this metabolic defect are:

a. Xanthomata.
b. Gaucher's disease of infants with enlarged liver and spleen with fatty infiltration of conjunctiva, choroid and retina.
c. Niemann-Pick's disease in infants with enlargement of liver and spleen and infiltration of sclera, choroid and retina and grey macular area with cherry red spot.

d. Amaurotic family idiocy (Tay-Sach's disease). Lipid degeneration of the cells of brain and retina with cherry red spot at macula.
e. Hyper cholestraemia

The ocular manifestations of Lipid Metabolic disorders can be:

a. Xanthoma of lids.
b. Fatty degeneration of cornea.
c. Lipaemia retinalis.
d. Coat's disease of retina.

PROTEIN METABOLIC DISORDERS

Defective amino-acid metabolism causes clinical conditions like cysteinuria and alkaptonuria. The former may be associated with ectopia lentis, secondary glaucoma, retinal detachment and optic atrophy. The latter mainly affects conjunctiva and cornea. It is interesting that gyrate atrophy of the choroid is also an inborn metabolic disorder due to high concentration of an amino-acid (orthinine) in blood. This is caused by deficiency of an enzyme which breaks down orthinine. The treatment is pyridoxine (Vitamin B_6).

Another condition which is hereditary and due to abnormal serum immunoglobulins, is myotonic dystrophy which may be associated with bilateral cataract and bilateral ptosis.

COLLAGEN DISORDERS

Collagen fibres are one of the three types of connective tissue fibres, the other two being the reticulin and elastic fibres. Collagen fibres usually form connective tissue bundles which are held together by the ground substance composed of sulphated and non-sulphated mucopolysaccharides. Collagen fibres on boiling form gelatine and are therefore different from the other two types of connective tissue fibres. They are formed from fibroblasts and are present in all organs with connective tissue.

The ocular manifestations of common collagen diseases are given below:

1. **Rheumatoid Arthritis**
   a. Keratoconjunctivitis Sicca, Sjögren's disease.
   b. Marginal and band-shaped corneal degeneration.
   c. Episcleritis, Scleritis, scleromalacia perforans, necrotising scleritis.
   d. Tenonitis.
   e. Anterior Uveitis.
   f. Complicated cataract.
2. **Lupus Erythematosus**
   a. Conjunctival atrophy and shrinkage.
   b. Recurrent erosions of the cornea.
   c. Deep keratitis.
   d. Marginal ulcers of cornea.
   e. Nodular scleritis.
   f. Irido-cyclitis.
   g. Choroiditis.
   h. Retinal perivasculitis.
   i. Papilloedema.
   j. Muscle palsies.
3. **Poly-arteritis Nodosa**
   a. Conjunctival haemorrhages.
   b. Nodular scleritis.
   c. Marginal ulcer of cornea.
   d. Posterior uveitis.
   e. Retinal exudates.
   f. Central retinal artery occlusion.
   g. Ocular palsies.
   h. Pseudo tumour in the orbit.
   i. Serous retinal detachment.
4. **Pseudo-xanthoma Elasticum**: Angoid streaks of the retina is the only likely ocular manifestation.

JOINT DISEASES

Collagen diseases, like rheumatoid arthritis, metabolic diseases like gout and bacterial infection like rheumatic fever, may be associated with ocular manifestations.

Gout with high uric acid in blood, may be associated with:
   a. Blepharitis.

   b. Conjunctivitis.
   c. Episcleritis.
   d. Uveitis.

Rheumatic fever which is streptodccocal in origin and is characterised by Aschoff nodules in heart, joints and blood vessels causing acute joint pain and fever may be associated with:
   a. Episcleritis.
   b. Deep scleritis.
   c. Tenonitis.
   d. Uveitis.

In addition, there are certain symptom complexes with ocular manifestations and joint disease. The common examples are:
a. Reiter's disease with
   i. Polyarthritis.
   ii. Urethritis.
   iii. Conjunctivitis.
   iv. Iridocyclitis.
b. Behcet's disease with
   i. Arthritis.
   ii. Ulcers in mouth, lips and genitals.
   iii. Thrombophlebitis.
   iv. Anterior uveitis.
   v. Vitreous haemorrhage.
   vi. Chorio-retinitis.
   vii. Optic neuritis.

SKIN DISEASES

Diseases of the skin may involve skin of the lids and extend to the epithelial covering of eye ball. Some of these may be severe and indolent in nature and pose difficult therapeutic problems. These are described here.

Pemphigus is a recurrent bullous condition of skin and mucous membranes with generalised exfoliation, auto-immune in nature with reduced lymphocytes. Ocular involvement may include conjunctival bullae, shrinkage of conjunctiva, symblepheron, conjunctival xerosis and corneal opacity.

Steven Johnson's disease (Erythema multiforme) is a vesiculo-bullous disease of skin and mucous membranes and may cause serious systemic symptoms. The disease may affect skin, conjunctiva, mucous membrane of mouth and genitals. The condition is usually a hypersensitivity reaction to bacteria, viruses and drugs like antibiotics and sulphas.

Ocular manifestations are severe in nature:
  a. Conjunctival ulceration with pseudo-membrane formation.
  b. Corneal ulceration and perforation.
  c. Heavy corneal vascularisation.
  d. Subconjunctival cicatrisation resulting in extensive symblepheron and obliteration of fornices.
  e. Kerato-conjunctivitis sicca.

Acanthosis nigricans: There are pigmented warts on skin which may suppurate and fungate. The palpebral conjunctiva may be pigmented and there may be multiple warty lesions on lid margins. The condition may change to malignancy.

Xeroderma pigmentosa: It is a familial and hereditary disease affecting children. There are pigmented lesions on the exposed parts of body, particularly on face. The disease extends into conjunctiva and cornea causing fleshy growths like false plerygia and lesions resembling malignant squamous epithelioma (Figs. 17.1 and 17.2).

Exfoliative dermatitis is an inflammatory condition of the epidermis caused by systemic disease or administration of drugs. There is generalised oedema of skin resulting in peeling of skin. The condition may involve skin of lid and may cause keratitis and symblepheron.

Psoriasis is a chronic skin condition with patches of scaly lesions. When generalised, it may involve the lids and cause chronic conjunctivitis, conjunctival xerosis and sometimes corneal ulcers and perforation.

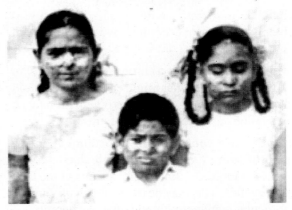

Fig 17.1: Xeroderma Pigmentosa affecting two sisters and a brother in the Family. (All of them died within four years, of taking the picture)

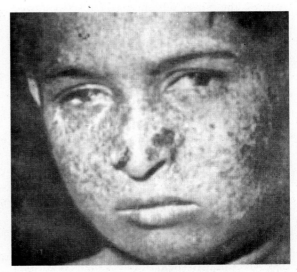

Fig 17.2: Xeroderma Pigmentosa. (Face of the brother showing pigmentary lesions, ulcer on nose and malignant lesion in right eye causing adhesion between lower lid and cornea

Ichthyosis: It is a hereditary disease causing dryness and thickening of skin. The ocular complications may be ectropion, lag-ophthalmos and exposure keratitis.

Impetigo: It is an infective condition due to staphylo or streptococcus infection. There are groups of blisters which leave behind crusts. It may be associated with blepharitis, ankylo-blepheron, chronic conjunctivitis and corneal ulcers.

Lupus vulgaris: It is a chronic condition of skin probably of tubercular origin causing tuberculoid lesions on the face. Ocular involvement may be ectropion and chronic conjunctivitis.

Molluscum contagiosum is a common condition of skin of viral origin, with characteristic small umbilicated superficial lesions of the face and eyelids. This may be associated with chronic follicular conjunctivitis and punctate keratitis.

FUNGAL DISEASES

Among the fungi which may cause systemic manifestations and involve the eye, are actinomyces bovis, aspergillus fumigatus, Candida albicans and Rhinosporidium. They may involve lids, conjunctiva, lacrimal glands and passages and may cause corneal ulcers, uveitis and neuro-retinitis sometimes resulting in orbital cellulitis and pan-ophthalmitis. The infection due to rhinosporidium may cause granulomatous lesions in the nose, throat, ear, genitals and lips and also in conjunctiva, lacrimal canaliculus and the lacrimal sac.

VIRAL DISEASES

There are a large number of systemic conditions of viral origin which may directly or indirectly involve ocular tissues. Some ocular conditions of viral origin have been described in appropriate places.

Other systemic viral diseases with ocular manifestations are described below:

Infectious Mononucleosis (Glandular Fever)

It is a virus disease with generalised lymphadenopathy. It may cause ocular complications like:
   a. Follicular conjunctivitis.
   b. Punctate keratitis.

   c. Dacryo-adenitis.
   d. Episcleritis.
   e. Uveitis.
   f. Retinal perivasculitis.
   g. Optic neuritis.
   h. Ocular palsies.

Infective Fevers

The common infective viral fevers affecting they eyes are measles, rubella, chickenpox, smallpox and mumps

Viral Fevers

1. **Measles is a common infective fever.** Children usually go through it unharmed. It may, however, cause ocular manifestations like:
   a. Conjunctivitis.
   b. Blepharitis.
   c. Keratitis.
   d. Tenonitis.
   e. Dacryo-adenitis.
   f. Choroiditis.
   g. Neuro-retinitis.
   h. Papilloedema.
   i. Ocular palsies.
      When associated with a severe degree of malnutrition, conjunctival xerosis and keratomalacia may be further complications. Virus encephalitis may cause severe generalised systemic reaction.
2. **German measles (Rubella):** Ocular manifestations are seen in new-born infants of mothers who suffered from this disease in the second or third month of pregnancy. The manifestations may be:
   a. Congenital heart disease.
   b. Deafness.
   c. Congenital cataract.
   d. Microphthalmos.
   e. Nystagmus.
3. **Chickenpox** (Varicella) is an erruptive fever caused by herpes zoster like virus and usually

runs a benign course but may however cause ocular manifestations which may be:

a. Conjunctivitis.
b. Phlycten like corneal ulcers.
c. Dacryocystitis.
d. Keratitis.
e. Iridocyclitis.
f. Neuro-retinitis.

4. **Smallpox** (Variola) is the severest of the infective fevers and an important cause of corneal blindness in developing countries. The disease has luckily been eradicated from many parts of the world. However the ravages already caused by it remained, for some time (Fig. 17.3).

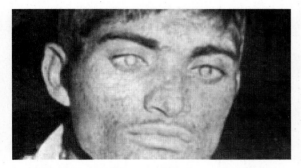

Fig. 17.3 This is what smallpox can do to cornea

The corneal involvement is caused by the specific dermato-tropic virus causing lesions in corneal epithelium which get secondarily infected resulting in gross corneal ulcers and scar formation. The resulting ocular manifestations are:

a. Pitted scars on skin of face and the lids.
b. Conjunctivitis.
c. Dacryocystitis
d. Corneal ulcers and consequently corneal scars like leucoma adherens, anterior staphyloma and phthisis bulbi.
e. Anterior uveitis.
f. Serous retinopathy.
g. Optic neuritis.
h. Ocular palsies.

5. **Mumps** is a fairly common condition in children which may sometimes cause meningitis, encephalitis and sterility in males. The ocular manifestations may be:

a. Episcleritis.
b. Tenonitis.
c. Deep keratitis.
d. Iridocyclitis.
e. Optic neuritis.
f. Conjugate ocular palsies.

PARASITIC DISORDERS

Parasitic diseases are much more common in tropical and developing countries. The parasites which commonly cause these conditions fall in two major groups—the intestinal parasites and parasites circulating in the blood stream.

Intestinal Parasites

The important intestinal parasites that can cause ocular manifestations are described below:

Taenia ecchinococcus is a tape worm and causes cystic lesions in the body with daughter cysts. The identification of scolices in the cyst wall confirms the histological diagnosis. These *hydatid cysts* may be in the lids, lacrimal gland, choroid, vitreous, retina and the orbit. The clinical features depend on the tissue involved. It is important to remember that ecchinococcus cyst should be removed intact because the cyst fluid is highly irritant to tissues and scolices if left behind can cause recurrence.

Ankylostoma duodenale which is a hook worm, is less common as a cause of ocular manifestation. The generalised systemic effect is anaemia and ocular manifestations are due to deficiency. There can be retinal haemorrhages and vitreous haemorrhages.

Cysticercus: Taenia Solium is a tape worm. The cystic lesions it causes are called *cysticercus callulosae*. These cysts can be seen in the lids, conjunctiva, orbit and sometimes intraocular tissues, choroid, retina and vitreous.

Giardia lamblia: This is a protozoan parasite and may, cause uveitis and macular lesions like central serous retinopathy.

Entamoeba histolytica: Although amoebic dysentery is a common disease in tropical countries, ocular effects are only rarely seen. It may cause exudative iridocyclitis, macular oedema and cysts.

Bacillary dysentery due to shigella can cause systemic effects like urethritis and arthritis. Ocular effects are anterior uveitis and conjunctivitis.

Non-Intestinal Parasites

Toxoplasmosis is a protozoan infection commonly congenital but may be acquired in some cases. Congenital toxoplasmosis is transmitted from mother during pregnancy and can cause hepatosplenomegally. Involvement of central nervous system may cause hydrocephalus and convulsions and later calcification of the lesions. It causes bilateral central chorio-retinitis and congenital cataract. A granulomatous lesion in the macular area of both eyes of a child or healed lesion seen in later age should always arouse possibility of congenital toxoplasmosis.

Acquired toxoplasmosis usually remains symptomless although it may cause lymphadenitis and fever. Central nervous system involvement may cause optic neuritis and optic atrophy.

Diagnosis of toxoplasmosis can be based on clinical findings, spots of cerebral calcification and laboratory tests like complement-fixation and immunofluorescence tests. A skin test and dye test are less reliable.

Leishmania Donovan is also a protozoal parasite transmitted through sandfly. It may cause local skin lesions called *tropical sores*, or *oriental sores*. The systemic infection causes Kalazar fever, which is associated with enlargement of spleen and liver. Ocular manifestations are rare and these are limited to the anterior segment causing conjunctivitis and keratitis.

Malarial parasites (Plasmodium falsiparum) is also a protozoal infection transmitted by a female anopheles mosquito and causes intermittent fever and splenomegally. Direct ocular manifestations are uncommon and these may be conjunctival congestion and sub-conjunctival haemorrhages. The important ocular manifestations are however due to anaemia . These may be retinal haemorrhages and optic neuritis. Malarial infection is often associated with recurrent attacks of herpetic keratitis.

Malignant malaria which causes haemoglobinuria is commonly associated with retinal haemorrhages.

Filaria Bancrofti is a parasite transmitted by mosquito and common in tropical countries. Systemic manifestation is elephantiasis of the legs caused by obstruction to lymphatic circulation. The ocular manifestations are very uncommon. Microfilaria may appear under conjunctiva or in uveal tissues. A microfilaria may be freely moving in the aqueous and vitreous. A blood smear for laboratory examination is always prepared during night with the patient asleep because the parasite is in peripheral circulation during night.

Schistosomiasis is caused by schistosoma haematobium causing systemic urticaria and granulomatous lesions on the skin. Ocular manifestations may be swelling of the lids and small tumours under the skin or in orbit. Associated cirrhosis may cause ocular manifestations like conjunctival xerosis.

Onchocerchiasis (river blindness) is a filarial infection caused by filaria volvulus and transmitted by a fly common in Central and West Africa and some parts of South America. In countries like Congo, villages had been blinded by the disease. Microfilaria may involve ocular structures causing conjunctivitis, sclerosing keratitis, exudative irido-cyclitis, choroiditis and optic atrophy.

DEFICIENCY DISEASES

Vitamin deficiencies and malnutrition are common in developing countries, affecting the poorer communities. Apart from poverty, dietary habits in certain populations may be responsible for malnutrition. Most clinical manifestations are multiple deficiency syndromes although there are certain clinical entities which are due to deficiency of a particular vitamin or dietary item.

Vitamin-A deficiency. Vitamin-A is found in highest concentration in carrots, green leafy vegetables, milk and butter, egg-yolk, fish liver, red palm oil, papaya, red plantains, jack fruit, ripe mango, green pepper, Persian dates, green chillies and corriander, cumin seeds, neem, cabbage, drumsticks, soyabeans and fenugreek (methi). This vitamin is synthesized and stored in liver. It is essential for the healthy condition of all epithelial linings of the body. Vitamin A is extremely important for synthesis of visual purple and hence for normal functioning of rod cells of retina.

The true ocular manifestation of Vitamin-A deficiency is night blindness which is reversible with administration of Vitamin-A. Deficiency of Vitamin-A is also an important component of multiple deficiency lesions like pigmentation of conjunctiva, conjunctival xerosis and kerato-malacia.

Vitamin-B$_1$ (Thaimine) is found in maximum concentration in beans, cereals and most nuts and dry fruits, meats, fish and yeast. It is important for carbohydrate metabolism. The systemic manifestations of Vitamin-B$_1$ deficiency are beri-beri and polyneuritis. The ocular manifestations are retrobulbar neuritis and peripheral palsy of the oculo-molor nerves.

Vitamin-B$_2$ (Riboflavin) is available in the same items of diet as B$_1$. A deficiency of Vitamin-B$_2$ causes seborrhoeic dermatitis and glossitis. Ocular manifestations of ariboflavinosis are superficial punctate keratitis and vascularisation of cornea. It is possibly associated with metabolism of lens.

A syndrome of angular stomatitis and angular conjunctivitis, (Kripatrick's syndrome) is often associated with riboflavin deficiency.

Nicotinic acid is present in high concentration in liver, yeast and ground nuts. The deficiency causes pellagra. The skin eruptive lesions may involve lids. Nicotinic acid, as a vasodilator of peripheral circulation is helpful in the treatment of conditions like pigmentary retinal degeneration.

Vitamin-B$_{12}$ and folic acid deficiency causes hyperchromic anaemia with achlorhydria. This deficiency is also associated with etiology of tobacco amblyopia. The ocular manifestations may be retinal haemorrhages.

Vitamin-C (Ascorbic acid). The best sources of Vitamin-C in food are citrus fruits, Amla (gooseberry), guava, vegetables like tomato, sprouting cereals, carrot leaves, coriander, drum-sticks, chillies (more in green chillies), karela (bitter gourd), cauliflower, turnip, papaya, pineapple and strawberries.

Vitamin-C is an important element for maintenance of intercellular cement substance and therefore of importance in tissue healing process including the post-operative healing after intraocular operations. Vitamin-C is an active participant in the anaerobic metabolism of the lens. Its concentration in the lens diminishes with advancing age and is, therefore, probably related to development of senile cataract.

The deficiency of Vitamin-C causes systemic scurvy. Haemorrhage under the skin, under the conjunctiva and probably in intraocular tissue may occur. This deficiency retards healing of corneal wounds and ulcers.

Vitamin-D (Calciferol) is present in highest concentration in animal fats and cod liver oil. It is synthesized naturally in the skin by sunlight and artificially by exposure to ultra-violet rays. Deficiency in children causes rickets and in adults osteomalacia. Because of its association with skeletal growth, it is probably related to etiology and progress of myopia.

Vitamin-E (Tocoferol). Vitamin-E is a constituent of cereals and animal tissues like liver. It is also present in wheat, rice, cotton seed and palm oil. The deficiency causes infertility in males and sterility and repeated abortions in females.

Vitamin-K is found in maximum quantity in green leaves. Its biological importance is its association with formation of prothrombin and reducing capillary permeability and therefore reduces haemorrhagic tendency. Its deficiency causes multiple haemorrhages in the system and ocular tissues.

Vitamin-P (Citrin). As a name suggests, it is found in maximum concentration in citrus fruits. It is important for the health of the capillary network in the body. Its deficiency causes capillary fragility and therefore systemic and ocular haemorrhages.

Hypervitaminosis

It is important to know that hypervitaminosis of some vitamins can also cause systemic and ocular manifestations.

Hypervitaminosis A causes irritability probably of cerebral origin and has been reported to cause papilloedema. Its excess during pregnancy may cause developmental ocular anomalies.

An excess dose of *nicotinic acid* causes symptoms of flushing and tingling on face and body due to vasodilatation.

An excess of *Vitamin-D* causing hypercalcaemia is known to cause zonular cataract.

An excess of *Vitamin E* during pregnancy can cause ocular anomalies like micro-ophthalmos and congenital cataract.

Multiple Deficiencies

The important deficiency syndromes are due to combined deficiencies of vitamins, proteins and calories. The two most important and serious deficiency syndromes are systemic kwashiorkar and ocular keratomalacia. In addition conjunctival pigmentation and conjunctival xerosis are also not pure Vitamin-A deficiency manifestations as used to be emphasised.

HEREDITARY DISEASES

Congenital and hereditary diseases are two different entities. Congenital diseases are those which are present at birth and may be hereditary or non-hereditary. On the other hand, hereditary diseases may be present at birth or may manifest later in life at any age. They are all genetically transmitted from parents to offspring through genes and chromosomes.

Congenital diseases which are not hereditary in nature are acquired during intra-uterine life and are caused by environmental influences like maternal syphilis and diabetes, malnutrition or exposure to radiation, infections during pregnancy like rubella or maternal toxoplasmosis, etc. Maternity in advanced age causing congenital anomalies is also the result of an important environmental influence. The list of congenital diseases is long and congenital anomalies in different ocular tissues are described in appropriate places.

Hereditary diseases on the other hand may be present at birth or become manifest in childhood or even later. Heredity is now being considered more and more important in etiology of many idiopathic diseases which are transmitted through genes and chromosomes from one generation to next.

The present concept of heredity is the original hypothesis of Mendelian law first conceived in the beginning of the twentieth century. Since then, the understanding of DNA molecule, the chemical constituent of genes and identification of chromosomes have made the understanding of the subject clearer and definitive.

Thousands of genes exist on each of the pairs of chromosomes. There are 23 pairs of chromosomes, 22 of which are autosomes and one pair sex chromosomes. The sex chromosomes in male is XY chromosomes and in female XX chromosomes. The daughters inherit one X chromosome from the mother and the second X chromosome from the father, while the sons have a Y chromosome from the father and X chromosome from mother. Most genes are carried by X chromosomes and only a few by Y chromosomes.

There are two modes of heredity transmission: the *autosomal* and *sex linked*, either of which can be dominant or recessive. In dominant transmission, the genetically affected parents transmit the disease in successive generations but not all the offspring suffer from the disease. In recessive inheritance, the offspring may become carriers and the disease may not become clinically manifest in every successive generation. The genetic defect is transmitted but may become clinically evident only after a gap of one or more generations. Thus apparently normal parents may have affected children or affected parents may have normal children.

Sex-linked inheritance is based on transmission of genes through the pair of sex chromosomes.

Good examples of sex-linked hereditary diseases are haemophilia and colour blindness where females are carriers and transmit the disease but the males are affected.

The element of genetic transmission and the hereditary nature of various diseases is described in the etiology of respective conditions. A few well-known ocular conditions due to chromosomal aberrations are given below:

a. **Chromosome pair 4-5:**
    i. Lacrimal duct block.
    ii. Coloboma iris.
b. **Chromosome pairs 6-12:**
    i. Lid anomalies.
    ii. Microphthalmos.
    iii. Strabismus.
c. **Chromosome pairs 13-15:**
    i. Anophthalmos.
    ii. Microphthalmos.
    iii. Colobomata.
    iv. Epicanthus.
    v. Ptosis.
    vi. Cataract.
    vii. Retinal dysplasia.
    viii. Retinitis Pigmentosa.
    ix. Retino-blasloma.
    x. Buphthalmos.
d. **Chromosome pairs 16-18:**
    i. Ptosis.
    ii. Epicanthus.
    iii. Squint.
    iv. Optic atrophy.
    v. Nystagmus.
e. **Chromosome pairs 21-22:**
    i. Mongolism.

MISCELLANEOUS SYSTEMIC DISORDERS

There are a number of systemic diseases causing ocular manifestations which do not fit in any category of diseases with a common etiology or common clinical features. They are described individually as follows:

Epidemic Dropsy: It is a tropical disease caused by the toxic alkaloid, sanguinarine in the grains of Argemone-mexicana which is a wild plant, the seeds of which are mistakenly or deliberately used to adulterate seeds of mustard. The oil of these adulterated seeds which is used for cooking, contains the toxic alkaloid. The alkaloid disturbs the carbohydrate metabolism of the body and causes generalised vasodilatation, serous effusion in the body cavities and peripheral polyneuritis. It causes secondary glaucoma of open angle type. It is endemic in some parts of eastern India. The glaucomatous process is arrested if ingestion of adulterated oil is withdrawn in the early stages of ocular pathology.

Sarcoidosis: It is a non-specific, sometimes fatal granulomatous disease and non-tuberculous in nature even though some features are like tuberculosis. A sarcoid nodule has a cellular character of a tubercle but is non-caseating in nature with absence of tubercle bacilli. The nodules may develop in lungs, lymph nodes, nervous system, skin and eyes. The ocular manifestations are:

1. Erythema nodosum in the skin of the lid.
2. Boeck's sarcoid in uveal tissue.
3. Episcleritis.
4. Nodules in lacrimal gland with consequent Sjögren's syndrome.
5. Uveitis.
6. Retinal periphlebitis.
7. Papilloedema.
8. Optic atrophy.
9. Ocular palsies.

Amyloidosis is a degeneration in chronic diseases of a suppurative or malignant nature with deposition of fibrillar amorphous material derived from reticulo-endothelial cells. The disease may damage kidneys and heart and may even be fatal. The amyloid deposits may involve structures like lids, conjunctiva, lacrimal gland, cornea, sclera, uvea and the orbit. Ocular manifestations may be proptosis, retinal haemorrhages and exudates, optic neuritis and ocular palsies. Exophthalmos and secondary glaucoma may also be caused.

Hodgkin's disease is a reticulo-endothelial disease, malignant in nature and primarily involves lymph nodes. It may also involve other tissues of the body. The ocular manifestations are:

i. Tumorous involvement of lacrimal gland.
ii. Proptosis due to orbital infiltration.
iii. Extra-ocular palsies due to muscle involvement.
iv. Retinal haemorrhage and exudates.
v. Optic atrophy.

Jaundice, which may be infective or obstructive. The ocular effects may be due to deposition of bile pigments, liver damage or due to osmotic changes in blood. The ocular manifestations, may, therefore be:

i. Discolouration of conjunctiva.
ii. Transient myopia.
iii. Conjunctival bleeding.
iv. Night blindness.

Pregnancy: This physiological condition can however be a cause of serious systemic damage and cause severe ocular manifestations. Normal pregnancy may rarely cause bilateral retrobulbar neuritis and blindness and may exaggerate existing diabetic retinopathy or flare up tuberculous infection. The most serious complication is in toxaemia of pregnancy which when it recurs in subsequent pregnancies, may leave behind kidney damage, hypertension and vascular retinopathy of toxaemia with haemorrhages, exudates and exudative retinal detachment. The ophthalmologist is required to guide the obstetrician whether fundus picture allows the pregnancy to continue or demands termination forthwith. Marked attenuation of arteries, exudates and haemorrhages with systemic hypertension is a composite picture which indicates prolonged nature of the pathology and organic damage to kidneys and therefore risk to mother's life. Termination of pregnancy is, therefore, indicated which if not done, may produce a living child but may cause death of the mother.

Renal disease: Renal pathology is important not only because of ocular manifestations in acute nephritis but also because of organic damage to the kidneys which causes renal hypertension.

Acute nephritis causes puffiness of face and oedema of lids. It may cause soft exudates and exudative retinal detachment.

Chronic kidney failure (nephrosclerosis) with renal hypertension causes hypertensive retinopathy which in no way differs from retinopathy of malignant hypertension with attenuation of arteries, soft exudates, superficial haemorrhages and papilloedema.

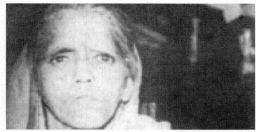

Fig . 17.4: Vogt-Koyanagi Syndrome showing vitiligo, Poliosis and Bilateral Chronic Uveitis

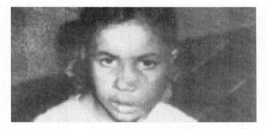

Fig . 17.5A: Large congnital capillary naevus on left of Face (Not yet caused buphthalmos)

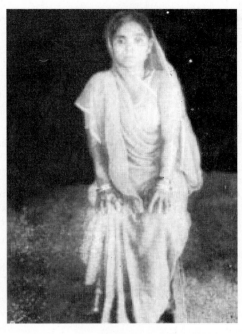

Fig. 17.6: Marchesani Syndrome. (Note the short limbs and stubby fingers. She had sphero-phakia and secondary glaucoma in both eyes)

SYNDROMES WITH OCULAR MANIFESTATIONS

Syndrome is an aggregate of signs and symptoms with characteristic constancy of clinical features. The following is a list of some important syndromes with typical ocular manifestations:

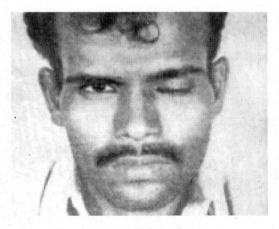

Fig . 17.7: Marcus-Gunn Syndrome (Looking straight—ptosis of left side)

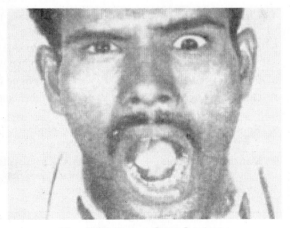

Fig . 17.8: Marcus-Gunn Syndrome (opening the jaw left upper lid retracts)

Syndrome	Ocular manifestations	Systemic manifestations
Anterior Uvea		
1. Behcet's syndrome	Iridocyclitis	a. Ulcerative stomatitis b. Ulcerative Urethritis.
2. Reiter's syndrome	Iridocyclitis Conjunctivitis	a. Urethritis b. Polyarthritis.
3. Vogt-Koyanagi Harada's syndrome (Fig. 17.4)	Chronic Uveitis Retinal Haemorrhage Exudative detachment commonly bilateral	a. Alopoecia b. Poliosis c. Vitiligo d. Deafness.
Endocrinal Syndrome		
1. Chiasmal syndrome	a. Typical bitemporal quadrantic or Hemianopic visual field defect b. Later optic atrophy	a. Endocrinal manifestations of hyper/hypopituitarism b. Radiological changes in Sella turcica.
2. Cushing's syndrome	a. Hypertensive retinopathy b. Exophthalmos c. Pigmentation of lids	a. Obesity b. Hypertension c. Diabetes due to pathology in adrenal cortex.
3. Laurence-Moon Biedl syndrome	a. Retinitis Pigmentosa	a. Obesity b. Hypogonadism c. Polydactyly d. Mental retardation.
Neurological Syndromes		
1. Adie's syndrome	a. Tonic pupil, dilated b. Poor light reflex c. Poor accommodation reflex	Tendon reflexes absent or diminished.
2. Benedikt syndrome	a. Ocular palsies on one side	Spastic hemiplegia on opposite side.
3. Carotico-cavernous	a. Ocular palsies b. Pulsatile proptosis c. Venous engorgement in ocular tissues	Disturbing noises in head.
4. Claude's syndrome	a. Ocular palsies on one side	Incordination and mid-brain lesions on opposite side.
5. Foster-Kennedy syndrome	a. Optic atrophy on side of lesion b. Papilloedema in opposite eye	Neurological evidence of tumour in anterior-cranial fossa.
6. Foville's syndrome	a. VI nerve paralysis on one side	Hemiplegia on opposite side
7. Gradenigo's syndrome	a. VI nerve and other ocular palsies	a. Suppurative Otitis. b. Extra-dural abscess on petrous bone.
8. Horner's syndrome	a. Uniocular ptosis b. Uniocular miosis	a. Unilateral anidrosis (less sweating) due to sympathetic nerve root lesion.
9. Meniere's syndrome	a. VII and VIII nerve palsies. b. Vestibular nystagmus c. Diplopia	a. Nausea b. Vertigo c. Deafness due to labrynthine disease, or internal ear.

Contd.

Contd.

Syndrome	Ocular manifestations	Systemic manifestations
10. Lowe's syndrome (Ocular cerebro-renal)	a Cataract b. Glaucoma c. Corneal opacitys	a. Mental retardation b. Renal failure.
11. Posterior-inferior cere-bellar artery syndrome	a. Cerebellar nystagmus on one side	a. Vertigo b. Ataxia c. Vomiting.
12. Petro-sphenoidal syndrome	a. Ocular palsies b. Proptosis c. Trigeminal neuralgia	a. Due to naso-pharyngeal carcinoma.
13. Weber's syndrome	a. Oculo-motor paralysis on the side of the lesion	a. Paralysis of extremities and face on opposite side b. Lesion in cerebral peduncle.

Miscellaneous Syndromes

1. Gronblad-Strandberg	a. Angoid streaks in retina	a. Pseudo-xanthoma elaslicum of skin of face.
2. Sjögren's syndrome	a. Kerato-conjunctivitis sicca.	a. Auto-immune disease b. Polyarthritis c. Dryness of mouth.
3. Stevens Johnson's disease (Erythema multiforme)	a. Pseudo-membranous conjunctivitis b. Symblepharon c. Keratitis d. Iridocyclitis	a. Vesicular dermatitis b. Bullae in mouth and genitalia c. Due to hypersensitivity reaction to bacteria, viruses and drugs.
4. Pemphigus	a. Conjunctivitis b. Corneal vascularization c. Symblepharon	a. Exfoliative dermatitis.
5. Sturge-Weber's syndrome (Fig. 17.5A, Fig. 17.5B Plate 13)	a. Capillary angioma of lids & conjunctiva b. Buphthalmos	a. Capillary angioma of face, meninges and brain may cause epilepsy.
6. Takayashu syndrome (Pulseless disease)	a. Transient Amaurosis b. Low pressure in ophthalmic artery	a. Cerebral ischaemia due to carotid artery narrowing.

Hereditary Syndromes

1. Howe's syndrome	a. Blue thin sclera b. Colour blindness c. Keratoconus	a. Hereditary b. Brittle bones c. Deafness.
2. Marfan's syndrome	a. Bilateral subluxated lens b. Myopia c. Spherophakia d. Secondary Glaucoma	a. Hereditary b. Polydactyly c. Arachnodactyly d. Long limbs e. Tall height.
3. Marchesani syndrome (Fig. 17.6)	a. Myopia b. Secondary Glaucoma c. Ectopia lentis d. Spherophakia	a. Hereditary b. Short fingers c. Short limbs d. Short height.
4. Marcus-Gunn syndrome (Figs. 17.7 and 17.8)	a. Ptosis when jaws closed b. Lid retraction when jaws opened	a. Congenital due to aberrant motor V and VII nerve connections.

18

Strabismus
(Squint and Orthoptics)

Eyes with a squint are a cosmetic blemish and have been known ever since recorded ophthalmic history. For centuries it was shrouded in mysticism and superstition. Even till the early twentieth century, patients did not seek treatment for fear of displeasing the gods. It is surprising that such an evident cosmetic defect was not treated for a long time.

The chronological history of squint is exciting. Hippocrates first noted cross eyes in children of cross-eyed parents. The use of a mask with two holes in front of the eyes to correct the squint was described by Paulus. Bonders in 1864 explained the relationship between accommodation and convergence and emphasized importance of hypermetropia in convergent squint. In 1903 Worth classified binocular vision in three grades and devised the four-dot test. Maddox emphasized treatment of abnormal retinal correspondence and Mary Maddox was the first to organise orthoptic clinic in London and with that, orthoptics became a subject.

In spite of all this background and knowledge of extra-ocular muscles, ophthalmic surgeons did not dare to interfere surgically because of poor knowledge of physiology of ocular movements and fear of uncertain results. Even when surgery developed, it was largely for cosmetic purposes and for grown up children. Consideration of visual recovery was insignificant. The surgical techniques then were largely limited to tenotomy of horizontal muscles.

The subject of squint and orthoptics, however, acquired importance after the rapid increase in incidence due to the stress and strain that expectant mothers went through during the Second World War and its aftermath. Additional forms of stress and strain continued in different forms after Second World War and the incidence of squint therefore continued to increase with the result that squint has become an important sub-speciality of ophthalmology.

A clear understanding of the subject and technical advancement have now made it possible not only to correct squint but also to restore good binocular single vision if treated adequately and at appropriate time. To achieve this, children with squint should be brought for treatment at the earliest after the parents note the squint. For best results, the treatment should be started at pre-school age and completed before the child is exposed to the strains of curricular studies.

ANATOMY OF EXTRA-OCULAR MUSCLES AND TENON'S SHEATH

It is important to first understand the anatomy and physiology of extra-ocular muscles.

The movements of the two eyes are a perfect example of co-ordination between the two eye balls. This co-ordination is essential for all the functions where two eyes have to work in such a way that the objects seen form images on corresponding retinal points so that these corresponding images are transmitted to the brain for final interpretation. The eyes in the resting condition are in a position of 5° divergence on either side but when looking straight, are kept parallel.

The two orbital axes are also not parallel to each other and yet the visual axes have to be parallel. This anomaly is rectified by the direction of the various muscles controlling eye movements and their points of origin and insertion.

The movements of the two eyes are controlled by six extra-ocular muscles in each eye, i.e., four recti and two obliques. These movements take place around three well defined axes. Upward and downward movements are on the *horizontal axis*, lateral and medial movements on the *vertical axis* and rotational movements round the *antero-posterior axis*. To facilitate understanding, the horizontal and vertical movements of eye ball are taken in relation to the centre of the cornea while the torsional movements are taken in relation to 12 O'clock point at the upper limbus This clarification is necessary because when the upper pole of the limbus rotates in, the corresponding lower point rotates out. Similarly, when the anterior pole of the eye ball moves down, the posterior pole moves up and vice-versa. (Figs. 18.1, 18.2 and 18.3).

THE FOUR RECTI AND THE TWO OBLIQUES

Medial Rectus

The muscle has a straight antero-posterior direction. It is the strongest and thickest of all

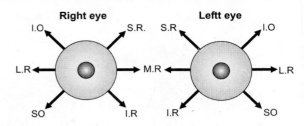

Fig. 18.1: Direction of Primary Action of Six Extra-ocular Muscles of each eye, (M.R—Medial rectus; S.R—Superior rectus; I.O—Inferior Oblique; L.R— Lateral Rectus; S.O— Superior Oblique; I.R—Inferior Rectus.)

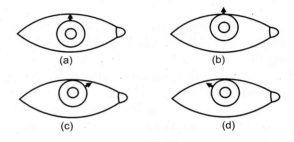

Fig. 18.2: Torsional Movements of Eye Ball in relation to 12 O'clock position at Limbus. (a) Looking straight; (b) Looking up; (c) Intorsion (d) Extorsion.

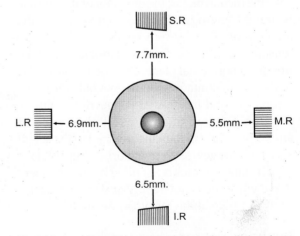

Fig 18.3: Insertion of four recti; Distance from limbus (note the obliquity of insertion line of the superior and inferior recti)

the extra-ocular muscles. It takes its origin from the fibrous annulus of Zinn at the apex of orbit and is attached in front, 5.5mm medial to the limbus in the horizontal plane. During its course

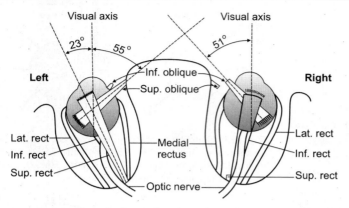

Fig. 18.4: Course of four Recti and two oblique Muscles indicating the obliquity in relation to Visual Axis. (The verticle recti form an angle of 23°, the superior oblique forms an angle of 55°, and the inferior oblique forms an angle of 51°)

the muscle, except at its insertion, is not in contact with the eye ball and has a tendency to retract into the orbit if tenotomized (Fig. 18.4).

The medial rectus is supplied by the inferior division of the 3rd nerve.

The action of the medial rectus is pure and simple adduction. The two medial recti when acting together bring about convergence.

Lateral Rectus

Like the medial rectus, the direction of this muscle is straight antero-posterior. It originates from the annulus of Zinn by two heads of origin. The muscle is attached in front, 6.9 mm lateral to the limbus in horizontal plane. During its course, the muscle is in contact with the eye ball for a few millmetres and has fascial connections with its surroundings with the result that even if tenotomized it still remains attached to the sclera and does not get lost into the orbit (Fig. 18.4).

The lateral rectus is supplied by the abducent nerve which does not supply any other muscle.

It is a pure abductor of the eye ball.

Superior Rectus

The superior rectus, which takes its origin from the upper part of the annulus of Zinn, is directed forward and laterally at an angle of about 23° to the visual axis and is inserted 7.7 mm above the limbus in vertical plane. During its course it passes

over the superior oblique muscle just behind the equator (Fig. 18.4).

The muscle is supplied by the upper division of the 3rd nerve.

Its action is of compound nature. It is a principal elevator of the eye ball and has a subsidiary action of adduction and intorsion. Because of the direction of its course, these actions depend on the position of the eye ball in relation to the visual axis. When the eye is in the position of abduction, the visual axis is parallel to the axis of the muscle and hence its principal action is elevation. When the eye is adducted which means the angle between the direction of the muscle and visual axis is increased, its main action is intorsion with practically no action of elevation. The superior rectus in conjunction with the inferior rectus has a small action of adduction also.

Inferior Rectus

Like the other three recti, the inferior rectus also takes its origin from the annulus of Zinn and like the superior rectus, is directed forward and outward at an angle of 23° to the visual axis. During its course from the medial to the lateral side, it overlies the inferior oblique (Fig. 18.4). The nerve supply of the inferior rectus is from the lower division of the 3rd nerve.

The actions of the interior rectus are like the superior rectus but opposite in nature with regard to vertical and torsional movements. It is a principal depressor in abduction and extorter in adduction (explanations given for superior rectus apply to these actions as well). However, it also has the subsidiary action of adduction in conjunction with the superior rectus.

Superior Oblique

It is the longest of all extra-ocular muscles. It originates from the bone above and medial to the annulus of Zinn and traverses forward, upward and medially and passes in form of a tendon through the trochlea or a pulley in the anterior and supero-medial part of the orbit and then is directed backwards and laterally to be attached to the sclera behind the equator between the superior and the lateral recti. During this backward course, it passes under the superior rectus muscle (Fig. 18.4).

It is supplied independently by trochlear nerve. The peculiarity of this nerve supply is that it enters the muscle belly from the upper surface with the result that after a retrobulbar injection of local anaesthetic, this muscle remains unaffected and, therefore, the intortional movement persists even though all other movements are paralysed.

The peculiar action of superior oblique is based on two important points. Unlike the recti, the direction of the effective part of the muscle, from the trochlea to its insertion, is backward and laterally and again unlike the four recti, it is inserted behind the equator. The principal action of the superior oblique is, therefore, intortion. The subsidiary actions are depression and to a lesser degree abduction.

Inferior Oblique

It is the shortest of the extra-ocular muscles. It takes its origin just behind posterior lacrimal crest from the orbital plate of maxilla. This is the only muscle taking its origin anteriorly. During its course laterally and posteriorly, it passes under the inferior rectus where it has a common sheath with it. The muscle is inserted under the lateral rectus and the nasal end of its insertion is very close to the macula (2.2 mm) (Fig. 18.4).

The inferior oblique is supplied by lower division of the 3rd nerve.

Action is based on the same anatomical considerations as the superior oblique. Its principal action is extorsion and the subsidiary actions are elevation and abduction.

Tenon's Sheath

It is a thin fibrous encapsulation of the eyeball performing the function of a synovial sheath of joints and providing the smooth movement of the eyeball. It extends from its attachment to the dural covering of the optic nerve behind up to its fusion with the conjunctiva near the limbus. It is reflected to cover the recti as they near their insertion. Two important anatomical facts are the thickness of the tenon's capsule in the lower part forming a hammock (ligament of Lockwood) which supports the eyeball and that at the sheathing of the lateral and medial recti, the Tenon's sheath is attached to the orbital tubercle on the lateral side and medial palpebral ligament on the medial side which act as *check ligaments.*.

Physiology of Convergence

Convergence is a binocular function whereby the two eyes converge for near work. Most of the convergence takes place for a distance of one metre or less. It is brought about by action of two medial recti.

The reflex for convergence is initiated by the desire to see near subjects clearly and is probably transmitted along the visual fibres of the retina to the occipital cortex. From occipital cortex, the reflex is mediated via peristriate area of the co-related cortex and is thence transmitted to 3rd nerve nuclei in mid-brain where the centres for both the medial recti are close to each other.

This area with decussation of fibres from both sides is called Perlia's nucleus. Efferent motor fibres from here go along the 3rd nerve supplying the two medial recti.

Convergence is measured in terms of the angle formed by joining the ends of the inter-pupillary line to a point one metre in front of the eyes. The angle subtended by each eye at one metre distance is called the one metre angle. This is inversely proportional to the distance from the inter-pupillary line. It can also be measured in terms of prism diopters.

Accommodative Convergence/ Accommodation Ratio (AC/A Ratio)

Accommodation, is the inherent power of the eye to focus and see objects clearly at distances from infinity to varying near points. The nearer the objects, the more the degree of accommodation needed. Accommodation is an uniocular function of each eye separately as well as both eyes together. It is measured in terms of diopters which is a unit of accommodation needed to see the object at one meter distance. When a person accommodates to see a near object clearly, it also causes the response of convergence of both eyes so that when he accommodates for near, he also converges.

This ratio of accommodative convergence and accommodation is called AC/A ratio. AC/A ratio is of clinical significance when evaluating a case of accommodative squint. This ratio varies with age, refractive error and muscle balance. It is also influenced by use of cycloplegic drugs.

SQUINT

To understand the subject of squint and orthoptics, it is necessary to understand various terms and conditions closely related to the subject. These are, therefore, described first.

Primary position: This is the position when both eyes are looking straight, with the head in erect position. In an emmetropic and orthophoric eye, both eyes are maintained parallel to each other by a subconscious effort which is needed because the eyes in a position of rest are slightly divergent and not parallel.

Poles of the eyes: There are two poles; the anterior and posterior. The former is centre of cornea and the latter is on the posterior pole of the sclera corresponding to the macular area.

Angle of squint: The angle of squint may be objective and subjective. The objective angle is one which is measured by the position of the corneal reflex in the squinting eye or by a cover test using neutralising prisms. The subjective angle is one which is measured by Maddox rod/ wing. Both types of angles can be measured on the synoptophore.

Binocular Vision

Binocular vision may be defined as the vision achieved by co-ordinating the two single images from each eye into one single mental impression.

Binocular vision is possible because visual fibres have a partial decussation at the optic chiasma so that visual fibres from each eye reach both sides of the cerebral cortex. Higher grades of binocularity are further achieved because of the association fibres between the two cerebral hemispheres interconnecting the centres on either side.

For binocular vision, it is essential that vision in two eyes should be equal or nearly equal or made equal with help of glasses. Any gross difference in the vision of two eyes or in the power of glasses of two eyes or size of images formed in two eyes are incompatible with good binocular single vision.

The examples of incompatible sensory obstacles are:
1. Corrected vision 6/6 in one eye and 6/18 or less in the other eye.
2. Difference in the power of glasses in two eyes of more than 2.5 dioptres.

3. Difference in the size of images of the two eyes of more than 30 per cent.

4. Aniseikonia, difference in shape and the form of images.

The above factors affecting the quality and quantity of vision are called *sensory obstacles* to binocularity.

In addition to sensory obstacles, there may be *motor obstacles* to binocularity when the parallelism of two eyes is disturbed, due to muscle anomalies where the visual image falls on the macula of one eye and away from the macula in the other eye. The image which is formed away from the macula is not clear and gets suppressed and hence there is no binocular single vision.

Binocularity may be affected by *Central obstacle*, e.g., psychological or mental trauma which disturb the cerebral functions of different grades of binocularity.

Man has acquired highest degree of binocularity which has the advantage of binocular single vision and appreciation of fusional depth of focus.

Binocular single vision may be divided into three grades:

1. **Simultaneous macular perception:** This is the ability to perceive simultaneously and superimpose two dissimilar images having a definite relationship. The images which fall on retinae of two eyes are perceived as one single image by the higher centres. A good example is the bird seen with one eye and the cage by the other eye and the two perceived as 'bird in the cage' as seen on synoptophore.

2. **Fusion:** This is the ability to fuse two incomplete pictures each of which has a common constituent. A good example of this is fusing together one rat without tail and one without ears. This is because half of the image is formed on the temporal retina of the right eye and nasal retina of the left eye and is transmitted to right hemisphere. The other half of the image forms on the nasal retina of the right eye and the temporal retina of the left eye and is transmitted to left hemisphere. The integration of these two images into one at the cortical level is called fusion.

3. **Stereopsis:** This is the appreciation of three-dimensional binocularity with the ability to fuse the images falling on two retinae of two eyes with a slight disparity in the lateral direction. This is again the function of higher centres and this is the highest grade of binocularity and gives appreciation of *fusional depth of focus*.

Methods of Testing for Binocular Vision

1. **Worth's four-dot test** is the simplest test. The four dots are two green, one red and one white. The patient sees through red and green goggles. A person with good binocularity will see all 4 dots but as 2 green, 1 red and 1 mixed. A person with absent binocular vision will see either 2 red dots through the red glass or three green through the green glass, the other eye being suppressed. A patient who has diplopia will see five dots.

2. **Friend** test is identical to Worth's four-dot test. A person with absent binocularity will see either FIN or RED.

3. **Maddox rod test:** A person with absent binocularity will either see the figures on the tangent scale or only the red line of the fixation light and will therefore not be able to judge the relation of one to the other.

4. **Synoptophore test:** This will not only indicate the presence or absence of binocularity but also determine the grade and type of binocularity.

Retinal Correspondence

Just as the fovea of one eye corresponds to the fovea of the other eye, there are corresponding points in the retina of each eye, those in the nasal area of one eye correspond to the points in the temporal area of other eye and vice-versa. All the objects whose images are formed on these corresponding points are located on an imaginary line in front of the eye called *horopter* and this condition is called *normal retinal correspondence*. When fovea of a straight eye and non-foveal area of a squinting eye form corresponding points and acquire common visual direction, it is called *abnormal retinal correspondence* (ARC). The abnormal retinal correspondence is, therefore, an abnormal binocular state in squinting eyes. Abnormal retinal correspondence is compatible with good visual acuity and binocularity in spite of squint, the angle of which is small. In ARC, the objective and subjective angles of the squint are different and this is an important diagnostic point. The difference between the two is called *angle of anomaly*. When the angle of anomaly is equal to the objective angle of the squint it is called *harmonious ARC*. When the angle of anomaly is smaller than the objective angle, it is called *unharmonious ARC*. Unharmonious ARC may be the earlier stage of harmonious ARC. The type of retinal correspondence normal or abnormal whether harmonious or unharmonious is possible to determine on a synoptophore.

The clinical significance of abnormal retinal correspondence is in a case of small degree of squint with good binocularity. The correction of squint in such cases is likely to introduce intractable diplopia and, in such cases, therefore, when the squint corrected, possibility of diplopia should be kept in mind which is often temporary. It is also important to understand the difference between abnormal retinal correspondence and eccentric fixation. The former is a binocular condition while the latter is uniocular.

Eccentric Fixation

In this condition, the image on retina is formed on a spot other than fovea on attempted fixation of a target. The new point tends to acquire the function of fovea. This point is called *false fovea or false macula*. Depending on the location of false fovea, the eccentric fixation may be *Para foveal, para-macular, centro-coecal or peripheral*. It is evident that the area of false fovea is relatively deficient in cones than the anatomical fovea. Therefore visual acuity in these eyes is sub-normal. The farther away the false fovea from anatomical fovea, poorer is the vision. It is important to emphasize that eccentric fixation is always a uniocular condition.

Eccentric fixation is more likely to develop when squint starts in early childhood and the squinting eye is not treated for a long time (Fig. 18.5).

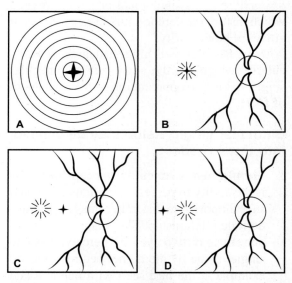

Fig. 18.5: Eccentric Fixation-Test with Ophthal-moscope (A) Star as in grid of ophthalmoscope (rings help in measuring degrees of eccentricity); (B) Foveal fixation—star at fovea; (C) Eccentric fixation in convergent squint—star between fovea and disc; (D) Eccentric fixation in divergent squint—star temporal to fovea.

Clinically a simple test to detect eccentric fixation is *light fixation test*. The patient is asked to look at the light with the squinting eye (the other eye being covered). If the patient fixes the light with the eye in an eccentric position, it indicates the presence of gross eccentric fixation. A lesser degree of eccentric fixation can be better detected with direct ophthalmoscope which has a star graticule incorporated in it. The patient is asked to look into the light of the ophthalmoscope and the observer notes the position of star shadow on the retina in relation to the anatomical fovea. If there is no eccentric fixation, the centre of the star and the foveal reflex coincide, but if there is eccentric fixation, the shadow of the star will be seen away from the foveal reflex. Other methods of detecting eccentric fixation are with the Euthyscope or Projectoscope.

Amblyopia

It is diminution of vision for which no pathological cause can be detected in the media or retina or in visual pathway up to the cortex and which cannot be corrected by any optical aid like glasses, contact lens, etc.

Types of Amblyopia

1. **Congenital amblyopia** which is usually associated with congenital anomalies like nystagmus and albinism etc.
2. **Amblyopia ex-anopsia** is also known as *disuse amblyopia*. This is also common in young age and can be caused by bandaging one eye for a long time, total congenital ptosis and occlusion of the eye, or any other cause depriving the eye of proper visual stimulation.
3. **Anisometropic amblyopia.** In a case in which two images in the two eyes are unequal and there is lack of binocular fusion, it leads to passive suppression of the weaker eye. A good example is *uniocular aphakia* in childhood and *hypermetropic anisometropia*. Amblyopia is much more common in hypermetropic anisometropia than in myopic anisometropia. Amblyopia can also develop even when both eyes have the same degree of spherical error but one eye needs an added

cylindrical correction or both eyes need the same amount of compound hypermetropic glasses but the eye with an oblique axis of cylinder develops amblyopia. The high incidence of amblyopia in hypermetropic eyes is due to its onset in early age and poor vision for near objects. Amblyopia may affect eyes with myopic anisometropia but it is uncommon because myopia develops after the age of 4 to 5 and near vision is good.

4. **Aniseikonic amblyopia** is where the images in two eyes are unequal in shape and size. A good example is an aniseikonic refractive state of the eyes (described in the chapter on Refraction—Rectinoscopy).
5. **Strabismic amblyopia** is a condition where the light focus in one eye is formed away from the macular area. This image is blurred and is actively suppressed. The vision in such amblyopic eyes may be as low as hand movements or as much as 6/12 or 6/18 but is poorer than the normal eye. The degree of suppression will depend on the age of onset of amblyopia, the degree of anisometropia and the duration of amblyopia.

Amblyopia is the result of visual suppression believed to be taking place at the cerebral cortex. Peripheral fields in amblyopia are not grossly affected but there is a general depression evident in relative scotometery and a central scotoma is present.

An electroretinogram is usually normal but an EOG and VER may show abnormal and delayed response.

Treatment of Amblyopia

The treatment of amblyopia depends on whether the amblyopic eye has central fixation or eccentric fixation. With central fixation, treatment is done by occluding the good eye and forcing the amblyopic eye to function. If the fixation is eccentric, then a trial occlusion of the good eye is done for 2-4 weeks. If during this period the fixation becomes central then the occlusion of the good eye is continued till the vision of the amblyopic eye improves to normal or near normal or after certain improvement becomes static. If the fixation does not tend to become central, then occlusion of the sound eye is stopped and an inverse occlusion to the amblyopic eye is given. This is done to eliminate the function of false fovea. This inverse occlusion is followed later on by pleoptics and reading through the red filter to stimulate anatomical fovea.

Occlusion

Occlusion is an accepted and rewarding therapy in treatment of amblyopia for restoring macular function. Occlusion may be conventional or inverse. In conventional occlusion, the good eye is occluded and the amblyopic eye with poor vision is forced to function. Occlusion may be total or partial. In total occlusion, eye is kept occluded during all waking hours. Occlusion is continued for as long as it is necessary. It is interesting how readily occlusion is accepted even by small children who may even sleep with the occluder on (Figs 18.6 and 18.7).

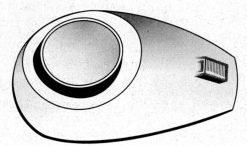

Fig 18.6: Rubber occluder

Total occlusion is best done with a rubber occluder which can be stuck to the spectacle glass by vacuum action, occluding the front as well as the side. In smaller children, an occlusion can be improvised with adhesive plaster, which does not have to be removed at night.

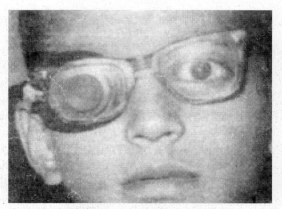

Fig 18.7: Occluder Fixed to spectacles

Partial occlusion has much less application and effect. It may, however, be the only choice in very small children. It is also indicated to equalise the vision of the two eyes where vision in the amblyopic eye is fairly good. Partial occlusion is done either by using atropine in the good eye or by putting a ground glass lens in the spectacle frame before the good eye.

Inverse occlusion as against conventional occlusion, described above, is occlusion of the amblyopic eye which has developed eccentric fixation and a false macula. The purpose is to inhibit the false macula. It is continued till the false fovea is suppressed and the anatomical fovea can be stimulated to take up fixation. This is followed by conventional occlusion.

When giving occlusion, vision of the occluded eye should be checked up every 1-2 weeks and the progress of the vision of the amblyopic eye should be noted. Occlusion should be continued till vision of both eyes has become equal or improvement in the amblyopic eye has reached its limit. The successful treatment of occlusion should be followed by orthoptic exercises or appropriate surgery to stablise the gain achieved by occlusion.

Alternate conventional and inverse occlusion should be continued if for some reason, suppor-tive treatment by exercises or surgery has to be delayed. Alternate occlusion is also indicated when vision in the good eye under total occlusion tends to deteriorate.

Prisms and Their Use

Prisms are used both for diagnostic and therapeutic purposes, The principle of their use is that rays of light passing through prisms are deviated towards the base and hence the object seen through a prism is displaced towards the apex.

Prisms are used for the following purposes:
1. Diagnostic.
2. Therapeutic.
3. Orthoptic.

1. **Diagnostic:** To measure angle of squint, latent or manifest. Prisms are used in increasing power till cover test becomes negative. Depending on whether the squint is horizontal or vertical, prisms are used either as base-in and base-out or base-up and base-down respectively.

2. **Therapeutic uses of prisms:** Prisms are prescribed to be incorporated in spectacle glasses but prismo-therapy is usually the last choice where the exercises are not fruitful or where surgery has left behind a small degree of squint either due to under-correction or over-correction. Prisms are sometimes prescribed for heterophoria to relieve symptoms. The principle of use of prism is the same as in diagnostic purposes, i.e., base-out for esophoria and base-in for exophoria. The same principle holds good for treating paralytic squint to avoid diplopia or to stimulate fusion.

   Small degrees of prisms is also prescribed in reading glasses for comfortable near work with decentring higher power of the lenses on the principle that 1 cm decentring in a one dioptre lens will cause prismatic effect of one prism dioptre. The same may be stated as 1 mm displacement in 10 D lens will cause 1 prism dioptre effect. In another way, the amount of decentring required may be calculated by dividing the desired prism effect by the dioptric power of the lens e.g. 2 prism dioptres lens = 2/10.0 is equal to 0.2 cm (2 mm) displacement.

3. **Prism for orthoptic exercises:** These exercises strengthen the muscle by making them act against the prism. For this purpose they are used with the base placed in the direction opposite to that used for prismotherapy and diagnosis. They are used base-in for convergence exercises and base-out for divergence effect. Similarly, in pleoptics they are used base-in for eccentric fixation to displace the image into the anatomical fovea.

AETIOLOGY OF SQUINT

Whatever the precipitating cause, there are always pre-existing factors responsible for development of squint. These factors are obstacles which come in the way of development of perfect binocularity and fusion and are thus responsible for development of squint. There are many types of such obstacles.
1. Sensory obstacles like errors of refraction.
2. Motor obstacles like faulty development or functioning of ocular muscles.
3. Central obstacles where there is failure to develop fusion at the higher centres.

   Among the common specific causes are:
   i. Uncorrected refractive states like hypermetropia, myopia, high astigmatism, anisometropia, abnormal AC/A ratio.
   ii. Obstruction to the light going into the eye by causes like ptosis, opacities in the media or occlusion by bandaging for some length of time.
   iii. Abnormal development of extra-ocular muscles or paralysis of the muscles.
   iv. Failure in the development of fusion.

   In addition, heredity plays an important role as a contributory factor.

   Most children are born without a squint. The eyes are prone to develop squint because of the obstructive factor which may be present. The precipitating cause like acute febrile illness, trauma or occlusion of an eye leads to breakdown of the balance which keep the eyes parallel. Once this balance breaks, the causative factors do not allow the eye to get back to normal position unless treated. With this breakdown, suppression factor in the squinting eye becomes dominant, breaking binocularity and thus making it more difficult to return to normalcy.

In young age, binocularity is in a phase of development and therefore the eye is in an unstable state. It is for this reason that onset of squint is mostly in young people. Once binocular vision is fully established, the chances of developing a concomitant squint are extremely rare.

The onset of concomitant squint is, therefore around the age of 2 to 3 years. It follows some temporary illness or trauma which does not mean that this has caused the squint but has disturbed the balance so that the eye which was prone to develop squint, actually develops the same.

Clinical Aspects of Squint

Clinically, squint may be latent or manifest. The former is called *heterophoria* and the latter is called *heterotropia*. If there is no squint either latent or manifest, it is called orthophoria.

Every case of concomitant squint should be examined in detail and evaluated on the basis of findings.

Examination and Evaluation of a Case of Squint

Critical assessment of a case of squint will go a long way in evaluating the prognosis and deciding the surgery indicated in a particular case. A routine procedure is described below:

History: To evaluate a case of squint, the patient's history is very important. The important questions to be asked are:
   i. Age of onset of the squint.

   ii. Mode of onset of the squint—slow or sudden.
  iii. Intermittent or constant.
  iv. History of acute illness or trauma or bandaging of one eye for some length of time.
   v. History of any treatment of squint, surgical or non-surgical.
  vi. History of squint in the other members of the family.

Examination of the Patient

1. **Distant inspection:** A look at the child is important to note an anomalous head posture and position of eyes in relation to each other. The uniocular or alternative character of squint, if present, may be noted. Incidentally nystagmus may also be noted.

2. **Visual acuity:** Vision should be recorded in each eye separately, both for near and distance, on standard vision charts. In pre-school children, the E-chart or C-chart are more practical to use.

3. **Ocular movements.** Eye movements should be critically observed for each eye separately and both eyes together in all 8 cardinal directions (Fig. 18.8).

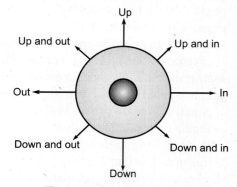

Fig. 18.8: Eight cardinal directions

In a concomitant squint of recent origin, eye movements are full in all directions. In long-standing cases where no treatment was done, the stronger muscle may develop contractures, particularly the medial recti. There may, therefore, be some degree of restriction of movement in the horizontal direction. The eye movements, however, are always defective in paralytic squint. There may be some anomalous movement in the squinting eye which has been previously operated for squint and develops adhesion due to faulty surgical procedure. Binocular movements will help in detecting common anomalies like over-action of the inferior oblique or similar aberration in other muscles.

4. **Cover test:** This is the most useful, informative and easy to carry out test. If performed with clear concept, it gives a sea of information. To get complete and dependable information, the test should be performed with the patient looking straight ahead and with the eyes turned in all eight cardinal directions of gaze one after the other. The test should be done with the patient looking at 6 metres and also at near object, 1/3 metre. It is important that the test should be repeated two to three times to ensure that the observations are dependable.

   Method of conducting the cover test. There are two parts of the cover test, uniocular *uncovering* and *binocular uncovering*. The former is also called *alternating cover-uncover test* and the latter is called *uniocular cover and uncover test*.
   a. **Uniocular cover and uncover test.** In this test one eye is covered and uncovered successively. Any movement of the eye on uncovering, if present, should be noted. If there is no manifest squint and the eye on uncovering moves in, it indicates *exophoria*. If it moves

out on uncovering, it is *esophoria*. If no movement is noted, the eyes are orthophoric, that is, there is no muscle imbalance. Similarly, vertical and cyclo elements can be detected.

   b. **Alternating cover-uncover test.** It is specially indicated when a manifest squint is present. One eye is covered, the position of the uncovered eye noted and then the cover is shifted to the opposite eye. Change in the position of the second uncovered eye is noted. If the patient has a manifest squint, the alternating cover test can indicate whether the squint is uniocular or alternating. If on uncovering, fixation returns to the same eye, it is uniocular. If each eye can maintain fixation in turn, it is an *alternating squint*. If there is a manifest squint but the alternating cover test indicates no movements, the interpretation is that the squint is an *apparent* and not real. If excursions of movement on uncovering is equal in each eye, the squint is a *concomitant squint*. If excursion is more in one eye than the other, it is a *paralytic squint*. If one eye, on uncovering, looks straight at the object while the other on uncovering fixes from the eccentric position indicates that one eye has *eccentric fixation*.

   If the cover test indicates the degree of esophoria or esotropia (internal squint) more for near than for distance it indicates *convergence excess*. If it is the reverse, it is *divergence weakness*. Similarly, in exophoria or exotropia, if it is more for near, it is a *convergence deficiency* and if the opposite, it indicates *divergence excess*. This information is valuable in deciding the type of surgery. During cover test, sometimes, nystagmus is discovered in the open eye when the opposite eye is covered although nystagmus was not present with both eyes open. This nystagmus which is discovered during the cover test, is called *latent nystagmus.*

c. **Cover test with neutralising prisms.** This test is to measure the degree of deviation. The cover test is repeated and increasing degree of prisms are placed in front of the fixing eye till the stage is reached that the cover test is negative. The prism is held base-in for a divergent squint, base-out for a convergent squint and base up or down in a vertical squint. The degree of prisms needed for neutralising the eye movements on covering and uncovering, gives the degree of squint in prism diopters.

To summarise, the cover test gives the following information:

i. If squint is present, whether it is apparent or real.

ii. Whether squint is latent or manifest.

iii Whether squint is uniocular or alternating.

iv. Whether squint is paralytic or non-paralytic.

v. Whether fixation is central or eccentric.

vi. Whether squint is convergence deficiency or divergence excess type.

vii. Detects latent nystagmus, if present.

5. **Measurement of angle of the squint.** There are various methods of measuring the angle of squint:

i. **Corneal reflex test (Hirchberg test):** The patient is asked, with both eyes open to look at a spot of light held 15 inches away. The position of the corneal reflex in each eye is noted. If the reflex is in the centre of the cornea in both eyes, the patient has no manifest squint. If the reflex in one eye is central and in the

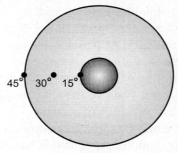

Fig 18.9: Hirschberg corneal reflex test in an average-sized pupil indicating approximate degree of squint

other eye is medial or lateral to the centre, the patient has a divergent or convergent squint respectively. This test also helps in excluding apparent squint due to facial anomalies. The distance of light reflex from the centre of the cornea gives approximate degree of squint. If the reflex in the squinting eye is at the limbus, squint is about 45°. If it is between the pupillary margin and the limbus, it is 20° to 25°. If it is at the normal pupillary margin, it is 10° to 15°. These figures are obviously approximate because the pupil size varies in different individuals. It may be noted that this test gives a rough estimation of degree of squint. The test can be erroneous in cases of facial asymmetry and asymmetrical pupillary position on the two sides

ii. **Measurement of the angle of squint** on a synoptophore or major amblyoscope. Measuring the degree of squint on the synoptophore has the advantage that one can measure the subjective angle of the squint based on the patient's own observations. One can also measure the objective angle in cases where there is no binocularity due to suppression in squinting eye.

6. **Type of Fixation:** It is important to know whether the squinting eye has central or eccentric fixation because it not only helps to assess prognosis of the case but it also

suggests efforts needed to revert the eccentric fixation to central fixation by appropriate means, if possible.

7. **State of binocularity:** It is also important to know whether some degree of binocularity, simultaneous perception and/or fusion, is present or not. The presence of some degree of pre-operative binocularity is necessary to indicate good visual prognosis after operation. If no grade of binocular vision is present, visual prognosis is unfavourable and uncertain.

8. **State of retinal correspondence:** Similarly it is also important to know whether retinal correspondence is normal or abnormal. A small squint with abnormal retinal correspondence is better not operated because of chances of post-operative diplopia. In higher degrees of squint with abnormal retinal correspondence, however, true fusion, stereopsis are not possible and squint correction is largely cosmetic and therefore no diplopia.

9. **Accommodative convergence/accommodation (AC/A) ratio:** This is also important because if the case has excessive AC/A ratio the patient may be treated on purely non-surgical lines or surgery may be supplemented by non-surgical measures.

10. **Refraction:** It is the most important examination to be done in all cases of concomitant squint. It is important to know if the eye is myopic or hypermetropic and whether there is any degree of anisometropia. In all cases of strabismus, assessing refractive state of the eye under complete cycloplegia with atropine ointment 1% applied thrice daily for 3 days or homotropine 2% solution eye drops every 15 minutes for 2½ to 3 hrs gives the information vitally needed to plan treatment.

Types of Squint

The different clinical types of squint are classified as follows:

1. Heterophoria (latent squint).
   a. Exophoria—Divergent latent squint.
   b. Esophoria—Convergent latent squint.
   c. Hyperphoria—Vertical latent squint.
   d. Cyclophoria—Rotational latent squint.
2. Accommodational squint and convergent deficiency.
3. Heterotropia (manifest squint).
   a. Uniocular concomitant squint.
      i. Esotropia—Convergent manifest squint.
      ii. Exotropia—Divergent manifest squint.
      iii. Hypertropia—Vertical manifest squint.
      iv. Cyclotropia—Rotational manifest squint.
   b. Alternating convergent or divergent squint.
4. Non-commitment (Paralytic squint).

Latent Squint (Heterophoria)

Latent squint is a condition where both eyes have an inherent desire for binocular single vision and remain parallel with effort required to fulfill the desire. If, however, the two eyes are dissociated by covering one eye, the eye goes into a position of squint. If the eye under cover converges, it is called esophoria. If it diverges, it is called *exophoria*. If the eye goes up or down, it is called *hyperphoria right or left* and if the upper pole of cornea under cover rotates in or out, it is called *incyclophoria* or *excyclophoria*. The latent squint can be measured with a Maddox rod for distance and a Maddox wing for near or more accurately measured by using neutralising prisms in the Maddox test (Fig. 18.10).

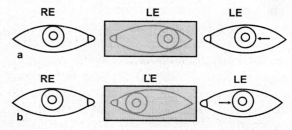

Fig 18.10: Cover Test Detecting Heterophoria (A) LE exophoric under cover, returns to primary position on uncovering; (B) LE esophoric under cover, returns to primary position on uncovering

In a normal population, some degree of latent squint is a rule rather than an exception. In fact, true orthophoria is very uncommon. Exophoria is more common than esophoria both in young as well as in old age.

Symptoms: Heterophoria being a common condition, always raises a question, whether the symptoms of eye strain are due to heterophoria or not. If heterophoria is fully compensated without effort, the symptoms are not due to heterophoria, but if it is not compensated and if there is a tendency for binocular vision to breakdown, even though it is temporary, muscle imbalance causes symptoms.

Latent squint is the second most important cause of ocular headache, next only to errors of refraction. In all cases of symptoms of eye strain where error of refraction does not explain these symptoms, the patient should be examined for muscle imbalance. If this is kept in mind, many patients will be saved from unnecessary reference to ENT surgeons or neurophysicians.

Symptoms are more common with exophoria than with esophoria because an exophoric patient has to make a constant effort to keep the eye parallel and this effort causes symptoms of eye strain like headache, tiredness and watering. Symptoms are usually common after office work, after going to a movie and after driving. Symptoms are more severe in heterophoria compensated with effort and less severe in uncompensated exophoria. Some patients complain of running together of letters and blurring of vision which coincide with a temporary breakdown of binocularity. Diplopia is sometimes complained of as a transient feeling when muscle balance breaks down. Some patients have difficulty in adjusting from distance to near and vice-versa.

In some cases, there is intermittent squint and this happens when muscle balance breaks down frequently.

Hyperphoria is much less common than eso- or exophoria. It is a condition where the eye under cover goes up, and hypophoria when it goes down, but for clinical purposes the terminology used is right hyperphoria when the right eye is at a higher level and left hyperphoria when the left eye is at a higher level.

Treatment of latent squint

There is a well-established procedure for these patients.

1. The patient should be examined for error of refraction under effective cycloplegia, using atropine in children below the age of 15 years and homatropine between 15 and 35 years. The error of refraction should be corrected with appropriate glasses, and patient advised constant use. Hypermetropia should be fully corrected in esophoria to relieve spasm of accommodation and under-corrected in exophoria. The vice-versa holds good when correcting myopia.

2. **Orthoptic exercises:** These should first be given to strengthen the weaker muscles so that binocularity can be maintained without extra effort. In most cases, 7 to 10 days' exercises on synoptophore may be followed by home exercises. Exercises are more effective in exophoria and less so in esophoria.

3. If exercises do not indicate response by appreciable improvement, an operation is necessary.

4. **Prisms:** If exercises do not overcome muscle imbalance and the patient refuses operation, relieving prisms may be prescribed, base-out for esophoria and base-in for exophoria. The principle is that we start with 1/2 of the total prism correction needed and this is divided equally between two eyes. In case of hyperphoria, exercises are least likely to be helpful and therefore prisms are more often prescribed and full correction is well tolerated. Whenever prisms are prescribed, repeated check-up is necessary to adjust the strength of the prisms.

In addition to the lines of treatment indicated above, patient's reading habits should be corrected if necessary and general health should be improved.

Accommodative Squint

To see a near object clearly, one has to accommodate and the eyes also have to converge so that clear image falls on macula in both eyes. Accommodation and convergence, therefore, work proportionate to each other. This mutual relationship is necessary for good binocularity and comfort in near work. If there is excessive accommodation, there ought to be excessive convergence but the inhibitory centre in the cortex prevents excess of convergence. If this inhibitory factor is inadequate, the excessive accommodation leads to excessive convergence which may result in *accommodational convergent squint.*

More accommodation for clear near vision is needed in hypermetropia. Accommodational squint is, therefore, more common in hypermetropic eyes. It usually becomes manifest about the age of 2-3 years when the child starts concentrating on near objects.

At this labile stage, any disturbance in the AC/A ratio is favourable for development of a squint.

Accommodational convergent squint may present different clinical grades:

1. When the squint disappears on wearing hypermetropic correction (Fig. 18.11)
2. When squint persists for near, even with hypermetropic correction.
3. When squint is present for distance and near both but the deviation decreases when hypermetropic glasses are worn.

Following examinations should be carried out in a serial order:

1. Record of vision with and without glasses for distance and near.

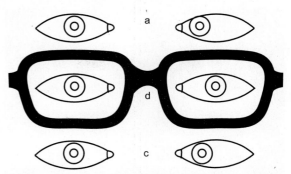

Fig 18.11: Accommodative Squint. (a) Internal squint; (b) With hypermetropic glasses, squint disappears; (c) Squint reappears on removal of glasses

2. Cover test for distance and near. This is not difficult even in small children by using a point of light and being tactful in handling.
3. Note light reflex on cornea (Hirschberg's test).
4. Test ocular movements in all directions.
5. Examination on synoptophore for assessing binocular function. This is difficult in very young or non-cooperative children.
6. Estimation AC/A ratio.
7. Most important of all in accommodative squint is estimation of refractive error under complete cycloplegia.

Accommodational squint, if diagnosed, and treated early, is in most cases curable without surgery. In fact, a child who develops an accommodative squint in early childhood about the age of one year, may grow out of it because as age advances, accommodation becomes less and, therefore, convergence becomes less. This should, however, not be taken for granted. The child should be examined from time to time. If not treated adequately and in time, binocularity may breakdown and squint may become constant (Fig. 18.12).

Treatment of an accommodative squint depends on its clinical grade. The line of treatment to be adopted is as follows:

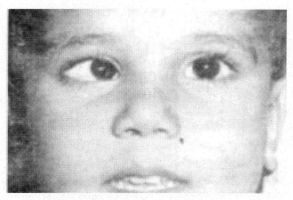

Fig 18.12: Accommodative squint in a child

1. **Correct the refractive error** at the earliest. Parents often object to use of glasses at too young an age. It is not difficult to prove the useful effect of glasses by disappearance of squint with glasses. It is interesting how a child 2½ to 3 years can go about with glasses on because he has subconsciously appreciated the gain in vision with glasses.

   Hypermetropic error should be fully corrected on the basis of retinoscopy values under cycloplegia. The use of glasses should be started before the effect of atropine has passed off. If however the child does not tolerate full correction, one may start with an under-correction and increase the power every 3 to 4 months. When accommodative squint is more for near, it is advisable to give bifocal glasses with under-correction for distance and full correction for near.

2. **Miotics:** The use of miotics is a well-established therapy for accommodative convergent squint. Sometimes miotics alone can correct squint.

The miotics by acting on the para-sympathetic nerve endings and the sphincter muscle, stimulate accommodative action of ciliary muscle and contract the pupil. Stimulation of accommodation and contraction of the pupil, both help in improving clarity of vision for near and thus reducing the need of accommodation from the higher centres which is closely related to convergence, so that if there is less central accommodation there is less convergence and hence less accommodative squint.

The best indication for miotic therapy is an accommodative convergent squint with small or no hypermetropic refraction when visual acuity is good and equal in both eyes and when AC/A is high.

Convergence Insufficiency

It has already been emphasised that eyes in a state of complete rest are slightly exophoric. It has also been explained that when doing near work, both eyes converge as they accommodate. This is a physiologically coordinated function. Convergence, therefore, is as important for near work as accommodation. If power of the medial recti muscles for simultaneous convergence movement is weak, it causes convergence insufficiency. This is a binocular deficiency because each eye may separately still have full movements in all directions of gaze. The simplest method of measuring convergence is the pencil test. A pencil held at 1/3 metre in front of the eye is slowly moved nearer towards the nose. The patient is asked to concentrate on the pencil point all the time. As soon as the single image becomes double, he should immediately inform the observer. At this point, the observer will also note that one of the two eyes moves out. The distance of the object from the eyes at this point is measured in centimetres. Normally convergence should not break earlier than 6 to 8 cm. Convergence can more accurately be measured on synoptophore with fusion grade and is recorded in degrees. Convergence of 20° or more is normal (Figs. 18.13 to 18.16).

Causes of Convergence Insufficiency

1. Most of the causes of convergence insufficiency are primary and idiopathic with or

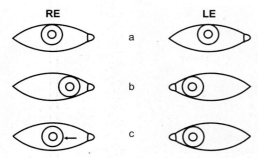

Fig 18.13: Convergence Test, (a) BE looking straight; (b) BE looking at near object, note convergent position (c) convergence breaks, right eye moves out

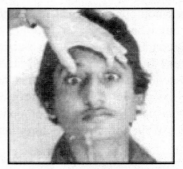

Fig 18.14: Convergence Test. Looking at a distance object

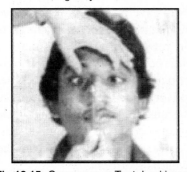

Fig 18.15: Convergence Test. Looking at a Near Object

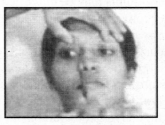

Fig 18.16: Convergence Test. (Looking closer than near point Convergence breaks and RE moves out)

without exophoria. The condition is usually precipitated by strain of near work or an illness.

2. Convergence insufficiency is commonly associated with presbyopia because with age, accommodation weakens and the patient tends to develop exophoria.

3. Uncorrected refractive errors or incorrect power of glasses cause blurring of near vision which disturbs the convergence-accommodation balance. This may result in convergence insufficiency.

4. Convergence insufficiency may also be caused by over-recession of the medial recti or over-resection of the lateral recti.

It is surprising how frequent convergence insufficiency is and how equally frequently it is overlooked as cause of symptoms of eye strain, specially on near work. The greater the demand on the eyes, poor visual hygiene, poor nutrition and stress and strain of fast life of the present era, could all contribute to the higher incidence of convergence insufficiency. It is, therefore, extremely important that in any case of eye strain, examination for error of refraction and muscle balance test should be followed by measurement of convergence.

Treatment: The line of treatment for convergence insufficiency is:

1. Correction of refractive error, if any, both for distance and near, on the principle of under-correction for hypermetropia and full correction of myopia.

2. Convergence exercises which should be started on synoptophore for a week or more followed by exercises at home. At home, the patient is asked to repeat the pencil test, overcoming diplopia by an extra effort and reduce the distance of the near point to desired range. Exercises

on synoptophore indicate before the week is out, whether the exercises will improve the condition or not. If there is no improvement by exercises, small and equal resection of both medial recti is indicated. If the patient refuses surgery, convergence deficiency may be compensated by prescribing prisms base-in for near only.

HETEROTROPIA (MANIFEST SQUINT)

Concomitant convergent squint (Esotropia). Convergent squints may be classified as:

1. Primary convergent squint from birth or early childhood.
2. Secondary convergent squint as in cases with corneal opacities or retinal pathology.
3. Consecutive convergent squint due to over-correction of a divergent squint.
4. Paralytic convergent squint as in 6th nerve, lateral rectus palsy.

The majority of uniocular concomitant squints are convergent in nature.

Unlike accommodational squint, a concomitant convergent squint is constant in nature and is present both for distance and near vision and also with and without glasses (Figs. 18.17 and 18.18).

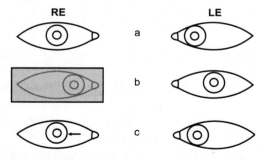

Fig 18. 17: Concomitant Convergent. Squint—Left Internal (a) RE fixing—LE convergent; (b) LE fixing—RE convergent under cover; (c) On uncovering, squint returns to LE

Concomitant convergent squint is mostly uniocular squint although alternating convergent concomitant squint is not uncommon. Visual

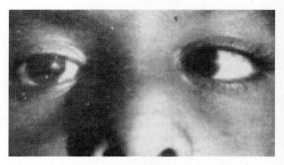

Fig 18.18: Left Concomitant convergent squint

acuity in the squinting eye is poor. There is a tendency to develop *suppression amblyopia* and *eccentric fixation.* Hypermetropia is the most common refractive error associated with it. Esotropia is however not uncommon in congenital high myopia where the child, to see at near point, has to converge and yet does not need accommodation because the difference between the far point and the near point in a high myopic is very small. Convergence is stabilised and he, therefore, develops esotropia.

In concomitant convergent squint the eye movements are normal and full but in long standing untreated cases, the contracture of medial rectus may develop and limit the lateral movements of the eye.

From the clinical and therapeutic point of view, it is important to group primary esotropia in three main groups:

1. Convergence excess type where deviation is more for near than for distance.
2. Divergence weakness type where deviation is more for distance than for near.
3. Basic type where deviation is equal for both distance and near.

Treatment: Principle of treatment follows the general lines which include:

1. Correction of the error of refraction and use of glasses as advised.
2. Treatment of amblyopia by occlusion as described earlier.

3. Orthoptic exercises if necessary, to overcome suppression.

4. Surgery, which may be recession of the medial recti alone or further supported by resection of lateral recti depending on the degree of squint or whether squint is convergence excess type or divergence insufficiency type. Sometimes surgery on two horizontal muscles of the same eye may not be enough to fully correct squint and in that case one of horizontal muscles of other eye may need to be similarly dealt with.

5. Orthoptic exercises should be continued post-operatively, to stabilise effects of operation and to develop and stabilise binocular single vision.

It is important to emphasize that treatment of squint should best be started and all lines of treatment should be completed before the child goes to school. These days of early school/nursery admission, treatment will need to be continued after the child has started schooling. The later the treatment, the lesser are the chances of developing binocular vision. Results are poor when the eye has developed eccentric fixation and the muscle has developed contractures.

Cosmetic correction of squint has so often to be undertaken in developing countries because the children are brought late and only when parents become conscious of the handicap from the social point of view. They bring the child to an ophthalmologist often for social rehabilitation. A cosmetic correction of squint will in most cases correct the alignment of the eyes but will not improve vision. Furthermore, the amblyopic eye will have a tendency to go back into squinting position in some cases.

Concomitant divergent squint (Exotropia). Divergent squints may be:
1. Primary divergent squint.
2. Secondary divergent squint.

3. Consecutive divergent squint.
4. Paralytic divergent squint.

Primary Divergent Squint

A primary divergent squint may be alternating or uniocular and may be intermittent or constant.

Alternating divergent squint is fairly common: Alternation is more common in divergent squint than in convergent. The characteristic feature is fixation with one eye at a time. Vision is usually equal and good in both eyes but no binocularity. There is often no error of refraction but when present, myopia is more common than hypermetropia. Myopic eyes have poor accommodation and therefore less convergence is needed for clear near vision and hence the eye tends to diverge, (Figs 18.19 and 18.20A and B).

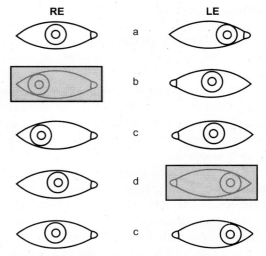

Fig 18.19: Alternate divergent Squint, (a) RE fixing—LE divergent, (b) RE covered—LE fixes, (c) On uncovering, LE retains fixation, (d) LE covered—RE fixes, (e) On uncovering, RE retains fixation

Treatment of an alternating divergent squint needs to be carefully considered. Neither occlusion nor orthoptic exercises can make any difference from the treatment point of view. While planning surgery, it is important to keep in

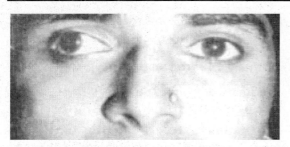

Fig 18.20A: Alternate Divergent squint, LE fixing— RE divergent

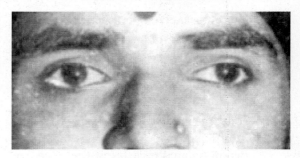

Fig. 18.20B: RE fixing—LE divergent

mind that there is a tendency to develop diplopia after full surgical correction.

Most of the alternating squints are usually more than 20° and it is important to evaluate whether the squint is:

1. Divergence excess type.
2. Convergence weakness type.
3. Basic type.

It is on this basis that the surgical line of treatment is decided.

Although a horizontal concomitant squint remains constant in all directions of the gaze, it is not necessarily always so particularly in vertical movements.

When a convergent squint decreases and divergent squint increases on looking up and on looking down the convergent deviation increases and the divergent deviation decreases, it is called a *V-phenomenon.*

On the other hand, when looking up, a convergent squint increases and a divergent squint decreases and on looking down the convergent deviation decreases and the divergent deviation increases, it is called an *A-phenomenon.*

Association of V or A phenomenon with a convergent or divergent squint is important from the treatment point of view.

It is therefore also important to assess presence of AV phenomenon because divergence with A phenomenon is due to convergence deficiency and therefore resection of the medial recti should be the first choice. Surgery can be recession of the lateral recti for divergence excess cases. The surgery should be equally divided on each eye. Post-operative orthoptic exercises should be given not only to help develop fusion but to prevent recurrence of squint.

Intermittent divergent squint: It is the precursor of a constant divergent squint if not treated early. The intermittence of squint is due to intermittent effort of convergence and accommodative convergence to overcome squint. The condition is, therefore, overlooked for quite some time till squint becomes constantly uniocular or alternating. So long as the intermittence persists, amblyopia does not develop.

The treatment of intermittent exotropia should start with orthoptic exercises particularly in cases of convergence weakness type. Exercises should be continued after surgery also. It is important that careful evaluation should be done to avoid over-correction by surgery which may cause intractable diplopia. It is better that any residual squint after recession of lateral recti should be corrected by prisms rather than operation on medial recti.

Uniocular divergent squint: This is rather uncommon. Uniocular myopia is a common association in primary cases. The degree of squint is usually constant in nature. There is less tendency to develop amblyopia. The correction of uniocular exotropia is by operation on both horizontal muscles of the squinting eye in one sitting. Only rarely the residual squint after surgery on the squinting eye may need a second operation on the horizontal muscles of the other eye (Fig. 18.21).

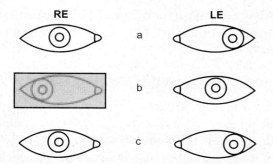

Fig 18.21: Concomitant divergent squint—LE divergent, (a) RE fixing—LE divergent, (b) LE fixing—RE divergent under cover, (c) On uncovering, squint returns to LE

Secondary Divergent Squint

It is usually uniocular. It follows the development of corneal opacity or a lens opacity or any other intra-ocular pathology causing diminution of vision in one eye. The eyes are usually exophoric and any gross disturbance of vision of one eye converts exophoria into exotropia of the weaker eye. If the causative condition is curable e.g. by a corneal graft or by removal of cataract with intraocular lens implant or contact lens, the exotropia may revert to exophoria and manifest squint may disappear (Fig. 18.22).

Consecutive Divergent Squint

It is usually the result of faulty surgery for correcting a convergent squint. A consecutive squint is, in most cases, amenable to surgical correction but it involves exploration for fishing out the improperly handled muscle and restoring it to its appropriate position.

Paralytic Exotropia

It is due to partial or total 3rd nerve paralysis. The unaffected lateral rectus tends to diverge the eye because the ipsilateral antagonist is paralysed. This is discussed in greater detail in the section on paralytic squint.

Vertical squint: A purely commitment vertical squint is extremely rare. Most-cases are associated with a horizontal component. The vertical squints are grouped in two categories:

1. When the vertical component is the primary defect and the horizontal element is secondarily introduced. The binocularity breaks. These squints are primarily due to paresis of one or more vertically acting muscles.

2. Secondary vertical squints are cases where the horizontal element is the primary anomaly and the vertical defect is secondarily caused by malfunction of one or the other vertical muscles. For example, in a convergent eye the inferior oblique has maximum elevation action in the adducted position and hence the inferior oblique develops overaction. The same applies to corresponding vertical muscles in a divergent squint.

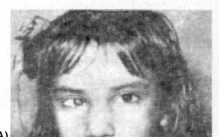
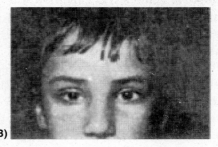

(A)   **(B)**

Fig. 18.22: Spontaneous recovery of squint following lamellar keratoplasty in a 7-years-old girl. (A) Before operation, (B) 70-days after lamellar grafting, in the right eye. Convergent squint that had followed corneal pathology disappeared, suggesting esopphoria turned into esotropia as a result of the uniocular pathology, which disapeared with improvement in vision following surgery

The best method to diagnose a vertical element in a horizontal squint is to do a cover test in all 9 cardinal positions. The angle of squint increases in the direction of faulty action of the vertical muscle. In primary vertical squint the horizontal squint is variable. Furthermore, binocular vision is more readily lost in primary vertical deviation than in secondary vertical deviation. In long-standing cases, however, with contractures in the direct antagonist muscle, evaluation may not be easy and dependable.

Treatment of vertical squint is surgical and orthoptics is only needed to improve convergence and binocularity. The principle of surgery in general is that correction of a primary horizontal deviation should be done first following which the secondary vertical anomaly can sponta-neously get corrected and no second surgery may be needed. In the primary type of vertical squint, both vertical and horizontal elements can be corrected at the same time provided of course the results of investigative evaluation are dependable. The surgery may include dealing with obliques and horizontal recti.

Microtropia: This is a condition where the eye is amblyopic to a varying degree with or without an eccentric fixation or with anomalous retinal correspondence but the degree of squint is so small that it cannot be detected by a cover test and when detected, is usually less than 5° and mostly esotropic in nature. This condition was earlier confused with amblyopia in non-squinting eyes. The condition though present since early childhood is rarely thought of till later in age. One of the tests for detection is the fuzzy appearance of certain letters of the words, e.g. missing the first letter or the last letter or there may be momentary disappearance of letters. A scotoma may be demonstrated on an Amsler's chart.

Treatment: As the condition remains undetec-ted for long, leading to amblyopia and eccentric fixation, the appropriate treatment is to prevent it by correcting error of refraction at the earliest age and orthoptic exercises to overcome amblyopia.

Non-Concomitant (Paralytic) Squint

Notwithstanding the fact that some small degree of paralytic element may be associated with many cases of concomitant squint in early stages of infancy, an evidently paralytic squint is much less common than a concomitant squint. As a paralytic squint is acquired later in life after binocular single vision is grounded, suppression and amblyopia do not develop. It is for this reason that diplopia is the most common and annoying feature of paralytic squint. Furthermore, suppression and amblyopia are less common in the paralysed eye also because head postures help in maintaining binocular vision.

The causes of paralytic squint are due to nerve palsy caused either by trauma, inflammation or new growths. A paralytic squint may be due to peripheral neuritis of the nerve supplying the muscle or due to the pressure effect on the peri-pheral nerve, e.g., the fracture of the apex of the orbit (contracoup fracture) or due to haemorrhage in the nerve sheath. A more serious cause is palsy due to an intracranial lesion, which may cause other neurological evidence as well. The lesion in the nerve may therefore be anywhere from the peripheral termination, along the peripheral trunk or at the nuclei in the mid-brain resulting in paralysis of the individual nerve or a muscle. The palsy of conjugate movements of the eye commonly seen in the supranuclear lesions does not cause squint.

A paralytic squint may be due to palsy of one nerve supplying one muscle which presents a simple clinical proposition easy to diagnose and easy to evaluate. A paralytic squint may however be more complex when more than one muscle is involved and diagnosis and evaluation are much more difficult.

The clinical examination of a case of paralytic squint requires the following examination:

1. Inspection to note degree of squint and to note any compensatory effort by the patient by turning the face, titling the head or elevating or depressing the chin. The inspection will also show the effort to overcome diplopia by closing one eye.
2. History of onset—sudden or slow, presence and direction of diplopia. History of any other systemic disease like diabetes, hypertension, etc.
3. Record of visual acuity.
4. Ocular movements, uniocular and binocular, keeping the head erect and face straight.
5. Cover test to note the difference in primary and secondary deviation.
6. Bielschowsky's head tilt test.
7. Diplopia charting.
8. Hess' screen study.
9. Complete neurological examination.
10. Investigations for any systemic cause, e.g., diabetes and hypertension.
11. Special tests like prostigmin test in transient and intermittent squint.
12. Electromyography.

Compensatory posture of the head and face: These postures are developed principally to overcome diplopia. The face is turned towards the direction of the action of the paralysed muscle which is also the direction of greatest separation of two images. The chin is elevated in palsy of the elevators and depressed in the palsy of the depressors. The head is tilted towards the paralysed side in elevator muscle palsies and towards the sound side in depressor muscle palsies. For ready reference, details are given in the table.

Visual acuity: It is important also because if vision in one eye is very poor due to any cause, patient may not have diplopia even though the squint is paralytic.

Ocular movements: A careful observation should be made when testing movements of each eye separately and both eyes together. The movement of each eye separately will indicate restriction of the movement in the direction of principal action of the muscle involved. A test of binocular movement will indicate conjugate movements and compensatory over-action of a contra-lateral muscle if any.

Cover test: In paralytic squint also this is significant and important because it indicates the difference between *primary deviation of the*

Table: Diagnostic features of extra-ocular muscle palsies

Muscle paralysed	Type of diplopia	Face turned	Compensatory posture	
			Chin	Head
Right lateral rectus	Horizontal uncrossed	to right	unaffected	unaffected
Left lateral rectus	Horizontal uncrossed	to left	unaffected	unaffected
Right medial rectus	Horizontal crossed	to left	unaffected	unaffected
Left medial rectus	Horizontal crossed	to right	unaffected	unaffected
Right superior rectus	Vertical crossed	to right	raised	tilted to right
Left superior rectus	Vertical crossed	to left	raised	tilted to left
Right inferior rectus	Vertical crossed	to right	lowered	tilted to left
Left inferior rectus	Vertical crossed	to left	lowered	tilted to right
Right superior oblique	Vertical uncrossed	to left	lowered	tilted to left
Left superior oblique	Vertical uncrossed	to right	lowered	tilted to right
Right inferior oblique	Vertical uncrossed	to left	raised	tilted to right
Left inferior oblique	Vertical uncrossed	to right	raised	tilted to left

paralysed eye and the *secondary deviation of the sound eye*. In non-paralytic squint, primary and secondary deviations are equal. In paralytic squint, secondary deviation of the sound eye is due to over-action of contra-lateral synergist. When the sound eye is covered, the paralysed eye tries to look straight even though it can not. This subconscious extra-effort is transmitted to the higher centres and the stimulus of extra-effort is then carried to the contralateral synergist of the opposite eye. This secondary deviation of the sound eye is therefore greater than the primary deviation of the paralysed eye. To elicit this, the alternate cover test is done in each eye in succession. The degree of movement of each eye on removing the cover indicates the degree of deviation under cover. The test has a fallacy that in long-standing cases of paralytic squint, contractures may develop in the contralateral synergist with the result that the primary and secondary deviation in such cases may not be very much different (Figs 18.23 to 18.25A–D).

Bielschowsky's head tilting test: This test is to find out which of the two vertical muscles, a rectus of one eye or the oblique of the other eye, is paralysed. To explain, an example is paralysis of the right superior rectus followed by the over-action of 'contralateral synergist', the left inferior

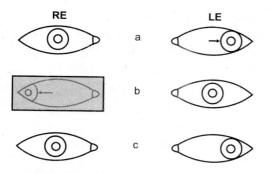

Fig. 18.23: Left Medial Rectus Palsy, (a) Looking straight, left divergent squint (Primary deviation); (b) On covering RE, LE fixes. RE diverges more than in (a) secondary deviation of sound eye; (c) On Uncovering RE, squint reverts to LE as in (a)

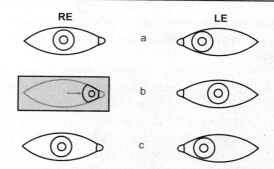

Fig. 18.24: Paralytic Squint—Left Lateral Rectus Palsy, (a) Primary position—LE convergent squint (primary deviation); (b) On covering RE, LE fixes. RE converges more than in (a), secondary deviation of sound eye; (c) On uncovering squint reverts to LE as in (a)

oblique. Consequent to the over-action of the left inferior oblique, there is under-action of the left superior oblique, the contralateral antagonist. The Bielschoskwy's test is to differentiate whether the palsy is in the right superior rectus or the left superior oblique. Both are under-acting in the example given above. Similar examples can be between the right inferior rectus and the left inferior oblique.

Bielschowsky's test includes forcibly tilting the head in the direction opposite to the head posture adopted to overcome diplopia. The eye which shoots up or down on forcible tilting of the head is the eye which has oblique palsy. The test is usually negative in palsy of the vertical rectus muscles.

It is important to emphasize that it is very uncommon for a single vertical muscle to be affected by paralysis except the superior oblique. More than one muscle is usually involved and to isolate the under or over-action of each muscle is a time consuming procedure but is of importance when selecting the muscle for surgery.

Diplopia charting: Diplopia is a prominent symptom of paralytic squint and the most annoying as well. Diplopia is seeing one object as two because one image is seen by the fovea of the normal eye and other image by the

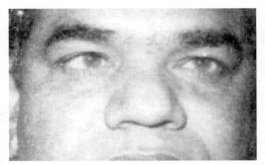

Fig. 18.25A: Paralytic Squint—Right Lateral Rectus Palsy. Looking straight—slight Convergence RE

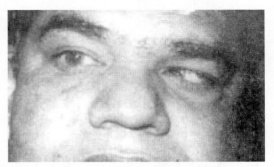

Fig. 18.25B: Paralytic Squint—Right Lateral Rectus Palsy. Looking Right—LE moves in, RE remains in Central

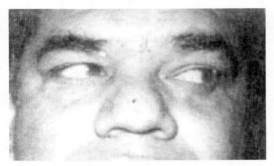

Fig. 18.25C: Paralytic Squint—Right Lateral Rectus Palsy. Looking Left—RE moves to the extreme

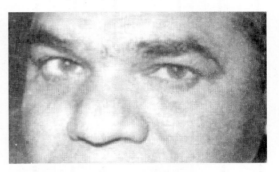

Fig. 18.25D: Paralytic Squint—Right Lateral Rectus Palsy compensatory turning of the Face to the Right to overcome diplopia

parafoveal area of the paralysed eye. Of the two images, one is a true image which is clearly defined and other is a false image and ill-defined. True diplopia is, therefore, binocular and disappears when one of the eyes is closed. When right eye image is left of the two images, it is *crossed diplopia* and when the right image is on the right side of the two images, it is called *uncrossed* diplopia . In divergent squint, the fovea is moved nasally and the image is, therefore, formed on the area temporal to the macula. This is projected nasally. The diplopia is therefore crossed. Similarly, in a paralytic convergent squint, it is uncrossed diplopia.

Diplopia charting is best done with a bar of light or a candle light held in front of the patient at a distance of one metre. The eyes are covered with diplopia goggles; a *red shield on the right eye* and a *green shield on the left eye.* The light is moved from the centre to the periphery in all 8 cardinal directions and the patient is asked to follow the light and to indicate whether red and green images are superimposed or they are separate from each other. If they are separate, he is asked to indicate the direction in which the separation is maximum. He is also to indicate whether the two images are on the same level or one is higher and the other is lower. In either case, he is asked to indicate in which direction the separation is maximum. The patient is also asked to indicate if one of the two images is tilted towards or away from the other. The observations are recorded on diplopia charts (illustrated below). It should be understood that charting of diplopia is not possible if vision in one eye is markedly reduced (Fig. 18.26).

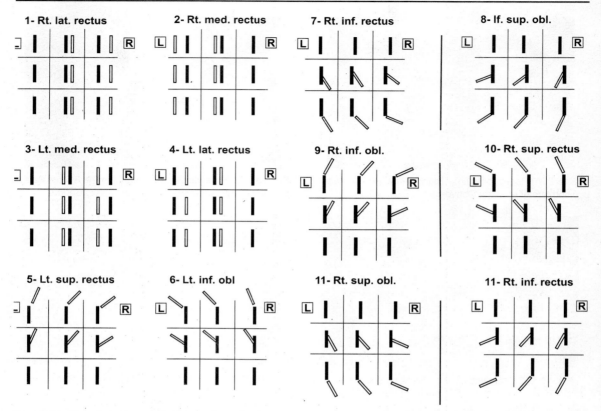

Fig. 18.26: Diplopia in Muscle Palsy. (L—Looking to left; R—Looking to right; Solid lines—true image; Double lines—false image. (1) Right lateral rectus palsy. Diplopia maximum looking to right. False image to the right—uncrossed diplopia; (2) Right medial rectus palsy. Diplopia maximum looking to left. False image to left—crossed diplopia; (3) Left medial rectus palsy. Diplopia maximum looking to right. False image to left—crossed diplopia; (4) Left lateral rectus palsy. Diplopia maximum looking to left. False image to the left—uncrossed diplopia; (5) Left superior rectus palsy. Diplopia maximum looking up and to right. False image above and to right—crossed diplopia; (6) Left inferior oblique palsy. Diplopia maximum looking up and to left. False image above and to left—uncrossed diplopia; (7) Left inferior rectus palsy. Diplopia maximum looking down and to right. False image to right—crossed diplopia; (8) Left superior oblique palsy. Diplopia maximum down and to left. False image down and to left—uncrossed diplopia; (9) Right inferior oblique palsy. Diplopia maximum looking up and to right. False image above and to right—uncrossed diplopia; (10) Right superior rectus palsy. Diplopia maximum looking up and to left. False image up and to left—crossed dipiopia; (11) Right superior oblique palsy. Diplopia maximum looking down and right. False image down and to right—uncrossed diplopia; (12) Right inferior rectus palsy. Diplopia maximum looking down and left. False image down and to left—crossed diplopia

Hess' screen study: It is an important investigative procedure in paralytic squint, more useful in the diagnosis of palsy of the vertical muscles. The Hess screen test is based on the principle of dissociating the two eyes by red and green goggles as in a diplopia test.

The internally illuminated Hess screen has red points of light at the crossing of the lines in such a way that there are eight points on the inner square and sixteen points on the outer square. The inner square is at 15° from the central point and the outer square at 30°. The patient wears diplopia goggles, red in front of the right eye and green in front of the left eye and sits at one half metre distance from the Hess' screen. He holds a green light torch in his hand.

Through the red glass he is able to see only the red light points on the screen while through the green glass he sees only the projected green light point from the torch so that what he sees with one eye; he does not see with the other eye. The two eyes are therefore dissociated. He is asked to project the green light over the red dots. If the two coincide, there is no palsy. If the two are away from each other, they indicate over or under-action of one or the other muscle. The distance between the two indicates the degree of over and under-action. Starting from the centre, the procedure is carried on to cover 8 dots of the inner square. The procedure is further extended to cover the 16 dots of the outer square. After recording with a red shield in front of the right eye, the procedure is repeated with a red shield in front of the left eye. The observations are charted on Hess' screen chart. The first is the chart for the right eye and the second is the chart for the left eye. The smaller field is the field of the paralysed eye and the larger field is that of the sound eye.

The principal advantage of Hess' screen is not only to find out which is a palsied eye but also discover under-action and over-action of the muscles. Like diplopia chart, this also is a permanent record of the progress of the condition.

Neurological examinations of all cases of muscle palsy are an essential part of investigations. It is important to determine whether the palsy is peripheral, nuclear or supra-nuclear and whether there is a focus of irritation or pressure in the course of the nerve involved.

Other investigative procedures include relevent haematological, serological or biochemical investigations keeping in mind the possible causes. Radiological investigations include X-ray of the orbital fissures, orbital venography and cerebral angiography, etc.

Electromyography is a useful procedure to test the functioning status of each muscle separately and the follow-up study will indicate whether the muscle is in the process of recovery or not. Electromyography is done by introducing a bipolar electrode into the muscle belly and the two poles are connected to an amplifier. The muscle is made to act and the electrical potential produced is recorded on a paper.

Except for the fourth and sixth cranial nerves which supply the superior oblique and lateral rectus separately, paralysis of any other lone individual muscle is very uncommon. In such cases it will need various investigative procedures to detect which muscle or muscles are involved and what is the effect of palsy on the ipsilateral antagonist, contralateral synergist as well as contra-lateral antagonist. This relationship of extra-ocular muscles is given as a guideline which will be helpful in detecting the effects and consequences of individual muscle palsies (Table). A majority of cases are due to lesions in the peripheral part of the nerve supply below the nucleus in the mid brain. Nuclear lesions can cause isolated muscle palsy but these are usually bilateral. Supranuclear lesions in the brain substance are characterised by conjugate movement palsy rather than paralysis of individual muscles.

The lesion may be within the brain substance before the nerve emerges from the brain, or in the cranial cavity during the course of the nerve or it may be extra-cranial till the nerve ends in the muscle. The lesion *may be traumatic, inflammatory, neoplastic or due to systemic diseases, metabolic, toxic or degenerative in nature.*

Trauma is an important cause of nerve palsy: The common mode being indirect or contra-coup fracture of orbit caused by a fall or hit on forehead. Among infections, viral infection is the commonest cause for isolated peripheral nerve palsies. Acute demyelinating diseases, more common in western countries are responsible for many cases of muscle palsies. Diabetes is an important metabolic disease causing peripheral

Table: Inter-relationship of extra-ocular muscles

| | Ipsilateal | | Contralateral | |
	Synergist	*Antagonist*	*Synergist*	*Antagonist*
Medial Rectus	Superior rectus Inferior rectus	Lateral rectus Inferior oblique Superior oblique	Lateral rectus	Medial rectus
Lateral Rectus	Inferior oblique Superior oblique	Medial rectus Superior rectus Inferior rectus	Medial rectus	Lateral rectus
Superior rectus	Inferior oblique Medial rectus	Inferior rectus Superior oblique	Inferior oblique	Superior oblique
Inferior rectus	Superior oblique Medial rectus	Superior rectus Inferior oblique	Superior oblique	Inferior oblique
Superior oblique	Inferior rectus Lateral rectus	Inferior oblique Superior rectus	Inferior rectus	Superior rectus
Inferior oblique	Superior rectus Lateral rectus	Superior oblique Inferior rectus	Superior rectus	Inferior rectus

neuritis and muscle palsy. Among the vascular lesions, the commonest are intracranial aneurysms pressing on the nerves as they traverse the intracranial cavity from behind forward. The aneurysm may be of internal carotid or branches of the circle of Willis. Intracranial neoplasms raise intracranial tension and cause palsy of the sixth nerve first. Localised intra-cranial tumours may cause palsies producing characteristic syndromes. *Recurrent palsies may be due to migraine and intermittent palsies due to myasthenia. Exophthalmic ophthalmoplegia due to thyroid and pituitary pathology cause slow and chronic palsies of the extra-ocular muscles.* Toxic causes include poisons like lead and alcohol.

Treatment of paralytic squint: The object of treatment from ophthalmic point of view is to neutralise diplopia and restore binocular vision. This is possible because the eye with a paralytic squint does not develop suppression or amblyopia. Treatment is also necessary to help overcome head postures, an important cosmetic factor. Like all palsies in the body, treatment should be first concentrated on the causative lesion by systemic therapy or by surgical removal. If, however,

muscle palsy is irrecoverable, surgery on the muscle or prismo-therapy should be considered. Before any surgery on the muscle is undertaken, it is important that enough time should be allowed for completing line of medical therapy and regeneration of the nerve before surgery is planned. The average period allowed for this is 9 months to one year. A paralytic squint should therefore not be operated in haste.

RELATED SYNDROMES

There are some clinical entities which are related to the anatomy and functioning of extraocular muscles and are therefore better described here.
Common among these are:
1. Duane's retraction syndrome.
2. Superior oblique sheath syndrome.
3. Strabismus fixus.

Duane's retraction syndrome: The clinical features of this syndrome are: on adduction, the eyeball retracts and as a consequence the interpalpebral fissure becomes small. Sometimes there is also a vertical displacement of the eye upward or downward in adduction (Figs 18.27A and B).

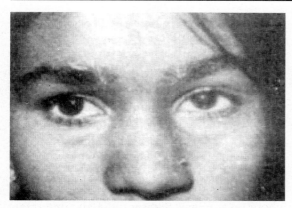

Fig 18.27A: Duane's Retraction Syndrome
(Looking Straight)

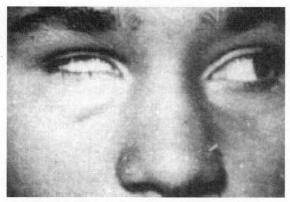

Fig 18.27B: Duane's Retraction Syndrome. (Looking left adduction of right eye, causes marked retraction of eyeball and consequent ptosis)

The morphological basis of this syndrome is that the lateral rectus does not relax during adduction. Hence the adductor medial rectus has to make an extra effort to adduct. This extra effort introduces some degree of upward or downward displacement of the eye. The retraction of the eyeball is caused by the backward pull of the three adductors when they are trying to overact. The narrowing of the palpebral fissure is purely mechanical due to the retraction of the eyeball.

It is a congenital anomaly possibly either due to the myogenic change in the muscle itself or due to anomalous nerve supply. The lesion may also be due to paradoxical innervation in the supra-nuclear area or in the medial longitudinal fasciculus.

Duane's syndrome may sometimes be associated with forward movement of eyeball and widening of the palpebral fissure on abduction.

The treatment is only for cosmetic purpose as the condition otherwise does not cause any symptoms. Surgery is recession of medial rectus and partial or complete tenotomy of lateral rectus along with excision of the fibrous bands of the lateral rectus.

Superior oblique sheath syndrome: It is a congenital anomaly and has the features of paresis of the inferior oblique muscle which is clinically indicated by absence of elevation in adduction. On the contrary, the eye tends to move down. There may be compensatory head postures with the face turned up and the head tilted to the same side.

Confirmatory diagnosis is by forced duction lest done under general anaesthesia. It is possible to displace the eye upward in adducted position. The anomaly is due to the fibrous sheath along the superior oblique muscle between the trochlea and its insertion. The treatment is entirely surgical but not satisfactory. Surgery includes removal of the fibrous sheath and replacing it by a plastic sleeve. It may be necessary to recess the contra-lateral superior rectus.

Strabismus fixus: This is a congenital condition where the eye is held fixed in adducted position with a severe degree of convergent squint. All eye movements are severely restricted. The condition is caused by thick fibrous bands restricting movements of the medial rectus and other muscles. The condition may sometimes be simulated by a long standing 6th nerve plasy with contractural changes in medial rectus. The treatment is very unsatisfactory. Recession of both medial recti may result in some improvement. Resection of both lateral recti may be added to keep the eyes in a central position.

The inferior rectus may also be fibrosed resulting in vertical fixus. The eye is then firmly held in a downward position.

ORTHOPTICS

Ortho is normal and optics is related to vision. The practice of orthoptics, therefore, means to help *restoration of normal binocular vision*. In the academic sense, orthoptics includes evaluation of a case of squint, its measurement and the state of binocularity. Orthoptics is further meant to give exercises with the purpose of helping development of single binocular vision (Figs 18.28 and 18.29, Plate 13).

Orthoptic exercises do not help patients give up glasses as it is so often believed. Orthoptics includes all methods of treatment except surgical for treatment of latent or manifest defect of binocular vision.

It includes investigative procedures like the cover test, Maddox wing test and Maddox rod test. The investigative procedures on a synopto-phore are *measurement of the degree of squint and state of binocular vision*. Orthoptics includes treatment either with a synoptophore or by home exercises. Orthoptics is a supportive therapy to surgery and glasses and not a substitute for either of them. The objectives of orthoptic treatment are:
1. Improve vision of the amblyopic eye.
2. Eliminate suppression.
3. Enhance range of fusion.
4. Control deviation.

Amblyopia is first treated by occlusion to equalise vision of two eyes and then anti-suppression exercises are given on cheiroscope in orthophoric eyes which is followed by fusion exercises on synoptophore. Increase in fusion range helps in control of deviation. It is important to know that orthoptic treatment is more rewarding when squint develops about the age of 2½ to 3 years of age. It is most rewarding in intermittent squints. The procedure is ineffective when the patient already has an established abnormal retinal correspondence.

Increase in fusion amplitude is the ultimate objective of successful orthoptic treatment. Fusion is the most important of all the three grades of binocular vision. The different methods of stimulating fusion and increasing its amplitude are convergence exercises either on synopto-phore or at home. Stereopsis is also important for good single binocular vision. This is achieved by suitable orthoptic exercises on synoptophore with appropriate slides. Similarly, special exercises with Haidinger brushes in synoptophore are indicated to overcome eccentric fixation. The Haidinger brushes act by stimulating the anato-mical fovea because the light passing through the blue filter of Haidinger brushes is perceived by cones only which are concentrated at the fovea.

In addition to synoptophore or major amblyo-scope, as it is called, other equipments used in orthoptic clinic for diagnostic and therapeutic purposes are:
1. Maddox rod.
2. Maddox wing.
3. Diploscope.
4. Ramy's separator.
5. Cheiroscope.
6. Worth's four-dot charts.
7. Red and green goggles.
8. Prism bar.

To be effective, the patient must be regular in exercises. To sustain the benefits achieved by exercises in the clinic, the patient should continue exercises at home. A periodical check-up in the clinic is also necessary to ensure that the bene-ficial results of exercises have not deteriorated.

Orthoptics is, therefore, a specialised subject and needs patience and time that are not always at the disposal of the ophthalmologist. This has, therefore, developed as a specialised section by itself needing a specially trained manpower called orthoptists (para-medical technicians) who work under the guidance of ophthalmologist. It is ultimately the ophthalmologist who completes the clinical examination and executes the line of treatment in which orthoptics is only a part. It is the ophthalmologist who refers the patient for orthoptic evaluation and exercises and the patient ultimately comes back to him for the final word.

PLEOPTICS

Pleoptics is the treatment given to cases of amblyopia with eccentric fixation.

The basic principle involved is to stimulate fovea to take up fixation and to establish co-ordination between the two eyes.

The various instruments available are:
1. Euthyscope.
2. Projectoscope.
3. Pleoptophore.
4. Centrophore.
5. Synoptophore.

The euthyscope and projectoscope work on the principle of after images while the synoptophore works on Haidinger brushes. The pleoptophore and centrophore can have either.

With projectoscope accurately localized foveal area 3° to 5° is protected with black spot graticule. Bright light of predetermined duration and intensity dazzles the surrounding retina while macular area is occluded by the black spot. The false fovea is inhibited and strong after image is produced by this technique. Black spot occluder is then replaced by a disc of white light and extra-macular area is protected by green filter light. An alternator in projectscope is activated to produce flashing light. Duration of light and dark phases is preset by dials on control unit of the instrument. The procedure stimulates true fovea to become superior to eccentric fixation.

Haidinger brushes are seen only in the foveal region and so their visualisation stimulates the central area.

Once the foveal area is stimulated, an attempt is made to establish coordination of two eyes in space. This is made by following the after image or Haidinger brushes. This gives very good results, (1) when occlusion alone fails, the best results are achieved, (2) when it is done in children at a younger age who have developed eccentric fixation e.g. after age of two years, (3) in children without any pathological lesion at the macula, (4) and when the angle of eccentricity is less than the angle of squint.

19

Lacrimal System

The surface of the eye ball must remain wet at all the times for comfort and proper functioning. The fluid which keeps the surface wet is provided by the lacrimal gland, the mucous secretion from the goblet cells of the conjunctiva and the oily secretion from the meibomian glands. Constant spreading of this mixture is facilitated by blinking of the eyelids. Most of the watery part of the secretion evaporates from the corneal and conjunctival surface. Only an excess passes through lacrimal drainage system to reach the nasal cavity where it is evaporated by the breathing process. If in excess, it appears as water from the nose as in weeping. It is only when the secretion is too excessive or there is blockage of the drainage system, that it flows over the lid margins on to the face. The lacrimal part of the tear fluid also contains lysozymes which have a very distinct anti-bacterial property.

ANATOMY

The lacrimal system is divided into the following anatomical structures (Fig. 19.1)

A. *Secretory system*
    a. Lacrimal gland.
    b. Accessory lacrimal glands (Krause).

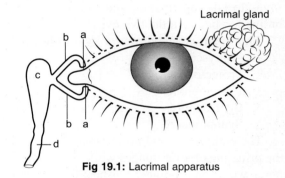

Fig 19.1: Lacrimal apparatus

B. *Drainage system*
    a. The puncta—upper and lower.
    b. Canaliculi—upper and lower.
    c. Lacrimal sac.
    d. Naso-lacrimal duct.

Lacrimal Gland

It is a tubulo-racemose type of gland situated in the bony fossa in the anterior part of the upper and outer orbital cavity just behind the orbital margin. It is covered by extension of septum orbitale anteriorly which is the lateral extension from the aponeurosis of the levator palpebrae superioris muscle. There is small palpebral part of the lacrimal gland. These glands of Krause are accessory lacrimal glands in the subconjunctival connective tissue in the outer part of the upper fornix.

The secretion from these glands is poured through fine ducts into the conjunctival sac mostly above the lateral palpebral ligament, but a few ducts also open below the ligament.

The lacrimal artery supplies the lacrimal glands. Lymphatics drain into pre-auricular gland. The nerve supply is derived both from the secretory para-sympathetic and vasomotor sympathetic systems. The para-sympathetic fibres come via the greater superficial petrosal branch of facial nerve, to which also join the sympathetic fibres via the deep petrosal nerve. These fibres together form the nerve of the pterygoid canal and reach the spheno-palatine ganglion in the pterygo-palatine fossa. The fibres finally reach the lacrimal gland via the lacrimal and zygomatic nerves.

Tear Fluid

The mucous secretion from the goblet cells and the fatty meibomian secretion get mixed with the lacrimal fluid by movements of the lid and the resulting fluid is called the tear fluid. It spreads over the surface of the cornea and the conjunctiva in the form of a trilamellar film which consists of the oily layer, watery layer and mucous layer. The superficial oily layer reduces the rate of evaporation and the mucous layer adsorbs on to corneal epithelium which helps maintaining smooth evenness of the corneal surface. The movement of the upper lid helps in the formation and reformation of this *pre corneal* film and in the process keeps the corneal surface, wet and free from dust particles etc.

Lacrimal Drainage System

The lacrimal drainage system extends from puncta through canaliculi, the sac and nasolacrimal duct opening into the lateral part of the inferior meatus of the nose. The system is activated mostly by action of orbicularis oculi muscle attached to the upper part of the sac fascia and to a small degree by the breathing process through nose.

The *upper and lower puncta* are situated at the medial ends of the two lid margins on top of a raised papilla. They are located at mucous part of the lid margin in line of the opening of meibomian ducts. The puncta are elevated from the marginal surface and are easily identifiable except when they are obliterated and may have to be looked for. The puncta can be easily presented to view by pulling the lower lid down or by everting the upper lid. The upper and lower canaliculi extend from the puncta till they enter into lacrimal sac either through a common dilated portion (ampula of Whaler) or by separate openings into the lateral wall of the lacrimal sac.

It is important to note the direction of canaliculi which is first vertical for about 2-3 mm and then turning sharply medially so that a punctum dilator or the lacrimal probe should first be introduced in the vertical direction and then turned medially.

The lacrimal sac is situated between the anterior and posterior lacrimal crests and is covered by the lacrimal fascia attached in front and behind to the lacrimal crests. The *medial palpebral ligament* crosses the upper part of the sac. The part above the medial palpebral ligament is called the fundus of the sac which is attached to the periosteal lining above. The medial attachment of the orbicularis oculi muscle passes in front of the lacrimal fascia, the upper fibres of which are attached to the upper border of the medial palpebral ligament, the fundus of the sac and the periosteum. A small strip of muscle called the Horner's muscle arising from the posterior lacrimal crest behind and below the lower canaliculus merges with the lower fibres of the orblicularis oculi muscle.

The following structures therefore have to be cut through to reach the lacrimal sac: (1) Skin,

(2) Sub-cutaneous tissue, (3) Fibres of orbicularis oculi, (4) Medial palpebral ligament and (5) Pre-lacrimal facia.

The angular artery and vein are in front and medial to the lacrimal sac and higher up turn laterally to anastomose with branches of the supra-orbital artery to form the *vascular arcades of the upper lid*. These blood vessels, unless carefully avoided, are likely to be cut during sac surgery and cause bleeding, which can be extremely disturbing.

The naso-lacrimal duct is continuation of lacrimal sac from above and is contained partly in a bony canal formed by the maxillary bone, lacrimal bone and the inferior concha. The duct opens into the lateral part of the inferior meatus of the nose. The direction of the naso-lacrimal duct is downwards, posteriorly and slightly laterally. This is important to keep in mind while passing a probe in the duct. When left free, the probe should stay in this direction. Failing to appreciate this point may result in the probe going into a false passage especially in young infants where probing of the lacrimal passages is commonly indicated.

The lowest end of the naso-lacrimal duct is narrowed by a fold of mucous membrane which acts as a valve. There are mucous folds in the naso-lacrimal duct also which have no muscle fibres. The thickening of these valves may give rise to physiological obstruction of naso-lacrimal duct where the patient complains of watering but when the fluid is syringed under pressure, it passes into the nose as against physical obstruction where the fluid regurgitates from the opposite punctum.

Development: The lacrimal drainage system develops from the solid column of cells from surface ectoderm which gets caught and invaginated by the approaching fronto-nasal and maxillary processes. The column of the ecto-dermal cells thus gets surrounded by mesoderm. The solid column gets canalized during the process of development. The upper sac, the canali-culi and puncta develop from the upper part and the lower sac and naso-lacrimal duct, from the lower part of the ectodermal column of cells. The canalisation starts from the upper end and proceeds downwards so that the lower part gets canalised last. This is usually complete just before or soon after birth. Even if it is not complete by the time of birth, the process continues and is expected to be complete by the end of third month after birth. This process of spontaneous canalisation after birth is interrupted if an inflammatory reaction is caused by infection.

Nerve supply: The lacrimal sac and duct get their nerve supply from a branch of the infra-trochlear nerve before it enters the infra-trochlear notch or canal.

It is important to inject anaesthetic solution just behind the notch for effective anaesthesia in a lacrimal sac operation.

Physiological process of movement of lacrimal fluid: The passage of the lacrimal fluid from upper fornix on the lateral side to drainage system on the medial side is facilitated by movements and the anatomical characteristics of the lid margin. The gravity also helps the fluid to come from the upper and outer part the lower and medial part.

The sharp posterior border of the lid margins creates a capillary action and helps in retaining the fluid in the conjunctival sac. The palpebral portion of orbicularis oculi muscle has a very important function in the active movements of the fluid. The muscle has a ligamentous attachment on the lateral side and bony attachment on the medial side and therefore when it acts, there is a wave of contraction from the lateral to medial side which facilitates movement of fluid from the lateral to the medial direction. The orbicularis oculi and Horner's muscle further help in creating a negative pressure in the lacrimal sac because of its action on the fundus of the sac so that whatever fluid reaches the inner angle of the eye is quickly sucked into the sac cavity.

There are two different views about this action:

a. Contraction of orbicularis oculi muscle causes a pull on the fundus of the sac creating a negative pressure and this helps lacrimal fluid to be sucked in the sac cavity. Relaxation of the orbicularis oculi muscle results in a rebound contraction of the upper sac thus pushing the fluid in the nasal cavity. Horner's muscle also probably helps in compression of the lacrimal sac.

b. The orbicularis oculi contraction compresses the upper sac and negative pressure is caused by muscle relaxation.

WATERING AND LACRIMATION

The lacrimal fluid that cannot pass into the nose through naso-lacrimal passage and cannot be taken care of by normal evaporation, will overflow over the lower lid margin and this condition is called watering of the eye. Lacrimal fluid overflow can be due either to excessive production when it is called *lacrimation* or it may be due to obstruction in the drainage system and this is called *epipora*. Although the terms are distinct, they are often mixed with each other.

Lacrimation which is an active process, may be caused by the following conditions:

1. Corneal irritation, inflammation or ulceration e.g. foreign body inturned eye lashes, exposure keratitis due to lagophthalmos, ectropion of lid margin or proptosis etc.
2. Conjunctival irritation, inflammation and ulceration.
3. Intraocular inflammations.
4. Reflex lacrimation due to irritation in nose and sinuses.
5. Emotional reactions like laughing and weeping.
6. Irritative lesions in the course of the nerve supply to lacrimal glands.

Epiphora: It is a passive overflow of the lacrimal fluid over the lid margins due to obstruction, malformation or malfunction of drainage channels anywhere between the puncta on the ocular side and opening of the naso-lacrimal ducts in inferior meatus on the nasal side.

The common causes of epiphora are:
1. Congenital absence of the lacrimal puncta.
2. Congenital non-canalisation or delayed canalisation of the naso-lacrimal duct.
3. Secondary occlusion, misdirection or damage to puncta and canaliculi.
4. Chronic dacryocystitis with organic blockage in naso-lacrimal duct.
5. Inflammation or growth affecting the inferior meatus of the nose.
6. Functional insufficiency for drainage of fluid into the nose.

It is important to remember that as long as the lacrimal passages are patent and there is free flow of lacrimal fluid from conjunctival sac to nasal cavity, the lacrimal passages remain in normal healthy condition. Like in running stream, the bacteria, if any, are not allowed to multiply and therefore cannot initiate an inflammatory reaction. If however there is blockage in the naso-lacrimal duct, the fluid remains collected in lacrimal sac and bacteria have an opportunity to multiply and cause an inflammatory reaction in the form of dacryocystitis. It is also important to emphasise that in normal circumstances the lower punctum and lower canaliculus are functionally more important because of gravitational factor. The upper punctum and upper canaliculus play an accessory role.

Examination and Investigation of a Case of Epiphora

1. Inspection of lacrimal sac area may show a localised swelling. The swelling is characteristically located below the level of medial canthus. Careful inspection may also reveal. presence of a fistulous hole or a line of scar of previous surgery.
2. The puncta should be identified and their position should be carefully noted. When the

lid margins are allowed to rest on the eye ball, both puncta should be touching conjunctival surface dipped in lakus lacrimalis in order to maintain capillary action.

3. *Position*, of lid margins and any scar on the skin round the medial canthus which can pull the punctum away from conjunctival surface, should be looked for.

4. *Pressure regurgitation test.* The lower lid is pulled down to bring the punctum in view. Firm pressure is applied over the sac area against the nasal bone and any regurgitation from either of the puncta, if present, is noted. It is also to be noted whether the regurgitating fluid is watery, mucoid, mucopurulent or sanguinous.

5. *Syringing the lacrimal passage:* This is a very important and useful procedure not only to detect obstruction but also to localise site of obstruction. Syringing should be done both from upper as well as lower punctum one after the other.

   Syringing is done with a round ended 24-26 gauge canula fitted on a 5 cc syringe filled with normal saline. Before the canula is introduced, the punctum is dilated with a blunt punctum dilator to facilitate introduction of canula, keeping in mind that the first part of the both canaliculi is in vertical direction and then is directed medially. The fluid is then injected and following observations are made. As the fluid is being pushed a careful watch should be kept on both the puncta to observe:

   i. whether the fluid is freely going into nasal cavity which is also evident as the patient swallows the fluid.

   ii. whether the fluid goes partially into the nose and partially regurgitates.

   iii. whether the whole fluid regurgitates, it is to be noted whether it is from the same punctum or from the opposite punctum.

   iv. whether the regurgitated fluid is watery, mucoid or purulent. It should also be noted

whether there is any regurgitation from any fistulous opening other than puncta.

The interpretations are:

   i. If there is total regurgitation and it is mostly from the opposite punctum, it indicates organic obstruction of the nasolacrimal duct (Fig. 19.2B). If fluid regurgitates from same punctum, it indicates obstruction in the same canaliculus. In such a case, syringing done through the opposite punctum will allow the fluid to pass into the nasal cavity provided the other canaliculus is patent. (Fig. 19.2A).

   iii. If the fluid passes into the nasal cavity with extra force on the syringe, it indicates physiological obstruction with non-organic blockage.

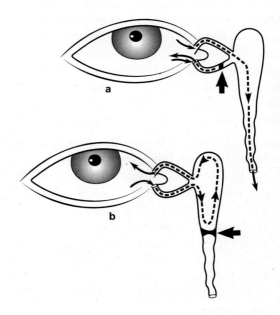

Fig. 19.2: Common sites of obstruction in lacrimal drainage channels. (A) Obstruction in lower canaliculus: Syringing through lower punctum-regurgitation through the same punctum syringing thro' upper punctum-patent (B) Obstruction in naso-lacrimal duct, syringing done through lower punctum, there is regurgitation through opposite punctum

Some surgeons prefer to use fluorescein or mercurochrome in the solution to facilitate its detection as it flows out of the nose or passes into throat. Syringing is a very simple procedure. It will be unfortunate if due to carelessness, the punctum or canaliculi are traumatised causing subsequent blockage. To avoid this, the point of the punctum dilator should not be too sharp and proper direction of the canaliculi should be kept in mind when introducing the canula. Syringing can be done in young infants without general anaesthesia by having the head held in position by the assistant. One should, however, not hesitate to take help of general anaesthesia if necessary. What is important is that the procedure should be correct and interpretation should be dependable. The one disadvantage of syringing under general anaesthesia is that the fluid might go in to the respiratory passage. Hence one should be mindful and careful and warn the anaesthetist in time.

6. *Dacryocystograghy*: This is a very useful procedure to determine size and shape of lacrimal sac and its communication with the nasal cavity. It is specially useful to identify a secondary sac (pseudo-sac) forming after an earlier dacryocystectomy operation. It also helps in identifying a fistulous tract if present and the patency or otherwise of the opening. in the middle meatus of the nose following a dacryocystorhinostomy. The procedure is simple. A radio opaque lipoidal or conray-280 thin oily fluid 1/2 cc. is injected in the lacrimal sac and a radiogram is taken immediately thereafter. One should be careful to swab any over-flow in the conjunctival sac to get proper radiological appearance of the sac. The X-ray may be repeated after few minutes to note if the fluid has passed into the nose to determine the tone of the sac and also to diagnose physiological obstruction.

7. *Radiography* of the bony canal of the naso-lacrimal duct if properly done can help in determining diameter of bony passage and decide whether the obstruction is soft tissue obstruction or bony closure.

8. *Nasal examination* is important in all cases to exclude any marked deviation of nasal septum or growth in inferior meatus of nose to explain the reasons for obstruction of nasal end of naso-lacrimal duct. Examination to exclude a gross infection in the nose and atrophic rhinitis is also important to prejudge the success or otherwise of DCR operation.

Diseases of the Lacrimal Drainage System

Congenital non-canalisation of naso-lacrimal duct. The commonest congenital anomaly is non-canalisation or delayed canalisation of the naso-lacrimal duct at birth or persisting even after birth. The child is brought with a history of watering since birth, in most cases, from one or both eyes. Syringing confirms that the obstruction is somewhere in the naso-lacrimal duct. No other investigations are usually necessary.

The active treatment depends on whether by the time the child is brought for the consultation, there is any secondary infection or not.

If there is no secondary infection, the parents should be advised to wait and watch and keep the eye clean. Antibiotic drops two or three times a day helps to prevent secondary infection. Syringing of naso-lacrimal passages done periodically hastens the process of canalisation.

If infection has already set in and the child has developed infantile dacryocystitis, there are three lines of treatment to be followed in succession.

A. If the child is less than three months old, syringing with an antibiotic solution should be done on alternate days for 15 days. The mother is also trained to empty the lacrimal sac by pressure against the bone, keep the pressure on, swab any discharge collected at the inner canthus, put a few drops of antibiotic solution at the inner angle and then release the pressure on the sac. The procedure will help sucking in the antibiotic solution and therefore help in fighting the infection. This should be repeated two to three times a day every day. In some children, infection may disappear and canalisation process is spontaneously completed.

B. If the child is more than 3 months old and if the above procedure has failed, probing of the lacrimal passages followed by daily syringing with an antibiotic solution may control infection and undo the obstruction. Probing may have to be repeated, if necessary, more than once.

It is important to emphasize that the epithelium of an infant regenerates quickly and can line the naso-lacrimal duct with a fresh epithelial layer once the duct has been made patent by probing which may remain patent for the rest of life. Probing is generally less likely to succeed in older children. Probing, in any case, is not possible if there is a bony obstruction in the naso-lacrimal passages and one should consider a dacryocystorhinostomy operation in due course of time.

C. If the child is one year or older, probing may be tried but with less chance of success. In a child with infantile dacryocystitis in that age group, one may have to consider a dacryocystorhinostomy operation.

The procedure of probing of lacrimal passages. Probing can be a simple procedure in careful hands and on the other hand, it can do more harm than good if the surgeon is unmindful of the accuracy of the procedure. The chief purpose of probing is to canalise the naso-lacrimal duct. Probing will also incidentally dilate the punctum and canaliculus as well.

Probing should always be done through the upper punctum and upper canaliculus for more than one reasons. Firstly, the direction of the upper canaliculus is more in line with the naso-lacrimal duct than the lower canaliculus. This being so, the actual procedure of probing is relatively much easier and less traumatizing through upper than through the lower punctum. Secondly, and a very important reason, is the possibility of structural damage to the lower punctum and lower canaliculus which are functionally more important than the upper. Probing which may have to be repeated and repeated syringing necessary thereafter may cause some trauma to the punctum and canaliculus with chance of its blockage resulting in epiphora, the very condition for which probing has been planned. Probing may therefore cause more serious damage to the punctum and canaliculus leading to fibrous obstruction with consequent undesirable results. From all points of view, therefore, the upper route should be the first choice and only if that choice is not available, should the lower route be used (Figs. 19.3).

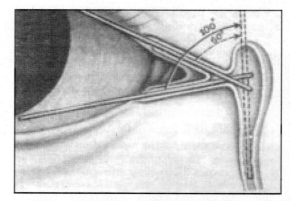

Fig 19.3: Lacrimal Probe in the Upper and Lower Canaliculi reaching up to the Sac Cavity. (The dotted line shows the position of the probe when it is pushed into the naso-lacrimal duct. Note that the probe in the lower canaliculus has to be turned through nearly 100° to be in line with the naso lacrimal duct, while the probe in the upper canaliculus has to be turned through 60° or less. Probing through upper canaliculus is therefore anatomically more appropriate and should be the choice of preference)

The procedure will be satisfactory if careful attention is given to the anatomical direction of the passages. After dilating the punctum, the probe is introduced first in the vertical direction and then turned inwards. One should feel the free passage of the probe through the canaliculus till the bony resistance is felt. Withdrawing the probe a little, it is now turned so as to direct it downwards with slight lateral obliquity and pushed down. The grip of the passage of the naso-lacrimal duct can be distinctly felt as it passes through it. It is pushed till it meets the resistance in the cavity of the nose. If the probe is now left to itself and if the upper end of the probe is directed slightly laterally it is indicative of the correct position of the probe in the naso-lacrimal duct. Any variation in this direction indicates that either the probe has gone into ethmoidal sinuses or slipped over towards the maxilla under the skin. Bleeding from the nose may also indicate false passage made by it. After ensuring that the probe is in the correct direction and position, it is moved up and down to make the patency effective (Fig. 19.4).

It is important not to use the thinnest size of probe. This should be reserved for canalising the punctum and the canaliculi only. One should better start with the second size probe followed by thicker sizes one after the other. Probing with three middle sizes should be enough for this purpose.

After probing, an antibiotic fluid should be syringed into the naso-lacrimal passage not only to wash down the debris but also to test the patency created by probing.

Probing in children should be done under general anaesthesia with intubation and packing of the throat to prevent blood or fluid going into the respiratory passage (Fig. 19.5).

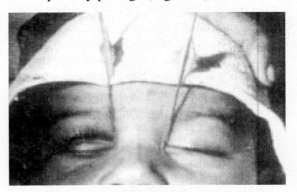

Fig 19.5: Lacrimal Probing in a Child under General Anaesthesia (The probes remain in correct position)

Other congenital anomalies

1. *The punctum may be absent.* If it is only at the surface, it can be opened with a sharp pointed punctum dilator. If the punctum does not remain patent, a small slit in the canaliculus on the conjunctival surface may provide an alternative route for fluid entry into the sac.
2. *Canaliculus* is non-canalised, it will be indicated by regurgitation of fluid through the same punctum. In cases where both canaliculi are obstructed, it will be difficult to determine the co-existing non-canalisation of naso-lacrimal duct. This can only be done by

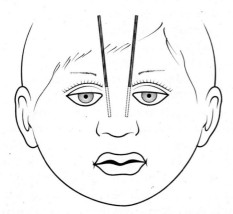

Fig 19.4: Lacrimal Probes in Correct Position after being pushed into the Naso-Lacrimal Duct. (Note the symmetrically divergent positions of the upper ends of the probes. This is essential to avoid false passage into the ethmoidal Sinuses medially or maxillary antrum laterally)

injecting fluid directly in the sac cavity either through the skin or the inner conjunctival fornix and noting whether the fluid passes into the nose or not. This can further be confirmed by dacryocystography.

An effective surgical procedure in case of a canaliculo-punctum block with a patent naso-lacrimal duct is to expose the lacrimal sac and incise its anterior wall. By everting the lateral lip of the incision, canalicular openings, single or separate, into the sac cavity are visualised. The canaliculus is probed and threaded from the sac side with 4-0 or 5-0 nylon thread to bring out the two ends through the two puncta at the inner canthus. The ends are tied leaving a loose ring of nylon thread. This is retained for some days and gently moved from time to time to shift the knotted end. Syringing can be done while the thread is in place which is cut and removed only when perfect patency with epithelialization is obtained.

3. There may be more than one puncta in either lid or there may be a fistulous opening through the skin. These need reconstructive surgery only if there is infection.

Physiological Insufficiency of Naso-lacrimal Passage

There may be epiphora even if the naso-lacrimal passages are patent as tested by syringing. Paralysis of orbicularis oculi muscle or hypertrophy of Hasner's valve at the lower end of naso-lacrimal duct are common causes of epiphora due to insufficiency factor.

1. The action of orbicularis oculi muscle on lacrimal sac and its role in the pumping action have been explained earlier. If there is palsy of the orbicularis and the fundus of the lacrimal sac is neither compressed nor pulled, the result is that the lacrimal fluid can neither be sucked into the lacrimal sac from conjunctival side nor pumped into nose through naso-lacrimal duct and hence epiphora.

2. If mucous folds in naso-lacrimal duct and Hasner's valve and the nasal end of naso-lacrimal duct are hypertrophied, the lacrimal fluid can not, in the normal process, pass through into the nose and this is called physiological a cause of epiphora.

Stenosis of Naso-lacrimal Passage

The sites where the naso-lacrimal passage can get blocked are the puncta, canaliculi, naso-lacrimal duct and sometimes the lacrimal sac itself. The pathogenesis of obstruction of naso-lacrimal duct has been described in detail earlier.

The lacrimal sac cavity closure is mostly due to intra-cystic neoplasm, congenital non-patency, injury, pericystic inflammations or tumours and a foreign body may sometimes also be responsible for stenosis of lacrimal sac cavity.

Stenosis of punctum and canaliculus can be due to any of the following causes:

1. As a congenital anomaly.
2. Post-inflammatory due to canaliculitis, bacterial or mycotic.
3. Traumatic lacerations either due to injury or improper probing.
4. Foreign body like an eye lash or a concretion formed locally.
5. Extension of the inflammatory process from lid or conjunctiva like trachoma or a lid abscess.

A canaliculus which has been involved in scarring following an injury in this area can be treated by opening the scar area, stricturectomy of the scarred part of the canaliculus and identifying the canalicular ends on either side of the scar. A polythene tube is now passed in both the ends, one coming out through the punctum and other into the sac and through the naso-lacrimal duct into the nose. The ends of canaliculus may unite over the tube and patency restored after the tube is removed.

The most common foreign body in the canaliculus is the eye lash. In most cases the pointed end enters the punctum and canaliculus and the bulbous end keeps pointing out from the punctum. Watering in these cases is also due to the irritation caused by the bulbous end when it touches the cornea as the eye is turned in. Treatment of this is to pull out the lash with an epilation forceps. Occasionally the eyelash may reach the sac cavity and cause local inflammatory reaction.

INFLAMMATION OF NASO-LACRIMAL PASSAGES

1. Canaliculitis

Inflammation of the punctum and canaliculus is usually an extension of the inflammatory process from the adjoining skin or the conjunctiva. Infection may however be prominently evident in the canaliculus. The common causes of canaliculitis are suppurative, mycotic or trachomatous.

a. **Trachomatous pathology** may extend from conjunctiva into canaliculi and even into the lacrimal sac, start an inflammatory process and cause watering due to obstruction of canaliculus. When the process heals, it may cause fibrous stricture and permanent closure.

b. **Suppurative canaliculitis**, an acute inflammatory lesion, may involve the punctum and canaliculus and present a clinical picture with a bead of pus seen at the opening of the punctum.

c. **Mycotic canaliculitis:** The infection by actinomycosis of the canaliculus is not uncommon. There is swelling in the canalicular area. The punctum is markedly prominent. A discharge from the punctum may be extruded on pressure. Commonly some degree of mild to severe conjunctivitis is present. In long standing cases, concretions may form in the canaliculus.

d. **Other infections:** Infection of punctum or canaliculus may also be caused by inflammation due to turberculosis, syphilis, herpetic infection and ulcerative and infective processes in the adjoining skin and conjunctiva.

2. Chronic Inflammation of Lacrimal Sac

Chronic inflammation of the lacrimal sac is a common eye disease. Its incidence is distinctly higher in persons with poor personal hygiene and recurrent inflammations in the nose, sinuses and conjunctiva. It is true that so long as the flow of lacrimal fluid is maintained through the lacrimal passage, any infection in the nose, sinuses or conjunctiva is not likely to get a foot hold in lacrimal sac. The same is true of bacteria often present in the lacrimal sac without causing any local reaction.

The initial pathology in chronic dacryocystitis is stasis of lacrimal fluid collected in lacrimal sac thereby providing opportunity for the bacteria to grow and multiply. The first step in the process is obstruction in naso-lacrimal duct. Many patients, therefore, first complain of watering and later of suppurative discharge.

If the obstruction in the naso-lacrimal duct does not lead to suppurative inflammation in the sac, fluid collects and enlarges the sac cavity. In this process the opening of the lacrimal canaliculi may also be blocked so that there is no communication of lacrimal sac on either side. This condition is called *encysted dacryocystitis (mucocele)*. This large sac may sometimes cause pressure atrophy of the thin ethmoidal bone and the sac may develop a communication with the nasal cavity through the ethmoid. In such a case, if pressure is applied on the full sac, fluid directly passes into the nose through this internal fistula.

So long as the inflammation is limited to the cavity of the lacrimal sac the sac may distend to a large size. If however, due to the thinning of the sac wall, trauma or any other factor, the infection within the sac extends into the pericystic tissue around the sac and under the skin, it excites an acute inflammatory process resulting in cellulitis and abscess formation in the sac region. This condition is called *acute dacryocystitis*. Pericystic abscess may burst on the skin and may result in the formation of a fistula on the skin with communication with the sac cavity.

Dacryocystitis is therefore chronic to start with and may secondarily lead to acute inflammation unlike most other suppurative inflammations in the body which are acute to begin with and may later become chronic in nature.

Pneumococcus is the commonest organism found in inflammed lacrimal sac. Other infections may however also be responsible, like tuberculosis, syphilis, leprosy, trachoma and mycotic infections.

Clinical Picture of Chronic Dacryocystitis

It has already been emphasised that chronic inflammation of the lacrimal sac is a primary chronic inflammation and not secondary to acute dacryocystitis.

Pathogenesis of chronic inflammation of lacrimal sac as stated before is based on obstruction to drainage and stasis of lacrimal fluid in the sac.

Symptoms of Chronic Dacryocystitis

1. Epiphora and discharge.
2. Small round swelling near the medial angle of the eye.
3. Patient complaining that pressure on the swelling causes regurgitation of fluid in the eye or through a fistula on the skin surface.

The swelling due to distended lacrimal sac when clinically evident, is characteristically situated below the level of the inner angle of the eye, because its extension upwards is prevented by medial palpebral ligament. On pressure, there

is regurgitation of fluid from both or one of the puncta. On careful examination, a scar of a previous surgery or a fistula may be detected. There is no sign of acute inflammation or tenderness on touch (Fig. 19.6).

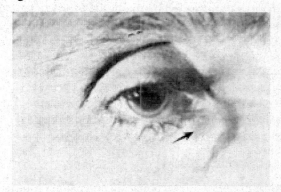

Fig 19.6: Chr. Dacryocystitis with a Fistula (Arrow). (Note the swelling in the sac area below the level of medial canthus)

Differential diagnosis: The other cystic swelling near inner angle of the eye can be a mucocoele from frontal sinus, ethmoidal mucocoele, a sabaceous cyst or a dermoid. The diagnostic features of a lacrimal sac swelling being below the medial palpebral ligament and syringing of the naso-lacrimal passage will clinch the diagnosis.

Treatment: The treatment is always surgical. The important considerations are:

1. An alternative passage should be provided for the contents of lacrimal sac to be drained into the nose to cure epiphora.
2. The constant presence of infection should be eliminated.

Dacryocysto-rhinostomy (DCR) is the operation of choice to establish a communication between the lacrimal sac and the middle meatus of nose by making a window in the bone and suturing the cut edges of the lacrimal sac to the naso-mucosal flaps. The surgery fulfills both the objectives. It should be remembered that it takes 4–5 weeks after a DCR operation for granulation tissue in the sac to resolve and for it to become infection free. Any intraocular surgery following DCR should therefore be done after an interval of atleast on month. A fistula, if present usually closes following a successful DCR operation. It may however sometimes need a separate excision.

Dacryocystectomy means removal of the sac including both canaliculi and the upper part of the naso-lacrimal duct. The operation eradicates infection but does not provide an alternative route of drainage for lacrimal fluid with the result that the operation is followed by persistent epiphora which, in most cases lasts a lifetime. There are reports that in some cases, there is a reflex adjustment between the need of the eye for lacrimal fluid to keep it moist and quantity of lacrimal secretion, so that epiphora may become less disturbing.

Where the sac has reformed after improperly done dacryocystectomy operation, the scope of DCR can only be decided by Dacryocystography. If there is a fair size of the sac present, a DCR may be possible. In cases where earlier DCR operation has failed, it can still be repeated after proper evaluation of the case by dacrycystography (Fig. 19.7).

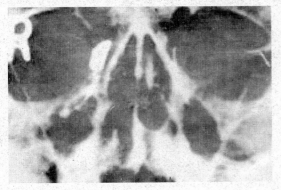

Fig. 19.7: Dacryocystogram (DCG) Showing lacrimal Sac of Normal Size and Shape.

Acute dacryocystitis: It usually follows chronic dacryocystitis and the inflammation is in the tissues around the lacrimal sac. Symptoms of acute inflammation like redness, tenderness are the prominent features. The swelling is much larger than the size of the sac. It extends downwards and laterally into the lower lid. It may even extend into the upper lid. The swelling may be diffuse with all signs of inflammation. Sometimes a pus point can be seen threatening to rupture through the skin. Glands in the submandibular area may be enlarged and tender.

For diagnosis, no attempt should be made for a regurgitation lest by pressing on the lacrimal sac nor should syringing be done to detect obstruction of the naso-lacrimal duct because both procedures are painful and not necessary for diagnosis. A very important diagnostic feature is the history of epiphora existing before the acute inflammatory process started.

If suppuration of acute dacryocystitis has already ruptured through the skin, the inflammation becomes sub-acute because the pus can flow out through the fistulous opening.

Differential diagnosis is from lid abscess and suppuration extending from orbital cellulitis or ethmoidal sinuses pointing through skin of the lower lid. Absence of proptosis and normal range of movements of the eye ball will exclude orbital cellulitis.

Treatment: The acute inflammation should be treated by conservative means such as fomentations, systemic antibiotic and anti-inflammatory drugs. These usually control acute inflammation within a few days. All cases of acute dacryocystitis will ultimately need a DCR or dacryocystectomy operation. This should be deferred till active inflammation has completely subsided. Operating too soon after the acute inflammation will cause severe bleeding from the tissue and will make the identification of the structure difficult.

If the sac is contracted with a small cavity, the appropriate course is to do a dacryocystectomy and the epiphora may be overcome by a *conjunctivo-rhinostomy.*

Tumours of the Lacrimal Passages

Neoplastic lesions of the naso-lacrimal passages arc very rare. The common benign neoplastic lesions are a papilloma of the canaliculus and polyps in the lacrimal sac.

More important, though rare, are malignant growths like epithelioma, carcinoma, round-cell sarcoma, lymphoma and melanoma. It is difficult to diagnose these lesions at an early stage. Enlargement of sac and solid character of the swelling may draw attention to their possibility. Regurgitation of blood stained fluid may also indicate the possibility. They become clinically evident only when they have reached advanced stage. A papilloma and a polyp may be amenable to local surgical removal. Solid growths will however need dacryocystectomy followed by irradiation, if indicated.

DISEASES OF THE LACRIMAL GLAND

There are two groups of diseases affecting orbital and the palpebral part of lacrimal glands.
1. Inflammatory group.
2. Neoplasms.

Inflammation of the Lacrimal Gland (Dacryo-adenitis)

Inflammations of lacrimal gland are rather uncommon and may be acute or chronic in nature.

Acute inflammations: The usual signs of inflammations are present in and around the outer part of the upper lid. There is usually localised acute conjunctivitis in the corresponding area.

Among important causes are metastatic gonococcal infection and mumps. The condition usually responds to appropriate therapy and does not leave behind any after-effects.

Chronic inflammations: Among common causes are tuberculosis, syphilis, actinomycosis and sarcoidosis. Trachomatous dacryoadenitis has been reported due to trachomatous lesion in the lacrimal gland ducts. It has also been emphasised that trachomatous virus may remain hidden in lacrimal ducts and may be a source of reinfection and exacerbations of trachomatous pathology from time to time.

Another chronic inflammatory disease of the lacrimal gland is *Mikulicz's disease*, a condition of unknown etiology involving a syndrome of enlargement of lacrimal and salivary glands with systemic lymphoid lesions.

Cysts and Tumours of the Lacrimal Gland

Cystic, lesions may be mucous cysts, parasitic cysts and dermoids. Among the tumours are pseudo-tumours, mixed cell tumours and adenocarcinoma, in addition to growths from different histological structures. All these present the clinical picture of growth in the lacrimal gland area. In the early stage the cysts and tumours first become evident when the upper lid is pulled up and a growth shows through the outer part of the upper fornix. This should be differentiated from prolapse of the orbital portion of the lacrimal gland. The prolapse is reducible while the growth is not. Mixed cell tumours may grow to an enormous size. The lacrimal gland may also be involved by a secondary metastasis from a primary growth elsewhere in the body. A biopsy may indicate the true nature of growth.

Systemic Conditions

The lacrimal gland may be involved in systemic diseases and one of the important ones is *Hodgkin's disease* with bilateral enlargement of the lacrimal gland.

Sjörgren's syndrome is a condition not uncommon to come across. The clinical features of Sjörgren's syndrome are kerato-conjunctivitis sicca, dryness of mouth and rheumatoid arthritis.

The eye symptoms are irritation, burning and frequent blinking. Some patients actually complain of dryness to eyes. The cause of symptoms is scanty formation of lacrimal secretion. In long-standing cases there may be filamentary keratopathy due to dryness of corneal epithelium. Schirmer's test indicates deficiency of lacrimal secretion Rose Bengal (1%) staining of the conjunctiva supports the diagnosis. The association of dryness in the mouth and arthritic symptoms confirm the diagnosis.

The ocular features of the disease are due to primary atrophy of the lacrimal gland followed by connective tissue replacement.

Treatment is very unsatisfactory and is therefore largely symptomatic. Artificial tear substitutes used frequently and for long time may keep the patient partly symptom free. If corneal involvement is causing unbearable symptoms, bandage contact lens (soflens) or epikerato-prosthesis may protect cornea and relieve symptoms to a large extent.

20

Orbit

The bony orbit is developed from the mesoderm forming skull and bones of face. The roof and the medial wall are developed from the fronto-nasal process and the floor and lateral wall are developed from the maxillary process.

The orbital space is a cavity which houses the eye ball. This cavity is directed laterally in front and medially behind. The large anterior opening is bounded by the orbital margins above, below and laterally, and the nose medially. The widest part of the orbital cavity is just behind the anterior margins.

Nature has provided many essential requirements for the safety as well as functioning of the eye in the orbit. The upper and lower anterior orbital margins are on a level just in front of the cornea and therefore protect the eye from impacts on face. The lateral orbital margin is, on an average, 16 mm behind the apex of the cornea providing a large temporal field necessary for human requirements.

The volume of the orbital cavity is about 30 cc as compared to about 7 cc of the eye ball which is suspended without touching the bony orbit but supported all round by fat and muscles. The average height of the anterior orbital opening is 35 mm and the average width is 40 mm.

The orbital cavity is surrounded by frontal sinuses above, ethmoidal sinuses medially, and maxillary sinus below. The zygomatico-temporal arch on the lateral side provides a communication with temporal fossa.

The walls of the orbital cavity are formed by **seven bones, namely frontal, zygomatic, the maxilla, lacrimal, ethmoid, palatine and sphenoid.** These bones form the walls as follows (Fig. 20.1).

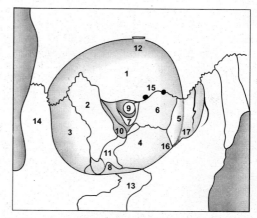

Fig. 20.1: Bony Orbital Cavity (1) Orbital plate of frontal bone; (2) Orbital plate of greater wing of sphenoid; (3) Orbital plate of zygomatic bone; (4) Orbital plate maxilla; (5) Lacrimal bone; (6) Ethmoid bone; (7) Lesser wing of sphenoid; (8) Orbital process of palatine bone; (9) Optic foramen between the two roots of lesser wing of sphenoid; (10) Superior orbital fissure; (11) Inferior orbital fissure; (12) Supra-orbital notch or groove; (13) Infra-orbital foramen or canal; (14) Whitnalle's orbital tubercle; (15) Ethmoidal formen for the nasociliary nerve and the ethmoidal arteries and nerve; (16) Origin of inferior oblique muscle; (17) Lacrimal fossa

Roof of the orbit	→	Orbital surface of the frontal bone.
Lateral wall	→	Orbital plate of zygomatic bone. Orbital plate of greater wing of sphenoid.
Floor of the orbit	→	Orbital plate maxilla.
Medial wall	→	Frontal process of the maxilla, lacrimal bone, orbital plate of ethmoid.
Apex of orbit	→	Lesser wing of sphenoid.
	→	Orbital part of the palatine bone.

There are two large fissures in orbital cavity and the optic foramen at its apex.

Superior orbital fissure: It lies between the two wings of the sphenoid bone and provides communication between the orbital cavity and the middle cranial fossa. It is divided into three parts by a fibrous annulus of Zinn (Fig. 20.2).

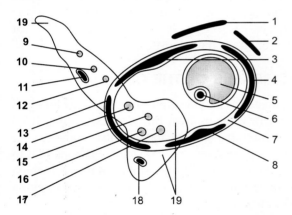

Fig. 20.2: Apex of Orbit. (1) Origin of levator palpebrae superioris; (2) Origin of superior oblique; (3) Origin of superior rectus; (4) Orgin of medial rectus; (5) and (6) Optic nerve and ophthalmic artery in optic foramen; (7) Fibrous annulus of Zinn; (8) Origin of inferior rectus; (9) Lacrimal nerve; (10) Frontal nerve; (11) Superior ophthalmic vein; (12) Trochlear nerve.(IV); (13) Origin of lateral rectus; (14) Upper division of III nerve; (15) Naso-ciliary nerve; (16) Abducent nerve; (17) Lower division of III nerve; (18) Inferior ophthalmic vein; (19) Superior orbital fissure

Within the central part and between the two heads of the lateral rectus muscle are the two divisions of the third nerve, the nasociliary nerve, the abducent nerve and the sympathetic fibres to the ciliary ganglion.

Above the annulus of Zinn pass the superior ophthalmic vein, the lacrimal and frontal branches of the fifth nerve and the troclear nerve. Below the annulus passes inferior ophthalmic vein.

Inferior orbital fissure: It is formed by the maxilla and palatine bones anteriorly and the greater wing of the sphenoid posteriorly. It is directed down and out and transmits infra-orbital nerve, zygomatic nerve and pterygoid plexus of veins. Fissure also provides communication with the pterygo-palatine fossa.

Optic foramen: It is the anterior end of optic canal and transmits optic nerve surrounded by its meninges, ophthalmic artery, sympathetic plexus and the lymphatics.

Other important anatomical features: At the medial part of the superior orbital margin is the supra-orbital notch which in some cases is converted into a canal by a fibro-osseous liga-ment. Through this the supra-orbital nerve and the corresponding vessels pass.

Behind the superior orbital margin and on the medial side is the attachment of the trochlea through which passes the tendon superior oblique muscle.

The infra orbital canal along the inferior border of the orbit transmits the infra orbital nerves and the corresponding vessels.

The ethmoidal foramina in the medial wall transmit anterior ethmoidal artery and nasociliary nerve.

In the anterior part of the medial wall is the lacrimal fossa formed by the frontal process of maxilla and the lacrimal bone bounded anteriorly by anterior lacrimal crest of the maxilla and posteriorly by posterior lacrimal crest of ethmoid bone. The fossa is occupied by lacrimal sac which continues through the naso-lacrimal duct to open into the inferior meatus of nose. The bony naso-lacrimal canal is formed by maxilla on the lateral side and the lacrimal bone and lacrimal process of the inferior turbinate on the medial side.

Orbital periosteum: The orbital cavity is lined by periosteum except in the large fissures and optic foramen, through which it continues to merge with the dura mater. The periosteum is adherent to the subjacent bone at the orbital margin, at the bony sutures and at the apex of the orbit. It can be easily separated from the bony walls except where it is adherent.

Contents of orbit: The orbital cavity is divided into 4 spaces. The sub-periosteal space and the sub-tenon's space are only potential spaces. The main spaces are within the muscle cone and outside the muscle cone. The space within the muscle cone contains important structures, *the optic nerve along with ophthalmic artery, the ciliary ganglion, the long and short posterior ciliary arteries and nerves and the nerves and blood vessels supplying the extra ocular muscles.*

The space outside the muscle cone is largely occupied by orbital fat which prevents shocks of concussion reaching the eye ball.

The lacrimal gland behind the orbital septum is situated in a fossa in the upper and outer part of the orbit just behind the upper and outer bony margin.

There is a thin involuntary muscle sheet about 1 cm broad in the posterior part of orbit covering the inferior orbital fissure and supplied by sympathetic nerve fibres. This is called the *Muller's muscle of the orbit.* The muscle in human beings is largely vestigeal and without any specific function, while in lower animals it is known to act as protruder of the eye ball.

The lymphatics of medial orbit are drained along the angular and the anterior facial veins into submandibular glands and from the lateral orbit into pre-auricular glands. The apex of the orbit drains into the deep cervical glands, via pterygoid plexus of veins.

The orbital outline and orbital spaces can be studied by radiological examinations. It is however important that both the orbits are exposed for comparative evaluation. It is also important to note that the sinuses surrounding the orbit are not fully developed till puberty and this fact should be kept in mind when evaluating X-ray plates. Special radiological procedures are necessary to determine the size of the optic foramen which is important in cases of optic nerve pathology. It is important to have for comparison the opposite optic foramen in view.

DISEASES OF THE ORBIT

Situated as it is, the orbit suffers from pathologies not only of its own but also extensions from surrounding sinuses and the intracranial cavity. Orbital involvement in systemic diseases adds to large number of diseases of orbit most of which are vascular, inflammatory and space occupying in character.

Vascular Lesions of the Orbit

The common vascular lesions which directly or indirectly involve the orbit are orbital haemorrhages, orbital varix and thrombosis of cavernous sinus.

Haemorrhages in orbit: These can be traumatic or spontaneous.

Spontaneous haemorrhages are due to haemopoetic diseases like haemophilia, leukaemia and scurvy. Arteriosclerosis and hypertension can sometimes cause an orbital haemorrhage.

Traumatic haemorrhage may be due to fracture of the orbital wall or middle cranial fossa and sometimes following a retrobulbar injection. When the haemorrhage is due to a bony fracture, it is usually subperiosteal while a haemorrhage due to retrobulbar injection is within the muscle cone.

The main clinical feature is proptosis of the eye ball which is irreducible. In case of haemorrhage in the muscle cone, the eye is pushed directly forwards while if there is a large subperiosteal haematoma the eye is pushed to the opposite side. There may be limitations of movement of the eye if the haemorrhage is large. An orbital haemorrhage may extend into the subcutaneous tissues of the lid and also under bulbar conjunctiva. If proptosis is severe and lasts longer it may result in exposure keratitis. Due to the pressure and pull on optic nerve, there may be a swelling of optic disc, haemorrhages on retina and pupillary dilatation. Depending on severity of haemorrhage and proptosis, there may be severe pain and loss of vision to some extent.

Haemorrhage tends to absorb unless the bleeding recurs. As the fluid part of the blood gets absorbed proptosis becomes less and symptoms and signs become milder.

Treatment is usually conservative unless proptosis is causing severe exposure. The haematoma tends to get absorbed and this may be helped by cold compresses and pressure bandages. If cornea is threatened with exposure, aspiration of blood through a large bored needle or as an alternative, decompression of the orbit may be necessary. A large haematoma within the muscle cone may get encapsulated in which case some proptosis persists and the picture of a cystic space occupying lesion of the orbit develops. A blood cyst if formed will need to be removed as is done for a cystic growth.

If investigations indicate a haematopoetic systemic cause, the same may be appropriately treated to prevent recurrence of orbital haemorrhage.

Orbital varix: This is a condition where dilated and convoluted veins develop in the orbit and cause a reducible proptosis which is usually unilateral.

Most cases of orbital varix are congenital in origin but may become evident only in later part of life.

Clinically, the condition starts as intermittent proptosis which becomes worse by bending. It also tends to increase during coughing or on severe exertion. The proptosis is reducible and non-pulsating. As proptosis is usually of moderate degree, there is no damage to cornea or optic nerve. Long-standing cases may develop loss of vision (Fig. 20.3A and B).

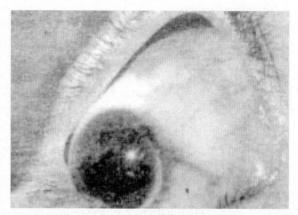

Fig. 20.3A: Orbital varix extending into the sub-conjunctival space. (Head erect)

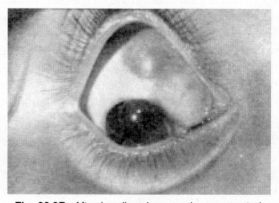

Fig. 20.3B: After bending down, varix exaggerated

Diagnosis of orbital varix is based on the finding that proptosis is reducible and increases on bending forwards. The absence of pulsation is also important. Venography may indicate degree of venous dilatation and the size of the area involved.

Treatment is very unsatisfactory. The patient should avoid postures and exertion which tends to increase the proptosis. Operative procedures like the injection of sclerosing fluid, ligation of superior ophthalmic vein or removal of the mass through Kronlein's approach are possible.

Arterio-venous fistula: A communication between the internal carotid artery and cavernous sinus is a well-known cause of a pulsating and reducible proptosis.

The carotico-cavernous fistula is mostly traumatic but may be spontaneous. Fracture of the base of the skull involving body of sphenoid and penetrating wounds of the orbit are common causes of arterio-venous communication. Spontaneous causes are an aneurysm of the carotid artery in the cavernous sinus or an atheromatous patch bursting into the cavernous sinus.

Communication between the internal carotid artery and cavernous sinus results in transmission of arterial pressure into the venous system thereby impeding the venous blood return due to positive pressure in veins as determined by ophthalmo-dynamometry. This is transmitted into the ophthalmic vein and other veins of the orbit. Even though the fistula may be on one side, venous engorgement and proptosis is bilateral because of the positive pressure transmitted to the opposite cavernous sinus through the sinus inter-cavernosus which communicates both the sinuses.

The clinical picture is typical. The onset is sudden and the patient is distressed by noises in the head. The manifestations are bilateral. There is bilateral proptosis and extreme engorgement of veins in the conjunctiva, lids and the forehead.

The proptosis is pulsating which can be easily felt. A bruit synchronous with arterial pulsation can be heard with stethoscope placed on the upper lid covering the eye ball. There may be marked chemosis of lids and the conjunctiva. The retinal veins are engorged and there is compensatory neovascularisation. III, IV and VI nerves may develop palsies in addition to other neurological manifestations.

Diagnosis is easy. Sudden onset and bilaterality of proptosis with bruit are diagnostic. Carotid angiography and orbital venography may clarify the anatomical morphology of the lesion.

Treatment by conservative means is unsatisfactory. Compression of the common carotid artery intermittently may help relieve symptoms when severe. The only sensible surgical approach can be the ligation of common carotid or internal carotid in the neck. The procedure can however cause a cerebral catastrophe and should therefore be tried after the compression test done preoperatively has indicated adequate blood supply to the brain through anastomotic channels. Ligation of the superior ophthalmic vein may help to reduce venous engorgement of the lids and the face.

INFLAMMATIONS OF ORBIT

Although an enclosed space partitioned in front by the septum orbitale above and below the eye ball, the orbit has communications alround through foramina, canals and fissures. It communicates with paranasal sinuses, it communicates with intra-cranial cavity and it communicates with pterygo-palatine fossa. Equally important are communications with the venous plexuses many of which communicate with the orbital veins. Inflammation of the orbit, therefore, in a majority of cases are extensions from surrounding areas. In addition, perforating injuries from front and acute intraocular inflammation extending into the orbit are other common sources of orbital inflammations. Furthermore, systemic infections can lodge infective focus in the orbit. The resulting condition is *orbital cellulitis, acute or chronic* and severe or mild.

External injuries, penetrating injuries introducing infection in the orbit, or infection consequent to an operative procedure may cause inflammations of the orbit.

Intraocular infections: Panopthalmitis following injuries or operations on the eye ball is associated with varying degrees of orbital cellulitis.

Infection in sinuses: Purulent sinusitis of ethmoids, maxillary sinus and frontal sinus can extend into the orbit either directly through the erroded bone or through a venous communication.

Infection from teeth: An acute infection in the teeth can travel into the orbit through the maxillary sinus or through the venous channels.

Infections from the face e.g. erysipalas, a streptococcal cellulitis from the skin can cause orbital cellulitis. An acute infection of lacrimal gland or lacrimal sac may similarly extend into the orbit. An acute suppurative infection of the lids, cheek, lips and nose can also cause orbital cellulitis.

Nasopharyngeal infections and other infections in the throat can extend into orbit through venous communications.

Intracranial inflammations: Like suppurative meningitis, extra-dural abscess, thrombosis of venous sinuses can extend into the orbit along the meninges of the optic nerve and superior orbital fissure or can extend through venous communications, just as the inflammations of orbit can extend into the intracranial space.

Primary inflammations of the orbit are rare and most of them are due to a systemic disease like tuberculosis, syphilis or emboli from infective sources anywhere in the body. Inflammations of the orbit may be acute and chronic.

Acute inflammations may be cellutilis, orbital periostitis, tenonitis of the eye ball and thrombophlebitis of the orbital veins.

1. **Orbital cellulitis:** This is an acute inflammation involving most of the contents of the orbit. Symptoms are severe with marked pain, swelling and fever. The signs of orbital cellulitis are fairly characteristic. There is marked swelling of the lids, chemosis of conjunctiva, proptosis and limitations of eye movements. The last two are important differentiating features from conditions like lid abscess, acute dacryo-cystitis, acute dacryodenitis or severe conjunctivitis.

   Orbital cellulitis may also cause optic neuritis, thrombosis of the retinal vein resulting in visual loss.

   If inflammation in the orbit is not controlled early and suppuration takes place, the orbital abscess usually points through the skin of the lower lid and may burst anteriorly.

2. **Orbital thrombophlebitis:** It is usually caused when infection is carried into the orbit either from cavernous sinus behind or from infections of face in front. The thrombophlebitis soon results in orbital cellulitis and presents a symptom complex as described above.

3. **Orbital periostitis:** It may be an extension from para nasal siuses or a metastatic infection from elsewhere in the body. There is severe pain and oedema of lids. Proptosis is of moderate degree and the eye is directed to the opposite side. The periositis may extend to involve the periosteum of fissures and foramina in the apex of orbit causing a clinical picture of *superior orbital fissure syndrome*. If an abscess is formed under the periosteum, it tends to appear anteriorly on the orbital margin and may result in osteomyelitis of the orbital bones and leave a fistulous tract.

4. **Tenonitis:** Acute tenonitis is commonly associated with pan-ophthalmitis. If inflammation is limited to tenon's space there is no proptosis but there is pain on movement of eye ball. The congestion due to tenonitis under the conjunctiva is deeply placed and abruptly ends about 2-3 mm from the limbus. There may be collection of pus in the Tenon's space which may extend along its reflections to recti muscles. If it extends posteriorly, it may cause optic neuritis and diminution of vision.

Complications and prognosis: Acute orbital cellulitis is a severe condition because it involves important structures of the eye and orbit and may cause irreparable visual loss. The complications may be listed as follows:

a. Optic neuritis, consequent atrophy.
b. Meningitis.
c. Intracranial abscess/cavernous sinus thrombosis.
d. Orbital fissure syndrome.

Treatment: Treatment of acute inflammation in orbit is intensive antibiotic therapy. The therapy should be started by intravenous route and then continued as intramuscular therapy. A broad spectrum antibiotic covering both gram positive and negative organisms should be the choice because bacteriological studies are not always possible.

Surgical drainage of pus is necessary when the abscess has pointed anteriorly and drainage should be through skin of lower lid. A subperiosteal abscess pointing along the orbital margin should be incised and drained. Suppurative tenonitis should also be drained but this is done through the conjunctiva. If response to antibiotic is not satisfactory and if complications are developing resulting in visual loss or the cornea is threatened with exposure keratitis, a careful exploration of the orbit to localise the orbital abscess may have to be undertaken.

Thrombosis of Cavernous Sinus

The cavernous sinus, one on either side of the body of sphenoid is not strictly a space containing blood only. Detailed anatomy and structures associated with the sinus has been described earlier.

The sinus is criss-crossed by fine fibrillar network therefore formation of a thrombus is readily facilitated. The communication of cavernous sinus anteriorly with superior and inferior ophthalmic veins and posteriorly with the lateral sinus makes it an easy victim for infections from different places and extensions of thrombus from feeding veins.

The common sources of infections are from face, orbit, adjoining meninges and mastoid air cells. An area on face from the inner angle of eye to the side of nose and upper lip is called the *danger zone* because any infection from this area can travel via the superior and inferior orbital vein into cavernous sinus. Therefore it was always considered dangerous to prematurely incise a stye, an acute dacryocystitis or a boil on the lip or the side of the nose because the incision may cut open a few dilated veins and infection may enter the cut end of vein and reach cavernous sinus leading to cavernous sinus thrombosis. Similarly, infection from mastoiditis may extend along lateral sinus and lead to thrombosis of cavernous sinus.

Clinical picture: The onset is sudden and progress is rapid. There is severe pain in eyes and forehead. There is a rise of temperature and the patient is acutely ill.

Signs are characteristic: There is oedema of the lids, congestion and chemosis of conjunctiva and proptosis which starts on one side and very soon extends to the opposite eye. 6th nerve paralysis is the earliest neurological manifestation while later on there may be palsy of all oculomotor nerves. The patient may develop symptoms of meningism and meningitis.

Diagnosis is based on the severity of condition, systemic reactions, bilaterality and early ocular nerve palsies. The important differentiating features from orbital cellulitis are early bilaterality, absence of tenderness and marked venous congestion.

Treatment: Antibiotic therapy should be given in massive doses of broad spectrum antibiotics combined with therapeutic doses of anti-coagulants like heparin. The choice of antibiotics should be the one which is effective against staphylococcus aureus because this organism is considered a common offending organism.

Chronic Inflammations of the Orbit

Most chronic inflammations of the orbit are primary and caused by systemic infections. These infections are:

- Syphilis
- Tuberculosis
- Actinomycosis
- Parasitic diseases
- Mycotic infections.

Syphilis and tuberculosis mostly involve periosteum of orbit and extend to involve the periosteal linings of the fissures and foramina. Gumma and hydatid cyst of the orbit may cause proptosis.

Other chronic infections may lead to chronic inflammation in orbit and manifest as slow proptosis, limitation of movement and formation of sinuses and fistulae.

There is however one condition which needs to be described under the category of chronic inflammations of the orbit and this is called pseudo-tumour of the orbit.

Pseudo-tumours of the orbit: Although the clinical manifestations are those of a tumour causing slow proptosis, the lesions are called pseudo tumours because some of these cases regress with non-specific therapy. Their response to steroids is an important point. Secondly operative exploration does not indicate any definite tumour mass but shows diffuse infiltration of orbital tissue. Thirdly, the biopsy of the tissue removed shows a chronic inflammatory reaction.

The clinical picture is that of an irreducible proptosis of slow onset. Proptosis may sometimes become severe even causing exposure keratitis and limitations of the movements of the eye. An ill-defined mass may be felt through the upper and, lower lids. In long-standing cases there may be a pale disc. Diagnosis of a pseudotumour on a clinical basis is very difficult. Biopsy may then indicate a chronic inflammatory reaction in the tissue. Tuberculosis and syphilis should be excluded. Parasites in stool and eosinophilia in blood should be looked for. Quite often diagnosis of pseudo-tumour is thought of when surgery is undertaken for a tumour and no tumour outline is found.

Treatment should be directed towards non-specific chronic inflammation. Empirical use of antibiotics and steroids may reduce proptosis in these cases.

In tropical countries with heavy incidence of tuberculosis, anti-tubercular therapy may help where nothing else has yielded results.

Surgical effort is usually unrewarding.

PROPTOSIS/EXOPHTHALMOS

Proptosis (Fig. 20.4A, Plate 13 and Figs 20.4B and 20.4C)

Proptosis is a *forward passive displacement* of the eye ball caused by a space occupying lesion of orbital space or the bones forming orbit while exophthalmos is an *active process* leding to increased prominence of the eye ball.

Causes of Pseudo Proptosis

1. **Enlarged eye ball as in buphthalmos, high** myopia. Unilateral high **myopia** often gives an impression of proptosis in one eye.
2. **Retracted lids:** Although the eye ball is in position, this gives an appearance of pseudo-proptosis:

3. **Shallow bony orbit:** A typical example is proptosis in oxycephaly. The clinical picture of all these conditions is evident in most cases.

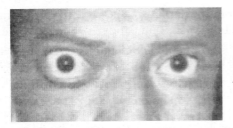

Fig. 20.4B: Proptosis. Axial proptosis Rt. due to a lesion in the muscle Cone

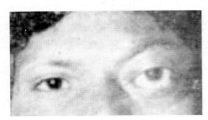

Fig. 20.4C: Eccentric Proptosis. left eye ball displaced fowards and upward due to lesion in the lower orbit

True Proptosis

This is always due to a space occupying lesion displacing the eye forwards. The normal position of the eye ball is evaluated in relation to the centre of the zygomatico-temporal arch forming the outer orbital margin. There are variations in this relationship in different races and in different individuals of same race. The anterior pole of the eye ball (centre of the cornea) is on average 16.0 mm in front of the level of lateral orbital margin, as determined by exophthalmometry. Anything more than 20.0 mm indicates definite proptosis. In uniocular proptosis, difference in the position of the two eye balls helps detection of even early proptosis, because any difference of more than 2 to 3 mm between the two eyes is, considered abnormal (uniocular high myopia excluded).

Proptosis may be sudden or slow. It may be constant or intermittent. It may be unilateral or bilateral. It may be pulsating or non-pulsating.

Causes of proptosis may be as follows:
1. Congenital causes like congenital cysts.
2. Traumatic—Due to an orbital haemorrhage, orbital emphysema, traumatic prolapse of the eye ball.
3. Chronic inflammatory condition like tuberculoma, gumma, sarcoidosis.
4. Vascular lesions like angioneurotic oedema, orbital varix, Arterio-venous fistula, retrobulbar haemorrhage and aneurysm in the orbit.
5. Cysts and tumours:
   a. **Cysts**
      i. Dermoid
      ii. Parasitic
      iii. Implantation
      iv. Blood cyst.
   b. **Tumours**
      i. Primary—of any tissues of the orbit
      ii. Direct Extension—from bones of the orbit
      iii. Secondary metastasis—from distant tumours elsewhere.
6. Systemic diseases:
      i. leukaemia
      ii. thyrotoxicosis
      iii. thyrotropic exophthalmos.
7. Among the osteopathies of the orbit causing proptosis are:
      i. Paget's disease (osteitis deformans).
      ii. Leontiasis ossea.
      iii. Fibrous displasia of bone.
      iv. Morgagni's syndrome
8. Metabolic diseases causing proptosis are:
      i. Hand-Schuller-Christian's disease.
      ii. Xanthomatosis.
      iii. Amyloidosis.

Bilateral Proptosis

One should first think of the following conditions in a case of bilateral proptosis.

1. Cavernous sinus thrombosis.
2. Arterio-venous fistula in cavernous sinus.
3. Leukaemia.
4. Thyrotoxicosis (Exophthalmos).

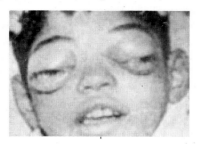

Fig. 20.5: Acute Leukaemia causing bilateral Proptosis, marked conjunctival chemosis and lid oedema

Pulsating proptosis may be caused by:

1. Arterio-venous fistula.
2. Aneurysm of ophthalmic artery.
3. Highly vascular tumour, like haemangioma. Reducible proptosis is typically seen in orbital varix.

Intermittant proptosis is usually due to:

1. Orbital varix.
2. Haemangioma.
3. Recurrent inflammation.
4. Recurrent emphysema.

Clinical features: Every case of proptosis should be evaluated under the following headings:
1. Unilateral or bilateral.
2. Direction of proptosis; straight forwards or to a side.
3. Constant or intermittant.
4. Reducible or irreducible.
5. Pulsating or non-pulsating.
6. Bruit present or not.
7. Change in the degree of proptosis, if any, on stooping forward or lying supine.
8. Any systemic cause.
9. Relevant laboratory investigations to exclude the possible cause.

Methods of examination and special investigations in a case of proptosis: Some are routinely done and some are indicated in special circumstances.
1. Inspection.
2. Palpation.
3. Auscultation.
4. Ophthalmoscopic examination to note condition of retinal blood vessels colour of disc, oedema of disc head, if any.
5. Exophthalmometery on both sides.
6. Plane X-ray of both the orbits.
7. X-rays of the optic foramen and orbital fissures of both sides.
8. Orbital tomogram.
9. Ultra-sonography.
10. Orbital pneumography.
11. Orbital venography.
12. Orbital arteriography.
13. Orbital biopsy.
14. Radio-active isotope uptake.

Prolapse of the Eye Ball

When the whole eye ball is suddenly prolapsed forward passing even beyond the level of lid margins, it presents an alarming picture but not as serious as it looks.

The common causes of prolapse or luxation of the eye ball are:
1. Blunt injury, the force being transmitted through the fornix. As the eye ball is pushed forward, the orbicularis develops a spasmodic contraction and the lid margins grip behind the eye ball preventing its spontaneous return.
2. Willful displacement is practised by individuals with a shallow orbit.

A sudden prolapse of the eye ball causes severe discomfort and pain due to the blepherospasm; demanding urgent attention to return the eye ball to its own place.

Intermittant prolapse can usually be reduced by patient himself by relaxing the orbicularis muscle. A little push may sometimes be necessary. If this is not possible a facial block or lateral canthotomy may make it easier and simpler.

Endocrine Exophthalmos *(Thyrotoxicosis—Grave's disease;* Fig. 20.6A and B).

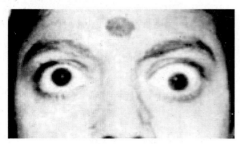

Fig. 20.6A: Thyrotoxicosis (Note prominence of the eye ball due to bilateral exophthalmos and retraction of upper lid particularly on left side)

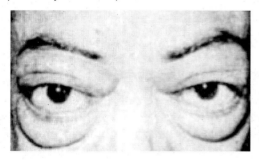

Fig. 20.6B: Thyrotropic Exophthalmos—Exophthalmic Ophthalmoplegia (Note the infiltration in upper and lower lids)

Exophthalmos is an active process leading to increased prominence of the eye ball. The whole symptom complex has for long been considered to be divisible in two parts. The first was called *thyrotoxicosis or thyrotoxic exophthalmos or Grave's disease.* It was attributed to hyperthyroidism. The second group was called *endocrine exophthalmos or thyrotropic exophthalmos or exophthalmic ophthalmoplegia* which was considered to be due to aberrant influence of the thyrotropic harmone of the anterior pituitary on the function of the thyroid. The disease is common and known for long. From gross proptosis as the only manifestation, it has become a complex syndrome. No disease has so many manifestations named after so many clinicians as thyrotoxicosis has.

This symptom complex is now considered to be two stages of the same disease; the first being oedema and cellular infiltration of orbital tissue and second being result of fibrosis in the muscles of eye ball and contents of the orbit.

The etiology of thyrotoxicosis has changed from the original concept of over production of thyroid hormone (thyrotoxin) to a thyrotropic factor of anterior pituitary stimulating higher thyroid function. The condition was therefore earlier called hyperthyroidism. It was later established that the pituitary secretes a hormone which influences function of thyroid gland. A number of substances have been extracted from anterior pituitary, the excess of which can cause over-activity of thyroid. Which of these substances is the most important has still not established. There is a view that the pituitary substance and its effect on thyroid function can be an autoimmune reaction, the thyroid being antigenic against the antibodies in the blood. The effect of hyperthyroid function either of its own or stimulated by anterior pituitary is increase in thyrotoxin in the blood and so also the protein bound iodine in the serum. Excess thyroxin in blood sensitises plain muscles to the action of adrenaline which is responsible for some of the clinical signs. Similarly, protein bound iodine brings about tissue changes responsible for exophthalmos.

These substances from the thyrotropic hormones of the anterior pituitary have been variedly named as thyroid stimulating hormone (TSH), Exophthalmos producing substances (EPS) and long acting thyroid stimulator (LATS).

Pathology. The pathological changes in the orbit are:

1. Extraocular muscles are enlarged many times.

2. Cellular infiltration with lymphocytes and plasma cells.
3. More fat and mucopolysaccharides in the orbital tissues.
4. In later stages, fibrosis in the muscles.

Clinical picture: Thyrotoxic exophthalmos and thyrotropic exophthalmos are now considered to be two stages of the same disease, and therefore the sequence of events starting as manifestations of thyrotoxicosis may end up as thyrotropic exophthalmic ophthalmoplegia.

Thyrotoxicosis is a condition more often affecting women than men. In most cases the condition is bilateral although manifestation in the two eyes may be unequal. It is however not unusual to come across unilateral manifestations only. Ocular manifestations appear in the following order as the disease progresses.

1. Upper lid retraction (Dalrymple's sign) due to over-action of Muller's muscle of upper lid which has a sympathetic nerve supply.
2. Lid Lag (Von Graefes' sign). As the patient looks down, the upper lid should also normally move down. If the upper lid does not follow the downward movement of the eye as is evident from the increasing exposure of the sclera above, the condition is called Lid Lag. Similarly, on looking up, the lower lid also lags behind (Griffith's sign).
3. Absence of folds on the forehead on looking up.
4. Infrequent blinking (Stellwag's sign).
5. Jerky movements of the upper lid on looking down (Boston's sign).
6. Deficient convergence (Moebius sign).
7. Oedema of lids and congestion of conjunctiva.
8. Pads of orbital fat appearing at the lower orbital margin through the lower lid.
9. Restriction of movement of the eye—ophthalmoplegia. Usually all the muscles are involved and in advanced stages, the eye ball is in a fixed position. The fibrosis

in the muscles does not permit even forced duction of the eye.
10. Marked chemosis and severe proptosis endangering corneal transparency because the lid cannot cover and protect cornea. In this stage, Bell's phenomenon is also absent and cornea remains exposed during sleep.
11. Pallor of optic disc and sometimes papillo-edema is due to increased intraorbital pressure pressing on the optic nerve.
12. Diminution of vision either due to corneal complications or due to optic nerve pathology.

When the condition reaches the stage of last four manifestations, it is labelled as thyrotropic exophthalmos or exophthalmic ophthalmoplegia.

In addition to ocular manifestations there are systemic disturbances like:

1. Loss of weight.
2. Tachycardia and nervousness.
3. Tremors in outstretched hands.
4. Enlargement of the thyroid gland.
5. Increased basal metabolism due to hypersecretion of thyroxin.

Diagnosis and investigation: In well developed case, diagnosis is written on the face. However, some investigations are necessary to confirm the same.

The important investigations are:

1. Estimate protein bound iodine in the serum.
2. Measure the uptake of radioactive iodine by thyroid.
3. Demonstrate thyroid antibodies.
4. Measure basal metabolic rate (BMR).

Treatment: Treatment is partly for ocular conditions and partly for thyrotoxicosis. It is curious that once exophthalmos has reached an advanced stage, it does not regress even though the systemic condition has been brought under control. The treatment should be under the guidance of a physician.

Treatment of thyrotoxicosis: With drugs, systemic aspects of thyrotoxicosis can be kept under control. The drugs which have been found useful are carbimazole and Thiouracil. These drugs inhibit release of thyroid hormone.

Radioactive iodine I^{131} or I^{125} is also a useful long acting therapy. The doses should be monitored because the over dosage can cause hypothyroidism and myxoedema.

Sub-total thyroidectomy, preferably in younger age group or where there is a relapse of the condition in spite of systemic therapy, should be considered.

Ablation of anterior pituitary has been recommended.

Treatment of exophthalmos. Steroids given orally in large doses are temporarily very effective but maintenance of the dose for a long time invites ocular and systemic complications. Steroids may preferably be used by a subconjunctival or retrobulbar injection for longer time.

Local eye drops like Guanethidine 5 to 10% or Bethenidine 10 to 20% solution used twice a day may help relieve lid retraction. These drugs act as adrenergic blocking agents. However, they have no effect on exophthalmos.

If proptosis is endangering the transparency of the cornea, the following surgical procedures may have to be undertaken depending on the severity of exophthalmos:

1. Lateral tarsorrhaphy or lateral canthoplasty.
2. Recession or aponurectomy of the levator palpabrae superioris may reduce retraction of the lid and thus help cover the cornea.
3. Decompression of the orbit.

CYSTS AND TUMOURS

Cysts and tumours of orbit are important causes of displacement of the eye ball. They may arise from tissues in the orbit, from the bony wall of the orbit or may extend from the surrounding tissues. In the orbit, the growths limited within the muscle cone cause a straight forward proptosis. Growths arising from or extending into the orbital space outside the muscle cone *cause* eccentric proptosis and so also the growth arising from bony orbital walls.

The cysts of the orbit may be grouped as follows:
1. Congenital micro-ophthalmos with a cyst.
2. Dermoid cysts.
3. Meningocoeles and encephalocoeles.
4. Blood cysts.
5. Parasitic cysts like hydatid cysts and cysticercus.
6. Cysts extending into orbit from the paranasal sinuses.

Tumours can arise from any of the tissues in the orbit. They may also extend from surrounding structures or there may be secondary metastasis from a primary growth elsewhere in the body.

The long list of tumours, can arise from every conceivable tissue in the orbit, the muscles, blood vessel, connective tissue, fatty tissue, optic nerve and its meninges, periosteum and the bony orbit.

Among the common primary tumours of the orbit are:

Vascular
1. Capillary angioma.
2. Cavernous haemangioma.
3. Haemangio-endothelioma.

Muscular–Rhabdomyosarcoma.

Optic nerve
1. Glioma.
2. Meningioma.

Orbital nerves–Neurofibroma.

Adenoid tissues
1. Lymphoma.
2. Lympho-sarcoma.
3. Leukaemia.
4. Hodgkin's disease.

Orbital bones
1. Osteoma.
2. Osteo-sarcoma.

Lacrimal gland
1. Mixed lacrimal tumour.
2. Adeno carcinoma of lacrimal gland.

Extension from intraocular tissues
1. Retinoblastoma.
2. Malignant melanoma.

Extension from surrounding structures
1. Mucocoeles from the ethmoids and frontal sinuses.
2. Sarcoma from the maxillary sinus.
3. Lymphosarcoma from the nasopharynx.
4. Meningioma from within the skull.

Secondary metastasis in the orbit from the primary elsewhere in the body
1. Carcinoma.
2. Sarcoma.
3. Melanoma.
4. Hypernephroma.

The pathological identity of most orbital cysts and tumours is made on exploration and biopsy. Some identity of their location may be possible by radiological procedures like X-ray plates, angiography or venography (Fig. 20.7, Plate 14).

Radiological investigations include:
1. Postero-anterior X-ray of sinuses and orbit in two positions.
    i. Nose and chin touching the plate.
    ii. Nose and forehead touching the plate.
2. Orbital tomograms for viewing the optic canal and size and shape of the soft tissue shadow.

Orbital angiography: This shows arterial network of the orbit and their displacement by any lesion. This is done by injecting the dye in the internal carotid artery.

Orbital venography: This is a helpful investigative procedure which demarcates the normal or abnormal venous channels in the orbit and their displacement, if any, by space occupying lesions.

Venography is done by injecting the dye in the angular vein or in the frontal or supraorbital vein.

A cerebral angiography may also help identifying lesions which have extended from intracranial cavity into orbital space.

Exophthalmometery: This procedure helps to determine the position of the anterior pole of the eye ball in relation to the outer orbital margin. Normally the anterior pole of the eye ball is on an average 16.0 mm in front of the lateral orbital margin. If it is more than 20 mm, it indicates proptosis or exophthalmos.

The position of the anterior pole of the eye ball in relation to the orbital margin can be roughly determined by placing a rule over the upper and lower bony orbital margins over the closed lid surfaces. Normally the rule should just touch the skin surface of the closed lids.

An estimation of the position of the centre of the cornea can also be done by simple inspection by looking down from over the head with the patient looking straight ahead. The apex of the cornea on each side can be compared and proptosis detected.

The position of the anterior pole of the eye ball can also be measured in millimeters with the help of a transparent millimeter scale. The scale is placed on the lateral orbital margin and the patient is asked to look straight ahead. The centre of the corneal curvature can be seen through the scale and noted against the millimeter mark of the sale. Exophthalmometry can be more precisely done with an exophthalmometer. The base of the exophthalmomometer is placed on the zygomatico-temporal arch at the lateral orbital margin and the patient is asked to look straight ahead. The position of the anterior pole of the eye ball in relation to the lateral orbital margin can be accurately measured simultaneously on both sides. There are various models of exophthalmometers. The simplest one is the one made of perspex scale with a bony support.

CT Scan, USG and Magnetic Resonance Imaging: Orbital space occupying lesions have always posed a diagnostic problem for ophthalmologists. Although a CT and Ultrasonography (USG) has been of tremendous help in the last decade so. It has limitations like USG for orbital apex lesions. CT scan being relatively non-specific for tissue characteristics and/or encapsulation of the lesion. Magnetic Resonance Imaging (MRI) has proved more useful and perhaps more superior in the detection of tissue character and delineation of orbital pathology (Fig. 20.8).

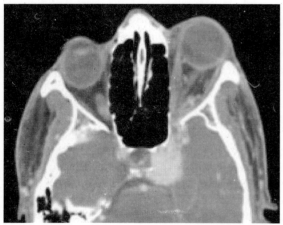

Fig. 20.8: Contrast enhanced axial CT scan of orbit showing orbital apex and thickened redial rectus *(Courtsy Dr. Saroj Gupta)*

PARA-ORBITAL PATHOLOGIES

The orbit is so closely related to paranasal sinuses, nasal cavity and the naso pharynx not only as an immediate neighbour but actually communicating with them. Many pathologies in these para-orbital structures involve orbit. It is therefore important that the ophthalmologist should be conversant with the interpretations of the investigative procedures of these areas. He should also not hesitate to take help of an ENT specialist not only in co-relating the findings but also in surgical procedures where both systems are involved.

Among the conditions in the para-orbital region that are significant to the symptomatology arising from involvement of orbit or the eye ball, following are of importance:

1. Sinusitis of maxillary sinus reflexly causes lacrimation or congestion of conjunctiva or may be a source of septic focus for anterior uveitis.
2. Sinusitis of frontal sinus may cause supra-orbital neuralgia.
3. A mucocoele of frontal or ethmoid sinuses may cause displacement of the eye ball.
4. Inflammations of ethmoids or nasal cavity may provide bacteria for causing conjunctivitis or may cause a blockage of naso-lacrimal duct, leading to dacryocystitis.
5. Dental infection may be a source of septic focus for anterior uveitis. Removal of a septic tooth without coverage of antibiotic has been known to cause optic neuritis or even orbital cellulitis.
6. Tumours of the para-nasal sinuses may appear either anteriorly and displace the eye ball or may invade the posterior part of the orbit and cause proptosis.
7. A sarcoma of antrum may extend into the orbit and cause upward displacement of the eye ball.
8. A malignant tumour of the nasopharynx may clinically attract attention first by causing proptosis or paralysis of 4th and 6th nerves.

Apart from these conditions specifically mentioned, one should always be on lookout for any pathology around the orbit if one can not locate aetiology or origin of ocular symptoms.

TREATMENT OF SPACE OCCUPYING LESIONS OF THE ORBIT

Treatment of a Primary Cyst or a Tumour

It is surgical, radiational, chemotherapeutic or a combination of more than one therapy. The choice will depend on whether it is a primary orbital growth, a benign or a malignant growth, an extension from the surrounding areas or is secondary metastasis from a primary elsewhere.

1. Exploratory aspiration.
2. Biopsy.
3. Removal of the mass.

Exploratory aspiration is indicated when a clinical examination clearly indicates the cystic character of the mass. A large bored needle is introduced from the side where a cystic mass is best felt. It may be introduced through the skin or fornix conjunctiva. It is safer to do it from the outer side either from above or below the horizontal line. The aspirated fluid should be examined in the laboratory for cellular contents and type of cells, biochemical character of the fluid. It may be cerebro-spinal fluid, a fluid of a hydatid cyst or blood from an angiomatous mass. It may be simple serous fluid from a mucocoele. Aspiration may temporarily reduce proptosis but the fluid is likely to recollect.

Exploratory biopsy: If the growth has extended anteriorly, removal of a piece for biopsy should not be difficult. After the removal of the mass, histological examination should always be done not only to know the nature of the tumour but the line of treatment indicated. Exploration in suspected malignant growths should be followed by radical surgery immediately after a frozen-section histology report.

Surgical removal of the orbital mass can be anything from a simple to an extremely complicated and destructive procedure. There are various surgical approaches depending on the location of the tumour.

a. *Lateral orbitotomy* through Kronlein's approach.
   This is the most satisfactory approach for growths in the lateral part of the orbit and apex of the orbit.
   An important structure which needs to be taken care of is the ciliary ganglion lying between the optic nerve and the lateral rectus muscle.

b. *Trans-frontal approach.* The procedure includes anterior craniotomy, lifting up the frontal lobe of brain and cutting open the thin bony roof of the orbit. The procedure is most suitably indicated for tumours of the optic nerve. It is obvious that this procedure should be undertaken jointly by the eye surgeon and neuro-surgeon.

c. *Direct approach.* It may be necessary from wherever the growth is nearest to the surface. It may be through the upper lid, lower lid or a medial approach.

d. *Indirect approach* to an orbital tumour may sometimes be needed either through maxillary sinus or through nasal cavity and the ethmoidal sinuses. This has necessarily to be done jointly with the ENT surgeon.

The above procedures are ideally suitable for orbital growths which have a well defined outline and are encapsulated. The treatment for proved malignant lesions are however to be approached differently.

The lines of treatment that are available for malignant growths are:

a. Removal of the mass.
b. Exenteration of the orbit.
c. Radiotherapy.
d. Chemotherapy.

It is difficult to give a clear cut outline of the indications of any of these procedures. The results of treatment largely depend on whether metastasis has already taken place. This, in many cases is not easy to determine. There are cases where a malignant growth was removed and the patient had no recurrence, while there are other cases where even exenteration was followed by local recurrence and systemic metastasis.

Exenteration of orbit is indicated where the malignant growth has extended and involved the various structures of the orbit. In such a situation, saving the eye is unimportant. It is more important to save life.

Exenteration of the orbit includes removal of eye ball, all the contents of orbit and entire periosteum lining the orbital cavity. If the growth has extended anteriorly, the lids may have to be sacrificed along with exenteration. In any case, exenteration is followed by skin grafts to line the orbital cavity and an orbital prosthesis at a later date.

Radiotherapy is by and large a post exenteration therapy. In radiosensitive lesions, radiotherapy alone may be enough although the eye may develop radiation cataract or other radiation effects.

Chemotherapy with antimitotic drugs is indicated to treat metastasis to prevent and treat local recurrence after surgery.

The sites for metastasis of orbital growths will depend on the pathological entity of the mass, its grade of malignancy and vascularity and also whether the growth is in the posterior or anterior part of the orbit. Metastasis may involve lymph glands draining the areas and these can be deep cervical glands, the pre-parotid glands and the sub-mandibular glands.

21

Injuries of
the Eye

Thanks to rapid industrialisation, both mechanical and chemical and to the high speed actions in industry and in social life, traumatology has become a speciality in ophthalmology. Ocular injury in fact is now the only major emergency needing urgent attention of an ophthalmologist.

Injuries of eye in the pre-industrial era were largely limited to domestic injuries. Sport and accident injuries and agricultural injuries needed routine attention and treatment. Even industrial injuries were limited in number and severity. Wars, however, brought in a temporary phase of war injuries needing specialised efforts from time to time.

So far as the eye ball is concerned, from clinical point of view the injuries are mainly of two types, *non-perforating* and *perforating*. They may be mechanical chemical and radiational injuries. There are more varieties of causes than the types of injuries. What is therefore important is not so much what caused the injury but what injury has been caused.

In the group of mechanical injuries are the domestic injuries, transport accidents, injuries due to sports, agricultural injuries, industrial injuries, war injuries and self-inflicted injuries. Birth injuries form a small-group of mechanical injuries.

In the group of non-mechanical injuries are burns and scalds, chemical burns, radiational burns, electrical burns, explosions and injuries due to toxic agents.

MECHANICAL INJURIES

Injuries to the Lids and Conjunctiva

1. Black eye due to subcutaneous haemorrhage is common. The blood may even extend to the skin of the opposite lid.
2. Abrasions and cuts of lids are due to blunt injury. These are usually against the bone and therefore commonly affect the lids against the orbital margins.
3. Lacerations of lids are mostly due to sharp implements. These lacerations could be anything from a small tear to an extensive loss of lid tissue.
4. Subconjunctival haemorrhage may be local or an extension from an orbital haematoma or even from a haemorrhage in the anterior cranial fossa.
5. Conjunctival tears.
6. Foreign bodies, may be single or multiple and of different varieties. The worst are gun

powder particles which may smear the face, lids, conjunctiva and cornea. The less common and the less harmful are the lead pellets from the shot guns.

Injuries of the Orbit

The posterior part of the floor of the orbit, the lacrimal and ethmoid bones in medial wall of orbit are the weakest parts of the orbit.

A. Injuries to the orbit may be concussion and compression injuries when the object hitting the orbit is bigger than the size of the anterior opening so that the primary impact is on the orbital margins. The impact causes sudden rise of intra-orbital pressure and as a result the weakest part of the floor of the orbit gives way. This is called a blow-out fracture of the orbit. The fracture of the floor may injure infraorbital nerve, inferior rectus and inferior oblique muscles. The orbital fat herniates through the break in the floor of the orbit.

The clinical features are:
1. Enophthalmos.
2. Vertical diplopia.
3. Infra-orbital nerve anaesthesia.

B. Contracoup fractures are also common following a blunt injury to the orbital margin. The force of impact is transmitted through the two processes, the zygomatic and maxillary of frontal bone resulting in a break in the thin part of the bone, near the optic foramen and superior orbital fissure. This may result in injuries to optic nerve and structures passing through superior orbital fissure. The clinical features may be sudden and total loss of vision due to a piece of bone cutting across the optic nerve in optic canal. Bony injuries to orbital fissure cause ocular palsies and ptosis.

C. An object smaller than the anterior orbital opening will hit the eye ball directly and cause concussion and contusion injury of eye ball.

D. Injuries of the orbit with objects which are not pointed and sharp commonly cause sudden displacement and rotation of the eye ball in the opposite direction. This may result in damage to optic nerve at its attachment to sclera because at the other end the nerve is firmly held at the optic foramen and optic canal by the attachment of the dural covering to the periosteum. The optic nerve fibres may get partially detached from the sclera or the optic nerve head may get avulsed.

The clinical picture will depend on whether there is tearing of the nerve fibres or *total avulsion of the nerve*. In the former the fundus picture is normal at first examination but develops optic atrophy in due course. When there is a complete avulsion of the optic nerve, there are haemorrhages round the disc, the arteries are thready and the optic disc area looks grey and empty.

E. Proptosis caused by orbital injuries is due to orbital haematoma. Most of the blood vessels are within the muscle cone of the orbit and the resulting proptosis is therefore axial. The haemorrhage may however be more extensive and may extend to the sub-conjunctival space and under the skin of the lids. The attachment of septum orbitale to orbital margin does not permit extension beyond the level of the orbital margin.

F. Prolapse of eye ball is another consequence of an orbital injury. As soon as the eye ball is displaced forward, the grip of sphincteric action of the orbicularis oculi prevents the return of the eye ball to its original position. It is surprising that there may be no visual loss even if the eye has remained in an abnormal position for hours because of the scope of the length of the optic nerve and the elasticity of extraocular muscles.

G. Emphysema of orbit is due to fracture of ethmoidal or frontal sinuses. This may extend forward under the skin of the lids. The crepitations felt by palpation, are typical.

H. Self-inflicted injuries by lunatics or criminals may vary from small local tissue injuries to gouging out eye balls with own fingers.

I. Injuries of the orbit may sometimes tear one or more of the extra-ocular muscles resulting in diplopia and the limitation of movements.

INJURIES OF EYE BALL

Prognostic as well as the treatment point of view, mechanical injuries to the eye ball should be described under two headings— non-perforating injuries and perforating injuries.

Non-perforating Injuries

i. **Cornea**
   a. Epithelial abrasions.
   b. Corneal oedema.
   c. Tears in Descement's membrane.
   d. Blood staining of the cornea due to hyphema.
   e. Pigmentary deposits on the cornea.
   f. Foreign bodies in the cornea.

ii. **Anterior Chamber**
   a. Hyphaema.
   b. Tears in Trabecular meshwork.
   c. Recession of angle of the anterior chamber.

iii. **Iris**
   a. Iridodialysis.
   b. Rupture of the sphincter.
   c. Traumatic mydriasis.
   d. Traumatic aniridia due to total irido-dialysis.

iv. **Ciliary Body**
   a. Ciliary spasm causing transient myopia.
   b. Tearing of longitudinal muscle fibres from scleral spur.

v. **Lens**
   a. Vossius pigment ring on anterior surface of the lens.
   b. Rupture of anterior or posterior capsule.
   c. Concussion cataract.
   d. Rossette lens opacity.
   e. Subluxation of the lens.
   f. Dislocation of the lens, anterior or posterior.

vi. **Vitreous**
   a. Vitreous haemorrhage.
   b. Vitreous detachment.

vii. **Choroid**
   a. Choroidal haemorrhage.
   b. Choroidal detachment.
   c. Choroidal rupture/tears.

viii. **Retina**
   a. Retinal haemorrhage.
   b. Retinal oedema.
   c. Retinal tears and dialysis.
   d. Traumatic retinal detachment.
   e. Macular oedema (Berlin's).
   f. Macular haemorrhage.
   g. Macular hole.

ix. **Optic disc**
   a. Tearing of the optic nerve fibres.
   b. Avulsion of the optic nerve.

x. **Sclera**
   a. Scleral rupture (Fig. 21.1).

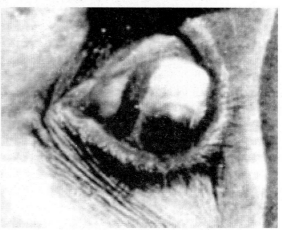

Fig 21.1: Contusion injury causing scleral rupture (iris lying under the conjunctiva)

xi. **Ocular Tension Changes**
   a. Instability of tension.
   b. Traumatic glaucoma.
   c. Traumatic hypotony.

Perforating Injuries of the Eye Ball

Perforating injuries of eye ball are by and large serious in nature. The seriousness depends on the site of perforation, tissues injured and the contents of the eye ball if expulsed. The site of perforation is either the cornea, the sclera or both. The tissues that can be expulsed are the iris, lens and the vitreous.

A. Perforating injuries of cornea:
   1. *Incised clean perforation* of the cornea with spontaneous closure of the wound and the restoration of the anterior chamber.

      This leaves behind a linear opacity in the cornea, which, if not in the central pupillary area, does not affect the vision.
   2. *Corneal perforation with iris prolapse* if untreated may result in a corneal scar with iris incarceration. Persistent hyphaema can result in blood staining of cornea (Fig. 21.2, Plate 14).
   3. *Laceration of the cornea with or without tissue loss* may result in any of the following:
      a. Ectatic scar.
      b. Cystoid cicatrix.
      c. Fistula.
      d. Total iris incarceration.
      e. Partial or total anterior staphyloma.
      f. Epithelial ingrowth causing epithelialisation of anterior chamber and secondary glaucoma.
      g. Extrusion of lens and vitreous.

B. Perforating injuries of sclera: The majority of scleral perforations are a continuity of corneal perforating wounds. Underlying ciliary body and choroid may show through the scleral wound though they do not usually prolapse out. However, these may be injured along with the sclera. The involvement of ciliary body and/or choroid is associated with intra-ocular haemorrhage. More extensive injuries may however expel all the contents leaving a collapsed eye ball.

It has been adequately emphasized that perforating injuries of the cornea and sclera should be promptly managed and repair undertaken at the earliest. Emergency penetrating keratoplasty will be a timely eye-saving procedure in the cases of lacerated corneal wounds. Even if a fresh donor eye is not available, a preserved cornea may be used as a stand-by to be replaced later by a fresh homologous graft. The scope and incidence of sympathetic ophthalmitis following perforating injuries is discussed in details in the chapter on Uvea.

C. Perforating injuries with retained intra-ocular foreign body: The gravity of perforating wounds of cornea and sclera is compounded if the injury is associated with retained intra-ocular foreign body. There is a large variety of foreign bodies which can penetrate and lodge inside the eye ball. Intra-ocular foreign bodies may be grouped as radio-opaque, and radio-luscent. Most of the metallic foreign bodies are radio-opaque while glass (except lead glass) and all non-metallic particles are radio-luscent.

The foreign bodies may be chemically active or inert. Glass, gold, porcelain, plastics and lead are chemically inert substances while iron, copper, silver are chemically active and if they are not removed in time, may cause siderosis and chalcosis resulting in permanent damage to vision.

Foreign bodies are also grouped as magnetic and non-magnetic. It is important to know that stainless steel is less magnetic than carbon steel.

Similarly, the magnetic character of many alloys will depend on the iron content.

Infection or sterility of the foreign body is another very important factor. Particles which fly at great speed from fire arms, from fast moving machines or a piece from a hammer, get sterilised due to heat produced in the beginning and during fast movement. Wood particles, are always infected.

Successful treatment of a retained intra-ocular foreign body demands its removal in most cases and at the earliest unless the removal is expected to cause more tissue damage than retention of the foreign body. The following steps are necessary in the treatment of retained intra-ocular foreign body.

1. *Confirmation of its presence* by radiography, foreign body locators or by ultra-sonography.
2. *Determining magnetic or non-magnetic character.* History is an important guiding factor. If a material identical to the foreign body is available, its magnetic character can be determined before removing the foreign body.
3. *Localising the foreign body.* This is an extremely important step. Removal of a correctly localised foreign body will cause less tissue damage and will avoid unnecessary fishing into the eye which can cause damage to tissues even if the foreign body is ultimately removed.

Radiography is the most dependable method for localisation. In case of a radio-luscent foreign bodies, however, localisation is less dependable. Herman's Foreign body locator (an electronic gadget) and ultrasonography can localise these foreign bodies. Among the many radiological investigations for detecting and localising an intra-ocular foreign body, one or more of the following are usually adequate:

i. A plain X-ray picture of the orbit, postero-anterior and lateral. This helps in identifying

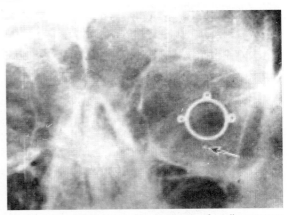

Fig. 21.3A: Radiological localistion of radio-opaque intra-ocular foreign body with a limbal ring. Antero posterior view. Foreign body outside the ringing

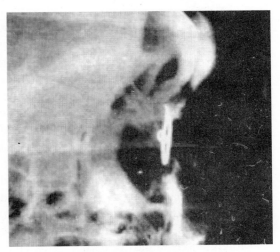

Fig. 21.3B: Side View showing the distance of foreign body from limbal ring

whether there is a radio-opaque foreign body.

ii. X-rays with a limbal ring. A 13 mm steel or silver wire ring is fixed with sutures just outside the limbus (Fig. 21.3A and B).

X-ray pictures of postero-anterior and lateral are taken with the patient looking straight ahead. These pictures indicate whether the foreign body is within the ring or outside the ring and the lateral picture shows how far behind the ring.

The postero-anterior and lateral picture are repeated with the eye looking up and then down with the face kept in unchanged position. If the foreign body shadow moves opposite to the movement of the ring, it is behind the centre of rotation and if it moves in the same direction, it is in front of the centre of rotation of the eye ball. The larger the displacement of foreign body, farther away it is from the centre of rotation. If the foreign body is outside the ring in the postero-anterior view, and there is no movement on movement of the eye ball, the foreign body is lying in the orbit outside the eye ball.

A more accurate measurement is further possible with the above procedure. A vertical line is drawn on the postero-anterior X-ray plate through the centre of the ring and the distance between this line and the foreign body is measured. Similarly, another line is drawn on the lateral picture from the centre of the shadow of the ring at right angles posteriorly. The distance between this line and the foreign body is measured.

These measurements can be transposed on a schematic eye on a graph paper and interpretations are made for localisation. This gives a better localisation of the foreign body in the eye ball.

iii. *Bone free radiography.* Although the above procedures are satisfactory in most cases, a foreign body may be obscured by dense bone shadow. Bone free pictures are taken by placing a dental film in the medial and the lower fornices with X-ray tube on the opposite side.

A magnet should not be used for diagnostic purposes because a free lying foreign body may be pulled towards the magnet causing damage to intervening tissues as well as displacement of the foreign body to probably a more difficult situation.

If ocular media are transparent, a detailed examination of fundus under full mydriasis may show the exact location of the foreign body. It will also reveal whether there are retinal haemorrhages or the foreign body is becoming encapsulated by fibrosis due to the inflammatory reaction.

iv. *Removal of a foreign body.* It should be a carefully planned surgery based on observations from the investigative procedures. It should be kept in mind that the removal procedure should cause the least damage to intraocular structures. Foreign bodies in the outer coat of the eye ball or those which are encapsulated are better not removed.

The procedure of removal of foreign body will depend on its location. The foreign bodies in the anterior chamber, iris and the lens are best removed through a limbal approach. For a foreign body in the posterior segment of the eye ball, the safest approach is through pars plana. A magnetic foreign body is best removed with a magnet through an incision in the sclera and the underlying choroid. Newer intra-vitreal illumination and instruments are available with which a non-magnetic foreign body can be removed under direct vision.

The complications caused by an intraocular foreign body.

1. *Intraocular haemorrhage.* This may be mild or severe. It may get absorbed or may leave behind organised bands or membranes which prevent restoration of sight, even if the foreign body is removed. Haemorrhage may cause *secondary glaucoma* and blood *staining of cornea.*

2. *Infection.* It is common with wood splinters, infected stone etc. When infection has advanced to stage of pan-ophthalmitis, removal of foreign body becomes a less important consideration.

3. *Sympathetic ophthalmitis.* It is a serious complication but luckily the incidence is far less than mentioned in the earlier

literature. It is true that from this point of view, a perforating injury with retained intraocular foreign body is worse than perforating injury alone.

CHEMICAL INJURIES

Chemical injuries are becoming more frequent due to the developments in chemical industry. Laboratory and domestic accidents are additional causes of chemical injuries. Homicidal use of acids to disfigure rather than kill a person is not uncommon. Careless use of drugs is not an infrequent cause of chemical injuries though not usually serious in nature. Chemical warfare also acquires importance in times of war.

There is a variety of chemical irritants, some causing only local symptoms while others leading to grievous damage to vision. By and large, the organic chemicals are less damaging than inorganic ones. Similarly, liquids cause more damage than gases.

Of the chemical agents, the two most important groups are the alkalies and the acids. The alkalies cause damage by fixing in the tissues while the acids destroy tissues. It is understandable that the body tissues being alkaline in nature, further rise in pH value by alkali burns will cause more damage and lasting effect. In addition the damage will depend on the liberation of H ions in case of acids and OH ions in case of alkalies that can combine with tissue proteins. The duration of the contact of chemical agents with the tissues is the most important factor (Fig. 21.4, Plate 14)

Vascular reaction is the most serious and damaging factor so far as the eyes are concerned and with particular reference to damage to the cornea. The vascularisation can be so malignant that it responds to no therapy, local or surgical. Worse still is the deep vascularisation which is most difficult to treat.

Preventive measures are the first essential requirement to reduce accidents. The treatment should be immediate and consists of neutralising the chemical removing as much of it as possible and preventing damaging effects of injury as far as possible.

Surgery needed includes plastic surgery of lids and keratoplasty of cornea. While plastic surgery can be undertaken soonest possible to prevent damage to cornea, the timing of corneal grafting is a debatable question. It should either be done as an urgent surgery before neovascularisation has set in or if this is not feasible, it should better be done after reducing vascularisation to the minimum possible.

Amniotic membrane transplant has proved useful to restore ocular surface. It decreases inflammation, scarring and neovascularisation. The membrane transplant performed soonest possible goes a long way to prevent stromal melting and reduces sequelae of chemical burn. It also helps revival and growth of surviving *stem cells*. Processed and preserved amniotic membrane tissue is available.

Conjunctival-limbal autograft either ipsilateral from unaffected site of same eye or contralateral from other eye can also be done. The graft lenticules comprising of limbal cornea-conjunctiva are secured at recipient sites with the epithelial side up and limbal edge at limbus of recipient.

In case an autograft lenticule is not possible to harvest as in bilateral extensively involved cases, homograft from close relative or cadaver kerato-limbal graft can be used. Immuno-suppressants have to be used. Live tissue from close relative is preferable to cadaver tissue.

Amniotic membrane/kerato-conjunctival stem cell graft procedures are satisfactorily practised in chemical burns, recurrent pterygium Steven-Johnson's syndrome, advanced Dry eye conditions and pemphigus.

THERMAL INJURIES

Thermal injuries are largely accidental in nature. Most of them are domestic accidents or suicidal and homicidal but industrial accidents are not uncommon.

The two groups of thermal injuries are fire burns and scalds due to hot liquids including molten metal. Thermal injuries can also be caused by electric burns and by freezing.

Fire burns: Damage to ocular structures is usually part of the general body injury. It may cause blisters on the lids, charring of the eye lashes and the eyebrows. Burnt material may enter the conjunctival sac but the eye ball usually remains protected by the lids and suffers relatively less damage.

Scalds: Domestic liquids like water, milk are common but less damaging agents to eyes because the lid is an effective protection. A very hot liquid in the conjunctival sac may cause conjunctival chemosis, necrosis and oedema of the cornea.

Molten metal burns are usually industrial accidents and can cause serious tissue damage because of very high temperature. A part or the whole of the lid may be disintegrated and the eye ball may be exposed.

Electrical burns: Electrical burns may be domestic or due to the lightning. In either case, the tissue damage is at the point of entry of current and the seriousness depends on the degree of voltage that passes through the body between the point of contact and the point of earthing. The burns of face may involve lids and rarely cornea. In lightning however, the temperature is so high that the tissues may be severely burnt. The high intensity of light exposure in lightning may however cause transient or permanent loss of vision due to macular burn if the person survives the accident.

Delayed effect may be cataractous changes due to the disturbance caused during the passage of current through the body.

RADIATIONAL INJURIES

By radiation is meant the passage of energy, visible or invisible from the source into the space. Sunlight can be a source of a wide range of radiational energy both in the range of visible spectrum as well as beyond the red and violet ends of the visible spectrum. A similar energy can also be produced by electro-magnetic units or by harnessing the energy of the atom. Radiational injuries can, therefore, be caused by:

1. Visible spectrum rays.
2. Ultraviolet rays.
3. Infra-red rays.
4. X-rays.
5. B-radiation.
6. Xenon light rays.
7. Argon laser rays.
8. Atomic radiation.

The biological effect of radiational energy on the tissues may be thermal (heat), abiotic (chemical) and ionising (biological).

Visible spectrum of sunlight. The visible spectrum extends from 3900 au wave length at the violet end to 7700 au wave length at the red end. Between these two ends the white light can be broken into a spectrum of colours mentioned in short as VIBGYOR (violet, indigo, blue, green, yellow, orange and red).

Beyond the visible spectrum on the violet end are the short wave rays, which include ultra-violet rays, X-rays and the cosmic rays. Beyond the red end of the spectrum are the long wave rays which include the infra-red rays, the radars and the television and diathermy.

It is important to know that the short wave rays, the ultra-violet rays, which are chemical rays, have more penetration power than the long wave rays, the infra-red rays are the heat rays.

By and large the cornea absorbs the infra-red rays and the lens absorbs the ultra-violet rays though not to the entire extent. Only a small part reaches the retina and therefore does not cause any tissue damage. Another important point is that the tissue reaction following exposure to infra red rays is quick while it is delayed following the exposure to ultra-violet rays.

There are two clinical conditions which are caused by sun light. They are a sunburnt macula or eclipse blindness and snow blindness. Other radiational injuries are caused by arc lights, furnace heat, xenon and laser rays, B radiation, X-rays and atomic radiation.

Eclipse blindness: This is due to looking directly at the sun during a solar eclipse for some length of time without any protection for the eyes. Normally, one is able to look at the bright sun only momentarily and photophobia protects the eye from damage. During a solar eclipse, however, one can look at the sun for a longer time and hence the damage to macula by concentrated infra-red rays.

Eclipse blindness is usually bilateral but may sometimes be unilateral. The symptoms include *photopsae* (flashes of light), *chromatopsia* (seeing coloured lights) and later *on a central scotoma*. Fundus changes include oedema of the the macula with micro haemorrhages. The condition tends to resolve but may take from few weeks to few months, but partial visual loss persists.

Prophylaxis by educative warnings is important. If an eclipse has to be seen, it should be seen through a heavily smoked glass. Ordinary sun glasses are not an adequate protection. It is better to see it indirectly where an image of the sun is seen on a screen.

Once the damage has been done, the treatment is unsatisfactory. Oral steroids and Vitamin C may be helpful in the early stages.

Snow blindness: It is due to damage by bright light reflected from snow at high altitudes in clear weather where the ultraviolet content of the sunlight is very high. It is, therefore, the ultraviolet high content of the bright light that causes damage to the outer eye. The immediate symptoms are *photophobia, foreign body sensation, lacrimation* and *blepharospasm.* This is followed by *conjunctival congestion and chemosis.* The corneal epithelium may become oedematous and may faintly stain with fluorescein. Most of these manifestations usually resolve in 48 hours. Protective glasses are important when one is likely to be exposed to environments which can cause snow blindness.

Arc lights: Welding arcs whether electrical or acetylene may have damaging effect on the eye when looked at from a near distance. The harmful effect is due to the heavy concentration of ultraviolet light. The transient symptoms are photophobia, lacrimation, diminution of vision and a temporary scotoma. There may be transient corneal oedema.

It is important that protective shields are used by workers and passers by should not look at the welding arc directly. Treatment is purely palliative and the symptoms do not last long.

The heat from the industrial units like steel and glass furnaces produce a typical radiational cataract which is a posterior cortical disc like, saucer-shaped opacity under the posterior capsule.

The heat rays passing to the retina are absorbed by the pigment layer and may cause macular burn.

Xenon light: This is the source of heat energy used for photocagulation of retina. The light is absorbed only by pigmented tissues. It, therefore, passes through the cornea, lens and vitreous without any tissue effects but it can cause burns of iris, ciliary body and the choroid. Xenon light is therefore used to cause aseptic choroidal inflammation and help retina get attached to the under-lying layers.

Laser: The word means 'Light Amplification by Stimulated Emission of Radiation (LASER).

The sources of LASER rays are Argon gas, Krypton gas, Diode crystal, Nd: Yag crystals. Except Nd: Yag, the rest of laser systems cause photocoagulation. Nd: Yag causes photo disruption.

Excimer laser system of helium and fluorine gas is used for photo-ablation.

Laser photocoagulation is used in retinal/vitreal neovascularisation and membranes, glaucoma iridotomy. Laser disruptions needed for posterior capsular thickening, pupillary membranectomy and recently laser phaco-surgery for cataract. Photo ablation by excimer laser is used in refractive corneal surgery.

X-rays *(Roentgen rays):* X-rays are electro-magnetic radiations analogous to gamma rays with great penetrating power through solid tissues and capable of causing destructive changes in living tissues. The tissue damage becomes clinically manifest some time after irradiation. The commonest ocular lesion is the post radia-tional cataract which is posterior subcapsular or posterior cortical. Another serious complication of X radiation is post-radiational malignant change. Most of the damaging effects are a result of therapeutic irradiation for malignant tumours. It is, therefore, important that protection with lead shields is always provided wherever the functioning eye is to be protected from harmful side effect of radiation therapy.

Other systemic side effects are burns of skin and damage to haemopoetic system causing aplastic anaemia and leukaemia.

Beta radiation: These are weaker rays than X-rays and have therefore less tissue penetration. The source of beta rays can be radium, radon seeds and Strontium 90. It is Strontium 90 source that is used for therapeutic purpose in ophthalmology. Beta radiation has a penetrating power of 2–3 mm only. The safest dose for ocular tissues is 1500 r at one place at one time and repeated not more than two to three times at two to three weeks interval. The total dose at one place should not exceed 4500 r. The most harmful though rare effet on the eye is radiational cataract.

The principal therapeutic indication of Beta radiation is to treat neovascularisation. It is important to emphasize that Beta radiation is most effective on newly forming blood vessels because of its inhibitory effect on endothelial mitosis. It has some effect on fine blood vessels but no effect on larger blood vessels.

Atomic radiation: The effect of atomic explo-sion is due to liberation of extremely high physical and radiational energy. The immediate conse-quence is due to *mechanical injury by blast, thermal injury due to heat* and *chemical injury due to ultraviolet light.* The long term ionising effect has been reported for years after explosion affecting the haemopoetic system (Fig. 21.5, Plate 14).

Ultimate Prognosis of Ocular Injuries

From the prognostic point of view, ocular injury may be from the mildest to a complete disor-ganisation of the eye ball. Prognostic evaluation is more important in injuries which can cause serious damage to vision. Such injuries may fall in any of the groups described, the concussion injuries, perforating injuries and injuries with retained foreign body. It is a very difficult exercise indeed to project ultimate outcome to any degree of dependability. The prognosis should, therefore, always remain guarded. Even when immediate prognosis may appear favourable, subsequent events of organisation and their effect on ocular tissues, like retinal detachment, may convert the earlier favourable prognosis to a bad prognosis. The prognosis may be more dependable after injury has been repaired, foreign body, if any has been removed and ocular reaction has subsided.

To summarise ocular injuries may leave behind the following after effects:

1. Scars in lids.
2. Entropion, Ectropion and trichiasis.
3. Conjunctival symblepharon.
4. Corneal opacities.
5. Leucoma adherens.
6. Partial or total anterior staphyloma.
7. Iridodialysis.
8. Irreversible mydriasis.
9. Unround pupil.
10. Traumatic glaucoma.
11. Lens opacities of varying shapes and sizes.
12. Subluxated or dislocated lens.
13. Vitreous retraction.
14. Retinal detachment.
15. Choroidal tears.
16. Optic atrophy.
17. Ocular palsies.
18. Enophthalmos.

Head Injuries—Effect on the Eye

It is not uncommon that an ophthalmologist is called to see a case of head injury; either conscious or unconscious, to guide a neurophysician or a neurosurgeon in his approach to therapy. There are generally speaking three groups of head injuries:

1. Concussion causing fracture of the vault or the base of the skull.
2. Cerebral compression due to oedema and haemorrhage.
3. Lacerations of the brain.

Clinical Features

Pupil: In unconscious patients, pupillary size and reaction are of utmost importance. In severe injuries, the pupil is initially small but soon dilates commonly on the side of the injury first. Pupillary dilatation on the other side also indicates a rise in intracranial pressure and this is a positive indication for decompression operation. Pontine haemorrhage is characterized by pin point pupils and ocular palsies.

The condition of pupil should be reviewed from time to time and therefore no mydriatic drops should be used for examination of the fundus in an unconscious patient.

Eye movements: In unconsciousness, the eyes are sometimes divergent. There may be irregular movements of eyes. These usually disappear when the patient regains consciousness. A gross damage to oculomotor nuclei or nerves results in permanent ocular palsies, the clinical change depending on whether the damage is supra-nuclear, nuclear or peripheral part of the nerve.

Proptosis: This is usually due to an orbital haemorrhage which often extends to the subconjunctival space and under the skin of lids. Carotid cavernous fistula following head injury can cause pulsating proptosis.

Loss of vision: This is often discovered after the patient regains consciousness. This may be due to contra-coup fracture involving optic nerve and chiasma, optic tracts, internal capsule, temporal lobe or occipital cortex. Cortical lesions may leave behind visual agnosia of different types. Visual field changes may vary from haemianopic defects due to chiasmal and tract lesions, quadrantic defects due to temporal lobe lesions and cortical blindness due to occipital lobe lesions.

Retinal changes: Large superficial exudates in retina may be caused by an extension of cerebral oedema or may be due to sudden raised intracranial pressure. There may be retinal haemorrhage due to back pressure in the veins. A sub-arachnoid haemorrhage may be associated with papilloedema and severe haemorrhage all round the disc.

22

Prognostic Evaluation

In ophthalmology as in all the other disciplines of medicine, the prognostic forecasting is more often forced by the patient than clinician himself volunteering prognosis of a particular disease or a surgical procedure. Most of the times, the clinician waits for the patient to ask the prognosis. In developing countries where medical practitioner still carries good faith and confidence of the patient, a casual remark that everything would be alright, brings on a smile on the face of the patient. In developed countries, however, the prognosis has to be a precisely calculated exercise and there is more emphasis on the pessimistic expression because one wants to make sure that the patient understands the worst that can happen. Furthermore the prognostic evaluation helps in pre-planning appropriate treatment or decide a specific surgical procedure. From all these points, assessing prognosis is an essential part of clinical examination and is often guided by experience, the status in the profession and knowledge of newer therapies and surgical procedures.

The prognosis in this era, where patients are becoming more legal minded should be expressed in very careful terms and should preferably be recorded on the case paper and explained to the patient with an addition that all diseases are not curable even though every effort will be made to achieve a good result. In the case of operative procedures, while indicating a favourable prognosis, warning of unexpected mishaps during and after operation, should always be indicated and preferably recorded on the case sheet and the patient should be asked to sign it after reading it or after it is read to him.

The prognosis in ophthalmology has to be from various different points of view:
1. *Visual prognosis* to assess whether the vision will improve, remain as before or may become worse.
2. *Prognosis for the integrity of the eye ball.* Whether the shape of the eye ball and its cosmetic appearance will be retained or not.
3. *Prognosis to life.* In conditions which can be a danger to life.
4. *Prognosis of individual* conditions.

VISUAL PROGNOSIS

It is only natural that every ophthalmic patient's first concern is restoration or improvement of vision. It is only rarely and in very painful conditions that the patient may emphasize on relief of symptoms irrespective of whether there is any gain in vision or not. Some may request for cosmetic improvement even if no visual improvement is expected. Even in these cases of unfavourable visual prognosis, however emphatically explained, the patient forgets it and expresses disappointment that even though relieved or cosmetically improved, his vision has not improved. It is therefore, extremely important that the visual prognosis should be indicated after careful evaluation and that too, the optimism should be rather guarded to keep a scope of margin for unexpected behaviour of the disease or unexpected operative or post-operative complications.

Visual prognosis may be immediate or distant and in either case, there are three possibilities as a result of the response of the disease to therapy or surgery. Vision may improve, it may remain as before or it may become worse.

Another important criterion is the residual vision if any, at the start of therapy or before operation. This will provide a comparison to the final visual acuity at the end of therapy or after surgery.

It is generally agreed that for a favourable prognosis, good retinal function and intact visual pathways are essential and this is best indicated by presence of perception and correct projection of light. Perception of light alone is not enough. The patient must be able to indicate the direction from which the light is projected on the eye. This means that perfect projection of light must be present from all directions. In a patient with good projection, the eye readily turns towards the direction from which the light is coming even before the clinician asks for the answer. This spontaneous turning of the eye is also a good indication of retinal function in small children where a question cannot be asked and an answer can not be expected. From prognostic point of view, projection is recorded as PR 1+, PR 2+, PR 3+, PR 4+ depending on from how many of the four directions the patient is able to give a correct answer. It is also important that when testing projection of the light, one should specifically record the quadrant in which it is present or absent. Dependability of this test varies from individual to individual.

It is not uncommon to come across a patient with bilateral mature cataract who refuses to indicate presence of projection of the light under the impression that he or she would be accepted for treatment only if total blindness is feigned. People with very low IQ or poor intelligence may sometimes behave similarly. In all such cases, the objective findings like pupillary reaction and ERG wherever possible, will be dependable guides.

Even though PR 4+ is the minimum requirement for indicating favourable prognosis, patients with PR 3+ and even PR 2+ may regain some vision though rarely, with treatment or surgery. This can happen in eyes with localised retinal damage due to some old pathology while remaining retina is in perfect functional order. One should, therefore, not be in a hurry to reject cases with PR 3+ but one should be dogmatic in firmly expressing that the *prognosis is uncertain*. This is of more practical importance in cases who are totally blind in one eye and the other eye has PR 3+ or PR 2+.

When there is some degree of residual vision, which may be counting of fingers to 6/60 or near about, the prognostic evaluation becomes all the more important because here diminution or loss of vision the patient already had, becomes a serious matter, both for the patient as well as for the clinician. One should avoid committing oneself, but the patient will need at least this much assurance that the existing vision will not be diminished by therapy or operation. The prognosis will depend on whether the condition is amenable to specific therapy and whether surgery, by general standards, is a safe surgery like cataract operation. When expressing prognosis, one should be mindful of unexpected total loss of vision as in the cases advanced glaucoma for surgery in the eyes with small tubular fields. Similarly, one should not be surprised when an eye which is given up as lost, may regain vision over a period of time.

INTEGRITY OF THE EYE BALL

Next to vision, the eyeball has the highest significance of being a very important factor in cosmetic appearance. Unless forced to, no patient would like to sacrifice his eye even if it is blind. Similarly, a patient would expect that even if vision cannot be restored, the shape and form of eye ball should be retained. There are however situations like an intra-ocular malignancy, when it is to save the life of patient rather than try to retain the eye ball is important and if that be the situation advice to the patient for enucleation should be based on very sound clinical judgement. Such an advice should be expressed in a language of persuasion explaining the seriousness if the advice given is not followed. The most stable indication of enucleation is the intraocular malignancy, the common ones being retinoblastoma or a malignant melanotic sarcoma. It is in these conditions that even an eye with some residual vision may have to be advised enucleation, a most difficult situation to convince the patient. One should not hesitate to get one's opinion and advice further supported by another ophthalmologist so that the hesitation of the patient can be overcome. Still more difficult situation arises when one eye has been enucleated and the only remaining eye also develops a retinoblastoma. Choice is, whether to make the child totally blind in both eyes by enucleation of the second eye and that too with a lingering uncertainty that metastasis may have already occurred before enucleation The general consensus, however, is that the malignancy in

the second eye should be treated by radiation or chemotherapeutic drugs, hoping for a remote chance of arresting the pathology and save the child from a life of iatrogenic total blindness.

The next condition where enucleation has for long been considered obligatory, is the removal of diseased eye which is likely to cause sympathetic ophthalmitis in the other normal eye. Enucleation of the exciting used to be advised before the onset of the sympathetic ophthalmitis in the opposite eye because of the fear that the patient may lose vision in both the eyes. Ocular therapeutics have so advanced that luckily sympathetic ophthalmitis has become much less common. Therapy now available, helps controlling inflammation of the exciting eye. Surgery is now possible that repair of an injured eye can restore anatomical integrity with much less fear of sympathetic ophthalmitis. Furthermore, steroids have made it possible to treat sympathising eye even after the onset of sympathetic ophthalmias.

The removal of an eye for fear of sympathetic ophthalmitis is, therefore, a rare indication. Condition, where it is positively indicated, is an injured eye with grevious tissue destruction and not even the remotest chance of restoration of any vision. These eyes end in phthisical atrophic condition with no vision and gross cosmetic defect.

Painful blind eye is another condition for which enucleation is advised without enough justification in every case. Not all blind eyes need be removed and not all painful eyes are resistant to pain relieving therapy. Enucleation is often indicated in blind phthisical or atrophic eyes for fear of malignant melanoma or sarcoma in these eyes. This may be true in white races where incidence of melanoma is much higher than in darker races. Such a fear is rather misplaced in tropical countries. It is important to bear in mind that an eye ball with normal anatomical attachment of extraocular muscles, is an ideal support for fitting a cosmetic prosthesis.

However, the eyes with severe ciliary congestion, marked tenderness and low tension which do not respond to therapy, are better enucleated.

Cosmetic enucleation is justifiable in certain conditions. A total anterior staphyloma or eyes with multiple ciliary and/or equatorial staphylomata, are the eyes which are cosmetically ugly looking and are incurably blind. Instead of doing a staphylectomy, it is better to remove the eye followed by an implant in the muscle cone. A better surgical procedure is to excise the anterior staphyloma, eviscerate all the contents of the scleral shell and place a spherical implant within the sclera followed by the closure of the scleral opening. This will provide an ideal cosmetic improvement permitting full movement of the artificial eye on the mobile scleral stump.

Evisceration has been indicated for panophthalmitis. In the pre-antibiotic era, an enucleation was contraindicated in panophthalmitis for fear of infection extending through the meningeal cut ends of optic nerve into the intracranial cavity.

PROGNOSIS OF CLINICAL CONDITIONS

Every clinical condition has to be prognostically assessed. It is important to know whether the disease process is likely to respond to treatment or whether it is a progressive condition and will end in failure of therapy. The patient's defensive system, local tissue response and the patient's cooperation in taking the treatment are such variable factors that uniform prognosis of each condition in each individual, is not an easy matter. One is largely guided by one's experience and experience of others. One should, therefore, make a cautious approach in volunteering a definitive prognosis not withstanding that some degree of optimistic assurance is always expected from the clinician.

In surgical procedures, however, prognosis can be relatively more definitive although a good surgical procedure may be adversely affected by an unexpected post-operative complication or misbehaviour of the patient. Even in these situations, a margin of safety should be kept and prognosis should be prefaced with "If all goes well".

The prognosis of individual conditions or operative procedures has been briefly indicated in their respective places. More detailed comments are, however, called for, for some conditions which an ophthalmologist has to commonly deal with. Some of these are discussed below.

Cataract

An ophthalmologist is faced with prognostic consideration from the moment the cataract as a diagnostic possibility is considered till not only the cataract is removed and successfully but long after that, because every subsequent event in the operated eye is attributed to surgery.

Complicated cataracts, pathological cataracts, subluxated or dislocated cataracts are a group which distinctly carry less satisfactory prognosis mainly because of the causative pathology which may prevent recovery of good vision.

Pre-operative prognostic evaluation in an eye with cataract has been discussed in detail in the Chapter on cataract. All those considerations should be constantly borne in mind and every effort should be made to keep good prognosis undiluted and giving 90% or more patients good visual recovery and symptom-free post-operative period.

Glaucoma

The assessment of prognosis in glaucomatous eyes is a difficult and uncertain proposition. The prognosis is further made more difficult in developing countries where glaucoma is often diagnosed when it has already reached an advanced stage.

Poor response from patient is also an important factor in missing the diagnosis of early glaucoma. Most patients stay at home under the mistaken impression that cataract is the main cause of defective vision in old age and they could wait till all vision is lost and cataract is mature. Even ophthalmologists often give a hurried diagnosis of the cataract without making a positive effort to exclude the early glaucoma.

Fate of glaucomatous eye in best of the circumstances has some uncertainty. It is not uncommon that therapy or operation may control intraocular tension and yet the eye may slowly end in blindness. This particularly is so when therapy is started or surgery is undertaken when the disease has already established its foothold.

The prognosis of glaucoma will, therefore, depend on the state at which it is diagnosed and the type of the glaucoma. It will also depend on cooperation of the patient for being regular in therapy and return for periodical checkup to evaluate the response of the disease to therapy.

Prognosis in angle closure glaucoma is favourable and more dependable to give, provided it is diagnosed before peripheral anterior synechiae are formed. Surgery, prophylactic or therapeutic which is more often required, usually restores the balance of intraocular tension and the eye retains normal tension and good vision. In eyes with extensive peripheral synechiae, however, the prognosis is unfavourable because although the recurrent attacks of congestive glaucoma may have been prevented by surgery, the condition may quietly progress to a chronic congestive stage and make the prognosis bad. In open angle glaucoma, the prognosis is relatively uncertain because there are cases on record where tension may become normal and yet progressive optic atrophy occurs inspite of adequate and regular therapy. The prognosis is more dependable in cases of early diagnosis and early therapy while it is more uncertain and unfavourable when treatment is started after glaucomatous cupping has already well developed and field changes have reached an advanced stage. The prognosis should be extremely guarded in a glaucomatous eye with gross peripheral field loss even though visual acuity may be moderate to good. These eyes can lose the remaining field and suddenly become blind following otherwise a good glaucoma surgery.

Prognosis can become very unfavourable if surgery is done on an eye with high intraocular tension overlooking the fundamental requirement that any glaucoma surgery should be done only when intraocular tension has been stablised to within normal limits even though temporarily.

Prognosis in glaucoma should therefore be always guarded and in established cases, uncertain. The best, one can indicate is to express the hope that the preoperative visual status of the eye MAY be retained. Patient should also know that in spite of the treatment, the end result may, in some cases be total loss of vision. The patient should religiously be regular in following local therapy whenever advised. He should be warned of danger of neglecting the follow-up examination.

Prognosis of glaucoma, therefore, depends on:

1. Type of glaucoma.
2. Stage at which therapy started or surgery undertaken.
3. The residual vision.
4. State of field of vision.
5. Response of therapy.
6. Patient's co-operation.

Squint

With better understanding of the physiology of the extra-ocular muscles and their coordination and more dependable investigative procedures available, the prognosis of squint can be more clearly expressed than in any other ocular condition. The prognosis has changed from a cosmetic prognosis to a functional prognosis. This has been made easier in communities who bring their children for investigation and treatment in the pre-school going age. More and more children are now brought not only for straightening the eyes but also for restoring full visual acuity so that the child in later age does not suffer from any social or economic handicap.

Concomitant squint: Prognosis of concomittant squint depends on many variables.

1. The age of the child at which the patient is brought.
2. Age of the onset of squint.
3. Degree of squint.
4. Whether the squint is constant or intermittent.
5. Whether it is influenced by the use of glasses.
6. Refractive state of the eye.
7. State of binocularity.
8. Whether retinal correspondence is normal or abnormal.
9. Pre-operative evaluation.
10. Changes in muscles, like contractures.
11. Readiness to alter plans after examining the muscle on operation table.

Most of these points are covered in the Chapter on Squint. It is, however, important to emphasize that howsoever good the pre-operative evaluation may be, there is always a chance however remote, of overcorrecting or under-correcting squint in some cases. It is a general rule that a divergent squint should be slightly over-corrected as these patients have poor convergence and patient's own efforts may not be able to retain perfect alignment, if not over corrected. For the same reason, an internal squint should preferably be under corrected.

It is important that in uniocular squint of 30° or more, full correction should not be expected even after the maximum recession or resection of both the horizontal muscles of the squinting eye and the patient should be clearly explained in advance that he may have to undergo surgery in non-squinting eye also at a later date.

It is also important from prognostic point of view that whenever the two eyes are operated, one muscle in each, the correction should be equally and evenly distributed in both the eyes as in alternating squint to prevent postoperative diplopia and to sustain balanced covergence.

It is important that a grossly amblyopic eye has a tendency to revert to original condition. Prognosis, in these eyes can be improved if amblyopia is preoperatively overcome by glasses, occlusion and exercises before surgery is undertaken. The amblyopic eye is always slightly overcorrected.

The prognosis in eyes with squint from birth is, however, less satisfactory because in these cases, macular area has not differentiated and macular function has not developed.

Prognosis of a paralytic squint is, however differently evaluated. The nerve supply of paralysed muscle has a tendency to regenerate in lower motor neuron lesions. One should, therefore reserve prognostic declaration and wait till there is no further scope for regeneration of nerves. This period may be from 9 months to one year. The prognosis in these eyes, therefore, depends on amount of residual power in the muscle and the degree of organic changes like contractures which commonly develop in ipsilateral antagonist. For the same reason, the surgery also carries a relatively uncertain prognosis. The prognosis is made worse when more than one muscle is involved as in the cases of external ophthalmoplegia due to third nerve palsy which is the nerve supply for the two vertical recti and one oblique in addition to the medial rectus.

Corneal Diseases

The prognostic evaluation of corneal pathology is mainly from two points of view, visual recovery and cosmetic improvement.

Corneal opacity in central part in front of the pupil obstructs the passage of light into the eye. Thinner corneal opacity causes visual loss not only because of the opacity, but because it causes irregular corneal astigmatism. It is not unusual to find that an eye with a paracentral dense, well defined corneal opacity may have fairly good vision while a thinner opacity may lead to gross visual defect.

One should be very careful in prejudging the prognosis of corneal ulcer particularly from the point of view of residual corneal opacity it may leave. The depth of the opacity and the extent of stromal involvement will influence prognosis. Perforation of the ulcer, however small, will always leave a through and through opacity.

It is a generally accepted criterion that younger the patient and more recent the pathology, more are the chances of its resorption. Older the patient and longer the duration of corneal pathology less are the chances of spontaneous resolution.

It may be emphasized that when corneal haze is due to oedema, the resolution is more complete, while if suppuration has taken place and healed with fibrosis, the opacity will be of a permanent nature.

It is also important that one should be able to clinically evaluate the thickness of the unaffected deeper layers of cornea to determine whether cornea is going to become ectatic. Perforated corneal ulcer with iris incarceration is likely to cause raised intra-ocular tension and lead to ectasia of corneal scar. In any case, a scarred cornea with disorganised pattern of corneal anatomy is weaker and may become ectatic even under normal intra-ocular pressure while a normal cornea with intact corneal architecture can withstand raised ocular pressure.

The prognosis of a corneal ulcer with perforation is made worse by forward movement of the iris-lens diaphragm which may cause anterior polar cataract and an irreversible secondary rise of intra-ocular tension. A sudden and large perforation may be disastrous for the eye because the lens may extrude and vitreous may get adherent to the corneal scar.

The prognosis of chemical burns of cornea is the most difficult to evaluate.

It depends on concentration of the chemical, the chemistry of the substance, the amount of tissue damage and the interval between the burn and institution of proper therapy. Intense vascularisation is a characteristic feature of the alkali burns and prognosis is made worse by simultaneous damage to surrounding conjunctiva and the chemical linkage between the alkaline tissues and the alkaline chemical. A peculiar feature of alkali burns is the recurrent nature of tissue break-down from time to time due to heavy concentration of collagenase in pathological epithelium.

Acid burns are more destructive. Strong acids can disintegrate the protective tissues in a matter of hours. Prognosis which is by and large, unfavourable will depend on whether the lid coverage remains undisturbed.

Among the *corneal dystrophies*, the most important from prognostic point of view is Fuchs' endothelial dystrophy with corneal oedema and bullous keratopathy. Being a slow process, developing over many years, the prognosis of corneal graft in these cases is by and large not bad. Associated rise of intra-ocular tension and secondary cataract however make the prognosis less satisfactory.

Another common condition causing corneal oedema and bullous keratopathy is *vitreous touch syndrome* in eyes with complicated aphakia or pseudophakic eyes. The prognosis is uncertain because the causative factor, vitreous in anterior chamber, is not easy to undo. Vitrectomy can however help rehabilitate some of these eyes.

Prognosis of staphylomatous eyes is very poor not only because inner structures of the eye are disorganised but also because of persistently high intra-ocular tension damages functioning capacity of retina and optic nerve. It is interesting to note that a staphylomatous eye may sometimes retain the perception projection of light for a long time but this does not improve the prognosis because the eye is a glaucomatous eye and disc is atrophic.

Retinal Conditions

The retina is the most important relay station in the visual pathways and, therefore, the prognostic evaluation of retinal conditions is entirely from visual point of view.

The retina has special features which make its prognostic evaluation rather difficult. The neural elements of the retina and the nerve fibres are an extension of brain tissue and therefore do not regenerate after damage. Like the brain tissues, the retina cannot stand total anoxaemia for more than a few minutes. The important layers of retina depend for nutrition not from its own blood supply but from the chorio-capillaries. Diseases of choroid easily extend into retinal tissues. Retinal layers have poor binding quality, and therefore, undergo oedema rapidly. Another very important factor is the functioning leadership of macular area which is the most sensitive part of retina. Moreover, many retinal pathologies are due to one or other systemic cause and prognosis of retinal conditions will, therefore, depend on prognosis of systemic causative disease.

The prognosis of retinal conditions first depends on location of pathology. Central lesions of macular area are more damaging to vision, both immediately and later on. A gross lesion destroying macular area leaves behind a vision of only 6/36 or 6/60 provided by the peripheral part. On the other hand, even a large pathological lesion in peripheral retina is compatible with 6/9-6/6 vision.

A fundus picture in some diseases may provide a much more dependable guide line to the physician as in *hypertensive retinopathy, renal retinopathy and toxaemic retinopathy of pregnancy.* Papilloedema in malignant hyper tension is a bad sign for vision as well as life. Permanent attenuation of arteries is indicative of renal damage. Changes at arterio-venous crossings are indicative of what may be happening in brain and elsewhere in in the body. Even though these are dependable guides, the prognosis should always be based on systemic clinical features and bio-chemical changes in the blood. It is, generally true that patients with malignant hypertensive retinopathy may retain good vision for a long time and in most cases they die before they become blind. Prognosis in these cases should therefore be the responsibility of the physician in-charge of the case.

Diabetic retinopathy is another very important ocular condition which has serious damaging effect on the vision. Diabetic retinopathy an important and fairly common cause of blindness in diabetics.

Juvenile diabetes causes many more diabetic retinopathies than senile diabetes. The visual prognosis is, therefore, much poorer in juvenile diabetes. These patients can be warned of the distant possibility of blindness. Once the retinopathy has reached a proliferative stage, poor visual prognosis should be writ large on the case papers. The most difficult part in this disease is the relatively little effect of control of diabetes on visual prognosis. Patients who have had fully regimented treatment for diabetes, may still end up in total blindness, in due course. Laser therapy has saved many eyes from ultimate blindness if the therapy is undertaken before proliferative stage of diabetic retinopathy.

The diabetic retinopathy influences the prognosis to life when it is associated with hypertension and renal damage, not an uncommon combination. These patients are exposed to the dangers, both of blindness as well as danger to life. Another fundus change in diabetics which is indicative of serious prognosis is the lipaemic condition of retinal vessels, usually due to ketosis in blood and therefore of serious omen for diabetic coma.

The retinal detachment is a local condition and the prognostic evaluation depends on the type and degree of retinal detachment and the condition of the eye before the patient develops detachment.

Many *myopic patients* often ask as to what are the chances of their developing detachment. *Not all myopics develop retinal detachments and not all retinal detachments are in myopics.* The prognostic answer to this question will depend on the degree of myopia, the history of detachment in the family and the results of careful examination of peripheral retina. It is interesting that retinal detachment is more common in eyes with moderate degree of myopia. High myopic eyes with extensive chorio-retinal degeneration rarely develop retinal detachment.

Examination of peripheral fundus by indirect ophthalmoscopy provides a better guide to prognosis in a particular eye. Areas of lattice or cystic degeneration and presence of any holes or tears suggest possibility of a subsequent retinal detachment.

The condition of vitreous is another guide to evaluate the possibility or otherwise of retinal detachment in a myopic eye. Importance should be attached when vitreous opacities which have been noted for a long time, suddenly increase in number and become coarser in character. Whenever there is one large dark chunk of vitreous floater, one should examine the periphery with greater care for the presence of tear or any other source in the retina. Vitreous loss or vitreous disturbance in cataract operation is an important consideration in evaluating chances of retinal detachment, potential are the eyes where disturbed vitreous is not adequately and properly managed on the operation table. The eyes with vitreous adhesions to the section are the ones which have a greater chance of retinal detachment.

Even though there are many such contributory factors to the causation of retinal detachment, many eyes are potentially and inherently pro-detachment and even a small insignificant precipitating cause may initiate the process. It is therefore, not safe to make too dogmatic an opinion whether a particular eye is likely or not likely to develop a retinal detachment. The prognostic opinion should, therefore, be always guarded.

Once retinal detachment has taken place in an eye, the prognosis will depend on different factors. A primary rhegmatogenous detachment carries a better prognosis than secondary detachment. Longer the duration of detachment, poorer is the prognosis. The vitreous retraction is a very unfavourable factor. Total or sub-total detachments are far more difficult to handle than sector or quadrantic detachments. The detachment in aphakic eyes is worse than the detachment in phakic eyes. The detachment with a detected hole is easier to settle than detachment where no hole is discovered in spite of careful repeated examination. Giant tears and multiple tears located at different antero-posterior levels make prognosis distinctly bad. A redetachment after first operation is a very difficult proposition and still more difficult if diathermy was used in the first operation.

The prognosis is good where hole is correctly localised on table and sealed. The prognosis is still better when retina is seen to have completely settled at the end of the surgery.

Even though prognosis can be fairly dependably evaluated on the basis of the above points, unpredictable post-operative tissue reaction may disturb the pre-operative evaluation. Vitreous reaction may delay the visual improvement. Traction bands may cause secondary tears and recurrence of detachment. Because of these and other uncertain factors, prognosis of detachment should be communicated with some degree of caution. Even though retina may be found well settled, visual improvement may take longer and this time factor should be kept in mind when indicating prognostic outlook. There is, however, no denying the fact that prognosis of retinal detachment has vastly improved in recent years. Except in complicated and unfavourable cases, reattachment of retina should be possible in 70–80 per cent of cases with good visual recovery in many of them.

PROGNOSIS OF OCULAR INJURIES

From the prognostic point of view, the ocular injury may be from the mildest to a complete disorganisation of the eye ball. Prognostic evaluation is, therefore, more important in injuries which can cause irreparable damage to vision. Such injuries may fall in any of the groups described, the contusion injuries, perforating injuries and injuries with retained foreign body. It is a very difficult exercise indeed to project the ultimate outcome with any degree of dependability. The prognosis should, therefore, always remain guarded. Even when immediate prognosis may appear favourable, subsequent events of organisation and their effect on ocular tissues, may convert the earlier favourable prognosis to bad prognosis. Importance of early reparative surgery has been discussed. It goes a long way in proper evaluation of ultimate prognosis.

23

Optics-physical and Physiological

Optics is a subject which deals with the passage of light through media of varying optical density. In normal atmospheric air of refractive index of 1.0, the light travels at a speed of 1,86,000 miles/sec, in straight lines. White light is a mixture of various colours and the spectrum of colours is called VIBGYOR (Violet-Indigo-Blue-Green-Yellow-Orange-Red) with violet light being at the short wavelength end and the red being at the long wavelength end of visible spectrum. Beyond the violet end of the spectrum are the ultra violet invisible rays like the X-rays, and gamma rays. Beyond the red end of the spectrum are the invisible infra red rays. The wave lengths of the light rays of the visible spectrum extend from approximately 3900 Au at the violetend to 7700 Au at the red end.

Refraction: Whenever light passes from one transparent medium to another transparent medium of different refractive density, the light rays are deflected. This is called *refraction*. If refracting medium is a glass plate with parallel surfaces, the emergent rays are parallel to the incident rays either in the same plane or in a different plane depending on whether the incident rays strike the plate at right angles or obliquely.

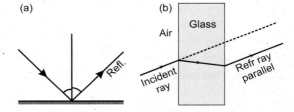

Fig. 23.1: Reflection and Refraction (a) Reflection from mirror surface (note that the angle of incidence and the angle of reflection are equal); (b) Refraction through a glass plate [Note the incident rays passing from lighter (air) to denser (glass plate) medium are deviated but come out parallel to the incident rays]

The higher the refracting density of the medium, the greater is the deflection of emergent rays.

Reflection: The phenomenon of light striking a polished surface and reflecting on the same side is called '*reflection*' of light. The angle of incident light rays on the polished surface is always equal to the angle of reflection.

Real and virtual images: An image which after reflection or refraction can be formed on a screen is called a *real image* and the image which cannot be projected on a screen is called the *virtual image*.

In ocular optics we are concerned with light passing through a prism or a concave or convex lens.

Prism: A prism is a refracting medium with a base and apex and obviously the two sides are not parallel. Light passing through the prism is deviated towards the base. The object therefore appears as if displaced towards the apex. A prism which displaces the image of an object situated at a one meter distance by 1 cm is a prism of one prism dioptre power.

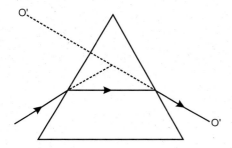

Fig. 23.2: Prism. [The incident rays after refraction are deviated towards the base. The object (O) seen through the prism is displaced towards the apex as O']

Lenses: A lens which has both surface convex or concave, is called a *biconvex or biconcave spherical lens*. A lens with one surface convex or concave and other surface plane, is called a *plano-convex or plano-concave lens*. A *cylindrical lens* is one which is formed from a cylinder of glass and is the lens which has power in one meridian and no power in the meridian at right angles. A cylindrical lens therefore acts only in one direction and the direction of action of cylindrical lens is at right angles to the direction of axis of the cylinder. It may be a convex cylindrical lens or a concave cylindrical lens (Fig. 23.3).

A lens which is a combination of a sphere and a cylinder, is called a *compound lens* which has less power in the direction of the axis of cylinder and more power in the opposite axis.

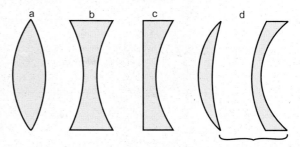

Fig 23.3: Type of lenses : (a) Biconvex lens; (b) Biconcave lens; (c) Plano-concave lens; (d) concavo-convex or minicus lenses

The combined power of two lenses arranged parallel to each other is an algebrical sum which is more than the arithmetic power of the two lenses added together. For example two convex lenses of 5 dioptres each in such a compound homo-centric system will be equal to 11.67 dioptres and the focal length of such system instead of 10 cms of 10 dioptres will be 8.57 cms. This homocentric system has clinical application in human eye ball in that the cornea and lens are two powerful converging systems placed homocentrically on the visual axis.

A convex lens is composed of two prisms base to base and is thicker in the centre and thinner at the periphery. A concave lens is as if two prisms are fused apex to apex and this lens is thinner in the centre and thicker in periphery. The centre of a convex or concave lens where the base or the apex of the prisms join is the *optical centre* and rays passing through the optical centre emerge undeviated. The straight line passing through the centre of the lens and the optical centre is called the *principal axis*.

The rays parallel to the principal axis entering above or below it, will obviously strike at an oblique angle whether the lens is convex or concave, and these rays will therefore be deviated from their normal course i.e. refracted by the medium. (Fig. 23.4 and 23.5).

The power of refraction of the lens is denoted as a dioptre: The rays passing through

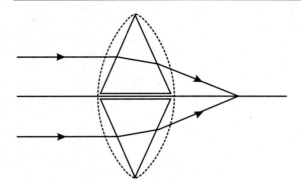

Fig 23.4: Biconvex lens. (Two prisms joined base to base constitute the biconvex lens)

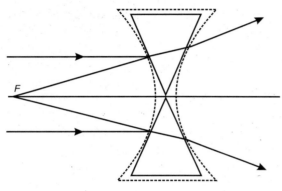

Fig. 23.5: Bioconcave Lens. (Two prism joined apex to apex constitute a biconcave lens

the lens of one dioptre (I-D) power will form a focus at a distance of one meter. This distance is inversely proportional to the power of lens, so that a two dioptre (2-D) lens will form a focus at 50 cms and 1/2 D lens will form a focus at two meters.

Refraction through a convex lens: A convex lens being composed of two prisms joined base to base and light rays passing through a prism being deviated towards the base, all rays passing through the convex lens above or below the principal axis will be converged to form a point of focus on the other side of the lens. A convex lens is therefore called a *converging lens*. The position and size of image will depend on the distance of the object from the lens. The object

from infinity will form an image at the focal length of the lens and the image will be inverted and real. It is also evident that if an object is at the focal length of the lens, the image will be at infinity. It is also evident that if the object is nearer than the focal distance of the lens, the image will be on the same side as the object and will therefore be a virtual image (Fig. 23.6).

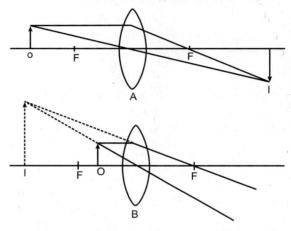

Fig. 23 6: Image through Convex Lens. (A) Object O beyond the focal length forms an image, I which is inverted, real and magnified on opposite side; (B) Object within the focal length forms an image which is erect, virtual magnified and on the same side

Refraction through a concave lens: As a concave lens is formed by two prisms joined apex to apex and as the light deviates to the base of a prism, the parallel rays from infinity will, after passing through a concave lens will be divergent and the image will therefore be formed on the same side as the object and will be virtual and erect. The concave lens is therefore called a *diverging lens* (Fig. 23.7).

Refraction through a cylindrical lens: A cylindrical lens is one which has power of refraction in one meridian and no refraction through the meridian at right angles. The image formed is linear and not circular.

If a lens has both, the spherical as well as cylindrical elements, both meridia will refract but

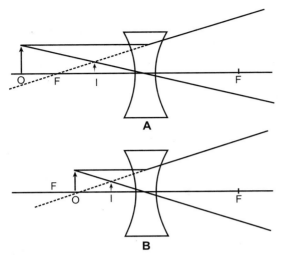

Fig. 23.7: Image through Concave Lens (A) Object O beyond the focal length forms an image, I which is erect, virtual and smaller, (B) Object within the focal length also forms and image erect, virtual and smaller

to different grades; the difference being proportionate to the difference in total power in each axis. For example, a combination of a 3D sphere and a 2D cylinder will have a power of 5D in one axis and 3D in the other axis. Such a lens is called a *compound lens.*

Determining the power of lenses: The power of the lens can be neutralised by an identical power of an opposite type of lens that is convex lens by a concave lens and vice versa. The neutralising lens should be placed in apposition to the lens under study. In high power lenses, the neutralising power should preferably be divided into two parts, each applied on either side of the lens under study. This will avoid errors in neutralisation.

For neutralisation, the lens under study should be held close to the observer's eye and an object three to four meters away is looked at. The lens is now moved in two directions at right angles to each other. The movement of the object seen in the two principal meridia will roughly give an idea of the power of the lens. The slower the

movement of the object seen through the lens, the higher is the power. This primary observation will also tell if it is a simple spherical lens, a simple cylindrical lens or a compound lens with a sizeable degree of the cylindrical element.

In a simple spherical lens, the movement of the object seen through will be the same in all meridia. If it is a simple cylindrical lens, the object will move in one meridian only and there will be no movement in the meridian at right angles. In such a situation the direction of the movement of the lens to be neutralised should be the same with the direction of the power of cylinder. In a compound lens, the movement will be slower in stronger meridian and faster in the weaker meridian.

If the movement of the object is in the direction opposite to the movement of the lens, it is a convex lens. If it is in the same direction it is concave lens. If the movement in one meridian is in the same direction and in the other meridian in opposite direction, it is a *mixed cylindrical lens.*

Neutralising lenses of opposite sign are now placed in contact with the lens under study in increasing powers till a stage is reached when movement of the object is absent in one or both meridia. If both the meridia are neutralised with the same lens, the lens under study is a spherical lens and the power is the same as the power of the neutralising lens but of opposite sign. The same will be the result when neutralising the active meridian of a cylindrical lens. If the movement is neutralised in one meridian only and the object continues to move in the other meridian, the lens under study is a compound lens.

A more powerful meridian should, therefore, be further neutralised with increasing power of a neutralising lens till the movement in that meridian ceases. The lens neutralising the first meridian gives the spherical component while the difference in the powers of first and second lens gives the power of the cylindrical component of the compound lens.

Denoting the axis of the cylinder: An international convention for the sake of uniformity has been established that the axis of a cylinder will be denoted only along the lower half of lens in the spectacle. As the figures start with zero to the right, in both lenses, the axis in the right eye will be 0–90° in down and out temporal sector and 90°–180° in down and in nasal sector.

Similarly the axis in left eye will be 0–90° down and in nasal quadrant and 90°–180° in the down and out temporal quadrant. It is evident that 45° will be down and out in the right eye and down and in the left eye while 135° degrees will be down and in, the right eye and down and out in the left eye.

The arrow shown on a prescription card should therefore be drawn corresponding to the axis along the lower half of 180°.

Lensometer: It is an instrument for quick neutralisation of lenses and probably more accurately. The lens is placed under the objective and by the provided adjustments, the spherical component and its sign, the cylindrical component and its sign and the axis of the cylinder can be read off the scale of the instrument. Computerised lensometers are now available. It is not absolutely necessary to have the lensometer. The method described earlier, if correctly practised, will give the results as correct as a lensometer.

PHYSIOLOGICAL OPTICS

The eye is truly an optical system: The refracting media, principal being the cornea and lens, refract light so that it focusses on the retina. The high refractive power of the cornea is due to light passing from *air* of refractive index 1, through the cornea of refractive index 1.33. It is further refracted when light passes through lens which has a still higher refractive index of a mean value of 1.4. The optical effect of this homo-

centric system is further augmented by the distance of 3.5–4 mm between cornea and lens. An additional increase of refraction is brought about in older age by the difference in refractive index of the nucleus and the cortex of lens which acts as if a biconvex lens is surrounded by two minisci.

The optics of human eye can, therefore, be constructed as shown in the following diagram of a reduced eye (Fig. 23.8).

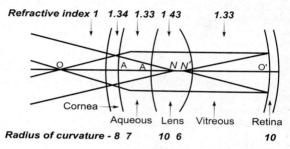

Fig. 23.8: Optical Data of the Homocentric System of Human eye (O—anterior focus of the e ball; O' posterior focus of the eye ball NN—nodal points)

The normal optics of the eye is influenced by other factors and these factors may be diffraction of light, chromatic aberration, spherical aberration, decentering and peripheral aberration. These aberrations are, by and large, overcome by small size of the pupil which allows light to pass into the eye only through the central part of the optical system and hence reduces the diffraction of light, peripheral aberrations and to some extent the spherical and chromatic aberrations (Fig. 23.9).

Chromatic aberration: It is an established fact that blue rays of short wave length light are retarded more by a refracting medium than the long wave length rays of the red end of the spectrum. The blue light rays, therefore, focus in front of the red rays. The middle spectrum of yellow rays focusses exactly on the retina. The eye is, therefore, hypermetropic for red rays and myopic for blue rays. The clinical effect of this

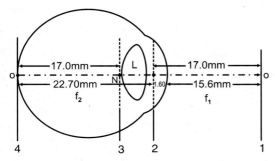

Fig. 23.9: Optical Data of the Homocentric System Transposed on a Human Eye Ball (1) Anterior focus of the eye ball; (2) Anterior principle plane (L-lens); (3) N-nodal point just behind the posterior surface of lens; (4) Posterior principle plane. (Note the following measurements: Anterior focus of eye ball is 15.6 mm from cornea and 17.0 mm from the anterior principle plane; principle plane is 1.6 mm behind the cornea; distance between the two principle planes is 22.7 mm; distance between the cornea and the anterior surface of lens is 3.6 mm and that between the anterior and posterior surfaces of lens is also 3.6 mm)

aberration is negligible because retina is more sensitive to yellow rays. In errors of refraction this defect can be overcome by using achromatic lenses which are formed by a combination of glasses of different refractive indices, for example flint glass of 1.7 and crown glass of 1.5 refractive index.

Spherical aberrations are due to inequality of refractive power between the central and peripheral lens. In the human eye, this defect is overcome by the size of the pupil so that light passes only through the centre of the lens. Even in a dilated pupil, spherical aberration is neutralised by the higher power in the central part of lens and lower in the peripheral part of human lens. In optical lenses, spherical aberration is neutralised by making the curvature of the anterior surface greater than the posterior surface as in meniscus and toric lenses.

Peripheral aberration: The image through the central part of the lens is clearer and more defined than the one formed through the periphery due to the aberrations described above. This is overcome by the smallness of the size of

the pupil and also the curvature of the retinal surface from behind forwards forming a hemisphere.

Decentering of lenses: It is important that in a homocentric combination of lenses, the centre of each optical system should be on the same line, which is called the *optical axis.*

In human eye, the optical axis cuts the corneal centre slightly down and out to the visual axis and these two axes from an angle of 5° at the nodal point. This arrangement in the human eye fits in with the situation of the macula which is two and a half disc diameters temporal to the disc margin and slightly below the horizontal plane.

Decentering is also very important in fitting of spectacle lenses. In large sized frames, decentering is important so that the optical centre of the lens corresponds to the centre of the pupil. The same is necessary when fitting glasses for asymmetrical face. Decentering of lenses is an essential part in fitting of bifocal and trifocal lenses because the optical centre of near segment of the lens should be decentered inwards. Decentering is also done when a prismatic effect is to be incorporated in a spectacle lens. One cm decentering in one dioptre lens gives one prism dioptre effect.

Optical System of Human Eye (Fig. 23.10)

1. *A nodal point is a point through which all rays pass to reach the retina.* This point is located just behind the posterior pole of the lens.
2. *Centre of rotation:* This is a point round which the eye rotates and is located in the centre of the eye behind the nodal point.
3. *Optical axis:* It is the line joining the centre of the cornea and centre of the lens and passes through the nodal point.

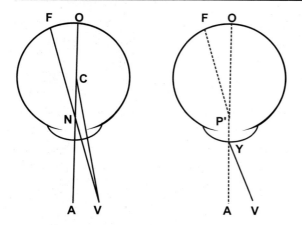

Fig 23.10: Optical axes of Human Eye Ball. AO–Optical Axis; VF–Visual Axis; VNA–Angle Alpha; VCA–Angle Gamma; VYA Angle Kappa (Clinical); P–Centre of Pupil; VPA–Angle Kappa (Geometrical); N–Nodal Point; C–Centre of rotation

4. *Visual axis:* This is a line joining the fixation object and the macula and passes through the nodal point. As already explained, the visual axis cuts the cornea slightly up and in to the centre of cornea while the optical axis cuts the centre of the cornea which is down and out to the point of visual axis. The visual and the optical axes cross each other at the nodal point. The angle formed at the intersection is called *angle alpha*. The angle is approximately five degrees and is called a *positive angle* when the visual *axis cuts* the cornea nasal to the optical axis as in most normal eyes. If the visual axis cuts the cornea temporal to the optical axis, it is called *negative angle alpha*.

5. *Fixation axis.* As the eye moves, it revolves round the centre of rotation. The line joining the point of fixation and centre of rotation is called the fixation axis. The angle between the fixation axis and the optical axis is called *angle gamma*.

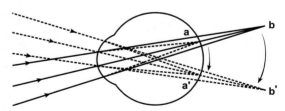

Retinoscopy and Errors of Refraction

24

The word is a misnomer because we do not see the retina as the term indicates. We only see the fundus glow produced by reflection of the light rays. However, as the term stands, by retinoscopy, we determine the refractive state of the eye. This is done by throwing light into the eye and observing the movement of the fundus glow in relation to the movements of the source of light. The source of light is usually a mirror through the central hole of which we observe the movements of the fundus glow. Generally we use a plane mirror, rather a very slightly concave mirror (Listers mirror) for retinoscopy. However, a regular concave mirror can also be used but the interpretations of the observations will be reversed. A self-illuminating retinoscope is often used.

OPTICS OF RETINOSCOPY

Retinoscopy with a plain mirror is based on the reflection of light from the mirror into the eye of the patient. With the movement of the mirror, the illuminated area of the fundus also moves. The relationship of the movement of the mirror and the illuminated area of the fundus depends on whether the eye is emmetropic, hypermetropic or myopic.

When a plain mirror is tilted, the reflected light follows the movement of the mirror and so also the illuminated area of the fundus. As the movement of the illuminated area of the fundus in emmetropic and hypermetropic eyes is in the same direction as the movement of the source of light, the fundus glow moves in the same direction as the movement of the mirror (Fig. 24.1).

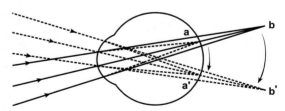

Fig. 24.1: Retinoscopy in Hypermetropic Eye. The rays emerging from the eye are divergent and appear to come from a focus behind the eye ball. If the illuminated area of the fundus moves from a to a' the focus moves from b to b' that is, in the same direction

In myopic eyes, the focus of the rays is in front of the eye and this moves in a direction opposite to the movement of the illuminated area of fundus. The fundus glow in myopic eyes therefore moves in the direction opposite to the movement of the mirror (Fig. 24.2).

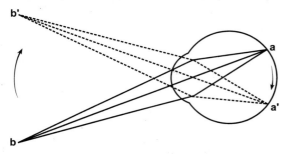

Fig 24.2: Retinoscopy in Myopic Eye. The rays (emerging from the eye are convergent and form a focus in front of the eye so that if illuminated area moves from a to a', the focus in front of the eye moves from b to b', that is, in the opposite direction to the movement of the illuminated area

When using a concave mirror, the optical directions are reversed and therefore the movements are opposite to those with a plain mirror. Further more, a concave mirror has the disadvantage that the light falling into the eye is brighter causing photophobia and the movements of the fundus glow are faster and therefore less convenient to neutralise.

Retinoscopy should be done at a distance of one meter between the observer and the patient. In order to do this, one should use a trial frame, but the disadvantage is that every time the lens is to be changed, the observer has to move forwards and backwards. The distance of one meter is arbitarily selected because theoretically the observer should be at infinity which is not practicable.

If a trial frame is not used, and the lens in front of the eye is held in the hand, it is not possible to maintain a distance of one meter even by stretching the head backwards. This is still more difficult for a short person. Retinoscopy with lens in hand is therefore done from a distance of 75 cm which does introduce a small though not significant element of error .

PRINCIPLES OF RETINOSCOPY

The principle of retinoscopy is to determine the power of the lens needed to neutralize the

movements of the fundus glow. This is called the point of reversal or the *point of neutralization*. At this point the retina of the patient and the retina of the observer are at conjugate focus with each other. At this point also the patient is made artificially myopic proportionate to the distance between the observer and the patient. This is 1 dioptre when the retinoscopy is done at one meter distance, 1.5 dioptre when the retinoscopy is done from 75 cms, 2.0 dioptres when done from 50 cms. It is important to explain why we say the patient is made artificially myopic. It is a physiological fact that the rays of light coming out of myopic eyes are convergent and form a focus in front of the eye. As the observer is sitting in front of the patient and the rays of the light coming out of the patient's eyes are forming a conjugate focus at the observer's retina in front of the patient, the patient is myopic at neutralisation point.

METHOD OF RETINOSCOPY

The observer sits in front of the patient at a distance of 1 meter or 75 cm. The eyes of the patient and the observer should be at the same level. The light source is behind the patient, or within the handle of retinoscope in cases of self illuminating retinoscopes.

For retinoscopy, the light source should not be very bright because that will cause photophobia and the patient may not be able to co-operate. To avoid reflection of the filament of the bulb giving uneven light, a frosted bulb is better as it will give diffuse illumination and therefore give a uniformly illuminated fundus glow.

A Lister's mirror is held by the observer in front of his right eye and light is reflected to the patient's eye while the patient is looking at a distant object in the direction of the observer's right'ear when the observer is refracting the right eye and beyond the left ear when refracting the left eye. This enables refracting the retina between the macula and the optic disc. It is important that patient should not look into the mirror because that will cause photophobia and make the pupil small if a mydriatic is not used (Fig. 24.3A and B, Plate 14).

The mirror or the retinoscope is now tilted in horizontal and vertical axes alternately. The observer seeing through the hole in the mirror or retinoscope, notes whether the movements of the fundus glow are with the movements of the mirror or against it. If the distance between the patient and the observer is 1 meter and the fundus glow moves with, the patient is either:

a. A hypermetrope.
b. Emmetrope.
c. Myope of less than 1 dioptre.

If the movements are against, the patient is a myope of more than 1 dioptre. If the fundus glow does not move at all, the patient has a myopia of exactly 1 dioptre. It is important to mention that if the fundus glow is dull, it indicates either a high degree of refractive error or hazy media that do not allow the light rays to pass through. If the rate of movement of fundus glow appears slow, it again indicates a high degree of error of refraction.

The movements of the fundus glow may be unequal in two directions and if this is so, it indicates that there is an astigmatic error either alone or in addition to a spherical error. It may also be that it moves against in one direction and with, in the meridian at right angles, the patient then is myopic in one axis and hypermetropic, emmetropic or myopic less than 1 dioptre in the other axis. Sometimes when the mirror is tilted in vertical and horizontal planes, the fundus glow moves obliquely to the movement of the mirror. In these cases the mirror has to be moved in the direction of the obliquity and then at the right angles to it. When this is noted, patient has an oblique *astigmatism* alone or in addition to a spherical error.

Having noted the brightness of the glow, the rate of movement and the direction of movement,

the observer proceeds to neutralise these movements with appropriate lenses held at the anterior focus of the patient's eye about 15 mm in front of the anterior pole. Starting from low power, the lenses are held in front of the patient's eye in gradually increasing power till the movement of the fundus glow just reverses. The lens used just before the last lens, is the lens required to reach a point of neutralisation. It is important that each axis is neutralised separately. The power of the lens needed to neutralise the movements in each axis is recorded in the form of a retinoscopy reading as for example:

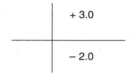

This shows that the vertical axis is neutralized by a convex lens of +3 dioptres and the horizontal axis is neutralized by a concave lens of –2 dioptres. In moderate degree of error of refraction, the lens power should be increased by 0.25 to 0.5 dioptres each time. In higher refractive states as indicated by dull fundus glow or slow movement of fundus glow, a jump of 1–2 dioptres is permissible.

For the purpose of description that follows, the calculations and evaluation of retinoscopy will be based on 1 meter distance with the use of a plain mirror.

At the point of neutralization from one meter distance, the patient is made myopic by one dioptre. In addition, the cycloplegic, paralysing accommodation, adds to this artificial myopia by 0.5 D in case of homatropine and 1.0 D in case of atropine. It is, therefore, necessary to add to the reading of retinoscopy –1.0 if retinoscopy is done without cycloplegia, –1.5 D if done with homatropine and –2.0 if done with atropine. The resultant common factor between the readings in the two meridia at right angles to each other is denoted as the spherical correction and the difference between the two is denoted as the cylindrical correction. The examples of retinoscopy reading and calculating the power of glasses needed by the patient are self-explanatory.

When to Use Mydriatic/Cycloplegic for Determining the Error of Refraction

The refractive state of the eye is constantly changing, depending on whether one is looking at distance or near. This is brought about by the process of accommodation. It is obvious that when the eye is actively accommodating, the retinoscopy reading will be inconstant and undependable. It is, therefore, important that retinoscopy be done with the eye in a state of rest and this can only be achieved by paralysing accommodation. Accommodation is stronger in younger people than in older people and is stronger in hypermetropes than in myopes, so that a stronger cycloplegic is needed for younger patients and hypermetropes. It is, therefore, generally accepted that retinoscopy in children is done after cycloplegia with 1% atropine ointment applied three times a day for three days. Homatropine 2% solution is used in adults upto age 35 years. In known myopes who have weak accommodation, homatropine drops may be adequate even in younger age. When using a cycloplegic, the patient should be fore warned of the temporary effect of the drug on vision particularly in near vision. When atropine is used, mydriasis cycloplegia lasts 10-12 days. When homatropine is used, the effect lasts 36-48 hours. The immediate effect of these drugs is stronger in hypermetropes than in myopes, so that the disability felt will be more severe in hypermetropes than in myopes. It is, therefore, extremely important that one should ask the patient his immediate commitments of near work before suggesting use of these drugs.

The fear of secondary rise of intra-ocular tension following use of a mydriatic should be kept in mind in older patients particularly when the anterior chamber is shallow.

It is also important to keep in mind that the effect of atropine cannot be neutralised. The effect of homatropine can and should however be neutralised with a drop of 2.0 per cent solution of pilocarpine. These drugs are equally effective in lesser dilution in light coloured eyes as compared to dark eyes.

Refraction with Mydriatic Alone

The commonest drug available for quick mydriasis is sympathomimetic, Phenylephrine Hydrochloride, used as 5-10% solution. The effect becomes maximal in about 25-30 minutes and passes off in 1½-2 hours. Phenylephrine in eyes with active accommodation will therefore be undependable for the spherical error of refraction. However, difference between the two axes will be satisfactorily evident. Refraction under phenylephrine can therefore fairly indicate the astigmatic component of the error of refraction and that in fact is the important element, because spherical error can be subjectively determined in a reasonably co-operative patient. Phenylephrine has distinct advantage that even though it causes mydriasis, it tends to lower tension of the eye because of its vasoconstrictive action, and can therefore be safely used in elderly persons. The quantity used for retinoscopy is so small that even if absorbed, the effect on blood pressure is insignificant. It can therefore also be used in hypertensive patients. However remote, the possibility of rise of tension following use of phenylephrine in pro-glaucomatous eyes must be kept in mind.

Retinoscopy without Mydriasis

It is possible to determine the refractive state of the eye with accuracy to a certain degree without

Without cycloplegia	Under Homatropine	Under Atropine
$+4.0 + (-1.0) = +3.0$	$+4.0 + (-1.5) = +2.5$	$+4.0 + (-2.0) = +2.0$
$+4.0 + (-1.0) = +3.0$	$+4.0 + (-1.5) = +2.5$	$+4.0 + (-2.0) = +2.0$
Prescription: + 3.0 Dsph	*Prescription:* + 2.5 Dsph	*Prescription:* +2.0 Dsph

$-4.0 + (-1.0) = -5.0$	$-4.0 + (-1.5) = -5.5$	$-4.0 + (-2.0) = -6.0$
$-4.0 + (-1.0) = -5.0$	$-4.0 + (-1.5) = -5.5$	$-4.0 + (-2.0) = -6.0$
Prescription: − 5.0 Dsph	− 5.5 Dsph	− 6.0 Dsph

$+2.0 + (-1.0) = +1.0$	$+2.0 + (-1.5) = +0.5$	$+2.0 + (-2.0) - 0.0$
$+1.0 + (-1.0) = 0.0$	$+1.0 + (-1.5) = -0.5$	$+1.0 + (-2.0) -1.0$
Prescription: + 1.0 Dcyl 180°		*Prescription:* − 1.0 Dcyl 90°

$$\frac{+ 0.5 \text{ Dsph}}{- 1.0 \text{ Dcy } 90°}$$

OR

$$\frac{- 0.5 \text{ Dsph}}{+ 1.0 \text{ Dcyl} \rightarrow 180°}$$

$+5.0 + (-1.0) = +4.0$	$-5.0 + (-1.5) = -6.5$	$-2.0 + (-2.0) = -4.0$
$+3.0 + (-1.0) = +2.0$	$-3.0 + (-1.5) = -4.5$	$+3.0 + (-2.0) = +1.0$
Prescription: $\dfrac{+ 2.0 \text{ Dsph}}{+ 2.0 \text{ Dcyl } 180°}$	*Prescription:* $\dfrac{- 4.5 \text{ Dsph}}{- 2.0 \text{ Dcyl } 180°}$	*Prescription:* $\dfrac{+ 1.0 \text{ Dsph}}{+ 5.0 \text{ Dcyl } 180°}$
		OR
		$\dfrac{- 4.0 \text{ Dsph}}{+ 5.0 \text{ Dcyl } 90°}$

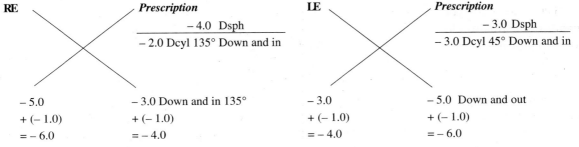

RE   Prescription

$$\frac{- 4.0 \ \text{Dsph}}{- 2.0 \text{ Dcyl } 135° \text{ Down and in}}$$

LE   Prescription

$$\frac{- 3.0 \text{ Dsph}}{- 3.0 \text{ Dcyl } 45° \text{ Down and in}}$$

− 5.0	− 3.0 Down and in 135°	− 3.0	− 5.0 Down and out
+ (− 1.0)	+ (− 1.0)	+ (− 1.0)	+ (− 1.0)
= − 6.0	= − 4.0	= − 4.0	= − 6.0

mydriasis. To accomplish this, the room should be darkened, the source of light should be dimmer and patient asked to relax his accommodation by looking at a distance of at least 6 meters. This will help to enlarge the pupil to some degree to permit retinoscopy procedure. It is important to emphasize that latent hypermetropia cannot be discovered without the use of cycloplegics. In younger age patients with active accommodation, retinoscopy observations without cycloplegia may change from moment to moment and make it difficult to reach a conclusion. There may be situations where the time factor demands that the patient is to be given prescription of glasses at one sitting. This is possible to a fair degree of accuracy in reasonably intelligent and co-operative patients. The power of glasses needed is first determined by subjective examination and then confirmed by retinoscopy under homatropine or phenylephrine. The procedure is time consuming and the time taken will depend on the type of error, intelligence and co-operation of patient.

DIFFICULTIES IN RETINOSCOPY

It is important that for a correct assessment of refractive state of the eye, refractive media should be clear. The opacity in cornea, lens or vitreous will make the assessment not only difficult but undependable too. Another difficulty is the irregularities in curvature of the cornea as in keratoconus or change in the refractive index of the lens as in nuclear sclerosis.

There are two types of anomalous movements of the fundus glow:

1. *Circular movement* around the centre of the glow as in keratoconus and lenticonus. It is difficult to determine a correct retinoscopy reading in these cases.
2. *Scissors shadow.* Where the reflex from the two peripheral sides moves towards the centre

in opposite direction to each other while the central reflex moves with or against depending on the refractive state of the eye.

These anomalous movements can be due to changes in cornea or lens, and are more often seen with a widely dilated pupil due to different refractive states through the centre and periphery. Ignore the movements of the periphery and concentrate on the movement of the central glow only and neutralise the same with appropriate lenses. The scissor movement can however be avoided by refracting through an undilated or moderately dilated pupil.

A dull fundus glow may give an impression that media are not clear. In all such cases, one should straight away start with the high power lens of 3-4 dioptres when the fundus glow will become brighter. If there are opacities in the media, this change in the brightness of the fundus glow will not occur.

VERIFICATION OF RETINOSCOPY

Years of experience are needed for performing retinoscopy correctly and speedily. One can dependably verify one's own retinoscopy readings. The following procedure may be adopted for the same:

1. On reaching the point of neutralisation, the observer may move the head forwards and backwards from the initial position by about 15 cms. If the observer moves forwards the fundus glow should start moving with and if the head moves back, the fundus glow should start moving against. If this is observed, the retinoscopy reading may be taken as correct.
2. By placing the appropriate lenses indicated by the retinoscopy reading, in the trial frame and repeating retinoscopy, if the fundus glow does not move in either meridian, the retinoscopy readings may be presumed to be correct.

SUBJECTIVE TEST

It is advisable to do a repeat examination after the effect of the mydriatic/ cycloplegic has passed off. Therefore, a subjective test which is called PMT (post-mydriatic test) more appropriately called, the post-cycloplegic test is done after varying intervals. If atropine is used, the patient is called 15 days after the last application of atropine. If homatropine is used, a subjective test is done not earlier than 48 hours. If phenylephrine is used, the examination may be done any time after 5–6 hours.

A final prescription may quite often be a compromise between the retinoscopy findings and the acceptance of the lenses by the patient. It is more often the acceptable spherical correction which may be different from what retinoscopy indicates. For example, in older people, a higher concave lens is needed in eyes with early lenticular changes or a higher convex lens is needed when the lens is unaffected. The accommodative state of the eye at the time of subjective test may partly be responsible for these variations. Cylindrical correction needed usually conforms to the correctly estimated retinoscopy readings.

While doing the subjective test, the position of the trial frame should be such that the lenses placed are at the anterior focal length of the eye. It is also important that aperture of the frame is so centered that centre of the pupil corresponds with centre of the lens. When the spherical element is the major part of error of refraction, one should first proceed with spherical lenses and find out the best visual acuity with the best acceptable lenses. Cylinders may then be added to the accepted sphere and again their axis and their power should be examined, guided by the retinoscopy readings. In cases of high astigmatic retinoscopic findings, a cylindrical trial may be done first and a small spherical correction if useful may be incorporated later.

It should be expected that visual acuity of an otherwise normal eye should improve to normal standard with appropriate combination of lenses If in spite of one's best efforts, vision does not improve in one or both eyes to the expected degree, one should consider the following alternatives:

1. Presence of amblyopia even in non-squinting eye if one eye remains unimproved.
2. Repeat retinoscopy even if it has to be done with a cycloplegic again.
3. Examine the anterior surface of cornea for its regularity with placedo's disc and also look for any faint corneal facet or a thin nebula which may have been missed.
4. Look for any opacities in the lens and vitreous and any fundus changes to account for the non-improvement of the vision.
5. Functional elements may also be kept in mind, for example, hysterics and malingerers.

While estimating the power of the sphere required, a Duochrome or FRIEND test may be of particular help in preventing over correction specially in myopia. The Duochrome Test presents letters printed on two parallel strips of red and green colour. The chart is internally illuminated. The test is used to finalise the spherical correction of the refractive error. In a normal eye, the red end of the spectrum focuses behind the retina and the green in front of it. For any condition of refractive error it is aimed to make the letters in both colours nearly equal in readability. With subjective correction in the trial frame, patient is asked to look at the green and red letters of the Duochrome chart 6 meters away. If green letters are clearer, a plus lens is added and if red letters are clearer, minus lens is added till clarity of red and green are equalized. The Duochrome test is a very practical and sensitive test for checking the spherical element of the error after astigmatic error if any is fully corrected (Fig. 24.4A and B, Plate 15).

For confirming the correctness of a moderate degree of cylindrical correction, the use of a cross cylinder is helpful. A *cross cylinder* is a lens mounted on a handle with a small sphere and a cylinder of double the power of sphere, with opposite sign. It has an effective power of +0.25 D cylinder in one axis and –0.25 D cylinder in the opposite axis. The handle is fixed at 45° to the two meridia. When a cross cylinder is placed in front of the accepted correction parallel and same sign as the cylinder in trial frame, it enhances the power of the cylinder. The same is reduced if the cross cylinder is placed with opposite sign parallel to the cylinder in trial frame. If cross cylinder improves vision further, slight adjustment of cylindrical correction is called for. The test may then be repeated till the cylindrical correction is finally determined (Fig. 24.5).

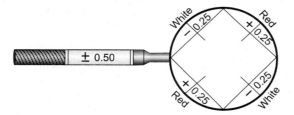

Fig. 24.5: Cross cylinder showing –0.25 Dcyl in one Axis and +0.25 Dcyl in opposite axis

To confirm the axis of astigmatism, an astigmatic FAN may also be used by rotating the axis of the cylinder in such a way that all the lines of the astigmatic fan become equally clear. When a particular set of lines looks clearer than others, the cylinder should be added at right angles to the clear lines. There are different models of astigmatic fans available and most of them serve the same purpose.

A *stenopic slit* can also be used to determine the spherical element in two directions at right angles to each other. The slit is put in one axis and the spherical correction is determined by adding or subtracting the sphere. The slit is then turned at right angles. The spherical element in that meridian is then determined by adding or subtracting the sphere. The stenopic slit therefore acts as a pin-hole in each direction separately.

Subjective evaluation for glasses in illiterate patients may sometimes be a frustrating exercise. Their response is the same whether the lens in front of the eye is +1.0 or +3.0 or whether the cylinder axis is at 90° or 180°. Their behaviour is particularly so for distance vision. One has, in such cases, to depend entirely on retinoscopy readings and final glasses prescribed on retinoscopy alone. The co-operation of these patients is slightly more dependable for testing by dots for near vision. Glasses accepted for near vision may therefore be a guide for distance correction which may be arrived at after giving due consideration to age, retinoscopy readings etc.

After determining the final correction of each eye separately, the patient should be given the opportunity of seeing with both eyes simultaneously to note any disturbance in binocularity. The final prescription for glasses can then be given. The correctness of the subjective examination whether before cycloplegia or as a postmydriatic test, always depends on the co-operation and intelligence of the patient.

In cases of young children where retinoscopy is always done under full cycloplegia of atropine, it is neither advisable nor necessary to do a postmydriatic test. Prescription of glasses can and should be given immediately after retinoscopy.

This is particularly important in children with high hypermetropia when full correction is not accepted once cycloplegic effect is over. It causes spasm of ciliary muscle.

It is therefore necessary to prescribe hypermetropic correction earlier and gradually build it up in following months. Sometimes it may be necessary to continue with mild cycloplegic drops during this period till full correction is accepted.

It is necessary to emphasize that when glasses of high astigmatic power are prescribed for the first time in adults, the eye may not accept the full cylindrical correction. In such cases, one may start with a lesser cylindrical correction and increase it in subsequent examinations at 3–6 monthly intervals. Some patients will accept only spherical correction and not tolerate any cylinders at all.

Whether the spectacles should be used constantly or intermittently, will depend on various factors to be described later when dealing with the individual refractive states of the eye. Similarly whether the same power should be used both for near and distance or a separate power is needed for distance and near will not only depend on the age of the patient but also on the degree of refractive error and the actual near work pattern of the patient.

The best visual acuity achieved with appropriate correction of lenses in each eye, should be recorded on the prescription card.

REFRACTING UNIT

Compact units are available with a magazine of lenses and prisms. This unit has the advantage that the lenses can be changed in power in rapid succession and therefore save time as compared to when subjective verification is done with the help of trial lenses set and a trial frame. Recently, more sophisticated equipment has been produced like auto-refractor units where the patient can sit at the unit and with little prior explanation, find out the power of lenses needed. The prescription by the auto-refractor should however be confirmed by subjective test and acceptance by the patient.

DYNAMIC RETINOSCOPY

Dynamic retinoscopy is determination of refractive state of the eye while the patient is seeing an object at the near point and is accommodating. This examination is, therefore done without cycloplegia and mydriasis. The result of this examination may be helpful in finding the difference in accommodation of two eyes and the near point may be assessed. In practice, however, these assessments can also be done by subjective verifications already described.

STREAK RETINOSCOPY

Unlike retinoscopy with the mirror, a streak retinoscope throws a slit light which can be turned in different meridia. This method is of particular advantage to determine power and axis of cylinder. Streak retinoscopy is done with a self-illuminating retinoscope in a dark room. The meridian which is at right angle to the streak is neutralised first. The streak is then turned at right angles and opposite meridian is checked by appropriate lenses as is done in retinoscopy with the mirror.

ERRORS OF REFRACTION

However perfect nature may have been, it is rare to have a truly emmetropic eye, i.e., an eye without an error of refraction. Further more, the refractive state of the eye is in a process of continuous change in childhood and again in old age.

Although not all are genetic in origin, the refractive states of the eye are the result of evolution from birth to good old age. The changes during evolution affect the two principal refractive media of the eye, the cornea and the lens. The eye ball at birth is 16 mm in diameter and grows to full size of about 24 mm by the age of 8–12 years. Although cornea grows to its full size by about the age of two years, the process of maturation continues till about the age of 10 years. The lens which is more spherical at birth changes its shape and size as it grows. The refractive index of the lens substance undergoes a definite change as nucleus forms about the age of 20–25 years. The nucleus further hardens as age advances, so much so that in older age due to change in the refractive index of the nucleus, it behaves as if the nucleus is surrounded by two meniscus lenses. These and other factors have to be constantly borne in mind when finally prescribing glasses and giving advice to the patient regarding the use of glasses.

An ophthalmologist is constantly faced with a question, why refractive errors of the eye have become more common among the present generation as compared to a few decades earlier. We should look at this proposition more critically and be able to answer a frequent question like this to the patient. It needs to be emphasised first that retinoscopy as a practical science developed only after the first treatise on physiological optics by Helmoltz published in 1856. The second relevant factor is the change in environments. Education in the 19th century and earlier in 20th century was a privilege of a few. Most people were content with the amount of vision they had, using some sort of magnifying aid for observing finer objects or finer letters. These two basic factors explain the lack of importance attached to refractive errors of the eye in the past.

However the fact remains that we are paying the price of advancement of education and the advances in technology, making greater demands on vision. The early schooling of a child puts strain on the eye in the phase of development. While 6 years used to be minimum age of joining primary school, there are schools today which will not admit the child after the age of 3 years. The nursery and kindergarten schools do inadvertently cause strain on the eye in that delicate phase of life. The use of finer writing materials as compared to the thick pens used earlier cause strain on the eye, an important factor for the higher incidence of refractive errors. Finer prints in the books for school children and a heavy curriculum, is no less important. It is because of these factors that the education

system in developed countries is getting more audio-visual oriented while in developing countries, the eye continues to be a victim of extra load and strain. Nutrition can be another important factor for higher incidence of refractive errors. If the body is not healthy, eye functions are likely to share the consequences of poor health. In addition to all these factors, heredity plays its important role. More the precipitating factors, higher is the incidence of errors of refraction. The less diluted the genes, the higher is the genetic transmission of the errors. Most of the smaller errors show a dominant transmission while larger errors like high myopia are recessive in character. Refractive errors also have a very definite racial predilection. Dependable studies have indicated that hypermetropia is more common in western countries and blacks, while myopia is distinctly more common in Chinese, Japanese, Indians and Jews.

The incidence of refractive errors is different in different age groups. In childhood upto the age of 8 years, hypermetropia is a dominant state of the eye. From the age of 10 years to the presbyopic age, incidence of refractive error is of myopia or myopic astigmatism. There is a hypermetropic shift after the age of 40 years and a myopic shift becomes evident after the age of 50–60 years because of the changes in the lens.

TYPES OF REFRACTIVE ERRORS

An *emmetropic eye* is a normal eye where the rays of light entering the eye are focussed on retina in all planes and vision of the eye is normal. Ametropia is state of the eye where the light rays focus either in front or behind the retina and the vision of the eye is less than normal. This can be due to different anomalies in the refractive system of the eye. When it is due to change in the length of the eye ball, it is called *axial ametropia*. When it is due to change in the curvature, it is called *curvature ametropia*. When it is due to the change in the refractive index or refractive power of the media, it is called *index ametropia.*

A majority of the errors of refraction are due to a change in the length of the eye ball. A change of 1 mm in the length of the eye ball introduces 3 diopters of refractive error. The axial length of the eye ball can therefore indirectly be determined by degree of refractive state of the eye. The posterior segment of the eye being embedded in the orbit, it is not possible to physically measure the dimensions of the eye in situ. This has however now become possible by ultrasonography.

Knowledge of actual length of the eye may be of importance when the refractive state of the eye cannot be made out due to opacity in media and yet we want to know the length of the eye ball specially for intra-ocular lens implant surgery when we want to know the exact power of the lens needed for the patient's eye ball (Figs 24.6 and 24.7).

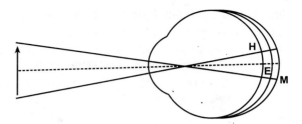

Fig. 24.7: Axial Length of Eye ball in errors of Refraction and Size of the Image (I) Myopic eye (M) is longer and hypermetropic (H) is shorter than emmetropic eye (E); The size of the image in myopic eye is bigger and in hypermetropic eye smaller than in emmetropic eye.

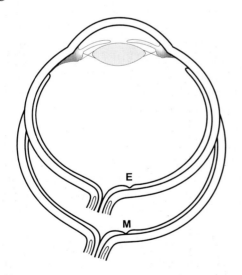

Fig 24.6: Myopic Eye elongated at the Posterior Pole

Refractive errors of the eye are usually consistent in nature, except that they change in character with age. A refractive state of the eye may sometimes be transient. Systemic disease process can bring about a temporary change in the refractive media of the eye. Most of these transient refractive errors are myopic in nature, the causes of which can be diabetes, liver disorders, chronic debilitating states, etc. Certain drugs may also bring about transient myopia like sulphonamides, arsenical, etc.

AMETROPIA

Ametropia is an abnormal refractive state of the eye. Ametropic errors may be of the following types:
1. Hypermetropia.
2. Myopia.
3. Astigmatism.
4. Presbyopia.
5. Aphakia.
6. Pseudophakia.

Hypermetropia

Hypermetropia is a condition where the light rays, without an accommodative effort, form a focus behind the retina. It is called axial hypermetropia when the antero-posterior length of the eye ball is shorter than the normal.

Hypermetropia in childhood is mostly axial in nature because of the short antero-posterior length of the eye ball at birth. This hypermetropia decreases as the eye grows and most such eyes become emmetropic by the age of 8–10 years. However, if the growth of the eye is slowed down, the antero-posterior length remains permanently short and axial hypermetropia persists into later age.

Types of Hypermetropia

1. Manifest hypermetropia.
2. Absolute hypermetropia.
3. Facultative hypermetropia.
4. Latent hypermetropia.
5. Total hypermetropia.

These different types can be determined clinically by use of a convex lens. The weakest convex lens with which the best visual acuity can be obtained gives *absolute hypermetropia.* The strongest convex lens tolerated and yet the visual acuity remains unchanged gives *manifest hypermetropia.* The difference between manifest and absolute hypermetropia is *facultative hypermetropia* because this part of hypermetropia is corrected by effort of accommodation, which is normally not used for distance. The retinoscopy reading under full cycloplegia will give *total hypermetropia* while the difference between total and manifest hypermetropia is called *latent hypermetropia.*

Hypermetropia can also be caused by pathological conditions of the eye like orbital growths, detachment of the retina and severe papilloedema. A micro ophthalmic eye will be a hypermicropic eye by virtue of its dimensions. Similarly, an aphakic eye is also a hypermetropic eye because of the absence of a highly refracting medium, the lens.

Clinical Features

Features of a hypermetropic eye are:

1. The eye is shorter in antero-posterior diameter, the far point is behind the eye ball.
2. The cornea is smaller in size.
3. The lens is more spherical.
4. The eye has a stronger accommodation.
5. If uniocular, it has a tendency to develop amblyopia.
6. The disc appears smaller and sometimes gives the appearance of what has been described as pseudo neuritis.
7. The macular area shows shot-silk reflexes.
8. These eyes are pro-glaucomatous.

As the image of a distant object by an uncorrected hypermetropic eye is formed behind the retina, a constant effort is made to bring the image forwards to the level of the retina to improve the clarity of the object seen. This is subconsciously done by the patient with accommodative effort so that in low or moderate degree of hypermetropia, the patient can maintain the clarity of distance vision with help of his own accommodation. The accommodative effort is acting all the lime. The symptoms of eye strain are therefore more persistent and more severe in hypermetropic patients and the condition is called *hypermetropic asthenopia.* When looking at a near object, a still greater effort of accommodation is needed which in moderate degrees of hypermetropia can cause a spasm of accommodation and this may compel the patient to hold the object close to the eye and this anomaly is called *hypermetropic myopia.* The use of constant and extra accommodation in hypermetropia also disturbs the AC/A ratio. The more the accommodation used, the greater is the convergence needed and this can lead to an accommodative squint to begin with but may become a concomitant convergent squint later. It is a common experience that amblyopia gets more frequently established in hypermetropic eyes. It is not only common in hypermetropia with uniocular squint but even hypermetropic eyes without concomitant squint may not improve to full visual acuity because of *amblyopia of arrest.*

Treatment: The eyes of children are developmentally hypermetropic therefore no correction need be given before the school-going age. Later only manifest hypermetropia needs to be corrected and should be checked every year under atropine preferably planned during the annual vacations.

A good rule is to give correction for full manifest hypermetropia plus l/4th of latent hypermetropia. As the age advances, the latent hypermetropia becomes less and less and therefore a lesser correction is needed. If there is spasm of accommodation as evident by accommodative squint, glasses may have to be prescribed even before the school-going age. In these children a full correction should be given. If however, the child is too young to wear glasses, prolonged use of cycloplegic may correct the squint for a temporary period till glasses can be used.

Full correction may not always be tolerated in the first instance. If necessary use of glasses should be started during the effect of atropine. It may even be necessary to keep the eye under a weak cycloplegic effect for a few weeks to prevent the spasm of accommodation in these cases. A full hypermetropic correction is also indicated when there is associated esophoria or esotropia. In higher degrees of hypermetropia, it may be necessary to give extra correction for reading and recommend use of bifocal glasses even in young age.

Myopia

Myopia is short sightedness of the eye. A myopic person is like a frog in a well with a small world of his own and more interested in near and close activities. Of all the refractive states, myopia has a distinct hereditary transmission in generations usually recessive in character. However it may be dominant and be present in consecutive generations.

In myopic eyes, parallel rays of light form a focus in front of retina, and hence the defective vision. Unlike hypermetropia, accommodation cannot improve vision because in myopia, rays have to be more divergent to form a focus on the retina. This can only be achieved by placing concave lens at the anterior focal point of the eye. Light rays coming out of the eye are covergent and form a focus in front of the eye so that the far point of the myopic eye is in front of the retina.

Clinical Features

a. The eye ball in axial myopia is longer than normal and the increase in antero-posterior length is at the posterior pole of the eye. The far point is in front of the eye and distance between the far and near points is short.

b. The eye may look prominent.

c. The anterior chamber is slightly deeper than normal.

d. The pupil is slightly larger.

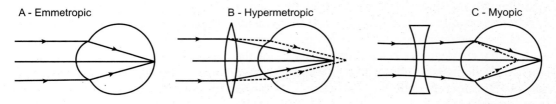

Fig 24.8: Refractive states of eye: (a) Emmetropic eye where parallel rays form a focus on the retina; (b) Hypermetropic eye where parallel rays form a focus behind the eye ball and by putting a suitable convex lens in the spectacle, focus forms on the retina; (c) Myopic eye where parallel rays form a focus in front of the retina which is brought on the retina by a suitable concave lens

e. The optic disc is distinctly larger in size with a temporal or annular crescent.

f. There is a shallow cupping.

g. The fundus background appears tessellated.

Clinically and Pathologically Myopia is of Two Types

1. *Simple myopia*, which is not associated with degenerative chorio-retinal changes.
2. *Pathological myopia* when in due course of time degenerative changes lead to severe deterioration of vision and complications.

1. **Simple myopia:** Myopia sets in usually around the school-going age, and increases as the body grows. The increase is usually arrested by about the age of 18–20 years in boys and 15–16 years in girls as the growth of body has reached the limit. Simple myopia is considered moderate up to 6 dioptres and high when more than six dioptres. The main symptom of myopics is defective vision for distance. Often the difficulty in seeing the writing on the black board in school is the first clinical symptom. A medical report from school may draw the attention of the parents. Sometimes, parents note that the child holds reading objects at a close distance. Uncorrected myopics have a habit of narrowing the palpabral fissure which helps them to improve the vision to some extent but this may cause symptoms of eye strain. Because of the poor use of accommodation, myopic eyes have a tendency to develop exophoria or exotropia.

2. **Pathological myopia:** If myopia continues to progress beyond the age of puberty, it is usually associated with degenerative changes in the retina. The degree of myopia has usually reached 10 diopters or more by puberty and may progress to as high as 20-25 diopters. Degenerative changes which involve posterior pole, macular area and the peripheral retina, may lead to further deterioration of vision, which cannot be improved with glasses. Large

patches of chorio-retinal atrophy with sclera shining through around the posterior pole are commonly seen in advanced stages of pathological myopia. Peripheral degenerative changes may lead to retinal detachment.

It was generally believed that myopic eyes are less prone to glaucoma, it is necessary to emphasize that glaucoma is not as rare in myopes as is often believed. The erroneous impression is because myopic eyes do not record higher grades of intra-ocular tension due to compensatory stretching of the coats of the eye ball. This is the reason why diagnosis of glaucoma is often missed in myopic eyes. It is usually a low tension glaucoma with an open angle and is best diagnosed by field changes and provocative tests. A myopic disc usually has a large temporal cupping and it can be a matter of critical evaluation of this cupping from the glaucomatous cupping.

Changes in the lens in high myopia are also a frequent association and these usually become clinically evident in older age. The eye may give an appearance of advanced cataract although the lens change is not as advanced.

The colour of the pupil in these eyes is typically brownish white. The lens change is characteristically nuclear, in the form of nuclear sclerosis, but no gross opacity. The differential diagnosis from immature cataract can always be confirmed by examination of the lens under mydriasis. Many eyes are operated for cataract under misplaced diagnosis unless ophthalmoscopy is done in all such cases.

The vitreous in high myopia is fluid in nature and often develops floating opacities. Black spots in front of the eyes are therefore another important symptom of myopic patients. Because of the fluid nature of vitreous, the supporting network usually breaks down and appears in the form of fibrillar or web-like opacities floating in front of eyes. There may be large floaters from degenerative patches in the retina in malignant myopia. Choroidal haemorrhage deep to the macular area may cause sudden diminution of vision and appear as a brownish red spot, called *Foster Fuchs' flakes*. Stretching of the outer coats can lead to ectasia of the sclera at the posterior pole which is called a *posterior staphyloma* which covers an area of 2-3 disc diameter. It can be clinically detected by ophthalmoscopy by finding a difference in the dioptric level of retina near and away from the disc.

Prognosis of myopia: The most important consideration from the patient's point of view is the unavoidable progress of myopia. The patient and parents should therefore be clearly advised that myopia is going to increase and that in most cases of simple myopia, the increase will be arrested by the time the body has grown to full size on reaching puberty.

The prognosis of pathological myopia, however, is always uncertain and in bad cases may lead to extremely poor vision which cannot be improved with visual aids. It is however interesting to note that the incidence of retinal detachment is less common in high pathological myopia as compared to moderate degrees of myopia.

It is also a well known fact that once a high myopic retina has developed chorio-retinal degenerative changes, it is incapable of undergoing any other pathological change such as vascular retinopathies. Thus a diabetic with high myopic changes rarely, if at all, develops diabetic retinopathy.

Treatment of myopia: Suitable concave lenses is the treatment for improving vision in myopia. Correction of –0.50 to –1.0 diopter may need to be used only when clarity of distance vision is important like in seeing a movie or driving. Any myopic correction of more than 1 diopter should be used constantly even though the patient can read without glasses. He should be advised to use the correction both for distance and near because it will increase the distance between the far and near point and hence relieve strain.

Patients needing higher degrees of myopic correction are however entirely dependent on lenses all the time. A full correction in myopia is usually avoided. It is better to sacrifice one line in distance vision because that will make the patient comfortable for near work. The higher the myopia, larger the under correction.

In an uncorrected myopic eye the image at the retinal level is larger. Correction by lens reduces it to the normal size. In over correction therefore and sometimes even in full correction, the patient sees the objects small. One should therefore be careful to ask the patient whether the size of the object has become smaller with the best correction and if so, an under correction is clearly indicated at least at the first stage. In high degrees of myopia, a separate prescription may be given for near work even before the presbyopic age. It may also be advisable to prescribe lenticular glasses with a flatter periphery to avoid prismatic effect when looking through the periphery of the lens.

A question is often asked whether non-use of myopic glasses will contribute to rapid increase in myopia and whether early use of glasses would have stopped the increase. There is no reason to believe that this is so. Myopics will feel more comfortable with moderately tinted glasses because of the larger size of the pupil.

Contact lenses have a definite place in optical correction of myopic eyes both from cosmetic as well as from visual point of view. High myopic lenses in spectacles may be difficult to tolerate. In some cases vision may not improve with glasses to a satisfactory level and in both these situations contact lenses may be a distinct advantage.

That the use of a contact, lens can reduce myopia is a misplaced concept and there is no evidence in support of this claim. Contact lens practitioners claimed that a technique called *orthokeratology* in which more and more tight fitting lenses are given at 3–4 month interval with the hope that it will flatten the cornea and reduce myopia. There is no reason to believe that this can bring about any lasting change in myopia. Furthermore, a tight fitting lens is uncomfortable to tolerate.

High myopes with degenerative changes where the vision is poor and cannot improve with ordinary lenses or with contact lenses, may be benefited to some degree with the use of special low visual aids. The indication of prescription of low visual aids is when the vision is reduced to less than 6/60, even with best optical correction. If a patient cannot afford a telescope type of low vision aids, a hand magnifier may be helpful.

Surgical treatment: Myopia being a common refractive state and still increasing in incidence in years to come, attention has been given for decades whether it can be cured rather than treated with spectacles. The removal of a physiological lens of +20.0 diopters to reduce a myopia of −12 to −15 diopters was for some time considered a therapeutic measure. Removal of lens in high myopia with degenerated fluid vitreous was associated with serious operative and post-operative complications. It even precipitated retinal detachment in some cases. This surgery therefore never reached a stage of general acceptance. Shortening of the antero-posterior length of the eye ball by *circumferential sclerectomy* just in front of the equator had also been tried by dare-devil ophthalmologists. It was never accepted as a surgical answer to myopia.

Scientifically more accepted but too sophisticated a procedure indicated even for moderate degrees of myopia is *keratomilieusis.* A lamellar button of corneal stroma of measured thickness after computerised calculations, is removed from the cornea of the myopic eye. This reduces the thickness and so the refracting power of the cornea and thus reduces the myopic error. *Radial keratotomy* as a simple surgical procedure at the anterior pole had fascinated many eye surgeons the world over. The procedure first conceived by Sato in Japan and later developed by Fyodorov in Moscow aims at flattening the cornea. Because of the limited change in the cornea the procedure has its own limitations. The resultant effect of this procedure, even though temporary, does not reduce myopia by more than 4–5 diopters.

Intra lamellar calculated stromal excision with excimer laser in optical zone is a procedure to reduce corneal thickness and thus reduce myopic refraction. Excimer keratomy for high astigmatism is also practiced.

In the last few decades, refractive surgery for myopia has been developed with use of laser (LASIK) for flattening the cornea.

Myopia being a progressive condition, causes concern to the patient and to parents for the future fate of these eyes. Although most myopes are in the simple category and do not lead to unremediable serious consequences, appropriate advice is necessary in cases of progressive and pathological myopes. Genetic inheritance of myopia is accepted and therefore marriages between myopic families should, if possible, be avoided. Glasses should be used from early age and changed from time to time. Care for visual hygiene is necessary. Good light and not holding the objects too close for near work is advisable.

In high myopia specially with degenerative changes, appropriate counselling is necessary in selecting the professional career for the reason that at the crucial time the patient may not be declared unfit for the job.

Astigmatism

Astigmatism is a refractive condition where the parallel rays entering the eye in two principle meridia do not form a focus at the same level. If one meridian is focussed at retina and the other in front of. retina, it is called *simple myopic astigmatism.* If the rays in both meridia focus in front of retina but at different levels, it is called

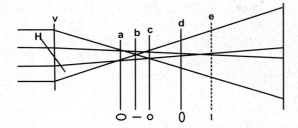

Fig. 24.9: Astigmatism—Sturm's Conoid. V—vertical meridian; H—horizontal merdian; (a) Compound astigmatism more in horizontal than in vertical meridian; (b) Simple astigmatism in horizontal direction; (c) Circle of least diffusion; (d) Compound astigmatism more in vertical axis; (e) Simple astigmatism in vertical direction

compound myopic astigmatism. If the rays of one meridian focus on the retina and the other behind retina, it is called *simple hypermetropic astigmatism* and if both focus behind retina but at different levels, it is called *compound hypermetropic astigmatism.* If one meridian focuses in front of retina (myopic) and the other meridian behind retina (hypermetropic) it is called *mixed astigmatism.*

The optics of astigmatism is best illustrated in the diagram which has been described as Sturm's conoid. The illustration shows the changes in the form of focus of light as the rays in two principal meridia at right angles to each other converge at different levels. At points where one meridian is focused and the other is not, the focus formed is a line, vertical or horizontal and represents simple astigmatism.

Similarly, the images are oval when the convergence and divergence of rays are unequal and represent, compound astigmatism. Where the convergence of the set of rays and divergence of other are equal, the image is circular.

Astigmatism alone or in association with a small spherical error is in most eyes a rule rather than an exception. Some small degree of astigmatism is invariably present which is called physiological astigmatism. It is due to two important physiological variants. First is the

increased radius of curvature of anterior surface of the cornea in the vertical meridian as compared to the horizontal meridian. The second factor is the slight rotation of the lens axis so that the nasal border of the lens is slightly in front of the temporal border and the upper border is slightly in front as compared to the lower border. This small physiological astigmatism also called *"astigmatism with the rule"* is corrected by a small plus cylinder in the vertical axis or a small minus cylinder in the horizontal axis. Astigmatism with the rule, usually reverses in old age needing a plus cylinder in the horizontal axis or a minus cylinder in the vertical axis.

If the two meridia of astigmatic refraction are in the vertical and horizontal axes respectively, it is *regular astigmatism.* If two meridia, though at right angles but are away from the vertical and horizontal meridia, it is called *oblique astigmatism.* If the two meridia are in oblique axis but not at right angles to each other, it is called *obliquely oblique astigmatism* or *bi-oblique astigmatism.* When the refractive state of the eye is such that it is not possible to refract either meridian due to anomalous movement seen on retinoscopy, it is *irregular astigmatism* and is mostly corneal in origin. It can easily be confirmed with the use of placedo's disc in which the concentric lines will appear distorted, irregular and wavy. Common conditions responsible for irregular corneal astigmatism are keratoconus, trachomatous cornea and corneal facets and nebulae.

Regular astigmatic error can be brought about by a number of factors. Most astigmatic errors are due to changes in curvature of cornea which is called *corneal astigmatism.* Change in the curvature of the anterior or posterior surfaces of lens can also cause *curvature astigmatism,* though it is much less common. Another important causative factor is the change in the refractive index of the lens which can induce *lenticular astigmatism.* This is particularly common in old age, when vision improves with a cylindrical correction for the first time, there having been no astigmatic error in the earlier age.

Retinoscopy in astigmatism: The assessment of correct astigmatism by retinoscopy demands good practice and experience. It is not uncommon to face difficulty in case of small astigmatic errors. Larger degrees of astigmatism however become evident as soon as the movements of the fundus glow are observed.

Clinical Features

It is evident from the above that the focus of rays in two meridia do not form at the same level and hence the visual clarity is different in the vertical and horizontal components of the objects seen. The commonest and most characteristic observation is that a patient can read lines of the chart but commits mistakes in each line leading to a visual record as for example 6/24 P, 6/18 P, 6/12 P. This can also be denoted as 6/12–3, 6/9–2 etc. On the other hand, a patient with a spherical error will read a few lines correctly and then suddenly say that he cannot read further. The effect of astigmatism is usually at right angles to the axis of the cylinder, so that if the astigmatism is in the vertical axis, the horizontal components of the letters look blurred. He therefore misreads some letters like F for T, D for O, etc.

Astigmatic error is a common cause of symptoms of eye strain. This is due to the patient using an accommodative effort to correct the error in one meridian and in doing so makes the other meridian more myopic or more hypermetropic. This continued effort though unsuccessful can give rise to severe eye strain. It is only natural to expect that symptoms are severe in hypermetropic astigmatism because accommodative effort is more in these cases. Symptoms of eye strain are usually less pronounced in a high degree of astigmatic errors because the eye does not make an effort to overcome it. A small degree of anomalous head posture may be present in cases of oblique astigmatism.

Treatment: The treatment consists of prescribing glasses with a cylindrical component not only appropriate in power but also the correctly prescribed direction of cylindrical axis. Glasses with astigmatic component should normally be worn constantly because as stated above, accommodation cannot compensate for the unequal error in two meridia. Astigmatism should always be corrected fully, subject to the tolerance by the patient. It should be borne in mind that sub-total correction of astigmatism may leave behind a small element which may cause more symptoms. Common complaints of patient if the cylindrical axis is not correct are slanting appearance of the ground and difficulty in judgement while going downstairs.

Most astigmatic errors are developmental in origin. A person who has not used astigmatic correction till adult age and is accustomed to the shapes and forms of objects as seen, may therefore not tolerate an astigmatic correction when prescribed for the first time later in age. A compromise has to be evolved wherein only so much astigmatic error is corrected as can be tolerated and 50 per cent of the undercorrection added as a sphere. Excimer keratotomy for high astigmatism has already been referred.

If retinoscopy indicates a cylinder of opposite sign in two eyes, it may be advisable to so transpose that the cylinder in both eyes should be of same sign, provided they are symmetrical in axis.

Irregular astigmatism due to the anterior surface of the cornea, is correctable only by contact lenses. Contact lenses are also a better alternative for eyes with high astigmatism or where the astigmatic lenses are not tolerated by the patient.

Presbyopia

Presbyopia is a variant of physiological state of the eye. There is difficulty in seeing near objects clearly in old age. It is a condition caused by two factors, viz., changes in the lens and weakness of accommodation. As age advances, the central part of the lens becomes harder. Simultaneously, the physiological activity of the ciliary muscle also becomes weak. The accommodative power of the eye is usually reduced to about 3 diopters of accommodation by the time an emmetrope reaches the age of 40–45 years. It becomes still less in older age but the eye never totally loses its accommodative power.

The patient usually tries to overcome the early stage of presbyopia by holding the object farther than the usual 13–15 inches, using brighter light for near work and extra accommodative effort.

Clinically, presbyopic needs help of glasses around the age of 40–45 years by which time the near point of the emmetropic eye recedes beyond the comfortable working distance. Premature presbyopia sets in hypermetropic eyes so that near glasses may be needed earlier. A myopic on the other hand has the advantage that he will need separate near correction at a later age depending on the degree of myopia. As the lens elasticity decreases and accommodation becomes still weaker, presbyopic glasses need to be stronger at regular intervals, depending on the elasticity and amplitude of accommodation of the individual. Some patients prolong this interval by a few months by shifting the position of the glasses on the bridge of the nose farther away from the eyes which increases the effective power of the convex glasses used for presbyopia.

Treatment: Correction of presbyopia requires the use of convex lenses. It is important that one should give only as much presbyopic correction as is needed to see objects clearly at a comfortable working distance of an individual. With the final lenses in a trial frame, the patient should be asked to move the near-vision chart a few inches forwards and backwards to ensure that he has a good working range. For comfortable near working, at least one-fourth of reserve accommodation will be helpful.

Spherical presbyopic correction should, in an ametropic eye, be an addition to distance glasses and should carry appropriate cylindrical component in the near correction also. Every presbyopic should therefore be tested for distance vision which, if less than 6/9 in each eye, should be refracted and correction for distance determined and only then the presbyopic correction added and prescribed. Patient is asked to use glasses both for distance and near. Whether an emmetropic patient should use a bifocal with no power in the distance segment or use presbyopic glasses for near work only, will depend on the type of work and profession the patient is involved in.

Aphakia

The term aphakia means an eye without the lens. It should however also include the condition when the lens is not present in the visual axis. The correct definition of aphakia will therefore be absence of lens in the pupillary area which includes surgical removal of the lens or that the lens is congenitally absent or the lens is dislocated into the vitreous and lies in a position away from the visual axis.

Treatment: As the strong refracting medium, the only treatment for aphakia is to provide an alternate correcting lens. The human lens that has been removed from the eye has an average power of 18–20 diopters. A proportionate high power correcting lens is necessary, which can be provided in a spectacle frame, a contact lens on the anterior surface of cornea or an intraocular lens inside the eye.

The most common spherical component of an aphakic correction in a previously emmetropic eye is +9 to +11 diopters. It will obviously be lesser in myopic eyes and larger in hypermetropic eyes. Most aphakic eyes have some degree of astigmatism of about 1.5 to 2.5 dioptres cylinder in the horizontal axis. This is caused by the flattening of the cornea in the vertical meridian by the healing process of the cataract section. This astigmatic element will be understandably less where cataract surgery is either decision and aspiration as in juvenile cataract or lensectomy operation through the pars plana. Small incision cataract surgery (SICS) reduces post-operative astigmatism to a great extent.

It is evident that aphakic eyes have no accommodation and therefore a separate correction is always needed for near work. The usual addition is +3.0 to +3.5 dioptres to distance correction. Bifocal and multifocal IOLs have been designed. Some surgeons have used them with gratifying results. No extra near correction is needed when such an IOL is implanted.

Contact lenses: The improvement in the quality of material and fitting of contact lenses has provided a better alternative to aphakic spectacles. A significant advantage of a contact lens in the aphakic eye is the reduction in the magnification of the object seen. The magnification of the object which is nearly 30% with the spectacle lenses is reduced to 9 to 11% with a contact lens. Contact lenses also have the advantage of giving full visual fields, avoiding prismatic effects, etc. A higher degree of binocularily is possible with contact lenses in uniocular aphakia, but it still cannot reach the degree of stereopsis because of the disparity of the sizes of the objects seen by two eyes.

Pseudophakia (Aphakia with Intra-ocular lens implant)

Ideal position is by introduction of an acrylic lens inside the eye and the resultant condition is called *pseudophakia.*

A posterior chamber lens will be exactly where the human lens is situated and therefore of greater advantage. An intra-ocular lens is nearest to overcoming disadvantages of a spectacle lens and a contact lens. Perfect binocularity with stereopsis in uniocular aphakia is possible only with an intra-ocular lens.

The power of the lenses needed can be determined accurately by ultrasonography and a custom-made intra-ocular lens can then be available for precision work. The magnification of the objects seen with an intraocular lens implant is insignificant to a degree of 1.9% only.

ANISOMETROPIA

It is a condition where the refractive state of two eyes is unequal. There can be various possibilities. One eye may be emmetropic and the other may be hypermetropic or myopic. Both eyes may be hypermetropic or myopic but unequal in power. One eye may be hypermetropic and the other myopic. One eye may be emmetropic and the other astigmatic. Both eyes may be simple or compound astigmatic but of unequal grade.

Vision in anisometropia will naturally be unequal without correction. In case one eye is myopic and the other hypermetropic, the hypermetropic eye may be used for distance and myopic for near and the patient may get comfortably adjusted to this situation. The eye with higher refractive error tends to develop amblyopia and squint from early childhood and this is more common with uniocular or unequal hypermetropic error of refraction.

An important consideration in hypermetropia is the size of the image presented to each eye. A difference of 0.25 dioptre causes a difference in size by 0.5%. It is generally true that a difference of more than 5% in the size of the images is not tolerated by the patient, and the weaker eye in such cases tends to develop amblyopia or squint. It therefore means that the eye will not tolerate glasses and maintain binocular vision if the difference between the correction of the two eyes is 2.5 dioptres or more. This is by and large true but binocularity has been known with higher difference, particularly in myopic eyes. Binocularity in myopic eyes is sometimes possible even with very large anisometropia if the weaker eye (higher myopia) is corrected by contact lenses.

Treatment: The prescription of glasses for anisometropia should be aimed at bringing the vision of both the eyes to equal level or as near as possible. This should, however, be compatible with the acceptance of the correction and the maintenance of binocularity. A higher degree of anisometropia, particularly in cases of high myopia in one eye are treated with contact lenses and better still is LASIK refractive surgery.

ANISEIKONIA

It is a refractive condition when the images formed on the retina of the two eyes are unequal in size and differ in shape. This condition could be due to the high degree of anisometropia as already described and this is called diopteric *aniseikonia*. More disturbing however is the unequal shape of the two images, which is due to unequal concentration and distribution of cones in the macular area, usually developmental in origin. This is called *morphological anisei-konia*.

The eyes have a capacity to overcome small degrees of difference in the shape of the two images by their power of fusion and stereopsis maintaining perfect binocularity. If however the degree of aniseikonia is of higher order, the patient is not only disturbed by the unequal shape of the two images but also manifests symptoms of eye strain.

Treatment: Aniseikonia can only be corrected by special lenses called *iseikonic lenses*. The special quality of these lenses is that it magnifies the object without a change in the dioptric power. These lenses are costly to manufacture and not ideally suited to all patients. The use of contact lenses is helpful only for dioptric aniseikonia and not for morphological aniseikonia.

The various forms and types of spectacle lenses may be listed as follows:

1. Distance or constant use lenses.
2. Lenses for near vision, presbyopic lenses.
3. Bifocal lenses which may be:
   a. Lens with a small round near segment.
   b. Lens with a small D near segment.
   c. Executive bifocal with a demarcated lower half for near.

   The near segment may be joined edge to edge or may be cemented on a distance piece. A good quality bifocal is one in which near button of flint glass (higher refractive index) is fused onto the distance lens. These are called invisible bifocals.
4. Trifocal lenses.
5. Multifocal lenses with gradient power.

All the above lenses can be made into lenses of various tints, the standard ones are:

1. A1—Light grey
2. A2—Light blue
3. B1—Light smoke
4. B2—Dark sun glasses colour
5. Pinkish colour.
6. Photochromatic lenses.

Bifocal lenses are best indicated for desk workers. Some people, however, prefer to take off and put on presbyopic glasses or even interchange separate near and distance glasses rather than use bifocals. For constant use of bifocals, the patient has to get adjusted and should avoid looking through reading segment when going downstairs. Final advice should, therefore, depend on patient's requirement and his attitude to use or not use bifocals. From the clinical point of view, it makes no difference whether the patient uses bifocals or separate glasses for distance and near.

Trifocal and multifocal lenses are specially indicated for people who have to see at close distance and long distance. Multifocal lenses are also good for professionals like doctors and lawyers who have to write, look at patient across the table and at the same time at distance objects. Progressive corrections are best for the purpose.

LENTICULAR LENSES

These are special types of lenses where the power is maximum in the centre but is reduced in the peripheral part of the lens to overcome the prismatic effect. They are specifically indicated for high myopic eyes.

Transposition of Lenses

By transposition of lenses is meant, conversion of one prescription of lens into another but with same resultant refracting power. The transposition may be simple and is commonly required to alter the quality of the cylinder in a compound lens from minus to plus or vice-versa. This is sometimes required to change the sign of cylinder so that it corresponds to the cylinder of the opposite eye because it is advisable that the sign of the cylinder in two eyes should be identical. It is also transposition where the sign of the spherical component may need to be changed either for the comfort of the eye or to make the lens lighter in weight. The ophthalmologist may need these transpositions when prescribing glasses and should, therefore, know and understand the optics of simple transpositions. A few examples will make it clear.

In compound lenses

$$1. \quad \frac{+3.0 \, \text{Dsph}}{-1.0 \, \text{Dcyl} \mapsto 180°} = \frac{+2.0 \, \text{Dsph}}{+1.0 \, \text{Dcyl} \uparrow 90°}$$

$$2. \quad \frac{+3.0 \, \text{Dsph}}{+2.0 \, \text{Dcyl} \uparrow 90°} = \frac{+5.0 \, \text{Dsph}}{-2.0 \, \text{Dcyl} \mapsto 180°}$$

In mixed astigmatism

$$3. \quad \frac{+2.0 \, \text{Dcyl} \uparrow 90°}{-1.0 \, \text{Dcyl} \mapsto 180°} = \frac{+2.0 \, \text{Dsph}}{+3.0 \, \text{Dcyl} \mapsto 180°}$$

or

$$\frac{-1.0 \, \text{Dsph}}{+3.0 \, \text{Dcyl} \mapsto 90°}$$

It is evident in (3) above that prescription (b) will be lighter in weight and should therefore be preferred but for presbyopic correction (a) will be better.

Toric Transposition

This is more often necessary for the optician when manufacturing a lens with base curve on one surface and the power on the other surface. For plus lenses a minus base curve is used and for minus lenses a plus base curve is used. A lens with a 1.25D base curve is known as a meniscus lens and one with a 6D base curve is known as toric lens.

There is a standard formula for toric transposition. The formula is based on the following steps for a given prescription.

1. Convert the prescription so that the sign of the cylinder is same as the sign of the base curve, if necessary.
2. Now subtract the base curve from the sphere of this prescription to get the numerator.
3. Write the first denominator as the base curve in the form of a cylinder of same sign with axis at right angles to the axis of cylinder of the prescription.
4. Add the second denominator which should be of a power which gives the difference in the two denominators equal to the power of the cylinder in the prescription. The axis of the second denominator should be at right angles to the first denominator.

Requirements for Refraction Clinic

A routine refraction clinic needs the following equipment:
1. Vision charts.
2. Trial frame.
3. Trial lenses.
4. Cross cylinder.
5. Retinoscopy outfit.
6. Ophthalmoscope.

Vision charts: The best vision charts are internally illuminated drums or illuminated sliding charts. The latter has the advantage that the patient sees only one line at a time and cannot easily memorise the chart. Moreover one can skip over the line and save time. Whether it is a drum or a sliding chart, there should be provision for a Duochrome test and an astigmatic fan either as a part of the drum or separately fixed. For examination of patients outside the clinic, in schools and in eye camps, vision charts on cardboard sheets are convenient to carry. There should always be a provision for 'C', 'E' or dots charts for illiterate patients. The chart should be in the regional language of the area in addition to English and Hindi charts for literate patients. It is only rarely that a picture chart may be needed for small children because most children at the age of 4–5 years can count and even read alphabets.

Reading charts should similarly be both for literates in different languages and in dots for illiterates.

Trial frames: It is important to have a trial frame which stays close to the eye and remains steady and has provision for the adjustment of the interpupillary distance as well as shortening and lengthening the side fittings on the ear to make it comfortable. An added luxury can be a provision in the trial frame of rotating the lens with a mechanical device as is provided in West German Oculus and Japanese trial frames. Sophisticated frames also have a provision for measuring the back vertex distance which should be indicated on prescription to help the optician for preparing an optically good pair of spectacles.

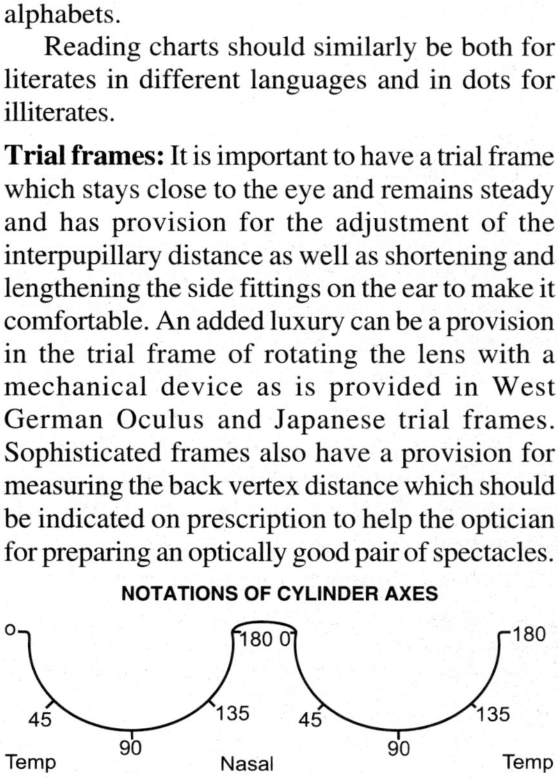

NOTATIONS OF CYLINDER AXES

Fig. 24.10: Axis markings on trial frame

Cross cylinder: This is a very useful and handy small instrument for confirming the cylindrical power of the lens in the prescription. The commonest cross cylinder and the one most frequently used is the one which has a combination of –0.25 Dsph and +0.5 Dcyl. The resultant action is equal to +0.25 Dcyl in one axis and –0.25 in the axis at right angles. Its use is described alongwith retinoscopy and the post mydratic subjective test.

Trial lenses: A set of trial lenses in a trial case is essential for retinoscopy and post-cycloplegic test. For retinoscopy, only a set of spherical lenses, both convex and concave, may be enough. It is however better if cylindrical lenses are also available because that helps in the confirmation of retinoscopy readings. For a post-cycloplegic test, however, a set of spherical lenses, cylindrical lenses and prisms are necessary. The trial case should also have a pin-hole disc, stenopic slit disc and a block disc. A good trial case should preferably have small aperture lenses so framed that they are easy to manually rotate in the trial frame. It is also important that the marking of the axis on cylindrical lenses be very accurate. The sets of convex and concave lenses should be easily identifiable even in a dark room. An illumination device in the trial case helps to pick up correct lenses during the procedure of retinoscopy and post-cycloplegic test.

Visual Aids

There are two different groups of visual aids needed: The first group are visual aids for specific purposes in well-sighted people. The second group are aids for people who are grossly visually handicapped and these are called low visual aids.

Visual aids for well-sighted people: Apart from spectacles for distance and near, special aids are often needed for specific purposes. A few among common such aids are:

1. Operating glasses or loups for the surgeons, which provide magnification of 2.5 to 6 times. The aids all have incorporated prisms to avoid strain of convergence.
2. Prismatic recumbent glasses for people who are non-ambulatory lying in plaster and who must read while lying flat.
3. Divers glasses: These allow vision under water. Water neutralises the power of the cornea and makes the eye highly hyper-metropic. Diver's glasses are made with a binconvex air lens in between the two glass miniscus lenses.
4. Adapting goggles with red filter glasses for working in dark room and yet avoiding the white light as in photography work.
5. Polaroid glasses for fishermen and drivers to offset the surface reflection from water or shining ground.
6. Protecting glasses for welders and workers exposed to welding arcs and molten metals. These glasses absorb 95% of infra-red and ultra-violet lights.
7. Lead glass for X-ray technicians for protection against radiation.
8. Sun goggles for protection against sunlight and solar eclipse.

Low Visual Aids (LVA)

Low visual aids are required for visually handicapped persons and where vision cannot be improved with regular lenses. The first requirements in such cases is that they should have some residual vision, preferably better than 2/60. The purpose of visual aids in such patients is to help them in reading and writing. Most of these aids are magnifying aids and the person using them has to get used to the method of use and the distance at which they should be used. These aids have the disadvantages that the field is restricted and the reading object has to be held steady.

The common conditions where low visual aids are needed are:

1. Myopic degeneration.
2. Diabetic retinopathy.
3. Chorio-retinitis.
4. Albinism.
5. Macular degeneration.
6. Retinitis pigmentosa.
7. Retinal detachment.
8. Optic atrophy.
9. Glaucoma.

Magnifying low visual aids that are commonly used are:

1. Magnifying spectacles.
2. Hand-held magnifiers.
3. Magnifiers on stand, un-illuminated or illuminated.
4. Telescopic glasses.
5. Stenopic pinhole glasses specially for cases with poor vision due to irregular corneal and lens opacities. These are also helpful in albinism because they help cutting off extra light. The pinholes are from 1 to 2 mm in diameter and help improvement of vision by making the image more defined and clear cut.

The type of low visual aid needed by a particular individual will depend on the need of the person, the amount of residual vision, the amount of improvement in vision with the aid and the economic condition of the person.

25

Congenital Anomalies of the Eye Ball

It is important to mention here that developmental defects include not only structural anomalies but scores of more subtle, chemical or functional abnormalities. Thus a number of pathological conditions are grouped as 'genetically determined error of metabolism' such as galactosaemia, affections of lipid metabolism or amino acids metabolism.

It is better to recollect here that the development of the eye ball also follows the general pattern of development passing through the period of *'embryogenesis'* during which a fertilised ovum becomes an identifiable embryo, a period of *'organogenesis'* when embryonic tissues differentiate themselves and future organs of the body can be individually identified and lastly the period of *foetal life* when further development; structural and functional, of the organs take place to complete the development of the foetus.

It is easy to understand that if a causative factor is present during the period of embryogenesis i.e., the period of the first four weeks, the deformity is gross and mostly incompatible with life if generalised. If localised, affecting only the development of the optic vesicle, the ocular anomaly is gross like anophthalmos, cyclopia etc. During the next four weeks, 4–8 weeks, a rudimentary eye ball has already formed and

individual structures are being differentiated. Any disturbance at this stage affects their development and results in anomalies like micro-cornea, microphthalmos with cyst, colabomata of uveal tract etc., which grossly affect function of the eye ball.

During the foetal period, that is from 8 weeks to birth, a detrimental influence can cause only a minor defect because a fully differentiated miniature eye ball has already formed.

The ocular anomalies occuring during this period involve individual tissues. These may be:
a. Generalised under-developed eye ball which is functionally normal.
b. Congenital cataract of different types.
c. Anterior chamber anomalies.
d. Angle of the anterior chamber anomalies.

Some of the common deformities clinically seen are described below:
1. Anophthalmos means complete absence of ocular tissues. The diagnosis of this condition is possible only by histological sections of orbital tissues. Clinically however, anophthalmos is a condition where the eye ball appears to be absent. Anophthalmos can be due to:
   a. Failure of the optic plate to form into an optic vesicle. This occurs before 2 mm stage and is the real anophthalmos called

primary anophthalmos. The rest of the forebrain develops normally. It is compatible with the normal development of rest of the body but blind life.

b. Complete failure of development of forebrain including optic plates from the neural tube causing *secondary anophthalmos.* This is not compatible with normal development. The foetus is usually a monster and does not survive.

c. A third type of anophthalmos may result from degeneration or atrophy of the optic vesicle soon after its formation. These are usually clinically seen as cases of extreme microphthalmos. A rudimentary eye ball-like structure or a very small pinhead sized cornea-like disc appears on a pea-sized nodule.

Anophthalmos, clinically, may be present bilaterally or may be unilateral with a microphthalmic or normal eye ball on the other side.

2. **Cyclopia:** This is an anomaly due to fusion of two optic vesicles. The fusion may be complete or partial to form a single eye ball in the centre. Complete fusion of two optic vesicles or formation of one single optic vesicle in the centre results in 'cyclopia'. True cyclopia is almost always associated with anomalies of anterior brain and mesodermal structures in median plain. These anomalies are not compatible with life because of involvement of brain and midline structure of the face and thorax.

3. **Congenital cystic eye:** The optic vesicle is formed but fails to be invaginated by surface ectoderm anteriorly and there is no formation of embryonic fissure on the lower medial surface. This results in persistence of optic vesicle cavity and failure of formation into a secondary optic cup. The conjunctiva and lids are formed normally but the eye ball tissues fail to differentiate and the distended vesicle occupies orbit to result in *anophthalmos with orbital cyst.*

Congenital non-attachment of retina. Partial invagination of the cup may take place. There may be a small lens anteriorly but the anterior wall of the optic vesicle (future retina) fails to appose posterior wall of optic vesicle (pigment epithelium). The congenital detachment unlike acquired detachment, extends even beyond the ora serrata.

4. **Colobomata:** Anomalies due to defective closure of embryonic fissure result in *typical colobamata.* The time of invagination of the optic vesicle and closure of the embryonic fissure is between 7–14 mm stage of development or the 4th to 5th week period.

Colobomata may be complete or partial, that is, along the whole extent of the fissure or only in part. The basic defect is non-closure of the fissure at the edges of which the retinal layers undergo an eversion. A number of defects occur depending on the extent of retinal eversion and degree of non-closure.

They are due to:
i. Non differentiation of retina in the area of open fissure.
ii. Everted retinal elements prevent pigment epithelium in the area.
iii. Choriocapillaris fail to develop in the area.
iv. Sclera remains thin.

The two layers of undifferentiated neuro-ectoderm undergo atrophy and fusion and line the sclera in the coloboma area in which there is no pigment epithelial layer and no choroid.

Clinical appearance: All the tissues associated with the embryonic cleft or only some of them, may be involved. When all tissues are, involved, the coloboma extends from optic nerve head posteriorly to the pupillary margin of the iris anteriorly. When only part of the extent of the embryonic fissure fails to close, the coloboma is limited and partial. There may be only *coloboma of iris, coloboma of iris and ciliary body or coloboma of choroid* of different grades with or without involvement of the optic nerve head.

Coloboma of the iris is clearly seen during routine examination of the anterior segment. It has to be differentiated from a sector iridectomy or an optical iridectomy in the down and inward situation to which it greatly resembles. However great the similarity, the collarette of the iris can be clearly made out to skirt the congenital coloboma following its shape and size while the same is seen abruptly ending at the cut edges of an iridectomy.

Coloboma of the ciliary body usually occurs as part of a complete coloboma. It is not easily seen on clinical examination. It is more often presumed than actually visualised, particularly when other colobomata are present. The presence of coloboma of lens and absence of zonule corroborate a most likely presence of ciliary body coloboma.

Coloboma of the choroid and retina is discovered accidentally on routine ophthalmoscopic examination or looked for expectantly when anterior segment examination has revealed an iris coloboma in a normal or microphthalmic eye or in case of a microcornea.

The appearance is striking. In the area of the coloboma, the normal pink red reflex of the fundus is completely replaced by a glistening white background appearance of sclera with clear cut margins showing varying degrees of pigmentation. Blood vessels crossing over the floor can easily be distinguished as those belonging to the retinal system. These vessels dip at the edge of the coloboma to reach the floor while a few choroidal vessels which are broad and irregularly antastomosing are on the floor of coloboma lying at a deeper level.

The chorio-retinal coloboma can be graded according to its situation and extent as follows:

i. A small round or oval defect anywhere in the line of the embryonic fissure from the infero-nasal disc margin to the inferonasal periphery. There may be more than one such defect with a bridge of more or less normal tissue between them. This is sometimes called a *bridge coloboma*.

ii. A coloboma extending from the periphery towards the lower nasal disc margin with normal retina and choroid between the posterior edge of the coloboma and the disc margin. The posterior edge is always convex towards the disc; the coloboma being broader peripherally.

iii. Convexity of the posterior extremity of coloboma enclosing the entire disc.

iv. The most minor grade of coloboma of choroid-retina is the presence of an inferior crescent at the disc or a lightly pigmented linear appearance in the line of the embryonic fissure with some amount of choroidal thinning.

Coloboma of the optic nerve is usually part of a complete coloboma of the embryonic fissure. A coloboma of the nerve head alone is rare. Abnormal entrance of the central vessels is common.

Visual acuity. Cases with partial coloboma of choroid discovered in routine ophthalmoscopy may not cause any gross visual disturbance. A negative scotoma is recorded on perimetry which is smaller than the size of the coloboma because normally functioning retina overlays the edges of coloboma. When coloboma is associated with other congenital anomalies like micro-cornea or microphthalmos and the eyes have developed squint or nystagmus, there is gross diminution of vision (Fig. 25.1, Plate 15).

5. **Anomalies in the size of the eye**. *Microphthalmos*. A smaller than normal eye ball has a functional defect also. The anomaly occurs due to influences affecting optic cup

and embryonic fissure and is therefore often associated with other anomalies. Rarely a small eye ball is structurally and functionally normal except for size. It is usually transmitted as a dominant heredity. The exact etiological factor cannot be determined in these cases. Heredity of different types, maternal environmental factors, Rh incompatibility, X-ray exposures, maternal infections have all been suggested as possible factors.

The next group of anomalies include individual tissues of the eye ball. Which fail to develop into normal structure and therefore function.

Cornea

Developmental anomalies of cornea may involve:
  i. Size of the cornea,
  ii. Curvature of the cornea,
  iii. Transparency of the cornea.

Size of the Cornea

a. *Megalocornea:* Also known as megalophthalmos. The diameter of the cornea is very distinctly larger than normal. A diameter of 16-18 mm has been recorded. Thickness of the cornea is normal. It has to be differentiated from buphthalmos by the absence of raised intra-ocular tension, absence of Descemet's tears and stromal oedema, absence of embryonic mesodermal tissues in the angle of the anterior chamber and normal function of the eye.

b. *Micro-cornea:* Micro-cornea is often associated with other ocular anomalies but occurrence of a slightly small cornea in an otherwise normal eye ball is not uncommon. Many eyes with a small cornea tend to be myopic with relatively increased corneal curvature and a normal sized lens which is bigger for the smaller anterior segment (Fig. 25.2).

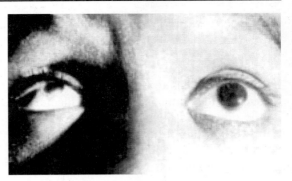

Fig 25.2: Micro-cornea BE and microphthalmos-RE

Curvature of the Cornea

a. *Cornea plana* is a condition when the corneal curvature fails to increase as compared to scleral curvature. Reduced curvature and resultant flattening of cornea causes a shallow anterior chamber. It also may be associated with corneal opacities.

b. *Keratoglobus:* The curvature of the cornea is increased to the extent that cornea appears globular and eye ball is of normal size. There is no remarkable increase in diameter but stromal thinning, particularly in the periphery many occur. It is usually stationary without any symptoms. Rarely there can be acute episode due to rupture of the Deseemet's membrane and oedema resulting in acute keratoglobus. It should be distinguished from Keratoconus.

c. *Keratoconus* where along with increased curvature, corneal thinning is central giving the conical appearance. Keratoconus very often causes ruptures in the Descemet's membrane resulting in oedema of stroma and hydrops. Keratoconus is a progressive condition. The increased curvature and thinning of the cornea gradually extend towards periphery and in well advanced cases, a paper thin conical cornea extends right upto the limbus.

d. *Posterior keratoconus* may also be present. The anterior corneal curvature is normal but the posterior curvature is increased resulting in the thinning of the cornea in the area. Diagnosis is usually on routine examination on slit lamp in a case of irregular astigmatism. Sometimes a *keratoconus posticus* is observed while dissecting hazy recipient cornea for lamellar grafting. It can cause an inadvertent perforation of the recipient bed.

Transparency of the Cornea

Congenital corneal opacities can be due to:
a. Developmental defects.
b. Intra-uterine inflammations.
c. Hereditarily determined abiotrophies.

Developmental defects: These can result due to effect on the developing cornea
  i. Delayed separation of lens vesicle from surface ectoderm which is the future cornea. In these cases a corresponding defect in the form of an opacity of lens may also be present.
  ii. The mesoderm may fail to develop normally to form iris stroma, corneal endothelium and corneal stroma. This may result in failure of development of corneal endothelium and descemet's membrane of the cornea resulting in an opaque stroma of cornea.

Inflammations: Intra-uterine inflammations of cornea and/or conjunctiva can result in a corneal opacity. The pathology is likely to be very similar to that occurring in childhood or adult life. A foetus may even have an anterior staphyloma or a vascularised opacity.

Heredity: These opacities, better called dystrophies, are bilateral, symmetrical and non-inflammatory. Many of them appear fairly late in life but some, e.g., congenital Fuchs' dystrophy may be present at birth. Hereditary transmission may be recessive or dominant.

Two other conditions need mention here:
Anterior embryotoxon is commonly called 'arcus juvenilis'. It is a ring like opacity similar to arcus senilis, just inside the limbus. It involves the anterior and midstromal layers of corneal periphery.

Posterior embryotoxon is a very prominent Schwalbe's line on posterior corneal surface which, unlike normal Schwalbe's line, is seen easily on a slit lamp. It forms a prominent projection on the posterior corneal surface into the anterior chamber near the angle. Strands of peripheral iris tissue may be seen attached to the line seen on gonioscopy.

Congenital sclero-cornea. The cornea appears like the sclera either only in the periphery so that the distinction between the sclera and cornea at the limbus is lost or the opacity may be diffuse and extend to the centre of cornea in which case there is gross visual loss. A peripheral scleralisation of the cornea does not cause any symptoms.

Limbal dermoid. Metaplastic changes during corneal development usually result in formation of limbal dermoid or very rarely fibrolipomatous nodules at the limbus.

SCLERA

Among congenital anomalies of sclera, blue sclera is frequently seen. It is normally seen in infants. The sclera shows a uniform bluish tinge which is not due to actual discolouration but due to the uveal pigment showing through a less opaque and thinner sclera. Other ocular tissues and functions of the eye are normal. It is perhaps due to defective scleral condensation resulting in the persistence of foetal collagen.

Congenital scleral ectasia involves the posterior pole of the eye ball. A normal nerve head with normal vessels appears to be situated in the floor of a pit which is often surrounded by a halo of atrophic choroid. It is neither a coloboma nor post-inflammatory ectasia. Ectasia occurs due to failure of mesodermal condensation which gives way. Normally too, condensation of the sclera at the posterior pole takes place the last.

Anterior Chamber (AC)

Congenital anomalies of anterior chamber, either absence of AC or presence of mesodermal elements in its angle or on the back of cornea can occur due to defective development of anterior mesoderm.

Defective development of anterior mesoderm can result in anomalies of the iris, anterior chamber and its angle and the cornea. Normally the mesoderm forms iris stroma, corneal endothelium and corneal stroma. The intermediate layer of mesoderm atrophies in due course to form the space of anterior chamber. Normally this atrophy process extends well into the angle of anterior chamber which facilitates drainage of intraocular fluid. However the atrophy process may stop short at different stages resulting in:

a. Strands of mesodermal tissue on the surface of iris often attached to the corneal endothelium which shows localised opacities.
b. Presence of hyaline membrane on the posterior surface of the cornea usually in the periphery extending into the angle. This is usually associated with defective mesodermal layer of iris also.
c. Persistence of foetal mesodermal tissue in the angle of anterior chamber.

Among the above three, the last is more frequent and of greater clinical importance in that it causes obstruction to drainage of aqueous due to mesodermal tissue in the angle and consequent failure of trabecular meshwork to differentiate; the result being buphthalmos. As aqueous drainage is obstructed, intra-ocular tension increases. The sclera being quite elastic at this stage, stretches with increasing intra-ocular tension enlarging the eye ball. As the tension continues to increase, tears in Descemet's membrane of cornea occur giving rise to corneal oedema. The typical clinical picture presented is an enlarged eye ball including the cornea which is diffusely hazy due to oedema. The anterior chamber when seen, is usually deep. A gonioscopy shows mesodermal remnants in the angle stretching from the corneal periphery to the root of the iris.

Iris

Congenital or developmental anomalies of the iris include:

a. Aniridia—absence of the iris.
b. Coloboma of the iris.
c. Holes in the iris—pseudopolycoria.
d. Defects in the pigment epithelium.

Aniridia: Although clinically it appears to be total absence of the iris, actually a rudimentary iris tissue is present receded behind the limbus and therefore not seen clinically but visible on gonioscopy examination.

Clinically, the pupil is as big as the cornea. The lens equator and sometimes even the zonular fibres are seen with oblique illumination. Aniridia is often associated with other anomalies particularly of the cornea like micro-cornea, corneal opacity etc. Aniridia has been reported as a strongly dominant transmission in successive generations.

The defect is due to failure of development of the rim of optic cup whereby the neuro-ecto-dermal scaffolding is absent and mesodermal iris fails to develop. Common complications in aniridic eyes is glaucoma because of associated angle anomalies.

Coloboma of iris: It may be part of coloboma due to failure or defective closure of the embryonic fissure or may be independent of it since the iris develops well after the closure of the fissure. This may be due to a notch caused by a persistent vessel at the rim of the optic cup. Such a coloboma of the iris may be associated with coloboma of the zonule and even the lens. A localised coloboma may result in an iris hole, a *pseudo polycoria*. Similarly peripheral coloboma rarely seen, resembles iridodialysis and is called an *iridodiastasis*.

Pupillary aperture may vary in size, shape and number. Difference in size of pupil in two eyes is called *anisocoria* while that in shape is known as *dyscoria* and more than one pupillary aperture is called *polycoria*. An eccentrically situated pupil is known as *corectopia*. A pupil may be a slit instead of a round hole.

Pigment epithelial anomalies of the iris may present clinically as simple eversion or ectropion of the pigment epithelium of the iris at the pupillary border.

Ciliary Body

Rarely, there are clinical manifestations of developmental defects of the ciliary body as part of a generalised ocular anomaly, such as coloboma or cyst of the ciliary body.

Choroid

A typical coloboma of the choroid has been described earlier. Choroideraemia is a defect due to progressive atrophy of the choroid and pigment epithelium of retina. It is a sex linked hereditary condition. Males are affected and females remain carriers. Visual handicap caused is gross because the rod and cone cells of the retina do not function in the absence of normal pigment epithelium and the choroid.

Retina

Developmental defects of the retina include:
1. Retinal dysplasia: Usually due to undifferentiated neuro-epithelial layers of the retina or presence of gliosis.
2. Defective night vision—Oguchi's disease—A condition of extremely poor dark adaptation. Structurally the cones predominate while the rods are practically absent.
3. Hereditary retinoschiasis is separation of retinal layers usually at the outer nuclear layer.

4. Medulated nerve fibres.
5. Tapeto-retinal degeneration:
    a. Primary pigmentary degeneration of the retina and its various forms.
    b. Many types of Chorio-retinal degenerations.
   These conditions are abiotrophic in nature and have been already described.

Developmental anomalies of the macula
1. Macular aplasia.
2. Macular hypoplasia.
   Both these occur in gross ocular anomalies like microphthalmos, coloboma, extreme albinism etc.
3. Congenital cyst of the macula. This usually shows a dominant heredity and considerable visual handicap.

Anomalous Functional defects of vision include:
1. Congenital night blindness.
2. Congenital colour vision defects.
   Both these functional defects exist with a clinically normal ophthalmoscopic picture.

Optic Disc and Nerve

1. Aplasia and hypoplasia of the optic nerve is rare and is usually in malformed eyes with deformities of the central nervous system.
2. Holes and pits in the optic disc.
3. Congenital crescent commonly inferior.
4. Congenital optic atrophy, usually associated with central nervous disturbances.

Lens

Congenital aphakia. Complete absence of lens is rare and can be due to failure of development of lens vesicle. More commonly, the lens develops but later degenerates with only traces of its structure left behind.

Other congenital anomalies of size, shape, position and transparency of the lens are not uncommon.

Anomalies of size and shape of the lens:

a. *Micro-spherophakia.* This is the most common anomaly. The lens is small in size and more convex as the name suggests. The diameter being smaller, the equator of the lens is seen with a dilated pupil. The eye is myopic because of greater power of refraction due to its spherical shape. A spherical lens is also responsible for higher incidence of glaucoma. The greater the anterior curvature, the greater are the chances of pupillary block. Because the zonular fibres stretch, subluxation and dislocation of the lens are not uncommon.

The anomaly is considered to be due to arrest of normal development around the 5th-6th month of foetal life. It is a recessive hereditary condition.

b. *Lenticonus.* A conical deformation in the centre of either the anterior or posterior surface of the lens may present clinically as anterior or posterior lenticonus. Anterior lenticonus is common in males while posterior is common in females.

Anterior lenticonus can cause a pupillary block when the pupil contracts round the protruding lenticonus. Usually the lens is transparent but polar opacities in the capsule and subcapsular zone are not uncommon.

The central area is highly myopic due to increased curvature in either type of lenticonus. Refraction in the periphery may be emmetropic.

Ophthalmoscopically and during retinoscopy, the area of the lenticonus is seen as a separate greyish central round zone with a normal red glow surrounding it. This is due to the high difference in the refraction between the central and peripheral parts and also due to the prismatic effect in the central area.

Delayed separation from the surface ectoderm is considered to be an etiological factor for anterior lenticonus. Theories postulated for causation of posterior lenticonus, do not satisfactorily explain the cause of the defect. These theories range from pull of hyaloid remnant, weakness of the posterior capsule resulting in localised herniation, anomalies of posterior vascular sheath of the lens to localised hyperplasia of the lens itself.

Diagnosis of lenticonus, anterior or posterior, is indisputably confirmed by a slit lamp examination under full mydriasis.

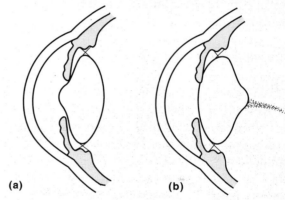

(a)   **(b)**

Fig 25.3: Lenticonus (a) Lenticonus anterior, (b) Lenticonus posterior with hyaloid remnant attached

c. **Coloboma of lens:** It may be associated with other coloboma or may occur as an isolated defect. The shape and size of coloboma vary. There is usually an associated defect in the zonular fibres. The fundus seen through the aphakic area is normal. The causative factor is considered to be a defective development of the ciliary region of the neuro-ectoderm from which the zonule develops.

Anomalies of Lens Position

A common clinical entity under this group is *ectopia lentis*. This is a displacement of a normally developed lens due to a defect in zonular fibres. The displacement is in the opposite direction from that of the poorly developed zonule.

It can occur as an isolated anomaly but more often it is part of a general systemic syndrome of mesodermal origin with skeletal manifestation such as Marfan's or Marchesani's syndromes.

The condition is bilateral. Clinically, the lens equator is seen in the dilated pupillary area. On ophthalmoscopic examination, the equator of the lens appears as a dark crescentic line separating the phakic and aphakic areas. Uniocular diplopia may be present if a normal undilated pupil is evenly divided into phakic and aphakic areas. Refraction through the phakic area is almost always myopic. A very probable complication is dislocation of ectopic lens into vitreous or anterior chamber, the latter causing a secondary glaucoma. When visual symptoms are disturbing, extraction of a transparent lens in young people has to be considered.

Anomalies of Transparency of the Lens

Congenital lens opacity is one of the most common developmental anomalies of the eye. It figures as an important clinical condition in ophthalmic practice and poses a challenge because of the necessity of critical assessment in a young child regarding type of opacity and surgical procedure if necessary.

Congenital lens opacities may be capsular, nuclear, cortical and sutural.

Congenital cataracts may be due to developmental aberrations primarily or due to a disturbing influence during intrauterine development of lens.

Some of these are genetically determined, some due to maternal abnormality and other hereditary. Autosomal dominant as well as recessive heredity have been reported. In many of these, metabolic and endocrinal factors are responsible, such as parathyroid hyperfunction. Toxic elements have often been blamed for a congenital lens opacity.

An important point to keep in mind is that whatever the detrimental influence on the developing lens, the result is that the fibres being formed and laid down at that particular stage of development become opaque. Once the factor ceases to exert its noxious effect, the lens fibres resume their normal development and are transparent. This is the reason that many of these lens opacities are localised and non-progressive.

In many of these congenital hereditary lens opacities, it is not the cataract itself that is genetically determined but the influence or disturbance that causes the lens opacity which is genetically deciding.

Capsular cataract: Anterior capsular opacity is more common. This is more or less a round opacity occupying pupillary area; thus being anterior polar also. The opacity itself may be flaky or dot like. Association of a persistent pupillary membrane is not uncommon.

Posterior capsular opacities are not common but when present, may be associated with a hyaloid remnant.

Anterior polar cataract: The morphology of anterior polar cataract varies greatly from a well circumscribed central opacity to a pyramidal opacity protruding into the anterior chamber. Cortex behind the opacity is normal. Sometimes a reduplicated lens opacity may occur so that the anterior polar opacity is separated from an identical deeper cortical opacity by a zone of clear fibres.

Posterior polar cataract is an uncommon developmental defect. It is often an acquired opacity due to posterior segment disease. However, posterior polar opacity of lens may be associated with remnant of the hyaloid artery. A progressive posterior polar opacity has been described which extends in radial spoles towards the equator of the lens.

Zonular cataract is an opacity limited to a specific zone of the lens. This is a typical example of lens fibres getting affected during a particular period due to a detrimental factor. The fibres of lens formed before and after this period are normal. Thus, the centre of lens and the anterior-most and posterior-most cortex may be transparent while the zone of fibres in between is opaque. These lens opacities can be pre-natal or postnatal, post-natal when the disturbance occurs early in infancy.

The characteristic of this type of lens opacity is that it is surrounded by a transparent peripheral lens.

Sutural cataracts: They are most often bilateral and always stationary. They rarely cause visual disturbance. Most of these conform to the morphology of different suture formations.

Anomalies of the Vascular System

Foetal vascular system: Persistence of foetal vascular system is anomalous because during normal development, these foetal vascular channels normally atrophy and disappear. If they do not, they may either persist as patent vascular channels or strands of tissue representing incomplete atrophy. These, when present after birth are:
1. Persistent hyaloid vessels.
2. Persistent vascular sheath of the lens.
3. Persistent pupillary membrane.

Persistent Hyaloid Vessels

Hyaloid vessels enter the developing eye ball through embryonic fissure and extend from optic nerve head posteriorly to end at the posterior pole of lens anteriorly. Normally, the whole system atrophies completely to leave no trace of itself. However, incomplete atrophy may result in remnants of main hyaloid vessels along the whole course or more commonly either at the posterior pole of the lens or at the optic disc.
a. When a hyaloid remnant is present from optic disc to lens, it may be a fine thread. It can be seen with ophthalmoscope and traced right from the disc to the lens or vice-versa. The anterior attachment to the posterior lens capsule is often discovered on routine slit lamp examination with a dilated pupil hanging freely in the anterior end of Cloquet's canal.
b. Persistence of the posterior end of the hyaloid artery is seen as a strand of tissue originating at the disc from the central artery or an actual extra vessel at the nerve head which extends into the vitreous. This may be associated with a varying degree of glial tissue. When it is associated with glial proliferation forming a pyramidal shaped tissue in front of the disc, it is called *Bergmeister's papilla.*

Persistent Vascular Sheath of Lens

Persistent posterior vascular sheath of lens is not common but when present, it clinically appears as a pseudoglioma. It has to be differentiated from retinoblastoma and retrolental fibroplasia.

Persistent Pupillary Membrane

Persistent pupillary membrane is failure of atrophy of anterior foetal vasculature. Few fine strands, white or variably pigmented, extend from the collarette of iris to the anterior lens capsule or right across to the opposite part of collarette.

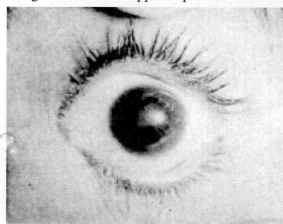

Fig. 25.4: Persistent Pupillary Membrane

These usually do not affect visual status of the eye. It is rare but possible that it may be in the form of a well-formed membrane across the pupillary aperture. This naturally will cause visual symptoms depending on its density and extent. The attachment on the anterior lens capsule may present a dot or pyramidal type of lens opacity.

Anomalies of the Retinal Vessels

These may be gross in a defectively formed eye ball and depend on the type of generalised ocular anomaly. The minor anomalies in functionally and structurally normal eye balls are compatible with normal functions and are more of an academic interest than clinical significance.

Anomalies of the branching of retinal vessels basically depend on the site in the optic nerve where the first branching of the central artery takes place.

Accordingly, a single central arterial trunk, two trunk, inferior and superior or four separate branches, two nasal and two temporal may be seen at the optic nerve head.

The vessels may be congenitally tortuous either in one area or all over the fundus.

Communication between retinal and ciliary systems of vessels is fairly common. Common clinical examples of these are:

a. **The cilio-retinal artery.** It emerges just inside the temporal margin of the disc and running temporally supplies the macular area. It is a branch from the circle of Zinn which encircles the optic nerve just behind the optic nerve head.

b. **The cilio-choroidal artery** arises from choroidal network, appears on the disc, sometimes on the nasal side, dips down again and disappears from the fundus after giving a few twigs to retina.

c. **The chorio-vaginal arterial vessels** arise from the choroidal vessels, appear at the disc margin and turn backwards to terminate in the pial-plexus of optic nerve.

Anomalies of Pigmentation

In all tropical races, along with dark skin, the iris is dark brown in colour unlike in Caucasian races in whom the skin is lighter and ocular structures like the iris, have a lighter colour, variably described as grey, blue, green, etc.

The pigmentation may not be uniform. *Heterochromia* is the term used to describe ununiform pigmentation. Hyperpigmentation of a patchy nature is better known as a *naevus*. If generalised and diffuse, it is called melanosis. This may also involve conjunctiva, sclera, iris, choroid (Fig. 25.5).

The optic disc may have pigment in a crescentic shape, usually prominent on the temporal margin. Ocular function is not disturbed.

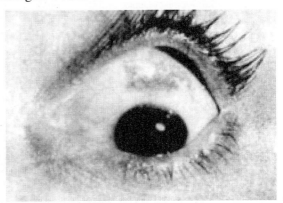

Fig 25.5: Scleral Melanosis

Heterochromia usually remains stationary. If and when a patch of hyperpigmentation shows signs of increasing in size or develops neovascularisation, it is a cause for worry. It is therefore important that ocular naevi should be periodically observed for such signs so as to suspect and detect signs of malignancy if any at the earliest.

Hypopigmentation: It is usually due to an inborn error of metabolism involving tyrosinase; an enzyme which normally converts dihydroxyphenylalanine (DOPA) into melanin. It is called *albinism* which may be diffuse and generalised or localised to ocular structures only.

The uveal pigment is variable even in normal individuals but the retinal epithelial pigment is more or less constant and its absence has therefore been considered to be a criterion of ocular albinism.

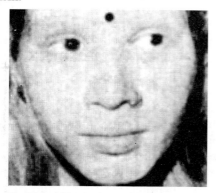

Fig 25.6: Albinism Ocular and Generalised Involving Hair, Skin, Iris and Choroid

Ocular albinism, as part of systemic albinism or localised only to ocular structures, presents clinically as white eye lashes, light-coloured iris, moderately dilated pupil through which fundus glow is seen, nystagmus and defective vision. On ophthalmoscopy and during retinoscopy, the thin non-pigmented iris transmits enough light to show fundus glow through. The optic disc is inconspicuous and can be identified by the retinal vessels converging on the area. Macular function is defective and therefore the nystagmus. Photophobia is a prominent symptom.

Generalised systemic albinism is hereditary. Ocular albinism as an isolated manifestation is sex-linked usually affecting males, females being carriers.

Anomalies of Eye Lids

Developmental defects of lids can occur at two stages:
1. Defective formation of the lid folds in the early stage of intra-uterine life, leading to developmental anomalies of the lids.
2. Anomalies of lid margin and differentiation of the lid structures.

Defective development of lid folds: The lid folds form after the lens vesicle separates from the surface ectoderm. These appear around 16 mm stage and continue to grow till around 32 mm when the upper and lower folds approximate and fuse. Developmental defect at this stage can result into:

i. *Cryptophthalmos:* The lid folds have failed to develop and a condition of ablepheron (absence of lids) results. The skin passes from the forehead over the eyes on to the cheek. It is usually associated with other facial anomalies and many times ocular anomalies also.

ii. *Microblepharon:* The lids are short in their vertical extent. The lids are so short that they fail to cover the eye ball.

iii. *Coloboma of lids* is a defect in the lids so that part of the eye ball remains exposed when the lids are closed. Usually the whole thickness of the lid tissue is involved. A common defect noted is a notch at the lid margin. However, the defect may extend into the whole vertical extent, though it is rare. Sometimes only the tarsal plate is absent while the skin and conjunctiva are present. In such a partial coloboma, the defect is neither apparent nor does it leave the eye ball exposed.

iv. *Blepharophimosis:* A small palpebral aperture due to shortening of the lids can occur as an autosomal dominant hereditary trait. Clinically, there is an appearance of ptosis with the superior palpebral fold abolished and the lid movements restricted.

v. *Mongoloid palpebral fissure* due to obliquity upwards of the outer canthus. These are often racial characteristics. Full Mongoloid facies has the following features:
   - Up and out obliquity of interpalpebral fissure.
   - Broad and flat bridge of the nose.
   - Protruding lower lip and a thick tongue.

Mongolism as a syndrome is a chromosomal pathology which is also associated with mental retardation, stunted growth and some skeletal abnormalities.

vi. *Epicanthus:* It is a fairly common developmental anomaly of autosomal dominant type. Clinically it presents as a semilunar fold extending vertically on the side of the nose with its concavity towards the inner canthus. The fold exists normally in foetal life during the third to sixth month to disappear later as the development of the nasal bone and lacrimal apparatus completes. It persists as a racial characteristic. It is always a bilateral anomaly. It may be associated with ptosis and some degree of blepharophimosis.

Epicanthus inversus is the opposite condition when the skin fold starts in the lower lid and extends upwards into the upper lid resulting in shortening of palpebral fissure. Congenital ptosis is a common association of epicanthus inversus also (Fig. 25.7).

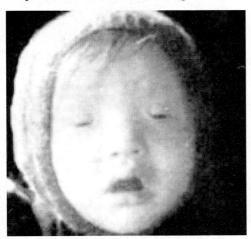

Fig 25.7: Bilateral Epicanthus Inverse Type

vii. *Epiblepharon or blepharochalasis* appears as a redundant skin fold in the lids, more commonly in the upper lids. It may overhang the upper lid margin to give an appearance of a narrow palpebral fissure (See Fig. 7.8).

Anomalies of Lids Margins

Lids have formed by approximately 35 mm stage and are fused till the 5th month when separation of lids starts. During the period of fusion, formation and differentiation of lid structures take place. The following anomalies can result during this period.

1. **Entropion:** Congenital entropion can be due to absence of tarsal plate or a spastic type of entropion due to hypertrophied marginal fibres of the orbicularis muscle.

2. **Ectropion:** Congenital type is rare but a secondary ectropion may be present along with microphthalmos or anophthalmos.

3. **Ankyloblepharon:** The lid margins remain fused together along part of their extent due to imperfect separation. The lids may remain fused either at the external canthus or inner canthus. In either case, the palpebral fissure is shortened. Defective separation may take the form of strands of tissue stretching between two lid margins and restricting their movement. This is called *ankyloblepharon filli formis.*

4. **Congenital hypotrichosis:** Total or partial absence of eye lashes is usually part of a condition affecting the eyebrows and scalp hair.

5. **Uncommonly long eye** lashes *trichomegaly* or multiple rows of eye lashes, *polytrichia* are other anomalies. It is a condition when there may be extra row of eye lashes at the posterior border of lid margin when they rub on the cornea. Another congenital condition is *dystichiasis* when there may be an extra row in the normal position of lashes.

6. **Congenital ptosis:** It is perhaps the commonest lid anomaly, partial or total, simple or associated with superior rectus paresis. It can also be associated with other lid anomalies

such as epicanthus, blepharophimosis and as part of the Marcus Gunn syndrome.

Developmental Anomalies of Lacrimal Apparatus

These can be classified structure wise:

1. **Lacrimal gland:** The lacrimal gland may be absent or there may be hypoplasia of the gland. Both of these result in absence or grossly deficient lacrimal secretion.

   Congenital cyst of the gland may exist. Depending on the *size,* the clinical picture varies from appearance of a tumour in the outer upper orbital region to proptosis and ptosis.

2. **Lacrimal passages:** The anomalies of the lacrimal drainage system can be:
   i. Absence of puncta; one or both.
   ii. Atresia of canaliculus.
   iii. More than one punctum.
   iv. Atresia of the lacrimal sac.
   v. Non-canalisation of the naso-lacrimal duct.
   vi. Congenital fistula of the lacrimal sac.

Anomalies of Orbit

It is not within the limits of this textbook to describe all the bony orbital defects or cranial defects affecting the orbits. The common orbital conditions of congenital origin are:

1. Orbital dermoids and teratoma presenting with proptosis.
2. Orbital involvement secondary to skull vault defect like craniofacial dysostoses.

   Most of the dysostoses which mean abnormal and untimely fusion of sutures of the skull, cause a secondary effect on orbits in their depth, size and shape. A normal eye ball in a markedly shallow orbit as in oxycephaly appears proptosed. The defect causes bony pressure on the optic nerves resulting in visual deterioration (Fig. 25.8).

3. **Hypertelorism:** Wider separation of the two eyes is an anomaly due to disproportionate growth of skull bones.

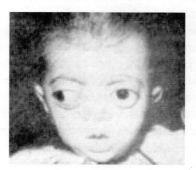

Fig 25.8: Cranial dysostosis. (Note proptosis due to shallow orbits)

Some Important Developmental Syndromes

1. *Marfan's syndrome:* Dominant heredity presenting the features of:
   a. Ectopia lentis.
   b. Long extremities.
   c. Arachnodactyly.
   d. Cardiovascular anomalies.

2. *Marchesani's syndrome:* This defect is the opposite of Marfan's syndrome. The extremities are short with well-developed musculature and short stubby hands and feet.

   The height is short. Ocular manifestations include spherophakia and microphakia resulting in lenticular myopia. Subluxation of lens may occur. Glaucoma of a secondary nature is often an associated feature. Spherophakia itself may cause a pupillary block glaucoma.

   The hereditary transmission is of irregular type, sometimes dominant and sometimes recessive. At times only skeletal features may be present without ocular manifestations.

3. **Van Der Hoeve's syndrome.** It manifests as blue sclerotic, brittle bones and deafness. Fractures with slightest trauma are usually the presenting feature. Heredity is dominant.

4. **Sturge-Weber syndrome.** It presents as: Capillary angioma of the skin of the face, usually unilateral involving the area of distribution of the first and second divisions of the fifth cranial nerve. Associated angiomatous involvement of skin elsewhere may also be present. Angioma may extend into conjunctiva. Even an intra-cranial angioma may be present.

The significant ocular complication is a secondary glaucoma due to vascularisation in the angle of the anterior chamber in some advanced cases resulting in buphthalmos.

Cerebral calcification may lead to gradual mental retardation or epileptic seizures.

Some developmental defects are not only structural anomalies but there are conditions which involve functional capacity of tissues. These are usually termed as inborn or genetically determined errors of metabolism.

Accordingly, we have disturbances of:
1. *Carbohydrate metabolism,* e.g., diabetes mellitus, galactosemia.
2. *Lipid metabolism,* e.g., amaurotic family idiocy (Neimann Pick disease), hyperlipaemic xanthomatosis.

26

Introduction to Immunology

The cells in general have some capability for recognition. In vertebrates, this function resides in a specialised system, the immunological apparatus. Like other organs, the immunologic system is specialised to perform its function in a highly proficient fashion. However, unlike most other specialised organs, the immunologic apparatus is not a localised structure, but is distributed throughout the body, an arrangement favourable for the kind of function assigned to it, namely, the *immunological surveillance*. The localised distribution of various lymphoid organ systems such as tonsils, lymph nodes, as a part of overall body defence system is somewhat comparable to the postings of army units in places of strategical importance. Because of a highly well-organised defence system, one rarely suffers twice from maladies such as mumps, measles, smallpox, whooping cough and some other similar infectious diseases. This is because, the first contact with an infectious agent (micro organism) imparts some MEMORY so that the body is effectively prepared to deal with any future invasion by that organism. Thus, it is obvious, that in a healthy individual, there exists a well-organised system to recognise the "non-self" (foreign). The first encounter with any such foreign non-self entities is recorded, and the event is stored in memory, and the body gets ready with the necessary arsenal to deal with the subsequent encounter that may arise in future. In the event of second encounter, because of the body's preparedness, the infectious agents do not succeed in causing the disease. Thus the body is rendered IMMUNE (protection) against subsequent infection.

The immunological defence apparatus comprises of 3 basic biological components. The *lymphocytes*, the *macrophages* and the *immunoglobulins*. These function in two systems, the *humoral* and *cellular*. These two wings of body defence system are independent, but their functions are well coordinated with complementary support from each other.

The *lymphocyte* is the primary cell involved in both the humoral and cell mediated immunological defence mechanism. The detection of various surface markers on the lymphocyte membrane as well as on the basis of the functional characteristics, they have been grouped into two categories called B and T lymphocytes.

The B lymphocytes derived from stem cells are differentiated in bone marrow. The B cells, about 15–20 per cent, are responsible for humoral immunity. When B lymphocyte encounters an antigen for which it has a receptor, it undergoes proliferation and morphologic changes giving rise to a characteristic cell called plasma cell. The plasma cell secretes large amounts of specialised proteins of immunological functions—the *immunoglobulins* or *gamma-globulins.*

Immunoglobulins (Ig). These are antibodies, protein in nature and produced by plasma cells. There are two groups of immunoglobulins, the humoral and the cell bound. The humoral antibodies are freely circulating in the blood and the cell-bound gamma-globulins are attached to the lymphocytes.

There are five types of immunoglobulins named as G, M, A, E, D.

Ig-G are the commonest type of gamma-globulins and comprise 80% of all types. They have a long latency and therefore act when exposed to an antigen for a second time as in cases where the first dose sensitises the tissues and the second dose causes tissue-immune reaction. Ig-G are particularly effective against bacterial activity by causing agglutination of bacteria thereby facilitating their phagocytosis.

Ig-M are the next commonest gamma-globulins. They are rapidly produced at the first contact with antigen but result in a short-term immunity of two weeks or so.

Ig-E is related to immediate hypersensitivity which causes anaphylactic reaction.

Ig-A acts in defence of surface conditions like skin diseases.

Ig-D is in very low concentration in serum and therefore of very little significance.

T-Lymphocytes. The stem cells which migrate to the thymus, transform themselves into *T-lymphocytes* under the influence of thymic factors form about 70 per cent of cells. It is during this transformation that they acquire characteristic T-cell surface markers and competence to mediate allograft cytotoxicity. The T-lymphocytes are responsible for cell mediated immunity (i.e., delayed skin reactivity, allograft rejection, anti-tumour immunity and cellular defence against fungi and viruses) and delayed hypersensitivity. They do not produce antibodies but react with the antigens and become 'killer cells'.

The macrophage, like the lymphocyte is produced mainly in the bone marrow. The main function of the macrophage is phagocytosis. Phagocytosis as a function is immunologically non-specific in the sense that it is governed by the physio-chemical properties of respective surfaces of foreign entities rather than their antigenic determinants. However, it is also observed that a particular kind of antibody attaches firmly to the macrophage, and confers it the ability to recognise certain antigens. Adherence of the particle to the macrophage cell membrane is a pre-requisite before the phago-cytosis is ensued. Both the process of adherence and phagocytosis are greatly facilitated by coating of particles with certain components of the serum, a process called *opsonisation*, meaning rendering palatable. Especially encapsulated micro-organisms such a pneumococci can be engulfed easily only after successful opsonisation. Following the adherence of the particle, the process of engulfment takes place with the help of extended pseudopodia.

However, some organisms such as Mycobacteria, Brucella and Salmonella can escape the onslaught and even show multiplication within the cells. It has been observed that some recurrent microbial diseases are associated with defects in phagocytosis and microbial killing by host phagocytes.

Nature and Function of Complement

Complement is a complex system of proteins, heat labile in nature, i.e., they lose their activity by heat to 56°C for half an hour, or by prolonged storage. There are at least 11 discrete serum proteins that have been identified as components of complement system. These are not antibodies. Immunisation does not increase their concentration. The components of complements are designated as C1, C2 and so on, the number following C refers to the sequence of discovery. Most of the current knowledge of complement system is derived from studies involving its ability to lyse sheep erythrocytes coated with antibody. The guinea pig serum is the best source of complements for diagnostic purpose.

The complement mediated reactions of host defence depends upon the operation of 11 components and designated in order of their reaction sequence with two exceptions. The Cl component is a macromolecular complex consisting of Clq, Clr and Cls and linked by calcium. The lytic activity of the complements in conjunction with specific antibody is dependent on the presence of ions such as magnesium and calcium. Basically the complement mediated lytic action is initiated first by binding of first component of the complement system (Cl) to the antigen-antibody (immune complex) complex, resulting in the activation of the subsequent component in the sequence. This in turn is able to act upon the next component and so on, producing a cascade effect with amplification.

AUTO-ANTIBODIES IN HEALTH AND DISEASES

The immunologic defence system of the body is designed in such a way that there are appropriate mechanisms to prevent the recognition of 'self components as 'Non-self antigens by lymphoid system. However, as it is now established that auto-antibodies (i.e., antibodies capable of reacting with 'self components) appear, although the pathologic significance of these antibodies in many cases is uncertain. Whatsoever may be the physiological or pathological significance, there seem to be a number of auto-antibodies in

normal persons as well as in individuals with various diseases. The term 'auto-immune disease' is used in these situations where it can be shown that the auto-immune process contributes to the pathogenesis of the disease.

Disease associated with auto-antibody production may range from strictly organ specific (e.g., Hashimoto's disease of thyroid) to disorders of more generalised character (e.g., systemic Lupus Erythematosus where both lesions and auto-antibodies are not confined to any one organ).

Sometimes the cross reaction or similarity between the antigenic determinants of endogenous components with that of exogenous antigens may provoke auto-antibody formation. For example, post-rabies vaccination encephalitis is a consequence of auto-immune reaction to the brain tissue initiated by heterologus brain tissue in the vaccine.

Another such example is that, in rheumatic fever antibodies produced against streptococcus also react with heart as there happens to be some similarity between streptococcal antigen and heart muscle component.

Very often the interaction of micro-organisms with surface antigens on the host cell membrane may provoke a vigorous response from host immune system resulting in the antibody production against pre-existing cell component.

TRANSPLANTATION IMMUNOLOGY AND HLA SYSTEM

It has been a cherished dream in medical science to replace the diseased organs by transplant of a healthy one. The most common tissue transplant that is being practised is blood transfusion where the unfortunate consequences of mismatching are well known. The successful organ transplantation surgery has been hindered by the presence of an antigenic system that acts as a major barrier, both in man and animal. The

Auto-antibodies in some of the human diseases

Disease	Antigens against which the antibodies are formed
Hashimoto's thyroiditis	Thyroglobulin
Primary myxoedema	
Thyrotoxicosis	Cell surface TSH receptors
Male infertility	Spermatozoa
Juvenile diabetes	Cytoplasm of islet cells in pancreas and cell surface
Multiple sclerosis	Brain
Phacogenic Uveitis	Lens
Sympathetic Ophthalmia	Uvea
Sjogren's syndrome	Duct epithelium of salivary and lacrimal glands
Myasthenia gravis	Acetyl choline receptor of skeletal and heart muscle
Auto-immune haemolytic anaemia	Erythrocytes
Systemic lupus Erythematosus	DNA, Nucleoprotein, Cytoplasmic soluble antigen, formed elements of blood clotting factor etc.
Rheumatoid arthritis	Ig-G

specific antigens involved in graft rejection, like any other components of a body can provoke intense allograft (Homograft) reaction in members of the same species but different genetic constitution as from one man to another man and this is due to a *major histo-compatibility complex (MHC)* in the system. As a matter of fact, among all the vertebrates, each species possesses a single MHC which dominates allo-transplantation reactivity. In man, there is one dominant group of antigens which provoke strong allograft reactions known as the HLA (human leukocyte antigen) system. In addition to HLA system, ABO group antigens and possibly the organ specific antigens are also considered as transplantation antigens.

There are four well-defined HLA antigens and these have been designated alphabetically HLA-A, B, C and D. The typing of HLA antigens is carried out by immunological methods such as *Microlymphocytotoxicity test* to determine the serologically defined antigenic determinants.

By making use of specialised immunological techniques, it was shown that -HLA loci A, B and C control distinct biochemical molecules that do not interact with each other.

The greatest clinical value of histocompatibility testing at present is the matching of donor and recipient pairs for tissue grafting. The tissues of major significance in transplantation currently are kidney, heart, liver, bone marrow, platelets and possibly the granulocytes. Co-relation between HLA matching and the success or failure of corneal transplants has also been reported, though the need of tissue typing for corneal grafting is limited to patients with heavily vascularised recipient cornea and where grafts have repeatedly failed due to tissue immune reaction.

Test for tissue typing: The procedure is matching donor-recipient antigens by observing reaction between donor and recipient lymphocytes in tissue cultures. This is done to identify the HLA against an anti-serum of known specificity. Blood sample of recipient is tested for HLA type. At appropriate time, the leucocytes of the donor are incubated with serum of the recipient with known antigen. If there is damage to the cells, it indicates incompatibility.

HYPERSENSITIVITY REACTIONS

Whenever there is an antigen-antibody interaction, there is a hypersensitivity reaction, systemic or local. The hypersensitivity reaction may be immediate or delayed depending on whether it is antibody mediated or cell mediated.

Immediate Hypersensitivity Reaction

There are three types of immediate reactions, type-I, II and III.

Type-I reaction. This is a reaction which appears within a few minutes. It is brought about by humoral antibodies freely circulating in blood belonging to Ig-E type. During the reaction, there is liberation of histamine and production of eosinophils. If the reaction is local in nature it causes urticaria, rhinitis, conjunctival oedema and spring catarrh, etc. The generalised type of reaction is associated with systemic vaso-dilatation, contraction of bronchiolar muscles and shock. Common example is sudden death due to hypersensitivity to a drug or respiratory crisis following insect bites.

Type-II reaction. This antigen-antibody reaction is dependent on complement which is initiated by Ig-G or Ig-M antibodies. The common examples of type-II reaction are incompatible blood transfusion and an early graft rejection. The antibodies fight the antigenic graft and in the process, destroy the same. Mooren's ulcer, endogenous uveitis and pemphigus are also considered to be diseases caused by Type-II reaction.

Type-III reaction. The reaction appears after some interval and is also mediated by Ig-G and Ig-M antibodies. Among the common examples are serum sickness, rheumatoid arthritis, hepatitis and lupus erythematosus.

Delayed Hypersensitivity Reaction

This type of reaction is cell mediated and the interaction of the antigen is with the antibodies in T-lymphocytes. The reaction appears after an interval of two weeks or more. Among the examples are the delayed graft rejection, sympathetic ophthalmitis, recurrent herpes, Vogt-Koyanagi syndrome and immune response to tumour cells.

In ophthalmology, tissue immune reaction is of significance in corneal graft surgery. Experiments done as early as 1911 were proved informative. Protein was injected intra-corneal in one eye and the traumatic reaction allowed to subside. A later injection of the same protein in opposite cornea produced a violent keratitis. Another experiment was similarly contributory. A corneal homo-graft was done in a rabbit. Subsequently, a piece of skin from the donor rabbit was implanted under the skin of recipient rabbit. This clouded the corneal graft. Experiments have also proved that all the cellular layers of cornea can be involved in tissue immune reaction. Epithelium, stroma or endothelium or all three may be involved. In spite of these experimental evidences, cornea has the privilege of being avascular and hence the successes in corneal grafting are far more than any other organ grafts.

Tissue-immune reaction in a corneal graft is initiated by the antigen on the surface of donor cells which sensitise the T-lymphocytes of the recipient. These sensitised lymphocytes undergo transformation and proliferation within the lymph nodes from where they are carried through blood and lymph circulation. This explains that vascularisation to the graft margin is essential for tissue immune reaction. It also explains the time lag between the grafting procedure and the appearance of tissue-immune reaction.

Even though infrequent, tissue immune reaction still continues to be an important cause of graft failure. Prevention of reaction is, more important than to control the reaction once established. Tissue matching, therefore, became an important consideration. It has been established that compatibility of blood groups of donor and recipient has very little influence on the incidence of tissue immune reaction. Histocompatibility of antigens, HLA of donor and recipient is more relevant. The polymorphism of HLA antigens is however very complex and therefore the difficulties in tissue typing. The time factor for determining the Histocompatibility of donor-recipient is another difficulty in making routine use of tissue typing in corneal grafting.

Treatment of Hypersensitivity Reaction

The immediate reaction is treated by adrenaline and cortico-steroids. Anti-histaminics may also be used. To prevent recurrence, desensitisation of the individual against the antigen may be helpful.

There are various immuno-suppressive agents. The ones commonly used are steroids, antimitotic agents and alkylating agents.

Steroids act by different modes as follows:
1. Lympholysis of B-cells.
2. Restrict lymphocytic immigration.
3. Inhibit vascular permeability.
4. Inhibit prostaglandin synthesis.
5. Reduce antibody synthesis.

Antimitotic agents like azothioprin or mercapto-purine reduce B- and T-lymphocytes but are toxic drugs and therefore very hesitatingly used.

The alkylating agents have depressant action on dividing cells, particularly B-lymphocytes.

Anti-lymphocytic globulins (ALG) are used as antilymphocytic serum which contains Ig-G antibodies and can destroy the antigen.

Immuran is less toxic and has been found to be useful particularly in overcoming corneal graft rejection. It is administered in daily doses of 100-150 mg by intramuscular route. If the therapy has to be continued beyond one week, a check should be kept on liver function, blood counts and platelet count.

27

Ocular Therapeutics

It is out of scope of this book to detail the numerous therapeutic agents and procedures. Advances come in vogue regularly in pharmacological agents equipments, surgical techniques and every other aspect. This has become possible with better understanding of physiopathology of diseases with laboratory/clinical research.

Pharmacological Agents

Drugs with specific role in ocular disorders, grouped according to their pharmacological action are discussed here.

Preferable routine of administration of drugs for ocular conditions is topical. Systemic administration of these has a limitation of crossing *blood-aqueous barrier* to reach intra-ocular tissue pathology.

Topical Application

a. **Solutions:** Drops are the most commonly used preparations in treatment of eye diseases. Their advantage is that they are easy to instill and easy to absorb. The only disadvantage is that aqueous drops are diluted by tear film and they do not remain in the conjunctival sac for a long time, being washed away by the lacrimal fluid. Therefore they require frequent instillations. Methyl cellulose is sometimes added to increase viscosity of the solution, thereby increasing its contact time in the eye. Oily solutions are also sometimes used as drops. Due to slow absorption and poor solubility in tear film, their action is prolonged but they cause some interference in vision.

b. **Ointments:** Drugs are used as ointments in a fatty vehicle. They have an advantage over drops in that they are in contact with the eye for a longer time and are slowly absorbed and their action is prolonged. Therefore less frequent applications are needed. They are particularly useful for application at bed time. Also there is less absorption from the lacrimal passages, minimising systemic side effects. This is important in children, particularly when using drugs like atropine. The disadvantage with ointments is that they form a thin film over cornea and obscure vision. The ointment may also cause contact dermatitis, mostly because of allergy. Ointments also inhibit mitotic activity of the corneal epithelium and hence are not a favourite mode of local therapy with many eye surgeons. Ointments with plastic base are more miscible and better than those with a vaseline or paraffin base.

c. **Hydrophylic contact lens application:** Soft contact lenses have the capability to absorb and slowly release the chemicals in solution. This property is used for sustained release of the drug into conjunctival sac and reducing the frequency of instillations of the drug. This method has recently been used for treatment of glaucoma with miotic drugs.

d. **Drug inserts in the conjunctival sac:** The drug is placed in between two permeable polymer membranes and is released in a constant amount over a set period of time. In this system the drug is continuously released into the conjunctival sac and so there is a uniform concentration of drug and the quantity of drug required is also reduced.

Presently this method is utilised in management of glaucoma with Pilocarpine inserts which are placed in the lower fornix. This is also a very good mode of administration of tear substitutes in dry eye conditions. The membrane is very soft and flexible and does not cause a foreign body sensation. The frequency of administration by this system has been prolonged up to once a week.

e. **Subconjunctival injection:** Injection of medicament into subconjunctival tissue is used in cases where a higher concentration of the drug is required in ocular tissues in a short time or when the drug is placed as a depot in the subconjunctival space for prolonged action. Another indication for subconjunctival injection is when topical applications cause local tissue allergy to the drug. Antibiotics, steroids and mydriatics are used by this route for a quicker and prolonged effect.

f. **Periocular and Retro-bulbar injection:** The drug can also be injected in the retro-bulbar space within the muscle cone behind the eye ball. Anaesthetic solutions are given by this route. Vasodilators, steroids and absolute alcohol (for relieving pain in cases of absolute glaucoma) are also injected retrobulbar.

g. **Intra-cameral and intra-vitreal injection:** Antibiotics are needed to be injected directly into the anterior chamber or vitreous cavity in cases of severe infections. Drugs to be injected into vitreous have to be diluted to minimise the reaction in vitreous which can sometimes do more harm than good. This route is however used only in severe intra-ocular infections which would otherwise destroy the integrity of the eye.

Iintravitreal steroids and antivascular endo-thelial growth factor (VEGF) drugs are advised for neovascular lesions like proliferative diabetic retinopathy and age related macular degeneration.

Factors Affecting Absorption of Drugs

Most of the drugs used topically have to penetrate the layers of the eye ball to reach inner structures for their therapeutic action. The various factors governing their absorption after topical application are:

a. **Tear film:** All the drugs instilled into the conjunctival sac first come in contact with tear film. Purely fat soluble oily solutions cannot penetrate cornea and conjunctiva. Water soluble drugs are therefore better.

b. **Permeability of drugs through the cornea:** The drug traverses by the simple process of diffusion and since cornea has a very high water content, water soluble drugs traverse through it easily.

c. **pH of drug:** Most of the drugs used for topical application are made isotonic to the tear film but variations from isotonicity do not harm the eye except that hypertonic drugs cause more irritation, lacrimation and are therefore less effective.

GROUPS OF DRUGS

Local Anaesthetics

Most of the surgical procedures in ophthalmic practice are done under local anaesthesia. Some diagnostic procedures may also need anaesthesia. Local anaesthetics can be used topically as surface anaesthetic agents for superficial procedures of short duration like tonometry, lacrimal syringing, removal of foreign body from cornea, suture removal, cauterization, etc. For more prolonged procedures, particularly for intra-ocular surgery they are used as infiltration anaesthesia for a facial nerve and retrobulbar block. The duration of action depends upon the concentration of the drug and the speed of removal of drug from the site by diffusion and circulation.

An ideal local anaesthetic agent should have following qualities:
a. Rapid onset of action.
b. Slow absorption and rapid elimination.
c. Sufficient depth and duration of anaesthesia.
d. Non-irritant.
e. Non-toxic to the corneal epithelium.
f. No local or systemic toxicity.
g. Reversibility of action.
h. Stable to heat.

Some Anaesthetic Drugs

Cocaine: It was the first drug to be used for local anaesthesia, introduced in 1884. It is a naturally occurring alkaloid and has a potent local anaesthetic effect on topical instillation.

It has a sympathomimetic effect also so that it causes some mydriasis. Cocaine however has a damaging effect causing oedema of the corneal epithelium with availability of better drugs, cocaine has been discontinued decades ago.

Procaine: It is one of the earliest synthetic drugs used as 1% solution for infiltration anaesthesia. Since it is poorly absorbed from the mucous membrane, it causes no surface anaesthesia. It was extensively used in ophthalmology as injection for facial and retrobulbar block in strength of 2.0%. The duration of anaesthesia is about an hour. To prolong its effect, it can be used along with epinephrine to produce local vasoconstriction and thus delay its absorption

from the tissues. Some patients are allergic to this drug and a pre-operative sensitivity test by intradermal injection should be done. It can cause severe systemic reaction if inadvertently injected into a vein. Safe derivatives of procaine are available. Procaine as such is therefore not used now.

Lidocaine (Xylocaine): It is a rapid acting local anaesthetic useful both for infiltration and topical application. It is twice as potent as procaine. It is used as 1–2% solution for infiltration anaesthesia and 4% as surface anaesthesia. It is also available as jelly. It has excellent penetration and rapid onset of effect, which can be enhanced and prolonged by addition of adrenaline if there is no contraindication of the latter. This also reduces the chance of side-effects by slowing absorption. It has got very few side-effects. Hypersensitivity reaction may sometimes occur characterised by hypotension, nausea, sweating, muscular twitching and convulsions. Anaphylactic reaction though rare is known.

Marcaine (Bupivocaine): It is a slower acting local anaesthetic. The advantage of Marcaine is its very prolonged duration of anaesthesia. It is also an analgesic. The anaesthetic effect is quick and lasts for 8 to 12 hours. Partial paralysis of extra ocular muscles lasts for 12 to 24 hours. The advantage of this drug is complete pain relief in the post-operative period. It is used in concentration of 0.5% solution. It is stable to heat. It causes some vasodilatation. Xylocaine and marcaine mixed in equal quantities is better.

Drugs Acting on Autonomic Nervous System

Drugs acting on autonomic nervous system include miotics, mydriatics and cycloplegics which are the most commonly used drugs for diagnostic and therapeutic purposes.

Sympathetic and parasympathetic systems supply the structures of the eye and have opposing actions to each other. The sympathetic fibres supply dilator pupillae muscle, longitudinal muscle fibres of ciliary body and Muller's muscle of lid. The parasympathetic system supplies sphincter pupillae muscle and circular fibres of ciliary muscle.

Drugs which enhance sympathetic activity are called sympathomimetics and drugs which inhibit the sympathetic activity are called sympatholytic drugs. Similarly, parasympathomimetic drugs produce effects of parasympathetic stimulation and parasympatholytic drugs inhibit parasympathetic activity.

Miotics

Miotics are drugs which produce constriction of pupil. These miotic drugs are of two groups according to their mechanism of action.
a. Direct acting (Cholinergic) which have an action similar to acetylcholine at the myoneural junctions.
b. Indirectly acting (Anti-cholinesterase). These drugs inhibit the action of cholinesterase enzyme (which destroys acetylcholine) thus prolonging the action of acetylcholine.

Important uses of miotics:
a. To neutralize effect of mydriasis.
b. To constrict pupil preoperatively in intraocular surgery like glaucoma surgery and keratoplasty.
c. To constrict pupil after lens extraction.
d. To lower intraocular pressure in both open angle and narrow angle glaucoma.

Directly acting miotics: The drugs commonly used of this group are:
  i. Acetylcholine 1% solution
 ii. Carbachol 1% solution
iii. Pilocarpine 1–4% solution

Acetylcholine: It is a chemical agent responsible for transmission of nerve impulses, naturally present at parasympathetic myoneural junctions and at ganglionic synapses. Since it is very unstable it is immediately destroyed by enzyme cholinesterase. Its duration of action, therefore, is very short—5–10 minutes. It is sometimes used directly as 1% drops into the anterior chamber to quickly constrict the pupil, after cataract extraction, during penetrating keratoplasty and after cyclodialysis. Because it is rapidly destroyed, it has very low toxicity.

Pilocarpine: It has been the most commonly used drug in treatment of glaucoma for a hundred years and continues to be the anchor sheet in the medical treatment of glaucoma. It is a naturally occurring alkaloid obtained from the leaves of 'pilocarpus jaborandi'. Synthetically, it is used as nitrate. It stimulates post-ganglionic parasympathetic receptors and causes miosis. It is effective in all types of glaucoma and has very few side-effects. Miosis caused by pilocarpine is a disadvantage in patients who also have central lens opacity. It is used only as drops in a concentration varying from 1-4% or even 6-8%.

It is effective in both narrow angle and open angle glaucoma and is commonly used in open angle glaucoma as 'miotic life' agent.

It also increases aqueous outflow facility by action on ciliary body and causing contraction of scleral spur. In eyes with high tension, pupil may not respond to pilocarpine. In such cases, use of diamox will facilitate action of pilocarpine. It is a vaso-dilator and so helps drainage through aqueous veins.

To prolong its action and to minimise frequency of application it has been used with hydrophilic soft contact lenses or as ocuserts.

Carbachol: It is a strong miotic agent and is used in concentration of 1–2%. Its duration of action lasts for 8–10 hours. It can cause ciliary spasm and headache. Its principal use is directly into the anterior chamber at the time of surgery where rapid constriction of the pupil is urgently needed. Unlike acetylcholine, it is not destroyed by enzyme cholinesterase and therefore its effect lasts longer.

Indirectly Acting Miotics

These drugs produce their effect by preventing destruction of acetylcholine by inactivating the enzyme cholinesterase. These drugs are therefore not effective when the nerve supply is blocked by the atropine group of drugs.

Commonly used drugs in this group are:
1. Eserine.
2. Prostigmine.
3. DFP.
4. Phospholine iodide.

Eserine (Physostigmine): Physostigmine is an alkaloid derived from the seeds of Calabar beans of physostigma venenosum. The drug produces stimulation of smooth muscles and glands supplied by parasympathetic. Atropine blocks its effect.

The topical application in eye produces miosis and spasm of accommodation. The miosis is rapid in onset and becomes maximum in about 30 minutes and the effect lasts for 2–3 days. It reduces intraocular pressure by increasing facility of aqueous outflow. The pressure reduction effect lasts for 4-6 hours. It was used mostly in narrow angle glaucoma. It has been used along with pilocarpine, for additive effect in acute narrow angle glaucoma.

It is used as eserine salicylate drops 0.25–0.5% or ointment 0.25%. It decomposes in bright light and heat and changes its colour to red. It should be stored in a dark and cool place and fresh solution should be prepared every week. Coloured solution should therefore be discarded.

Headache, ciliary spasm and twitching of lids may occur for a short time after instillation of the drops. The patient should therefore be asked to sit and wait for a few minutes after the drops of eserine. Prolonged use may produce follicular hypertrophy of tarsal conjunctiva. The drug is hardly used now since better anti-glaucoma agents are available.

Neostigmine (Prostigmine): It is a sympathetic analogue of physostigmine. Its principal use is as an injection of 0.5 mg as a therapeutic test for and in smaller oral doses as treatment for myasthenia gravis. It can also be used as a miotic in patients allergic to eserine.

Di-Isopropyl flurophosphate (DFP): It is a very potent and irreversible inhibitor of cholinesterase. The drug produces systemic effects of parasympathetic stimulation and should therefore be used with discretion.

Local instillation in the eye produces intense and prolonged miosis which lasts for several days. Accommodative spasm is also very severe. Action may last up to 2 weeks.

It was used in concentration of 0.05-0.1% as eye drops in the treatment of acute glaucoma when short acting miotics fail to control intraocular pressure.

Its side-effects include headache, ciliary spasm and vaso-dilation of conjunctival and iris vessels. Systemic side-effects include colic pain, diarrhoea and a fall in blood pressure. It is not used now.

Phospholine iodide: It is a potent and long acting miotic. It is used as 0.06 or 0.125% drops. It is an effective alternative where weaker miotics do not act. It has also been used in treatment of accommodative esotropia. Because of its cataractogenous effect, its use in glaucoma is mostly limited to aphakic eyes. Side-effects include headache, ciliary spasm, iris cyst and anterior subcapsular opacity of the lens.

Cyloplegics

Cyloplegics are drugs which cause paralysis of accommodation. Accommodation is brought about by the contraction of the ciliary muscles which are supplied by parasympathetic oculo-motor nerve. Cycloplegic drugs act by inhibiting the action of acetylcholine at parasympathetic nerve endings in the ciliary muscle. These drugs are therefore called parasympatholytic drugs. Along with cycloplegia, these drugs also cause dilatation of the pupil because the sphincter pupillae muscle is also supplied by the parasympathetic oculomotor nerve.

Commonly used cycloplegic drugs are

a. Atropine.
b. Scopolamine (Hyoscine).
c. Cyclo-pentolate.
d. Homatropine.

Atropine: It is a very potent mydriatic and cycloplegic. It is a naturally occurring alkaloid extracted from Atropa Belladona plant. It is used as Atropine Sulphate.

Actions in eye: In 1% concentration as drops or ointment, mydriasis starts in 30–40 minutes and maximum effect is reached in 3–4 hours. Cycloplegic action takes a little longer to start than mydriasis. The cycloplegic effect gradually wears off in 10–12 days but mydriasis lasts a few days longer. Like all cycloplegics, hypermetropes with stronger accommodation are disabled more than myopes by the effect of atropine. There is no drug to counteract the local effect of atropine. Atropine is a vaso-constrictor.

Uses in ophthalmology: Because of its action on pupil and ciliary muscle, atropine has wide range of uses in ophthalmology, both for diagnostic and therapeutic purposes.

a. **Iridocyclitis.** It is a drug of choice in the management of iridocyclitis. It acts by following mechanism:
    i. By producing cycloplegia, it reduces pain which is due to spasm of ciliary muscle.
    ii. By dilating pupil, it prevents formation of posterior synechia and also helps breaking of recently formed posterior synechiae.
b. **To dilate pupil** post-operatively after intra-ocular surgery like extra-capsular cataract extraction, needling and aspiration of congenital cataract, keratoplasty, etc., to prevent post-operative iridocyclitis.

c. **For retinoscopy:** It is used as a cycloplegic for retinoscopy in children below the age of 15. It is particularly important in hypermetropes and patients having accommodative esotropia.
d. **For partial occlusion** of the sound eye in treatment of amblyopia exanopsia.
e. **For relieving accommodation** spasm as in accommodative squint.
f. **For regular use before general** anaesthesia where it prevents vagal inhibition and reduces bronchial secretions.

Preparation and doses: It is used as 1% drops or 1% ointment. Atropine as an injection is used as 0.65 mg of atropine sulphate in 1 cc. Atropine is major component of compound mydriatic solution which also includes adrenaline and procaine.

Side effects and contraindication: Because of prolonged cycloplegia, blurring of vision and photophobia persist for several days after atropinisation. Local allergic reactions are not uncommon causing allergic dermatitis of lid skin which subsides on discontinuation of the drug.

Systemic side-effects may occur due to absorption from ocular tissues and through nasolacrimal passages. Children are particularly sensitive to atropine. Symptoms are dryness of mouth, flushing of skin, pyrexia, tachycardia and fall in blood pressure. Central nervous system stimulation causing convulsions can occur in children.

Symptoms of atropine poisoning may be mistaken for acute febrile illness, particularly in children. An antidote of atropine is physostigmine given by parenteral route. Barbiturates may be needed to suppress convulsions in children.

Scopolamine (Hyoscine): It has an action similar to atropine but the duration of action is shorter than that of atropine. It is used as 0.5% drops in patients who are allergic to atropine. Its cycloplegic effect is also of shorter duration. It is a good substitute where the patient is sensitive to atropine or develops allergic reactions to atropine and at the same time mydriatic and cycloplegic action on the eye is urgently required.

Cyclopentolate (Cyclogel) marketed in India as Cyclomid, is another alternative to atropine. Used as 1% solution it is both a mydriatic and cycloplegic. It is quicker in action than atropine and cycloplegia lasts for a shorter period, not more than 24 hours. Although it is good for refraction in children, cycloplegia is still not as complete as with atropine.

Homatropine: It is a synthetic ester similar to atropine but of lesser potency. It is used as homatropine hydrobromide solution in concentration of 2.0%. Cycloplegia starts in 20-30 minutes and reaches the maximum in one and a half to two hours. The effect lasts for 24 to 36 hours. It is commonly used for retinoscopy in the age group of 15–35 years. Its effect can be neutralised by eserine and pilocarpine. It is used for a mydriatic test in glaucoma suspects. It is also an alternative, though less satisfactory, in patients who are sensitive to atropine.

Mydriatics

Mydriatics are drugs which dilate the pupil. Dilatation of pupil is required for many diagnostic purposes and also as a therapeutic measure. The various indications for use of mydriatics where cycloplegia is not necessary are:

  i. For retinoscopy in patients, above the age of 35.
  ii. For examination of media and fundus.
  iii. For slit lamp biomicroscopy.
  iv. For doing fluorescein angiography and angioscopy.
  v. For photocoagulation therapy.
  vi. In patients with small central lens opacity, a mydriatic is used to improve vision till surgery is undertaken.
  vii. Pre-operative before cataract operation.

  viii. Post-operatively after intraocular operative procedures.

The mydriatic drugs act by two mechanisms and are accordingly divided into two groups:
A. **Parasympatholytic drugs.** These drugs also affect ciliary muscles. So they also produce cycloplegia.
B. **Sympathomimetic drugs.** These drugs act by stimulating the dilator pupillae muscle. They have no or minimal action on ciliary muscles. Cycloplegia is not a feature of these drugs.

The commonly used drugs of this group are:
  i. Adrenaline,
  ii. Phenylephrine.

Adrenaline: It is a hormone produced by the adrenal medula. It produces effects of sympathetic stimulation.

When instilled in the eye in concentration of 1 in 1000, it produces vaso-constriction of blood vessels of the conjunctiva. Vaso-constriction is followed about an hour later by vasodilatation. It also produces dilatation of pupil but this action is weak. It reduces intraocular pressure. This lowering of intraocular pressure is produced by its vaso-constrictive effect on the ciliary body thereby reducing formation of aqueous humour.

Systemic reactions can be caused by the drug like tachycardia, increase in blood pressure, broncho dilatation and visceral vaso-constriction.

Ophthalmic uses:
1. *Vaso-constriction:* (i) Used along with local anaesthetics. It prolongs their action by delaying absorption. (ii) It is used to control bleeding from small capillaries during surgery. (iii) It is sometimes used to differentiate conjunctival from ciliary congestion. Superficial conjunctival vessels blanch within 5 minutes on instillation of adrenaline while the deeper ciliary congestion persists.
2. *Mydriatic effect:* It is used along with other mydriatics to help dilate the pupil quicker at the time of surgery.

3. Anti-allergic effect in allergic conditions of the eye used in diluted form.

Side-effects: Prolonged use of drugs may result in pigment deposition on conjunctiva.

Systemic side-effects may occur due to absorption of the drug either through nasal passages or on injection along with local anaesthetics. These include tachycardia, tremors, headache and rise of blood pressure. Adrenaline should, therefore, not be used or used with caution in elderly patients. It should not be used in hypertensives.

Phenylephrine (Neosynephrine, Drosyn): This is a sympathomimetic drug which causes wide mydriasis and moderate vaso-constriction. It is used as drops in concentration of 5-10%. Mydriasis usually commences in 10-15 minutes and is fully effective in 25-30 minutes and lasts for one and a half to two hours. It is common to note that before full dilatation, the pupil acquires a vertically oval shape.

It is used to dilate pupil for retinoscopy and fundus examination in older patients. Used along with homatrophine, it is a much more effective mydriatic than when either of them are used separately. This combined use may be needed in aphakic eyes and in iritis with posterior synechia.

It also causes a slight fall in intra-ocular pressure in normal eyes and in cases of open angle glaucoma.

OCULAR HYPOTENSIVE AGENTS

Various drugs are used for lowering the intra-ocular pressure.

According to their mechanism of action, these can be divided into the following groups:

A. **Drugs reducing secretion of aqueous humour:** (i) Carbonic anhydrase inhibitor like diamox. (ii) Sympatholytic drugs (beta blocker)—timolol maleate. (iii) Sympathomimetic agents like adrenaline and epinephrine (Discussed in the section on mydriatics).

B. **Hyperosmotic agents:** (i) I.V. Agents: mannitol. (ii) Oral Agents: (1) Glycerol. (2) Sorbitol.

C. **Drugs increasing the aqueous outflows:** Parasympathomimetic agents like miotics (discussed earlier in the chapter).

Carbonic Anhydrase Inhibitor

Acetazolamide (Diamox): It is a sulpha drug. It is the most commonly used drug in glaucoma therapy. It inhibits carbonic anhydrase enzyme which acts as a catalyst in the formation of aqueous humour from ciliary epithelium. The enzyme carbonic anhydrase is also present in the kidney and the drug therefore also produces diuresis. Action at two different sites is independent of the other. Potassium depletion occurs with this drug and therefore when used for a longer time, potassium should be supplemented as potassium chloride. Agranulocytosis is another toxic effect and the white blood cell count should be checked when giving heavy doses for longer time.

Orally, it is given as tablets of 250 mg four times a day. The action reaches its peak by 2 hours and effective concentration lasts for 4 to 6 hours. When needs to be given over long periods, a maintenance dose may be determined in each individual case.

Diamox sequels for oral administration are available for slow action and less frequent administration. An intravenous injection of acetazolamide 500 mg reduces intra-ocular pressure within 5 minutes and is hence useful in acute attacks of glaucoma and prior to surgery.

Uses: It is used along with miotics to reduce intra-ocular pressure in glaucoma. It is commonly use for short-term control of glaucoma. It may be used as a long-term therapy in smaller doses where surgery cannot be undertaken or is contra-indicated.

It is used pre- and post-operatively in intra-ocular surgery, cataract and corneal grafting, to keep intra-ocular pressure low. It has also been used in the management of flat anterior chamber after surgery. In cases of massive hyphema, it is used to keep intra-ocular pressure low thereby avoiding complication of blood staining of the cornea.

Side-effects. Tingling in hands and feet is a common complaint of patient taking diamox, It is of no significance. Gastro-intestinal upset is another side-effect and a major cause for discontinuation of therapy. The symptoms vary from vague abdominal discomfort to severe nausea, vomiting and diarrhoea.

Frequency of micturition because of its diuretic effect may be quite disturbing to some patients specially at night.

Because of potassium depletion, use of Diamox is contra-indicated in cases of adrenal insufficiency. It is also contra-indicated in patients with amoebic liver. Patients sensitive to sulphas will be sensitive to Diamox also.

Topical carbonic unhydrase inhibitor, Dorzolamide 2% drops has been in use as an adjunct to other local therapy.

Hyper Osmotic Agents

The drugs of this group reduce intra-ocular pressure by increasing osmotic pressure of the plasma in relation to the aqueous humour. Because these drugs are effective for a short period of time, they are suitable for tiding over the acute rise of intra-ocular tension. They may be given in addition to Diamox in very high grades of intra-ocular tension.

Hypotensive agents may be drugs given by intravenous or oral therapy.

Intravenous infusions: These agents are given by intravenous route and the total dose should be administered in 1 to 2 hours depending on the degree of tension rise and how quickly tension needs to be controlled.

Mannitol: It is the most commonly used osmotic agent and has the least side-effects. The maximum effect on intraocular pressure is achieved after one hour and lasts for about 6 hours. The dose for adults is 1.5 to 2 gm/kg body weight in 20% solution. In children, it is given as 10% solution. The rate of administration is usually from 50 to 60 drops per minute. It may be given at a faster rate when quick lowering of tension is desired at the time of intraocular surgery.

Oral agents:
i. *Glycerol.* It is an oral hyperosmotic drug of choice. It is given in dosage of 1 to 1.5 gm/kg body weight. To make it palatable, it is taken in fruit juice. Intraocular pressure drops within 30 minutes and the effect lasts for 3 to 4 hours. Headache, nausea, vomiting are the common side-effects. Because of its high caloric value, it should be used cautiously in diabetic patients.
ii. *Sorbitol.* It is chemically similar to mannitol. Its use does not increase blood sugar level, so it can be safely used in diabetic patients. Sorbitol with I.V. mannitol may be a good combination.

Sympatholytic agents: Timolol maleate is a beta blocking agent which is used for lowering intraocular pressure. The exact mechanism of action is not known but probably it decreases aqueous formation. It does not have any effect on size of pupil. Timolol is used in concentration of 0.25–0.5% once or twice a day. Having been extensively used in recent years, some side-effects have been noted. Bradycardia, nausea and vomiting, mental depression and skin rashes have been attributed to timolol even though used topically as eye drops. Timolol should not be used in asthmatics at it can precipitate an attack. A transient myopia may be caused by the drug. Timolol is still not a front line drug like pilocarpine and though a good advance in glaucoma therapy, it should be used with discretion. Although

Timolol is an advancement in glaucoma therapy, an effective pilocarpine therapy should not routinely be replaced by Timolol.

Other beta-blockers available are betaoxolol 0.25%, levobunolol 0.25-0.5% and carteolol 1% solution. Each of these has some advantage in cardio-pulmonary disease and duration of its hypotensive action.

Sympathomimetic agent: Epinephrine is an adrenaline derivative and particularly indicated for open angle glaucoma with central lens opacity. Epinephrine due to its small mydriatic effect allows the patients to work while a miotic does the opposite.

Epinephrine is known to increase incidence of cystoid macular oedema when used in aphakic eyes. It causes local sensitivity like blepheritis both in phakic and aphakic eyes and also cardiovascular effects in elderly patients.

A new derivative is now being tried—DPE (Dipivalylepinephrine) which is effective in much smaller concentration, can diffuse through the cornea and it is much less toxic.

CORTICOSTEROIDS

The advent of corticosteroids has revolutionised the field of ocular therapeutics. Because of their strong anti-inflammatory effect, they find a wide range of uses in the management of ocular inflammations.

The discovery of adrenocorticotropic hormone (ACTH), a pituitary hormone which stimulates adrenal cortex to secrete cortisone was the starting point of steroids family.

Most of the steroids used are synthetic. The steroids in common use belong to two groups, the prednisolone group and the fluorinated steroid group. The prednisolone group comprises of prednisone and prednisolone, the dose of each of which is 5 mg tablet one/two tablets four times a day. This group causes sodium retention. Among the fluorinated steroids are Triamcelone,

Betamethasone and Dexamethasone, the dose is 0.5 mg tablets four times a day. The advantage of fluorinated steroids is that they do not cause sodium retention.

The cortico-steroids with their relative anti-inflammatory action and sodium retaining activity are given below:

Name of Preparation	Equivalent oral dose	Relative anti-inflammatory effect	Relative sodiumretaining activity
Cortisone	25 mg	0.8	0.8
Hydro-cortisone	20 mg	1.0	1.0
Prednisone	5 mg	4.0	0.8
Prednisolone	5 mg	4.0	0.8
Dexamethasone	1 mg	25.0	0.0
Beta methasone	0.6 mg	25.0	0.0

ACTIONS OF STEROIDS

Cortico-steroids have a strong anti-inflammatory effect. They reduce capillary permeability, decrease cellular exudation and reduce tissue infiltration. They inhibit fibroblastic activity thereby reducing scarring following inflammations. They also inhibit post-inflammatory neovascularization and retard regeneration of epithelium and endothelium.

It is to be remembered here that cortico-steroids have no effect on causative factors of the disease process. They only protect the tissues from damage due to inflammatory process during acute phase till the disease is controlled by other methods. They do not have any reparative effect on structural damage which has been already caused. The effect of corticosteroids can be described as *an umbrella which though it protects against the rains, neither clears the clouds nor dries the part already wet.* Thus, if the infective process is not eliminated by proper therapy, the disease process resumes its normal course and sometimes with even greater severity after the cessation of steroids.

As an anti-inflammatory agent, steroids are very beneficial in ophthalmology for protection of delicate tissues of the eye from the damaging effect of acute inflammation thereby preventing a visual catastrophe. However, if misused, they can do more harm than good. The patient may get rid of one disease and acquire another.

Methods of Administration and Dosage

Corticosteroids can be used in ophthalmic practice either by local administration or by the systemic route. The choice of method depends upon the tissues involved. Local therapy is more effective in anterior segment disorders including diseases of conjunctiva, cornea, sclera, iris and ciliary body. Sometimes local therapy has to be supplemented by systemic route to achieve quicker effect. The advantage of local therapy is that a higher concentration is achieved by lower doses, easy application and absence of systemic complications. Sub-conjunctival injections and retrobulbar injections help to achieve higher concentration. A sub-conjunctival depot injection of Hydrocortisone may be given for a prolonged effect. The drug is slowly released and is effective for 2 to 4 weeks.

Systemic therapy is required for posterior segment lesions like choroiditis, chorio-retinitis, optic neuritis, etc. Systemically, the drug can be given either by oral or parenteral routes.

Doses: Commonly used topical corticosteroids are suspensions or solutions. Cortisone and hydrocortisone are insoluble and therefore are used as suspension in 1–2.5% concentration. Soluble dexamethasone is used as 0.1% solution repeated 4–6 times a day or more depending on the severity and urgency of the therapy. It is better to use soluble preparations for acute conditions and insoluble suspensions for chronic conditions or when prolonged use is desired. This applies both for eye drops or ocular injections. The dose for systemic therapy depends upon the severity of the disease and the type of preparation used. In cases of severe inflammations, even 60–80 mg of prednisone may be given daily. After

the disease process has been arrested and a regression observed, the dose should be reduced gradually over a period of time. Sudden withdrawal of steroids may result in relapse of the condition or cause symptoms of adrenal insufficiency. A good rule for systemic use is to give a high dosage for shorter periods with a tapering withdrawal.

ACTH: Administration of biological adrenocorticotropic hormone (ACTH) is indicated as a starting steroid in some conditions to be followed by systemic corticosteroids. The best ocular indication is optic neuritis as an extension of meningitis. 20–40 units by injection twice a day is the optimum dose. ACTH cannot be given orally.

Uses of Steroids in Ocular Diseases

Corticosteroids find a wide range of uses in ophthalmology. They are useful in most inflammatory, allergic and traumatic lesions of the eye.

Inflammatory lesions: Steroids are helpful in most non-pyogenic inflammations of the eye; particularly in stromal keratitis, iritis, choroiditis, papillitis and retrobulbar neuritis.

Allergic conditions: It is used for the treatment of contact dermatitis of the lids, allergic blepharitis and conjunctivitis. In cases of vernal conjunctivitis, it is very useful in reducing symptoms during the active phase of the disease. It is also effective in phlyctenular conjunctivitis and keratitis, interstitial keratitis, episcleritis. It is the drug for treatment of tissue immune reactions after corneal grafting.

Collagen disorders: Corticosteroids have been found to be effective in collagen disorders affecting body and the eye i.e., in Boeck's sarcoidosis, temporal arteritis, sclero-malacia perforans, rheumatoid arthritis, etc.

Traumatic conditions: Corticosteroids are used to prevent scarring specially in chemical burns. It is used in treatment of traumatic macular oedema. Post-operatively, it is often used to reduce inflammatory reactions after various intraocular surgeries.

Complications of the Use of Corticosteroids

Although corticosteroids give dramatic results in certain ocular conditions, they are not without complications and side-effects. Non-judicious use of steroids may be deleterious to the eye. Steroids are aptly called a *'double edged sword'*.

Local complications:
1. Corticosteroids delay process of wound healing.
2. Prolonged used of Corticosteroids may produce a clinical picture similar to chronic simple glaucoma because it reduces aqueous outflow facility due to changes in trabecular mesh work.
3. Prolonged use may also cause posterior sub-capsular lens opacities which later may involve whole lens.

Systemic complications:
1. Because of derangement in carbohydrate metabolism, steroids may cause temporary increase in the diabetic status.
2. Due to increased mobilization of fat, prolonged use of steroids causes a moon face appearance and other features of Cushing's syndrome.
3. Due to electrolyte imbalance of sodium and water retention, it causes oedema, increase in body weight and rise of blood pressure.

Contraindications: *Systemic.* Steroids are contra-indicated in cases of peptic ulcer, diabetes mellitus and hypertension. It should also be avoided in patients having an active or recently healed tuberculosis as it may reactivate the disease.

Local: It is contra-indicated in Herpes simplex keratitis and fungal infections. It should also be used with caution in patients who are glaucoma suspects. In fact steroids have been used as a provocative test for confirmation of diagnosis of glaucoma. In case of bacterial infections of cornea or conjunctiva, therapy should be with antibiotics and only when acute infection is under control, steroids if needed, may be added.

ANTI-VIRAL AGENTS

The anti-viral drugs available at present are effective mainly against Herpex simplex. A brief account of these are given below:

IDU (5-iodo-2-deoxy uridine). IDU was the first anti-viral agent found to be effective in Herpes simplex keratitis. IDU is an anti-metabolic analogue of thymidine. By replacing thymidine from nucleic acid, it prevents synthesis of DNA and thus prevents viral synthesis. IDU is used as drops in the concentration of 0.1% and as ointment in strength of 0.5%. The drug has poor ocular penetration. To get maximum response, the solution is instilled every 2-3 hours till corneal staining disappears. The ointment is used at bed time. Early discontinuation of the drug may cause relapse of disease process. The solution should be in dark bottles and stored at cool temperature.

Uses: It is used topically for Herpes simplex keratitis. It is most effective in dendritic keratitis where the lesion is in the epithelial layers of the cornea. It is not very effective in stromal keratitis, chronic disciform keratitis and herpetic iritis.

There are no serious side-effects or absolute centra-indications for IDU therapy. The drug is, however, toxic to the tissues. Moreover the virus is known to develop drug resistance. It may therefore not be effective in all cases.

Vidarabine (Vira-A). It is a less toxic and a more effective anti-viral agent than IDU. It acts by stopping the growth of the viral DNA chain. It is effective in Herpes infections resistant to IDU. It is also effective in the treatment of herpetic iritis. It is used as 3% ointment 3-4 times a day.

Viroptic (Triflurothymidine) It is a newer addition to anti-viral therapy. It is a DNA inhibitor agent used as 1% solution eye drops instilled every 2-3 hours. It has been found effective when the lesions do not respond to IDU or Vira A.

Acyclovir (Acycloguanosine)

It is safe and effective in most forms of simplex as well as zoster infection. It inhibits viral DNA and has a better penetrating power thus is effective in stromal pathology. It is available as 3% ointment and oral tablets of 200 mg.

Interferons, immunoglobulins and cytosine arabinoside are agents known for their antiviral effectivity.

ANTI-FUNGAL AGENTS

Many corneal ulcers which are resistant to routine antibiotic therapy, turn out to be mycotic in nature.

The commonly used anti-fungal agents are as follows:

Amphotericin-B. It is a fungistatic agent derived from *streptomyces nodosus*. It is effective against Candida and Aspergillosis. In India it is available as Fungizone for intravenous drip which can be diluted for eye drops or subconjunctival injection.

Topically it is used as 0.5 per cent solution prepared in glucose or distilled water. It should not be prepared in saline as saline precipitates the drug. In ointment form also it is used in concentration of 0.5%. It can also be given subconjunctivally in doses of 0.125 mg in 0.5 ml but subconjunctival injections are painful.

Intravenous administration is needed for intraocular infections. Initially, 50 mgm dissolved in 5% dextrose is given by intravenous infusion repeated once a day. 5 mgm of heparin mixed in the infusion will prevent local vein thrombosis.

The drug is quite toxic in therapeutic doses. It should be used only in hospitalised patients. Initial side-effects include chills, headaches, fever and anorexia. Locally thrombophlebitis at the site of injection may develop.

Because of its renal toxicity, it should not be used in patients with renal diseases. Blood urea estimation should be done prior to and during the therapy with Amphotericin-B.

Nystatin (Mycostatin). It is an antifungal agent, soluble and well tolerated. It is effective mainly against Candida infection. It is used as 3% ointment or eye drops in concentration of 10,000 units/ml. It is available as Nistin ointment. Sub-conjunctival injections of 5000 units are also effective and well tolerated. The drug is very toxic if given systemically.

Pimaricin: It is an antifungal effective against aspergillus, candida fusarium and cephalosporium. It is used as 5% suspension or 1% ointment topically every 2 hours. It is not irritative and is well tolerated. It is insoluble in water, has poor ocular penetration, so it is not effective in intraocular infections. Debridement of necrotic tissues before its use, enhances its effect.

Imadozole antifungal drug series includes *miconozole, clotrimazole, ketoconazole, econazole* and *fluconazole*. Most of them are effective against candida, fusarium and cladosporium etc. Preparations are available for topical and systemic use.

Silver sulphadiazine has also been used in aspergillus and fusarium infections.

ANTIBIOTICS

Since the discovery of first antibiotic "penicillin", many antibiotics have been chemically synthesized. The use of these drugs has proved very beneficial in various infective conditions of the eye.

At present, there are numerous antibiotics available with varying spectrum of activity against most bacteria. These antibiotics can be divided into the following groups:

1. *Antibiotics mainly effective against gram positive organisms:*
   - Penicillin
   - Erythromycin

2. *Antibiotics mainly effective against gram negative organisms*:
   – Streptomycin
   – Polymyxin B
3. *Broad spectrum antibiotics effective against both, gram negative and positive Bacteria:*
   – Ampicillin—amoxycillin
   – Carbenecillin
   – Tetracyclin
   – Framycetin
   – Neomycin
   – Gentamycin.

Penicillin: Penicillin was the first antibiotic discovered by Alexander Fleming and John Florey who produced the first strain from the mould of penicillium. It was however Florey and his colleagues who extracted penicillin in 1939. Since its discovery, many new semi-synthetic and synthetic derivatives of penicillin have been prepared with varying advantages over others. Regular crystalline penicillin-G is effective against gram +ve bacteria only but newer derivatives are effective against gram –ve bacteria also. Some organisms like staphylococcus aureus produce an enzyme called penicillinase. Penicillin-G is therefore not effective against them. Newer penicillins have been developed which resist the action of penicillinase and therefore are active against more bacteria than penicillin-G.

There are three groups of penicillins.

The first group includes:
1. Penicillin-G
2. Procain Penicillin } for Injection
3. Potassium penicillin—V for oral use.

The second group is the penicillinase resistant group which includes:
1. Oxacillin
2. Cloxacillin } They are all effective against gram+cocci including staphylococcus aureus.
3. Floxacillin

The third group comprises broad spectrum penicillins like:

1. Ampicillin
2. Amoxycillin
3. Carbenicillin

Effective also against gram negative organisms like influenza bacillus, E-coli, proteus and pseudomonas Aerugenosa. This group however is hydrolized by penicillinase.

The oxacillin group is therefore most effective against all gram positive organisms and the broad spectrum penicillins against gram negative organisms also.

Modes of use: Penicillin is used as drops in the concentration of 10,000 units/cc. The frequency of drops depends upon the severity of infection varying from every 5 minutes to 6-8 times a day. It is also used as ointment in the concentration of 5000-10,000 units/gm.

Sub-conjunctival injections are given in concentration of 1–5 lac units/ml. By this method, a high intra-ocular concentration is achieved. The effect can be prolonged by adding five drops of 1:1000 adrenaline solution in each injection. Being an acidic solution, it causes severe tissue reaction.

Systemically it is given intramuscularly in doses of 5–10 lac units once or twice a day. For intraocular infections, systemic administration of penicillin is effective only in high concentrations as it has a poor penetration into eye through blood-aqueous barrier.

Toxicity: The external application of the drug in any concentration is non-toxic to the eye but local skin allergy to penicillin is quite common. The most serious complication, however, following parenteral administration is hypersensitivity reaction which may cause sudden anaphylactic shock and even death. Steroids, antihistamines and adrenaline 1:1000 may be given intravenously in the management of anaphylactic shock.

Ampicillin: It is a synthetic penicillin with a broad anti-bacterial spectrum. It is effective against gram +ve and gram –ve bacteria. It is given orally in dose of 250–500 mgm every

6 hours. The same dose may be given intra-muscularly or intravenously in severe inflammations. This drug has a better penetration across the blood-aqueous barrier so that it is useful in intra-ocular infection. It is one of the least toxic drugs, with practically no side-effects. Occasionally hypersensitivity reaction like penicillin may occur. *Amoxycillin* and *carbenicillin* are newer additions to the ampicillin group.

Other Broad-Spectrum Antibiotics

Gentamycin. It is one of the commonly used antibiotics in ocular infections. It is effective against many gram –ve organisms like Pseudomonas, Klebsiella, E coli, etc. It is also very effective against most strains of staphylococcus.

Topically it is used as 0.3% drops. Sub-conjunctival injections 20 mg/ml are given in intra-ocular infections and as prophylactic at the time of intraocular surgery. Systemically, it is given in doses of 1–3 mg/kg body weight intra-muscularly in divided doses.

This is one drug which has been used as intra-vitreal injection in cases of endophthalmitis. But it should be given in very small quantity. Gara-mycin is supplied as 40 mg per ml. 0.1 ml (4 mg) is diluted 10 times which makes 0.4 mg per ml. 0.1 ml of this solution with 0.1 ml of Dexame-thasone is injected in the centre of the vitreous chamber after aspirating 0.2 ml of vitreous fluid. The effect lasts upto 48 hours and there is minimal vitreous reaction. A higher concentration is retino-toxic.

Caphaloridine is a newer generation of effective antibiotic and can be given intra-vitreally in a dose of 0.25 mg in 0.1 ml solution.

Streptomycin: It has a wide anti-bacterial spectrum. It is effective against many gram +ve and gram –ve organisms. It is the effective drug against tuberculosis. It is given intramuscularly 1–2 gm daily. As topical administration, it does not penetrate the intact cornea in therapeutic concentrations. On prolonged parenteral use, it has a damaging effect on the eighth cranial nerve leading to tinitus, vertigo and deafness. It may be used as eye drops (25 mg/cc) for conjunctival and corneal infections by susceptible organisms.

Tetracycline: The tetracycline group of antibiotics includes chlor-tertracycline, oxy-tera-cycline. They are broad spectrum antibiotics and are effective against wide variety of gram +ve and gram –ve bacteria. They are also effective against some large viruses including those causing trachoma, inclusion conjunctivitis, lymphogranuloma venerium, psittacosis and molluscum contagiosum.

Systemically, they are given in doses of 1–2 gm daily in divided doses. For topical use 0.5% ointment or suspension is applied.

It is one of the safer antibiotics with low toxicity. Loss of appetite is a common effect. Nausea, vomiting and diarrhoea may occur due to their effect on intestinal flora.

Chloramphenicol: It is a broad-spectrum anti-microbial agent. Because of its quick absorption and easy penetration through the cornea and the blood-aqueous barrier, it was one of the most effective antibiotics used in intraocular infections. It is effective against many gram +ve organisms.

Systemically, it is given in doses of 1–2 gm a day orally or by parenteral route. Topically, it is used as 0.5% drops and 1% ointment. It is a drug with side-effects which include aplastic anaemia, agranulocytosis and optic neuritis which are noted on prolonged use of chloraem-phenicol.

Most broad spectrum antibiotics given orally reduce normal bacterial flora in intestines causing diarrhoea. Vitamin B complex should therefore always be given along with the oral antibiotic therapy.

Scores of antibiotics have become available over last two decades. A major category is that of **cephalosporins** having a wide spectrum of bacteriocidal activity. They are used topically as well as systemically. Adverse/side effects are infrequent with most of these drugs. Prolonged use may cause changes in blood counts, renal and liver function. However, these are reversible when the drug is discontinued.

Locally Used Antibiotics

Neomycin: It is a broad spectrum antibiotic effective against a wide variety of gram +ve and gram –ve organisms. It is particularly effective against pseudomonas and proteus group of organisms. It is used topically as 0.5% drops and is well tolerated. Local sensitivity to Neomycin causing conjunctival congestion and skin reaction is becoming more common. It is toxic to corneal epithelium and should not be continuously used for long periods.

Framycetin (Soframycin): It is also a broad spectrum antibiotic only for topical application. It is useful against pseudomonas group of organisms. It is used as 1% drops or ointment. It is non-irritative and non-toxic for topical application.

Polymyxin-B: It is a potent antibiotic against gram negative organisms. It is particularly useful in pseudomonas infections which may not respond to other antibiotics. Because of its toxic effects on kidney and nervous tissue, it is not used systemically. It is used as 0.1 per cent solution or 0.2% ointment locally.

Bacitracin is a good supportive agent along with other antibiotics as local therapy. It is used in 1000 units/cc as solution for eye drops.

Tobramycin 0.3% solution as eye drops is another antibiotic effective against larger range of gram positive and gram negative bacterial infections.

Chemotherapeutic Agents

Chemotherapeutic agents are chemical substances which have an anti-microbial effect. These have been used since a long time in the field of medicine. Since the discovery of the first sulphanilamide, many new agents have been found which are useful for their anti-microbial effect.

Of these, the commonly used drugs in ophthalmology are Sulphonamides for trachoma, Sulphones for leprosy and para-amino-salicylic acid and Isoniazide for tuberculosis.

Sulphonamides are bacterio-static agents with wide spectrum of activity. Many such drugs have been isolated with different kinds of anti-bacterial activity and side effects. With the discovery of antibiotics, the use of Sulphonamides has, however, been greatly reduced.

They prevent the utilisation of para-amino-benzoic acid by the bacteria and cause their immobilisation and therefore facilitate their phago-cytosis. They are ineffective in the presence of pus. Although they are effective against quite a few bacteria, they are largely used in ophthalmology as anti-trachoma local and oral therapy.

Sulphonamides are administered by the oral route. Systemic Sulphonamides are of two types—short acting *and* long acting.

Short acting sulphonamides include sulpha-diazine, sulphamerazine, etc. They are given in an initial dose of 1 gm and then a maintenance dose of 250 mg 6 hourly. Long acting sulphon-amides are sulphadimethoxine and sulphametho-xpyridiazine. They are given in an initial dose of 500 mg followed by a maintenance dose of 250 mg twice daily.

Sulphacetamide which is a soluble salt, is used locally as drops in concentration of 10–20% while in ointment form it is used as 5% ointment.

Co-trimoxazole first marketed as Septran is a combination of trimethoprim and sulphame-thoxazole, a non-antibiotic but anti-bacterial drug which has wider spectrum of effectiveness. It acts both as a sulpha as well as a broad spectrum antibiotic and the dose is two tablets twice a day.

Each tablet contains 80 mg trimethaprim and 400 mg of sulphamethoxazole. The drug is a suitable substitute when system develops resistance to antibiotics.

Side effects of sulphonamides: Sulphonamides have many undesirable side effects. The most common toxic effect is skin rash in form of dark patches. Sensitivity to sulphas has been known to cause bullous formation on skin and mucous membrane and cause a condition like Steven Johnson's syndrome. They can cause haemolytic anaemia and agranulocytosis. Renal complications are not uncommon because of the crystallization of sulphonamides causing haematuria and crystalurea. With sulpha therapy, the patient should be instructed to take plenty of.fluids to prevent crystal formations.

Sulphones: Sulphones are used for treatment of leprosy which should be advised in consultation with the physician.

PAS (Para amino salicylic acid). It is an anti-tubercular drug. It is used along with other anti-tubercular drugs like streptomycin and isoniazide because of its additive effect and also to reduce the chance of development of drug resistance.

Isoniazide (INH): It is an anti-infective agent derived from nicotinic acid. It is effective against tubercle bacilli. It is used in combination with other anti-tubercular agents.

Combination preparations (Forecox) for tuberculosis are available which include *Refampisin, isoniazide, pyrizinamide* and *ethambutol.*

Immuno-Suppressive Agents

Immuno-suppressive agents have been commonly used in various organ transplants to prevent rejection phenomenon. They are also used to suppress certain neoplastic growths. These drugs have been classified into various groups:

A. Corticosteroids.
B. Anti lymphocytic Serum.
C. Anti Metabolites, like:
 • Azothioprine (Immuran).
 • 6-mercaptopurine
D. Alkylating agents:
 • Thio-Tepa.
 • Triethylmelamine.
 • Cyclophosphamide (cytoxone).

Cyclosporin—2 percent solution in olive oil has been found effective and free from systemic effects when used topically.

A. **Corticosteroids** are potent immuno-suppresive drugs, most effective, most readily available and least toxic. Their pharmacology and therapeutics have been already discussed.

B. **Anti-lymphocytic serum:** It is a strong immuno-suppressive agent which is prepared by injecting the human lymphoid tissue into the horse. It mainly acts by suppressing the cell mediated immune response. It has been used to prevent tissue immune reactions after organ transplant surgery. In ophthalmology, it is used for preventing an immune reaction after corneal grafting and in uveitis. It is given by injection. Side effects include serum sickness and anaphylactic shock.

C.&D. **Anti-Metabolites and Alkylating agents** are more often used for malignant growths and their use, therefore, in consultation and guided by surgeon, physician and gynaecologist.

Non-steroid Anti-inflammatory Drugs (NSAID)

These drugs are needed particularly when steroids are contraindicated in acute inflammatory conditions such as iridocyclitis, posterior uveitis and in diabetics. These are salicylates, phenylbutazone, aminophenol, indomethacin, ibuprofen, flurbiprofen. Indomethacin and flurbiprofen are available for topical use also.

Visco-elastic Substances

These have been in use in ophthalmic surgery for over three decades. The first one to come in market was 1% Healon (sodium hyaluronate). It is non-toxic, non-inflammatory having good visco-elastic property. It used to be expensive and had to be imported.

Alternative substitutive preparations later became available such as methyl cellulose and hypomellose in 2% viscous solution. They have viscosity but no visco-elasticity. Chondroitin sulphate in combination with sodium hyaluronate (VISCOAT) is a good visco-elastic agent. A number of viscoelastic preparations are available, most containing 2% methyl cellulose as main constituent.

All visco-elastics are very important in intra-ocular surgery for maintenance of anterior chamber and more so for protection of corneal endothelium from surgical trauma. They have made intra-ocular surgeries easy and tension free by avoiding intra-operative complications.

DYES

Fluorescein is a dye which finds many uses in various diagnostic and surgical procedures in ophthalmology. It is used as a sodium salt and is water soluble. It produces a greenish colouration in alkaline medium.

Uses

1. **For the detection of corneal epithelial** defects. Fluoresceine staining is one of the simplest and most valuable methods of detecting corneal epithelial defects. By this procedure, epithelial defects of cornea are clearly visible as bright green patches. For staining, fluorescein is used in concentration of 1–2%. A drop is put in conjunctival sac and any excess of it is washed away after 1–2 minutes with normal saline.

   If fluoresceine solution is allowed to remain in the conjunctival sac for 3-5 minutes, it can penetrate through the corneal epithelium into the superficial corneal stroma.

2. **To test the patency of lacrimal** passages either by syringing with a weak fluoresceine solution or by just instilling 2% fluoresceine solution into the conjunctival sac and asking the patient to lie flat for a few minutes. The patient is then asked to blow his nose into a handkerchief. If the lacrimal passages are patent, the cloth will be stained green.

3. For **detecting a wound leak** in cases of the shallow anterior chamber following surgery.

4. For **applanation tonometry**, it is used to visualize applanated area and determine the point when reading is noted.

5. In **the fitting of hard contact lenses.** It helps in finding the area of lens-cornea contact in a tight fit and areas of fluorescein pooling suggesting a more curved lens.

6. **During corneal surgery** to stain the trephine mark for centering the trephine to be used.

7. **For studying corneal film and tear film break-up** (TFBT or BUT). It is the most important non-invasive means to study formation and maintenance of tear film. This is a very useful test for diagnosing particularly borderline DRY EYE cases. After staining the tear film with a fluorescein strip, it is examined on a slit lamp under a cobalt blue filter. The time taken to develop dry patches on corneal surface is noted. These appear as cobalt blue geographic areas surrounded by fluorescein green.

8. **Fluorescein angioscopy and angiography:** Fluorescein is used intravenously for procedure of fluorescein angiography. Fluorescein angiography gives information regarding various lesions of retina, choroid and optic nerve. By the same procedure,

fluoresceine is used for angioscopy with direct ophthalmoscope where a fundus camera is not available.

For fluorescein angiography, it is used, 10 cc of 10% or 3 to 5 cc of 20% solution given intravenously.

Fluorescein as such has no side effects on topical use except that in the solution, bacterial organisms like pseudomonas pyocyneous can easily grow.

Fluorescein is better used as strips impregnated with 4 per cent fluorescein. The advantage of strips is that there is no danger of contamination of fluoresceine, as fresh strip is used for every patient.

Complications may sometimes occur after intravenous use. They include nausea, vomiting, headache and sometimes hypersensitive reactions. The dye discolours the skin yellow and is excreted through kidneys imparting a deep yellow colour to the urine. The patient should be informed and reassured about it beforehand. Allergic reactions like urticaria may also be noted. Sometimes anaphylactic shock may occur therefore emergency measures should be readily available where fluorescein angiography is done.

Rose bengal: This dye has the property of staining devitalised conjunctival and corneal epithelium red. It is used in concentration of 0.1% solution or prepared strips. It is useful in diagnostic use for kerato-conjunctivitis sicca and neuroparalytic keratitis.

Methylene blue: It has been used for irrigation of lacrimal sac before sac operations. It helps in identifying the sac as the mucosal lining is stained blue. It is of particular help when doing a dacryocystectomy in eyes with fistula or when a secondary sac is being excised after the failure of the first surgery.

ENZYMES

Alpha-chymotrypsin—Zonulysin

It was pancreatic enzyme and like trypsin, is a proteolyctic enzyme. It was used in ophthalmology because of its action on zonules of the lens which are lysed by it. The solution once prepared is unstable and must be stored in a refrigerator and used within one month.

When the anterior chamber is irrigated with a solution of alpha-chymotrypsin in concentration of 1 : 5000 for 2–3 minutes, the zonular ligaments are broken down and lens lies free over the anterior vitreous face and can be easily extracted without any traction. It is particularly helpful in cases of young adults where the zonules are stronger and traction of lens delivery may have an adverse effect on the region of ora-serrata.

Alpha-chymotrypsin is contraindicated in very high myopic cases with fluid vitreous as there is danger of lens getting dislocated into the posterior segment after zonular ligaments have lysed. Zonulysin has been reported to diffuse through the vitreous and reach retina. Degenerative changes in the retinal layers have been reported. It can also cause enzymatic glaucoma following cataract operation. Intracapsular extraction is not practiced for more than two decades now since IOL after extracapsular is in vogue. *The drug therefore is not used at all.*

Hyaluronidase is an enzyme which hydrolyses and depolymerizes hyaluronic acid and mucopolysaccharides. Removal of these two substances from connective tissues greatly increase permeability of injected fluids. The hyaluronidase enzyme is therefore used to hasten absorption of various fluids injected into the connective tissue spaces.

It is used along with local anaesthetics for quickening and enhancing their effect of facial block, retrobulbar anaesthesia and peribulbar akinesia.

It also hastens absorption of sub-conjunctival haemorrhage, absorbs inflammatory exudates and blood from the anterior chamber. It has also been used for retarding progress of pterygium and reduce chemosis. It has no serious side effect. Its use is contraindicated in infective and cancerous conditions for fear of spreading the infection or malignant cells.

Fibrinolysin

It is proteolytic enzyme which breaks down fibrin and helps in the absorption of blood from the anterior chamber. Fibrinolysin breaks fibrin into non-coagulable fragments and thus help in dissolving clots. It also inactivates fibrinogen and therefore has anti-coagulant properties.

Fibrinolysin irrigation of the anterior chamber in concentration of 2000 units/ml helps in breaking down blood clots and absorption of blood. It is more useful in cases of fresh clots. It is useful in cases of massive hyphema associated with secondary glaucoma.

Because of its anticoagulant properties, it has been used in the treatment of occlusion of the central retinal artery.

Streptokinase

It is produced by haemolytic streptococcus. It dissolves blood clots and fibrinous portions of the exudates (thrombolytic). It is antigenic and may produce allergic reactions. Because of its toxic effects, its use in ocular conditions is restricted.

Urokinase is a better derivative as it is not antigenic. It is available in vials of 25,000 units in powder form and the dose is 1,50,000 units in a day given by intravenous route.

PROSTAGLANDINS

Prostaglandins have generated a lot of interest and excitement in the field of pharmacology. Although it was isolated as early as early 1930, its synthesis and full potentials came to light around 1960.

Initially it was thought to be secreted by the seminal vesicles but it has now been confirmed that they are found almost in every tissue and body fluid and have effect on many body functions even in very small doses. It has been demonstrated that prostaglandin is not a single compound but are a group of substances with a 20 carbon unsaturated carboxylic acid with a cyclopentane ring. Depending upon configuration of cyclopentane ring, various groups of prostaglandins have been isolated, E, F, A, B, C, D. Each group is again divided into further subdivisions. The prostaglandins have numerous effects on various body functions like vasodilatation, thrombolytic action by inhibiting aggregation of platelets, relax bronchial muscles and contract uterine muscles and therefore abortificient. It also has an effect on gastric and pancreatic secretions, urinary tract, central nervous system, autonomous nervous system and endocrine system.

In the field of ophthalmology, they have been found to play a role in inflammations of the uveal tract. Role of prostaglandin in glaucoma therapy has been discussed.

SOME OTHER DRUGS IN USE IN OPHTHALMOLOGY

Anticoagulants

1. **Heparin** is an anticoagulant normally present in mast cells in the body. It acts on all three stages of coagulation. As a drug, it is given by intravenous infusion, 20,000 units/litre in 24 hours or by intramuscular injection 5000 units every 4 hours. Protamin sulphate 1% solution by slow infusion is its antagonist. It may be given in early stages in cavernous sinus thrombosis or thrombosis of central retinal vein. The therapy should be monitored by repeated bleeding coagulation time and prothrombin blood level which should not be allowed to fall below 25% of normal (30 seconds prothrombin time). Further more, any surgical procedure during the therapy has the danger of severe bleeding.

2. **Dicoumarol:** This is an oral anticoagulant and depresses prothrombin level in blood. It

can cause bleeding from various tissues. The effect can be counteracted by Vitamin K.

In urgent situations it is better to start with heparin, followed by an oral anticoagulant.

OTHER THERAPEUTIC MEASURES

Diathermy

Diathermy is a procedure by which heat is generated in the tissues of the eye by passage of a high frequency current through a conductor. Heat applied directly through conduction or through radiation does not reach deeper tissues because tissues are poor conductors of heat and considerable amount of heat is taken away by circulating blood. It is not so in cases of heat generated by electrical current. This procedure of diathermy finds use in many ophthalmological disorders.

Surgical diathermy: In this procedure, the purpose is to coagulate the tissue by heat generated. If the active electrode is a cutting one, it can act as knife and simultaneously coagulate bleeding vessels.

Surgical diathermy was used in treatment of retinal detachment, intra-ocular neoplasms and glaucoma surgery (Cyclo-diathermy and Cyclo-anemization). Other uses include destruction of small growths of the lids and destruction of lashes in trichiasis. The current needed for destroying the eye lashes is 3–4 milli amperes and for the coagulation of deeper tissues between 40-60 milli amperes.

Cryotherapy

Cryotherapy is tissue coagulation by application of intense cold. Cryotherapy has found many therapeutic uses in ophthalmology.

The first use of cryotherapy was in the form of carbon dioxide snow for conjunctival growths and warts.

Cryotherapy entered into routine clinical practice, specially in ophthalmology in 1961 when Krawawicz developed metal probes for intracapsular cataract extraction.

Once the use of cryo was determined to be better than forceps for cataract extraction, it was important to find material which will be non-inflammable, non-explosive, inert, with a low freezing point and inexpensive. The gases from this point of view are freon, carbon-dioxide and nitrous oxide. Freon can produce freezing temperature of $-30°$ and is therefore adequate for cataract extraction. Carbon-dioxide and nitrous oxide produce temperature at the tip of the probe up to $-70°C$ which is necessary for retinal and ciliary body procedures. Medical carbon-dioxide is not readily available while freon is available even at smaller towns and nitrous oxide in all operation theatres with Boyle's anaesthesia apparatus.

Cryotherapy of retina is better than diathermy because the former causes no tissue necrosis, no vitreous shrinkage and re-operation after cryo is easier than after diathermy. The appropriate method is to apply $-30°C$ temperature for 2–3 seconds for cataract extraction and $-50°C$ to $60°C$ temperature for 5 seconds for retinopexy and $-70°$ to $80°C$ for 15–20 seconds for glaucoma therapy.

Uses of Cryotherapy in Ophthalmology

1. *Lids.* Cryotherapy is used for destruction of xanthelasma, haemangioma and lipomata. It is useful for trichiasis when applied on eye lash roots. The roots atrophy and the lashes fall off. There is no re-growth later.
2. *Cornea:* Cryotherapy has been used for the treatment of herpes simplex keratitis. It acts by coagulating the infected epithelium and killing the causative organisms.
3. *Cataract surgery:* The use of cryo probes in intracapsular extraction of cataract was of great advantage. It had almost replaced use of forceps for extractions of cataract.

The cryoprobe, when applied to the anterior capsule of the lens, freezes the anterior cortex up to 2–3 mm depth. An ice ball is formed giving a firm attachment between the probe and the lens which can then be easily delivered. The advantage of cryo over the forceps was that no pressure is required while the adhesion between the probe and the lens takes place. It minimizes the chances of vitreous loss. Secondly, as the capsule adheres and not caught, chances of rupture of the capsule are almost negligible. This method was of utmost value in hypermature morgagnian cataract and cataract with a friable capsule as in intumescent cataract.

4. *Glaucoma:* Cyclo-cryotherapy is similar to cyclodiathermy in which ciliary body is partially inactivated by applying cryoprobe over sclera corresponding to ciliary body underneath. The advantage of cyclocryotherapy over cyclodiathermy is that it does not require any cutting procedure. A cryo probe can be applied transconjunctivally. Moreover it can be repeated without any danger of necrosis of tissue.

5. *Retina:* Like diathermy, cryotherapy is used for producing chorio-retinal adhesions in retinal detachment operation. It is also used to treat benign peripheral retino-choriodal lesions like silent holes, microcysts and areas of lattice degenerations. Pre-equatorial cryotherapy has been found to be useful in treatment of vitreous haemorrhage and diabetic retinopathy.

6. *Other indications* include epithelialisation of the anterior chamber after cataract operation, iris prolapse, vitreous prolapse, pterygium, herpetic corneal ulcer, fistula and in the procedure of keratomilieusis.

Photo-Coagulation

It has been known since ancient times that looking directly at sun, particularly at time of a solar eclipse causes blindness. With invention of the ophthalmoscope, it was proved that diminished vision was due to macular burn by infra red rays of solar light. The same principle has been applied in development of photocoagulation therapy. When a high intensity light is focussed on to retina, it is absorbed by the pigment epithelium and heat is generated at the site. This causes a local aseptic inflammation which produces chorio-retinal burns and adhesions.

There are three types of photo-coagulation therapies available at present. Their characteristics are given below in a tabulated form:

Uses of photocoagulation

1. *Retinal disorders.* It has been used in various retinal disorders; the most important being diabetic retinopathy. The therapy is also used to seal posterior retinal holes. Central serous retinopathy and macular holes are other retinal conditions. Neoplasms like small retinoblastoma and choroidal melanoma in the early stages are good indications for photocoagulation. Vascular lesions like angiomatosis and periphlebitis are also treated with photocoagulation.

2. *Iris:* It has been used to reconstruct pupil in cases of updrawn pupil after surgery or trauma. Peripheral iridectomy, trabeculectomy as also capsulotomy of after cataract can all be done with a laser without operative intervention.

Complications of photocoagulation

Retinal haemorrhage may occur due to rupture of a blood vessel. Retinal shrinkage due to scarring after too much photocoagulation may give rise to secondary traction detachment of the retina.

Radiotherapy

Radiation has been used for treatment of various neoplastic conditions of the body for long. This

	Xenon coagulator	*Hruby laser*	*Argon, laser krypton and yag*
Type of light	*Poly chromatic*	Mono chromatic	Mono chromatic
Wave length	400–1600 nm	694.3 nm	457.9–514 nm
Minimum spot size	150–200 microns	80 microns	50 microns
Effect on blood vessel	No effect	No effect	Absorbed by blood pigment

therapy was not in the field of ophthalmology because of the damage it caused to normal ocular tissues along with destruction of growth for which it was used. With development of special instruments and various techniques of radiation and also protective devices, the undesired effects of radiation have been brought to a minimum and radiation used in minimum doses to get the maximum benefit precisely at the site of lesion is now possible without damaging normal surviving tissues.

Three types of radiations are used in the field of medicine and all these also find use in ophthalmology:

1. X-rays.
2. Gamma rays.
3. Beta rays.

X-rays are electromagnetic waves produced by applying a high potential current to the electrodes inside a vacuum tube. The X-rays can be of various energies and power of penetration. Low voltage X-rays are used for superficial surface lesions as their power of penetration is limited. High voltage deep X-rays are used for intraocular and intra-orbital growths.

Gamma rays are also electromagnetic rays and are produced by various radioactive isotopes like cobalt and radium. They are used for malignant growths; pre- and post-operative.

Beta rays are obtained from radio-active sources like radium and strontium 90. They have a very limited penetration and are useful in superficial benign lesions of eye.

Radiation can be given by various methods like *external application*, radio-active implants, *intracavity* radiation and injection or *ingestion of radioactive isotopes*.

Uses of radiotherapy in ophthalmology: Radiotherapy may be used in ophthalmology for both neoplastic and non-neoplastic lesions.

A. Non-neoplastic lesions. The main purpose of radiation therapy in non-neoplastic lesions of the eye is to promote healing by resolution of inflammatory process, to reduce the vascular engorgement and reduce vascularisation of the cornea. Radiotherapy is used only when other recognised methods of treatment have failed to produce the desired effect. The various non-neoplastic lesions for most of which beta irradiation is used, are Mooren's ulcer, corneal vascularisation after keratoplasty, spring catarrh and recurrent Plerygium.

B. Neoplastic Lesion
1. *Haemangioma:* Haemangioma occuring in infancy may resolve spontaneously. Sometimes they require treatment when they are in exposed parts of the body with danger of frequent trauma or haemorrhage. Superficial X-ray therapy by a single dose is given and this may be repeated after a year if necessary.

2. *Malignant lesions:* Radiation therapy of malignant lesions is undertaken either as a curative procedure alone or along with surgery or as a palliative treatment when the disease has widely spread with distant metastases. The various tissues of the eye and adnexa requiring radiation therapy are: (i) Retinoblastoma when binocular, better eye is treated with radium therapy after enucleating the worse eye. Post-operative irradiation is also indicated after

enucleation or exenteration procedures, (ii) Other tumours treated with irradiation are epithelioma of lids, limbus and lacrimal gland, (iii) Orbital malignant tumours like lymphosarcoma.

The latest modality in ocular therapy is Anti-vascular endothelial growth factor. It was demonstrated that in animal models and human specimens of choroidal neovascularisation. Vascular Endothelial Growth Factor exists which is capable of inducing neovascularisation. Hypoxic retinal pigment epithelium produces VEGF inducing endothelial proliferation. This meant inhibition of VEGF for prevention and therapy of neovascularisation, a pathological angiogenesis in ischaemic and inflammatory diseases.

Anti-angiogenic therapy was first thought of for cancer in form of Bevacizumab (Avastin) which is a humanised monoclonal antibody directed against active forms of VEGF-A. It prevents interaction between VEGA-A and its receptors on endothelial cells. Anti VEGF agents were introduced for ocular neovascular diseases, important are obviously Age related macular degeneration (wet ARMD) and diabetic neovascularisation, both conditions result in gross visual loss in older age group of patients. Similarly, neovascularisation due to retinal venous occlusive disease too can benefit. Available anti VEGF drugs are Avastin (Bevacizumab) and Lucentis (Ranibizumab). These are used as intravitreal injection, 1.25 mg in 0.05 cc, repeated 6 weekly. One limitation is the cost of the drug.

28

Community Ophthalmology

Community is a group of people with common rights and common interests. They live in common environments, have common health problems and therefore need community approach for health care. More than 75% of India's population lives in 6,00,000 villages in the country which are distinctly divisible into regions on the basis of climate, eating habits and social customs. There are however common factors like illiteracy, ignorance and superstition. Added to these is the ever increasing population which on one side demands greater community effort for national problems and on the other makes it more difficult to reach the target.

Community health in general and community ophthalmology are closely interlinked with the living habits and socio-economic factors. These well knit groups of population live in unhealthy environments and have unhealthy personal hygiene. Worse still, customs and traditions are so deep rooted that people are not easily receptive to preventive and curative measures.

With developments in medical science and internationalisation of community health, these communities of rural population cannot be left to themselves. The specific factors which disturb the dynamic equilibrium between man and his environment has to be restored to prevent disease.

Community ophthalmology like child health is important for the economic growth of community and the country. A healthy child is going to be a healthy man and become member of a healthy nation. A blind child will be a liability to the family, community and the country and even to the international fraternity. It is estimated that, even at the rural economy level in India, it will cost 10,000 million rupees to maintain the present totally or economically blind persons through a moderate span of life. It is therefore understandable that blindness has not only to be prevented but wherever possible, be cured. Community approach to eye care is therefore vitally needed to cover the length and breadth of the size of a country like India.

A survey, not only of the magnitude of the problem but also of the quality, is the first requisite for prevention of blindness and restoration of sight to the visually challenged. The last national survey conducted in India from 1971 to 1973 on a statistically controlled random sample basis has yielded the following information:

1. That, of the 9.5 million visually handi-capped persons; 3.7 million are totally blind in both eyes; 3.6 million are economi-cally blind; and 2.2 million are blind in one eye.

2. That 55% of the blindness is caused by cataract; 20% by corneal diseases; 5% by glaucoma; and 20% due to other ocular diseases.

There are 45 million persons who have less significant ocular health problems and suffer from some degree of visual handicap due to errors of refraction in school children and hazards due to rapid industrialization, etc.

Comparable figures of the prevalence of blindness in some of the developing countries as of 1981 are given in the following Table:

Global	0.4%
Developing countries	0.1–4.3%
China	0.1%
Argentina	0.12%
Brazil	0.15%
Peru	0.2%
Iran	0.8%
Bangladesh	0.9%
Burma	1.0%
Chile	1.0%
Iraq	1.0%
Venezuela	1.0%
India	1.5%
Afghanistan	2.0%
Phillipines	2.1%
Pakistan	4.3%

Whatever the veracity of these data, the fact remains that India has one of the highest incidence of blindness in the developing world and it is to be only expected because India is also the second highest populated country.

These statistical data are however a good guide line to plan projects with different emphasis on different factors.

PROBLEM OF RURAL EYE CARE

Community ophthalmology in a country like India is not entirely a medical problem. It is a socio medical problem interlinked with economic development, literacy and general health. A piecemeal approach therefore is less likely to yield lasting results. To be effective, it has to be a composite effort of Economics Ministry, Education Ministry, the Social Welfare department and of course the Ministry of Health. It has to be budgeted accordingly. From ophthalmic point of view, the approach has to be a total eye care approach including preventive ophthalmology, curative ophthalmology and rehabilitation of the incurably blind.

PREVENTIVE OPHTHALMOLOGY

Prevention is better than cure is an old age most appropriately applicable to ophthalmology. Differently said, it costs 1/10 to prevent a disease than what it takes to cure a disease. Although immediate relief to those who are visually handicapped is important, preventive measures are as important, if not more.

To prevent blindness, prophylaxis has to be at all levels and on all points and this includes:
- Personal prophylaxis
- School prophylaxis
- Community prophylaxis
- National prophylaxis
- International prophylaxis.

Personal Prophylaxis

1. Personal hygiene is an important factor in prevention. Clean body and clean eyes are extremely important.
2. Clean clothes, separate napkins for bath, face ash for each member of the family and avoiding habit of using sari ends for wiping the eyes of children, are important.
3. Working mothers should not dope their children with opiates because the drugged children are unmindful of flies sitting on the eyes and face which bring or carry infection.
4. The kajal and surma in the family members should not be applied with the same stick.
5. Reading habits of children should be supervised by the parents so that the child does not read in poor light, does not hold the object too close and adopts proper posture while reading. T. V. should be seen from a distance of at least 10 feet.

6. Animal sheds should be away from the living rooms.
7. Customs, traditions and taboos should be fought.
8. Any ocular symptoms, specially after 40 years of age, should not be casually ignored and a timely visit to the medical person will help getting guide lines of proper directions.

School Prophylaxis

1. Teachers can make a big contribution in prevention of blindness. They should have training in ocular hygiene.
2. Teachers should note wrong reading habits in any child under his/her care and report to the parents.
3. Child with infected eyes should not be allowed to attend the school till cured.
4. Any nutrition programme in school children should be seriously implemented.
5. An yearly examination of the eyes of school children is important to detect eye defects at the early stage. *It will be still better if at the entrance to the school, a health book of the child is started and maintained with periodical health check up till the child leaves the school.*

Community Prophylaxis

Community owes to itself that they live in clean environments and are free from disease as far as possible.
1. The village streets should be kept clean. The drains should be cleaned daily. Manure dumps should be away form the village.
2. Clean water for drinking and bath should be provided by disinfecting wells and ponds.
3. All means should be adopted to reduce fly incidence.
4. Community educational programmes should be organised from time to time on prevention of eye diseases.
5. Any epidemic, like epidemic conjunctivitis, should be promptly reported and the preventive measures should be faithfully adopted.

Nutrition

Eyes will be healthy if the body is healthy. Quite often dietary habits can be improved and nutritious items can be added to the food without a strain on economy which is important for poor communities of rural areas.

Green leafy vegetables are in abundance in villages only if they are taken in good quantity to provide adequate Vitamin A to prevent xerophthalmia, a major factor in causation of corneal blindness.

Cereals, as a poor man's meat in diet, are important more so in predominantly rice eating communities. It will give enough proteins for wear and tear of the tissues and overcome an important deficiency factor in the causation of keratomalacia.

Milk produced in the villages should first be for the children of the house than for the marketing in the cities.

Mass Communication

It is of utmost importance that the people should be educated to help themselves in these measures. All mass media of communication should be used to reach this information to the most peripheral parts of the country. Chapters on prophylaxis in the school textbooks will help educate children from very young age. Educative lectures through social organisations and cinema slides in the rural areas will be useful to bring to the masses the importance of prophylaxis. Radio, T.V. and newspaper media are equally important as these services have reached remotest part of the country.

Relief of Blindness

An active programme is necessary for those who are already blind or visually handicapped. Existing blindness has to be cured. Incurably blind have to be rehabilitated. Continued efforts are needed to treat those who may become blind later on. In a country like India, big in size and massive in population, an integrated national programme alone can tackle the heavy incidence of blindness. In any programme like this, public cooperation and enthusiastic participation is vital along with precise planning of the programme. International organisations like WHO, UNICEF, The Royal Commonwealth Society for the blind, Christofel Blinden Mission and Oxfam are a great source of vital support in implementation of these national programmes. Since the last few years International Agency for prevention of Blindness (IAPB) is active the world over.

Rehabilitation of Blind

Once a patient cannot be visually improved by surgical or non-surgical means, he needs to be rehabilitated to make his life tolerable and to some extent purposeful. The purpose is not only to improve him psychologically, free him from dependence on others for daily chores, but also make him a self earning member of the society that his liability to the society and the community is reduced to the minimum.

Those who are blind from birth or early childhood, are more easily amenable to rehabilitation if the process is started in early age. They are psychologically also better placed because they have never enjoyed good vision and therefore they do not know what they have lost. On the other hand, persons who become blind in adult age, are more difficult to rehabilitate.

The process of rehabilitation should be started at early age so that the child is saved from developing undesirable attitudes. The parents should be convinced that blindness in their child is incurable and should accept that the child has to be brought up as a blind child. They should plan the future of the child keeping these unavoidable facts in mind. It is surprising how pleasantly a child may get adjusted to the situation, if the approach is proper.

Rehabilitation includes the following:
1. *Mobility training:* This is the first part of training to make the blind less dependent on others. Use of *white cane* is an internationally recognised procedure. The blind uses the cane to free himself from dependence for walking. White cane in the hand of a person is an indication to the sighted persons to give the blind person priority on the road and also help him in a more difficult situation.
2. *Education.* Even though blind, education is an important part of rehabilitation. It not only improves him psychologically, it raises his intellectual status, makes his life purposeful and helps him to become economically self dependent. Madam Louis Braille did a great service to the blind community by developing alphabets based on touch system.

   Enough literature is available in Braille and the blind become enlightened by reading the extra-curricular Braille books. It is evident that Braille teachers have also to be trained as teachers.

   Thought has been given whether the school for blind children should be separate or they should study in schools along with sighted children. The consensus is growing that if the latter was possible, it will help better understanding of the blind by the sighted children. With proper psychological development and good opportunity of education, blind people have acquired highest qualifications and have proved that they are as good as sighted persons with some degree of limited handicap.

   Teaching in music has always been an essential part of educating the blind. Every blind school, should therefore, have opportunity of educating the blind children in various subjects of music.
3. *Sports:* Physical activity of blind being relatively limited, provision for sports is more important than even for sighted children. This

A	B	C	D	E	F	G
H	I	J	K	L	M	N
O	P	Q	R	S	T	U
	V	W	X	Y	Z	

BRAILLE ALPHABET

English Alphabets in Braille. [Note that every alphabet is based on varying combinations of not more than six dots (three pairs). Like the alphabets, punctuations are also covered by different arrangements of dots in three lines.]

should be provided in all schools and a competitive spirit should be introduced.

4. *Occupational rehabilitation.* A blind should and can become independent, if given proper training and proper opportunity.

The occupational training should be oriented to the background of the blind child. Agricultural training would be most appropriate for rural blind provided they have land and do not become an agricultural labour. The only such rehabilitation centre in India is at Phansa at the Maharashtra-Gujarat border.

Industrial training is the commonest training given to the blind the world over. The commonest jobs a blind can do are:

1. Weaving.
2. Caning.
3. Carpentery.
4. Small industrial productions.
5. Telephone operators.

Multipurpose training projects are therefore needed where a blind child can be trained, depending on his aptitude and his capacity.

An important requirement of occupational training is the employment opportunities for all those trained. It may be an employment in industry or self employment. In the industry, jobs need to be reserved and the sighted people around should be helpful. Blind people can work in variety of industrial units, particularly where safety mechanisms are incorporated in the machines, specially for use by the blind.

Rehabilitation of the blind is acquiring more and more importance and newer methods are being developed. Electronic gadgets may help the blind to a better mobility. Newer industrial units may provide greater and safer opportunities. The blind should become better members of the society than they are and the responsibility of sighted community is very great indeed if lacs of incurably blind people have to have a more purposeful life.

National Programme

A national programme has been prepared by Government of India to establish permanent facility for Eye Health Care as an integrated part of general health services extending to the peripheral level. This programme provides organisation at the peripheral level, intermediate level and the central level.

The peripheral level includes provision of a community health worker, multipurpose worker and an ophthalmic assistant at the Primary Health Centres and Sub-Centres.

The intermediate level provides for facilities for eye treatment at the subdivisional hospitals and district hospitals which have been identified and provided equipments and staffing facilities.

At the central level the organisation included upgrading of medical colleges and developing regional eye institutions. The whole programme is coordinated at National level by Apex Institute, the RP Centre of Ophthalmic Sciences, New Delhi.

Apart from implementing this long term national plan, mobile rural eye care services will need to be continued for many years to come to clear the back log of cataract patients. These services have extended to most parts of the country and form an important item in the 20 year National Programme for control of blindness which invisages 20/20 vision by year 2020.

Eye Camps

An Eye Camp is a mobile organisation where the ophthalmologist goes to the patient rather than the patient coming to the ophthalmologist. It provides periodical visits to the rural areas where blindness is heavy. India pioneered rural eye camps more than 70 years back and credit goes to Dr Mathuradas Pahwa of Moga, Punjab, who travelled all over the country and performed an estimated one million cataract operations during his long innings of ophthalmic career. He left behind a legacy which became a source of inspiration to the successive generations of ophthalmologists.

Eye camps are a necessity in all developing countries where population is heavy and eye diseases prevalent. Regular eye care facilities are not available in rural areas and poverty, ignorance, physical handicap and psychological fear prevent the blind going to the distant eye centres.

Eye camp organisation is a co-ordinated action which involves the following steps:

1. **Community initiative:** Community representative of the area concerned approaches the urban ophthalmic organisation inviting them to hold an eye camp in their area.
2. **Pre-camp publicity:** A wide publicity is necessary during one to two months preceding the eye camp about the date and place pf the eye camp so that largest number of patients can avail of the service in that area.
3. **Planning at the eye camp centre:** This includes:

a. Forming a local Eye Camp Committee representing the local administration like the Panchayat, active social workers and philanthropists.
b. Preparing volunteer cadre.
c. Selecting the site of the eye camp in consultation with the ophthalmologist.

Eye camps in the past have been more oriented to quantity than quality. There is no reason to continue the same. Eye camps have covered large parts of the country by medical colleges, ophthalmic institutions, eye relief organisations and by individual eye surgeons.

It is an extremely important consideration for all concerned that an eye camp should only be diagnostic camp in identified areas where the services are required. To maintain scientific standards it is better that these diagnostic camps are organised to facilitate better patient care. It is suggested that a medical college or an ophthalmic institute or a non-governmental eye relief organisation adopt a Taluka/tehsil. Ophthalmic personnel should visit the area regularly, diagnose operable cases of cataract, glaucoma etc. and get them to base hospital/institute for surgery which should be commensurate with present developments. This provides a standard surgical service to rural population. It is also important that the diagnostic services must not concentrate on cataract alone. Equipments like tonometers, ophthalmoscope, trial set and frame, mydriatic solution etc. for diagnosis of glaucoma, posterior segment disease, refractive error should be carried to the site in addition to vision charts, light torches etc.

Case selection for cataract surgery should be meticulously done. Every patient with doubtful diagnosis of cataract should be dilated for examination with ophthalmoscope for confirming diagnosis of cataract or assessing posterior segment pathology. It is extremely important that diagnosis of cataract should not be presumed simply because the patient, an elderly one, complains of defective vision or on torch examination, the pupil appears grey.

All diagnostic services in rural areas should be more broad based to include examination of school children for visual defects as well as any anterior/posterior segment pathology. An optometrist in the team is desirable. Educative information with emphasis on prevention and communicable eye diseases should also form an important part.

Rural camp services organised by governments, international agencies voluntary organisations like Lions, Rotarians and other service clubs, eye institutes/hospitals and individual eye surgeons have done a commendable service to the community.

Index